ANNUAL REVIEW OF PUBLIC HEALTH

EDITORIAL COMMITTEE (1995)

ANNUAL REVIEW OF PUBLIC HEALTH

VOLUME 16, 1995

GILBERT S. OMENN, *Editor*

University of Washington

JONATHAN E. FIELDING, *Associate Editor*

University of California at Los Angeles

LESTER B. LAVE, *Associate Editor*

Carnegie Mellon University

ANNUAL REVIEWS INC.   4139 EL CAMINO WAY   P.O. BOX 10139   PALO ALTO, CALIFORNIA 94303-0139

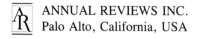

ANNUAL REVIEWS INC.
Palo Alto, California, USA

International Standard Serial Number: 0163–7525
International Standard Book Number: 0–8243–2716–0

Annual Review and publication titles are registered trademarks of Annual Reviews Inc.

⊗ The paper used in this publication meets the minimum requirements of American National Standard for Information Sciences—Permanence of Paper for Printed Library Materials, ANSI Z39.48-1984.

Annual Reviews Inc. and the Editors of its publications assume no responsibility for the statements expressed by the contributors to this *Review*.

Typesetting by Kachina Typesetting Inc., Tempe, Arizona; John Olson, President; Marty Mullins, Typesetting Coordinator; and by the Annual Reviews Inc. Editorial Staff

PRINTED AND BOUND IN THE UNITED STATES OF AMERICA

PREFACE

The goals of public health are not limited to public sector activities to improve and maintain health. Rather, public health aims to protect and improve the health of the public. Comprehensive health promotion requires attention to all factors that determine the health of a population. Many of these are outside the traditional domain of public health and are areas in which public health professionals have limited exposure.

In the United States, economically disadvantaged populations have high rates of morbidity, disability and mortality. Health is undermined primarily by poor educational attainment, lack of economic opportunity, high rates of teenage childbearing, and exposure to violence. To improve the health of these populations, we might learn from developing countries, where research shows that the most important determinants of health are formal maternal education, per capita income, and nutrition, plus the range and quality of core public health services.

For the more economically advantaged, we spend a disproportionate amount of our national wealth on health services, yet over 50 million Americans will spend part of this year without health benefits. Major causes of ill health—overnutrition, physical inactivity, preventable injuries, and environmental exposures—receive insufficient attention. If the nation were committed to investing in areas that could demonstrably improve health, why would over 80 million Americans live in areas without fluoridated water? We do not have a strategy that prioritizes investments based on what determines health status of populations.

Public policy debates on issues without obvious connections to health often miss implications for health. Lawmakers and others who influence public policy at the federal, state, and local levels need to be educated that low fees for cattle grazing on Federal lands decrease the relative price of animal fat compared to other nutrients, that failure to increase gasoline taxes to levels of other industrialized countries increases pollution and contributes to destruction of the environment with attendant health effects, and that programs that prevent youth violence should not be derided as "social pork."

Annual Review of Public Health addresses advances in understanding many determinants of health, but stretches beyond the boundaries of any single *Annual Review* title. We therefore urge our readers to consider the many complementary articles in other *Annual Review* titles such as Anthropology, Energy and the Environment, Genetics, Ecology and Systematics, Nutrition and Psychology. And certainly we encourage you to read widely in this volume, which reflects the breadth of public health sciences and public health practice.

JONATHAN E. FIELDING
GILBERT S. OMENN
LESTER B. LAVE

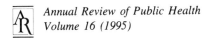
Annual Review of Public Health
Volume 16 (1995)

CONTENTS

SOME RELATED ARTICLES IN OTHER *ANNUAL REVIEWS*

From the *Annual Review of Genetics*, Volume 28 (1994):

The Hyperphenylanlaninemias of Man and Mouse, CR Scriver RC Eisensmith, SLC Woo, and S Kaufman

Mammalian PAX Genes, ET Stuart, C Kioussi, and P Gruss

Evolution of HOX Genes, FH Ruddle, JL Bartels, KL Bentley, C Kappen, MT Murtha, and JW Pendleton

Germline p53 Mutations and Heritable Cancer, D Malkin

Genetic and Phylogenetic Analyses of Endangered Species, SJ O'Brien

The Genetics of Wilms' Tumor—A Case of Disrupted Development, ND Hastie

Genetic Variability of the Human Immunodeficiency Virusa: Statistical and Biological Issues, F Seillier-Moiseiwitsch, B Margolin, and R Swanstrom

From the *Annual Review of Medicine*, Volume 46 (1995):

Repetitive Motion Injuries, PE Higgs and SE Mackinnon

Class II Antigens and Disease Susceptibility, GT Nepom

Hypertension in the Elderly, NM Kaplan

The Changing Face of Tuberculosis, RE Huebner and KG Castro

Alcohol in the Elderly, M Dufour and RK Fuller

Marrow Transplantation from Unrelated Volunteer Donors, C Anasetti, R Etzioni, EW Petersdorf, PJ Martin, and JA Hansen

Risks of HIV Infection in the Health Care Setting, VJ Fraser and WG Powderly

Hepatitis C: An Overview, BN Bhandari and TL Wright

Genetics of Colon Cancer: Impact of Inheritance on Colon Cancer Risk, RW Burt, JA DiSario, and L Cannon-Albright

The Nuclear Hormone Receptor Gene Superfamily, RCJ Ribeiro, PJ Kushner, and JD Baxter

From the *Annual Review of Nutrition*, Volume 15 (1995):

The Evolution of National Nutrition Policy, DA Kessler

Retinoids as Teratogens, DR Soprano and KJ Soprano

From the *Annual Review of Psychology*, Volume 46 (1995):

Understanding Human Resource Management in the Context of Organizations and Their Environments, SE Jackson and RS Schuler

From the *Annual Review of Sociology*, Volume 21 (1995):

ANNUAL REVIEWS INC. is a nonprofit scientific publisher established to promote the advancement of the sciences. Beginning in 1932 with the *Annual Review of Biochemistry*, the Company has pursued as its principal function the publication of high-quality, reasonably priced *Annual Review* volumes. The volumes are organized by Editors and Editorial Committees who invite qualified authors to contribute critical articles reviewing significant developments within each major discipline. The Editor-in-Chief invites those interested in serving as future Editorial Committee members to communicate directly with him. Annual Reviews Inc. is administered by a Board of Directors, whose members serve without compensation.

For the convenience of readers, a detachable order form/envelope is bound into the back of this volume.

STATISTICAL ISSUES IN THE DESIGN OF HIV VACCINE TRIALS[1]

Carl Schaper and Thomas R. Fleming
Department of Biostatistics, University of Washington, Seattle, Washington 98195

Steven G. Self
Program in Biostatistics, Fred Hutchison Cancer Research Center, Seattle, Washington, 98104

Wasima N. Rida
Division of AIDS, NIAID, Bethesda, Maryland 20892

KEY WORDS: HIV vaccine, vaccine efficacy, field efficacy, surrogate marker, behavioral intervention

ABSTRACT

HIV vaccine trials present significant challenges related to trial endpoints, vaccine efficacy measurement, and the role of nonvaccine interventions. Infection is a valid endpoint for detecting sterilizing immunity. But if the vaccine prevents AIDS without preventing infection, infection may be a misleading surrogate. Appropriate endpoints must be defined for other mechanisms of vaccine action. Direct, indirect, behavioral, and biological effects all determine vaccine efficacy. False security among HIV-vaccine recipients may make negative behavioral effects an important component of vaccine performance. Both biological potency and a more comprehensive program effectiveness should be measured. These goals may require unblinded designs or community randomization. Nonvaccine interventions are currently the only HIV-prevention strategy. Support for larger scale implementation requires more rigorous evaluation that is less dependent on self-reported behavioral changes. The vaccine trial cohorts provide a unique opportunity to cost-effectively evaluate behavioral interventions.

BACKGROUND

Acquired immune deficiency syndrome (AIDS), which is caused by the human immunodeficiency virus (HIV), has been reported to the World Health Organization (WHO) in 411,907 people in the United States and 985,119 worldwide as of June 30, 1994, but the WHO estimates that the actual number of AIDS cases worldwide is closer to 4 million (95). Estimates of current HIV infections range from greater than 13 million (9) to greater than 19 million (69). The WHO estimates that by the year 2000, 30 to 40 million individuals will have been infected since the beginning of the pandemic. As yet there is no cure for the disease.

HIV/AIDS research has included development of therapeutic interventions aimed at individuals already infected and preventive interventions aimed at individuals not yet infected. Therapeutic interventions investigated so far consist of treatments with drugs and biologics and therapeutic vaccines. Preventive interventions under investigation include prophylactic vaccines and nonvaccine interventions designed to reduce infection risk for uninfected individuals. Currently, no single one of these intervention types is capable of halting the epidemic.

A number of therapeutic interventions have been developed that inhibit the activity of the virus. Despite some successes in advanced AIDS patients, the overall success has been meager (58). Zidovudine (ZDV), an anti-retroviral drug, is the treatment that has been most extensively tested. It has shown success in extending the lives of advanced AIDS patients (36). In patients with early or no symptoms, however, it slows the progression to AIDS (37, 53, 92) but does not appear to improve overall survival time (1, 53). The initial results of the Concorde trial (1) have caused the medical establishment to reevaluate the role of ZDV in the fight against AIDS (26, 43, 80).

Two other anti-retroviral drugs have been widely examined in clinical trials. Didanosine (ddI) and zalcitabine (ddC) have been compared to ZDV and each other in a variety of trials (2, 35, 42, 60). There are settings in which ddI and ddC have been established to be effective, but they are still not close to being cures for AIDS. Combination therapies are also in the early stages of testing (24), but early results (34, 73) have not been impressive. Clumeck (22) reviews the current use of anti-HIV drugs.

An alternative approach for inhibiting the activity of the virus is the use of therapeutic vaccines. Since late 1988, a number have been evaluated in clinical trials (59, 93). Most have proved to be safe and many have induced immune responses to HIV. However, the responses seen so far have been on biological measures such as antibody responses rather than clinical measures such as prevention of symptomatic AIDS-defining events and death. At present it is still unclear whether the biological responses will translate into clinical efficacy. Since most of these trials are small, it will be some time before the efficacy of these therapeutic vaccines can be assessed.

There has been more success treating and preventing the opportunistic infections that take advantage of the HIV-infected individual's weakened immune system. Prior to the advent of prophylaxis, most HIV-infected individuals had pneumocystis carinii pneumonia (PCP) episodes (18) and up to 40% developed mycobacterium avium complex (MAC) (19). By significantly decreasing the risk of both PCP and MAC episodes, successful prophylaxis has had an impact on the morbidity and mortality of the HIV-infected community. For other AIDS-defining opportunistic infections, a wide variety of drugs is being tried for prophylaxis (46), although the bulk of these are still in the testing phase.

The cost of treatment and care of HIV-infected individuals is extremely high. In the United States, it has recently been estimated that the cost of treating an HIV-infected individual from the time of infection to death is approximately $119,000 (56) and that $10.4 billion will be spent in 1994 treating all HIV-infected individuals (55). In the developing world where most existing cases are and most new cases are expected, this level of expense is out of reach of most individuals and governments. The search for treatments that inhibit the activity of the virus and prevent opportunistic infections remains of utmost importance. However, the challenges in developing such treatments and the cost of their use make it imperative that strategies for prevention of HIV infection also be explored.

The AIDS epidemic has spread rapidly since it was first identified. The rate at which epidemics spread is governed by the basic reproductive number, R_0, which measures the expected number of individuals who become infected from a single infected individual in a completely susceptible population (4, 29). If R_0 is less than 1, the epidemic will die out because each infected individual is giving rise to fewer new infected individuals. Using data available through the mid-eighties, Anderson & May (4) present basic reproduction numbers for HIV that range from 2 to 11. These high rates help explain the rapid progress of the virus. HIV/AIDS prevention research is aimed at lowering these basic reproductive numbers to stop the onslaught of the epidemic. Two prevention strategies are the development of efficacious prophylactic vaccines and the development and implementation of effective nonvaccine prevention strategies.

The first generation of prophylactic vaccines is currently undergoing Phase I and II clinical trials, which are devoted primarily to testing vaccine safety and immunogenicity. Almost 30 (93) vaccine candidates are currently in clinical trials, of which 2 are in Phase II trials. These were anticipated to be the first vaccine candidates available for full-scale Phase III efficacy testing. However, based on various data available from the Phase I/II trials, animal studies, and cross-neutralization studies, the AIDS Research Advisory Committee recommended on June 17, 1994, that the National Institute of Allergies and Infectious Diseases (NIAID) not go ahead with immediate Phase III testing of these two vaccines. There are currently no other vaccines in NIAID-sponsored Phase II trials. In its June 17, 1994, press release, the NIAID estimated that it would take between one and three years to gather the data necessary before they could propose expanded trials of suitable vaccine candidates.

There is still tremendous uncertainty about many areas of HIV vaccine development, of which we mention five. First, there are questions about the appropriate composition of the vaccine. Both of the initial Phase II candidates are based entirely on the gp-120 envelope protein of the virus. However, numerous other approaches (33, 54, 83, 93) are also undergoing clinical or preclinical testing, including other vaccines based on recombinant subunits of the virus, DNA vaccines, as well as vaccines based on whole killed viruses or live attenuated viruses. Second, there are questions about how the vaccine should be presented to the immune system (3, 11, 47). Novel adjuvants are being evaluated to increase the magnitude, breadth, and duration of immune responses. Third, there are questions regarding what component of the immune system to stimulate and how to elicit long-lasting immune responses. This uncertainty relates to whether it is necessary to stimulate both the humoral and cell-mediated arms of the immune system and whether it is necessary to elicit both systemic and mucosal immunity (10, 11, 45, 71). Fourth, a major question relates to how to achieve protection against a wide variety of strains of the virus (11, 45). HIV exhibits extensive genetic variation, particularly in its most antigenic region. Recent reports have suggested that while vaccines in various stages of testing have shown some success in protecting against strains of HIV similar to that used to make the vaccine, little success has been recorded in protecting against different strains, particularly the "wild" strains to which most people are exposed worldwide (25). Addressing the issues related to HIV variation is currently a major focus of basic scientific research. Fifth, concerns regarding the safety of the vaccines include fears that the vaccine may in fact increase susceptibility to infection, or possibly worsen the impact of HIV once an individual has become infected (70). Safety fears are also the primary reason why early efforts have concentrated on vaccines based on envelope proteins and other recombinant subunits of the virus rather than live attenuated viruses or whole killed viruses.

These uncertainties make it imperative that the early vaccine trials, even if not providing sufficiently efficacious vaccines for widespread use, should at least provide information relative to these questions. They also necessitate increased focus on rigorous evaluation of nonvaccine prevention methods since these are currently the only weapon in HIV prevention and will be so for some time.

HIV infection can be prevented. Most HIV infections around the world result from high-risk behavior, so effective nonvaccine interventions that reduce high-risk behavior could theoretically lower HIV-transmission rates. A wide variety of nonvaccine interventions has been investigated in different communities (7, 38, 57), including needle-exchange programs, promotion of the use of barrier methods such as male and female condoms, use of topical virucides and microbicides, as well as more general health services and counseling programs. However, few nonvaccine interventions have received rigorous evaluations. Fisher & Fisher (38) note that "exhortations to intervene and recommendations for interventions far outnumber credible interventions that have been subject to statistical evaluation." Coates (23) notes that there is a "remarkable dearth of information on the effectiveness of behavioral change interventions" and Kelly & Murphy (61) observe that "the paucity of carefully evaluated studies of AIDS risk behavior change interventions is immensely troubling." Vaccine trials could provide an excellent opportunity to undertake rigorous controlled evaluation of nonvaccine interventions.

The trials raise ethical issues related to informed consent, exploitation of third-world and other vulnerable populations, potential risk increases for participants caused by perceived immunity to HIV, and possible discrimination against trial participants in areas such as health insurance, employment, and travel. Substantial effort is going into attempts to solve these difficult ethical questions (84); these efforts are not discussed here.

A final issue that potentially affects the feasibility of mounting vaccine-efficacy trials is the fear of government in the populations that will be needed for evaluating the vaccines (68). These considerations also motivate some of the statistical issues in designing the trials.

Because of the challenges in development of interventions for prevention of HIV infection, and the effort that will go into implementation of the pivotal field trials, the methods used to design and analyze these trials must be appropriate and must allow for reliable assessment of the proper role of these interventions. We review some of the more important issues in trial design and analysis.

CHOICE OF ENDPOINTS

A vaccine could have three basic mechanisms of action that would confer benefit to the individual: (*a*) it could prevent an individual who comes into contact with HIV from becoming infected at all, thus providing "sterilizing immunity;" (b) it could allow individuals to seroconvert but not have chronic infection, hence allowing only "transient infection;" and (c) it might not prevent chronic infection, but instead could prevent or delay the onset of AIDS and the death of the individual. One further mechanism of vaccine action that might not confer direct benefit to the vaccinated individual but might have considerable public health consequences is reduction in an infected vaccinee's level of infectiousness.

The goal of vaccine research is development of a vaccine that saves lives or at least provides some tangible benefit to individuals who become HIV-positive in spite of being vaccinated. Since potential benefits could arise from a vaccine that works according to any of the mechanisms described above, the methods used to evaluate vaccines should be able to detect success according to any of these mechanisms. This would require using death or onset of symptomatic AIDS-defining events as trial endpoints, but, since the incubation period for the virus is so long, this would result in very long trials. Because it may be unrealistic to wait for results from such long-term trials, surrogate endpoints such as HIV infection may need to be used.

A surrogate marker is usually a measure of biological activity that is meant to substitute for a measure of efficacy, where effects on efficacy endpoints should unequivocally reflect tangible benefit to the participant. These measures of biological activity can usually be determined over a shorter period than the measures of efficacy. However, some serious problems are associated with using surrogate markers; these have been discussed in different medical contexts (32, 39, 40).

Prentice (77) provided a criterion for what constitutes a valid surrogate: an endpoint that yields a valid test of the null hypothesis of no association between the treatment and the clinical endpoint. This criterion is satisfied if the surrogate fully captures the effect of the treatment on the endpoint, and is informative about the clinical endpoint. Unfortunately, it is rarely possible to establish that markers satisfy the Prentice conditions (39). An example is provided by CD4 lymphocyte counts, which were used as surrogates in HIV/AIDS clinical trials of nucleoside analogs. Although CD4 counts predict time to death in a natural history setting, intervention-induced changes in CD4 counts are not generally predictive of intervention-induced changes in survival time or in time to AIDS (27, 40, 67); CD4 count is therefore a less than ideal surrogate.

Most discussion relating to the evaluation of prophylactic HIV vaccines in definitive field trials has focused for two principal reasons on the occurrence of an initial infection (30, 87) as the measurement endpoint, which is appropriate for evaluating the sterilizing immunity mechanism of action. First, the nature of HIV's attack of the immune system and the ability of HIV to persist in host-cell DNA might make it impossible for a vaccine to cope with the virus once it has become established (64). Second, the time to initial infection is a well-defined endpoint that can be readily documented and that will be observable in a three-to five-year clinical trial with high enough frequency to make evaluation feasible. However, most effective vaccines for other diseases have not prevented initial infection but have allowed only transient infections to occur (64). If, rather than providing sterilizing immunity, the vaccine allows only transient infection, suppresses chronic infection, or reduces infectiousness, using initial HIV infection as the endpoint could lead to false-negative conclusions. As a result, a vaccine that prevented everyone from developing AIDS but did not prevent initial infection would possibly be discarded as worthless. Since AIDS rather than HIV infection is the problem, we could be discarding the solution to the problem by focusing on the initial infection. Motivated by these considerations and studies of vaccines in animals that have shown reduced viral burden even though they have not prevented initial infection, the appropriateness of initial infection as the endpoint is being questioned (24, 83).

Defining endpoints that allow initial infection but measure some other protective property requires a definition of what constitutes protection for an individual with an initial infection. A vaccine might be considered a success according to this endpoint if it allowed an initial infection but resulted in no detectable virus in subsequent serial viral cultures or PCR assessments after a period of, say, three to six months. Using transient infection as the trial endpoint will require the development of sensitive culture or PCR techniques able to detect low levels of virus. However, no technique is completely sensitive and so, for example, endpoints based on assays for transient infection must be interpreted as suppressed levels of virus rather than complete clearance of infection. It remains to be seen whether levels of virus that are suppressed by vaccine action translate into delay or prevention of symptomatic AIDS-defining events and death.

Although there are undeniable weaknesses with the use of either sterilizing immunity or transient infection as trial endpoints, the need to use surrogate markers in vaccine trials is much more acute than in treatment trials because the true endpoint of interest is further into the future. Acknowledging these weaknesses, continued long-term follow-up of all individuals will be essential to determine whether reduction in the rate of HIV infection translates into tangible benefits such as reduction of symptomatic disease or increases in survival time. Extended follow-up of all participants would pay special attention to those becoming infected, and where necessary record linkages to AIDS and death registries would be used to determine the effect of the vaccines on the real endpoints of interest, either onset of symptomatic AIDS or death. Meanwhile, better markers are being sought (90) and more reliable uses of surrogate marker information are being explored. The latter includes research into using marker information as auxiliary information, rather than as replacement endpoints, to improve efficiency of clinical trials (39–41, 65).

MEASURING VACCINE EFFICACY

The extensive literature on assessing vaccine efficacy, which goes back to Greenwood & Yule (49), has focused largely on efficacy measurement in vaccination programs rather than randomized field trials (74). We review the literature relevant to the situation of a randomized field trial. Throughout, we assume that a suitable endpoint has been specified.

Effects of Vaccination

The effects of vaccination are best understood by examining the factors that determine the risk of infection during some time period, from the perspective of an individual called the index participant. Because certain unsafe acts are riskier than others, the overall infection risk will depend on the various types of risk activities in which the index participant engages. However, to simplify exposition, we assume a single type of risk activity. The infection risk depends on the following four parameters: the number of unsafe contacts in the time period; the fraction of unsafe contacts with infected individuals; the probability that an infected individual transmits the virus at a single contact (infectivity probability); and the probability that an uninfected individual acquires the virus at a single contact with an infected individual transmitting virus (susceptibility probability). Note that the risk of infection increases as any one of these parameters increases. The product of the first two determines the number of contacts with infected individuals and of the second two determines the probability of HIV transmission on a single contact with an infected individual. Of the four parameters, the susceptibility probability and the number of unsafe contacts are specific to the index participant, whereas the fraction of contacts with infected individuals and the infectivity probability reflect the environment in which the index participant is active.

The intended effect of a vaccine is to provide biological protection against the virus. However, the act of vaccination may have the additional unintended effect of changing the vaccinee's behavior if he or she perceives immunity to the virus as a result of being vaccinated. If the index participant is the only individual in the population who is vaccinated, then the vaccine can affect the risk of infection for that participant only through effects on the two index participant–specific parameters. These effects constitute the direct effects of the vaccine for the index participant. However, if the index participant is part of a vaccination program, the vaccine could affect the risk of infection for that specific participant through effects on all four parameters. Then the effects for the index participant consist of the direct effects on the index participant–specific parameters, and the indirect effects on the parameters reflecting the environment in which the index participant is active.

The direct biological effect of the vaccine on risk of infection for the index participant is its effect on the susceptibility probability. The direct behavioral effect is on the number of unsafe contacts in which the index participant engages. The effect of vaccination on the infectivity probability represents an indirect biological effect. The effect of vaccination on the fraction of the index participant's contacts with infected individuals represents a combination of indirect biological and behavioral effects because either the vaccine's biological or behavioral effects could prevent infection in the index participant's partners. From the perspective of the index participant, the indirect biological and behavioral effects are experienced simultaneously. Together they make up what is typically called herd immunity.

Measurement Objectives

In an actual vaccination program, the vaccine's direct, indirect, biological, and behavioral effects all play a role. Since it is anticipated that the initial vaccines will be significantly less than 100% effective, behavioral changes could induce effects that would be an important component of overall program effectiveness. In particular, if individuals increase their exposure in response to vaccination, a vaccine that is not fully effective could result in an increase of HIV infections even though the biological activity of the vaccine is positive (85). Therefore, a measure of *program effectiveness* that accounts for the vaccine's biological and behavioral effects, as well as all direct and indirect effects, should ultimately drive decisions about the use of the vaccine in clinical practice.

One drawback of including behavioral effects in a measure of vaccine success is that they will depend on the particular community in which the vaccine is delivered. For example, the changes in risk behavior among gay men who know that they are receiving the vaccine may be different from those of injecting drug users (IDUs). Measures of program effectiveness estimated from vaccine trials will reflect the particular environment in which the trial is offered. Since the trials will be undertaken in the highest-risk communities, the behavioral effects of the trial will approximate these effects in the communities most at need of the vaccine. However, the behavioral effects may be different in lower-risk communities not participating in the trial. The behavioral effects may also change as better nonvaccine intervention programs are discovered. Therefore, in addition to having measures of program effectiveness, it will be important to obtain some measure of the vaccine's effect that is less influenced by the particular population in which the program is provided. Such a measure might concentrate entirely on the direct biological effect on the susceptibility probability—in other words, on the *biological potency* of the vaccine.

Two principal measurement objectives are therefore needed in comparative HIV vaccine trials:

- the effect the vaccine would have on the spread of HIV if used in a vaccination program; and,
- the effect the vaccine would have on reducing the susceptibility probability.

We use the terms *program effectiveness* and *biological potency,* respectively, to characterize these effects.

Greenwood & Yule provide criteria for evaluation of vaccines: in the context
of HIV vaccine trials, the participants must be alike in all material respects;
and the effective exposure to HIV must be identical among the vaccinated and
unvaccinated participants.

For estimating either program effectiveness or biological potency, random
assignment of individuals to the vaccine and the control groups in a randomized
field trial will satisfy the first of these criteria. The measure of biological
potency attempts to estimate direct biological effects controlling for all indirect
effects as well as direct behavioral effects. Therefore, the second condition is
appropriate for estimating biological potency. The combination of randomization and blinding of participants to their vaccine status will meet the second
criterion. For measuring biological potency, it will be necessary to ensure that
unblinding does not occur, since unblinding could cause changes in the behaviors in the two arms of the trial and result in confounding of biological
effects with exposure differences (52).

For measuring program effectiveness of an HIV vaccine, the second criterion
is not appropriate. This measurement should ideally include all direct and
indirect effects, including the direct effect on risk behavior for a participant
in a vaccine program. To measure the direct effects related to behavioral
changes, the conditions in a vaccination program must be simulated as closely
as possible. If a vaccine program were undertaken, individuals would know
they were receiving the vaccine. Thus, it would be inappropriate to conduct a
blinded randomized trial because individuals, if they remain blinded, would
not know their vaccination status and would not make the same behavioral
changes as if they did know their status. Therefore, the evaluation of program
effectiveness will require the use of unblinded randomized trials. Since measuring biological potency requires a blinded trial, whereas measuring program
effectiveness requires an unblinded trial, both measurement goals cannot be
met with the same simple trial. The actual design of trials will therefore depend
heavily on the relative importance of the different measurement goals.

Estimability of Measurement Objectives

Although we have just argued the need for blinded and unblinded randomized
field trials to assess a vaccine's biological potency and program effectiveness
respectively, neither quantity will be fully estimable in the type of blinded or
unblinded vaccine trials currently being planned. We discuss how biological

potency and program effectiveness are related to the respective estimable quantities of *vaccine efficacy* and *vaccine field* efficacy.

PROGRAM EFFECTIVENESS   Haber et al (50) point out that, even for an un-blinded trial, the effect of herd immunity is not measurable in a cohort study such as a field trial in which the individual is the unit of randomization, because both the vaccinated and unvaccinated groups experience the same indirect effects. Even if the vaccinated and unvaccinated groups could be separated, a vaccine trial consisting of a small fraction of the total contact population is not a realistic environment in which to calculate estimates of the type of herd immunity that might be expected in a full-scale program. A vaccine's beneficial effect could substantially be through a reduction in infectivity of breakthrough cases rather than through reduction in susceptibility. To obtain direct evidence of such effects on infectivity, one would need to design trials that capture both indirect and direct effects of the vaccine. These could be large-scale pre-marketing controlled field trials with essentially contained communities as the unit of randomization. Such trials might need to be of long duration if the vaccine does not reduce infectivity of individuals who are in the community and already have HIV at the time of trial initiation.

We denote the direct behavioral and biological effects measurable by an unblinded randomized vaccine trial as the *vaccine field efficacy*. Although this parameter is not equivalent to the program effectiveness parameter, it will capture that component of the vaccine's effects with the greatest potential to undermine the biologic potency of the vaccine, namely the direct behavioral changes. A primary weakness will be its insensitivity to detecting vaccines that would reduce the spread of HIV by reducing infectivity rather than sus-ceptibility.

BIOLOGICAL POTENCY   When the effective exposure to HIV is identical be-tween the vaccinated and unvaccinated persons, Greenwood & Yule define *vaccine efficacy* (*VE*) by:

$$VE = 1 - AR_v/AR_u,$$

where AR_v and AR_u are the attack rates in the vaccinated and unvaccinated groups, respectively. The attack rate is defined to be the probability of becom-ing infected. Note that $\{1-AR_v/AR_u\}$ would yield vaccine efficacy in a blinded trial and vaccine field efficacy in an unblinded trial that has individuals as the unit of randomization.

The use of randomization and blinding in a vaccine trial would result in approximately comparable exposure to the HIV virus in the vaccinated and unvaccinated groups. However, to estimate biological potency, it would be necessary to adjust for the *specific* amount of exposure experienced by the individual trial participants, not just to ensure comparable exposure (51). For HIV vaccine trials, amount of exposure means number of unsafe contacts with an infected individual transmitting virus. Because individuals will not know whether a partner is infected with HIV and transmitting virus, it will be impossible to accurately estimate exposure to HIV. Since adjustment would have to take place at the individual level, even if the two groups have comparable but heterogeneous exposure such as might be expected in a randomized blinded trial, the *VE* measure defined above will only approximate the biological potency.

Although alternatives to the *VE* measure have been proposed (50), these depend on assumed underlying models. As pointed out by Greenland & Frerichs (48), *VE* as defined above "is of straightforward utility in evaluating the benefit of a vaccination program, regardless of the model of effect." A further argument in favor of using the *VE* measure is that when the probability of infection from a single contact is low, as is the case with HIV (15), the *VE* statistic provides a reasonable approximation to the biological potency parameter.

Heterogeneity in Susceptibility and Vaccine Effectiveness

Another issue that arises in HIV trials is the heterogeneity in different individual's susceptibility to acquiring the virus from a single contact. Considerable evidence from various partner studies indicates that susceptibility to HIV varies across individuals (15). Svensson (89) considers variability in susceptibility and examines situations that could lead to either overestimation or underestimation of vaccine efficacy.

Heterogeneity can also arise in effectiveness of the vaccine. Smith et al (88) describe two models for the imperfect action of the vaccine: (*a*) the vaccine reduces the susceptibility probability for all individuals in the population by a fixed quantity but does not totally eliminate risk; or (*b*) the vaccine works perfectly for a fraction of the population and not at all for the rest. Any number of mechanisms of vaccine action between these two is also conceivable. Vaccines can also fail in the "duration" of protection they offer (72). The different ways in which a vaccine fails can have quite different effects on epidemics (50, 72, 88).

Developing an understanding of vaccine action could have useful implications for future vaccine development. It might be possible to identify measures of immunogenicity that are correlated with occurrence of HIV infection. By comparing biological and immunologic parameters of trial participants for those who do with those who do not become infected, we might obtain leads as to the type of immune responses that future vaccines should aim to stimulate (78). However, one should be very cautious about the reliability of such leads. These measures of immunogenicity might simply be markers identifying the intrinsic heterogeneity in different individual's susceptibility to acquiring the virus. For example, occurrence of a specific type of antibody response might simply provide identification of participants intrinsically at low risk of HIV infection rather than evidence of a causal mechanism by which the vaccine achieves a protective effect.

EVALUATING NONVACCINE INTERVENTIONS

Currently, nonvaccine interventions are the only tool for preventing HIV infection. At least for some individuals, they may remain the only prevention strategy for the near future since early HIV-vaccine candidates are unlikely to provide universal complete protection, and may never do so given the variation in the virus. The objective of nonvaccine interventions is to modify people's behavior to eliminate or at least reduce their risk of infection. These interventions vary as to their target audience, their promotion strategy and whom they use to communicate the message (31). Most interventions consist of some combination of suggested behavioral modifications, including recommendations for complete elimination of certain activities such as suggestions of sexual abstinence, or modification of existing behaviors through the use of technologies such as condoms or spermicides.

The complexity of nonvaccine interventions has presented many challenges for their evaluation. These challenges have made rigorous evaluation difficult and rare (23, 38, 61). Although numerous interventions have received evaluation with seemingly positive results (7, 38, 57), there remains ambiguity because of the evaluation method (38). We focus on two common shortcomings of existing evaluation of nonvaccine interventions—specifically, the observational nature of the studies and the endpoints used—and discuss the role of vaccine trials in addressing these shortcomings.

Study Design

Ideally, nonvaccine prevention interventions should be evaluated in a randomized, controlled field trial (RCT). All too frequently, RCTs have not been viewed to be feasible either due to perceived difficulties with achieving compliance/noncompliance of a prescribed behavior or because of beliefs that the intervention would provide some benefit without causing any harm. Observational studies provide an alternative approach to using RCTs and have had a long history in epidemiology. Unfortunately, because of lack of a randomized control group, "it is rare ... for a single study to provide convincing evidence of causality" (14); numerous studies reporting similar results are required before reliable conclusions might be reached.

An example of the need for observational studies is provided by the evaluation of latex condoms as an intervention technology. It would be difficult to identify a setting in which randomization could be used to determine condom use. Also, early studies provided positive although limited evidence in support of latex condoms as a device for reducing infection risk. Many studies over many years were required to establish efficacy for condoms. While Weller concluded on the basis of 16 studies up to mid-1990 that "a consistent association across studies remain[s] to be demonstrated" (94), two large European observational studies (28, 81) have recently demonstrated a strong association between infection and lack of consistent condom use. These and earlier studies form the basis for the CDC's statement that "condoms are highly effective for preventing HIV infection and other STDs when used consistently and correctly" (20).

Observational studies served a useful role in evaluating the efficacy of condoms, but the results from such studies have been less reliable for most other interventions. For example, an evaluation of pre- and post-HIV test counseling (75) suggested possible negative effects, although the conclusions of this observational study are unclear (44, 76) and must be considered along with numerous other evaluations of counseling, many of which have yielded positive results (57).

The evaluation of the spermicide, nonoxynol-9, provides another example of a technology for which efficacy remains uncertain. An observational study (96) was conducted to evaluate the effect on seroincidence rates of nonoxynol-9 administered in the form of vaginal suppositories. The investigators designed an observational study rather than a RCT because they felt "ethically bound to offer spermicides to all participants" based on the belief that use of the suppository would provide some protection from HIV. The study demonstrated a reduction in risk from the use of the nonoxynol-9 vaginal suppository. However, it is difficult to infer causality from this seemingly positive result because this study had no randomized controls and women were using condoms in addition to nonoxynol-9. Contrary findings were obtained in a placebo-controlled RCT of a commercially available nonoxynol-9 contraceptive sponge (66). Data from this trial indicated slightly higher rates of HIV infection associated with nonoxynol-9 use; however, the investigators noted two important issues that limit the generalizability of their results (66). First, the failure of the intervention may be due to the delivery mechanism, in this case the sponge, rather than the nonoxynol-9. Second, a number of women on the nonoxynol-9 arm of the trial experienced lesions in the vaginal mucosa, which may increase susceptibility to HIV. It is suspected that these lesions may be due to high doses of nonoxynol-9, and a lower dose might therefore be more efficacious.

Further examples of RCTs being used to evaluate nonvaccine interventions do exist (63, 82), but most have not been evaluated using RCTs (7). In some settings there may appear to be ethical reasons in favor of observational studies, nevertheless extreme care is required when determining whether it would be ethical to withhold an intervention from control arm participants; inappropriate reliance on observational studies could lead to negative consequences being undetectable, while at the same time could greatly weaken the strength of any positive results. Nonoxynol-9 as delivered in the RCT appeared to increase vaginal lesions and thus caused harm. These negative effects on the vaginal mucosa and on risk of HIV infection would have been much more difficult to detect in an observational study. In such studies, effects of a modest size, either positive or negative, can be difficult to ascribe to the intervention because they may be of the same order of magnitude as methodological biases that can arise in even the most carefully conducted observational study.

RCTs are the gold standard for evaluating interventions due to many well-known advantages that relate to the unbiasedness and reliability of such evaluations. Some examples of interventions that might be evaluated in a RCT include needle-exchange programs for IDUs and approaches for reducing HIV-infection risk from sexual intercourse through the use of mechanisms over which the female partner has control. In the latter setting, trials could include evaluation of female condoms, or of new delivery methods and dosing of nonoxynol-9 or, alternatively, of other spermicides such as gramicidin, which has shown a 1000% increase in anti-HIV activity relative to nonoxynol-9 in recent in vitro studies (12, 13).

Endpoints

Nonvaccine interventions aim to reduce the risk of symptomatic AIDS-defining events and death by reducing the risk of HIV infection. Thus, prevention of HIV infection might be an appropriate study endpoint in most definitive RCTs. However, alternative endpoints would be required when evaluating nonvaccine interventions that may have serious negative consequences, especially if these are not related to the occurrence of HIV. One example is the use of formula-feeding instead of breast milk as an intervention in developing countries for preventing HIV transmission from HIV-infected mothers to their babies. The use of potentially contaminated water in formula, and the loss of immunogens usually passed through the mother's breast milk, can have very serious negative consequences, including death, for the baby. Symptomatic disease and infant mortality must be considered to be key elements of the primary endpoints in such a trial.

Trials using HIV infection as the endpoint will typically be of long duration and require large numbers of participants because the endpoint of HIV infection is a rare event, even in communities at high risk (7). This fact previously has led to widespread use of self-reported changes in risk behavior as surrogate endpoints for evaluating nonvaccine interventions. Reviews list many examples of nonvaccine interventions with promising results as measured by self-reported endpoints (7, 38, 57). Unfortunately, the well-recognized difficulties associated with self-reported data (17, 79) have caused ambiguity in study conclusions (38).

As is usually true with surrogates, self-reported endpoints should not be used as primary endpoints in definitive trials. However, they remain an essential component of the evaluation process. In trials providing a definitive evaluation of the effect of nonvaccine interventions on the risk of HIV infection, self-reported risk-behavior endpoints provide valuable insight into participant compliance and into the impact of the intervention on behavior. Self-reported endpoints are also the appropriate primary outcome measures in smaller Phase I/II or screening evaluations (7), which are designed to rapidly screen promising interventions for potential evaluation in large definitive Phase III field trials. Because of their importance, there has been extensive research in recent years to improve the reliability of self-reported endpoints (91).

Some studies have attempted to overcome certain problems associated with self-reported changes in behavior. Changes in sexual behavior and injecting drug use have been measured by redeemed condom coupons and number of needles exchanged (38). Both suggest adherence to the behavioral recommendations, but neither is a perfect measure of actual adherence. In an evaluation of pre- and post-HIV-test counseling, Otten et al (75) use the presence of STDs as a measure of risk activity. This is useful in being not only a marker of sexual activity, but also an objective efficacy endpoint that represents occurrence of symptomatic disease and that is known to be correlated with occurrence of HIV infection.

To motivate much-needed implementation of interventions on a scale large enough to have significant public health impact (62), evaluations must demonstrate that "new infections have been averted by such change" (7). Since such support will likely be based on some cost-benefit analysis (7), with benefits measured in terms of prevented HIV infections, "hard" evidence is needed on the efficacy of the interventions. To increase rigor and gather harder evidence, it has been recommended that evaluation of nonvaccine interventions be undertaken in the same three-step process that is used in drug trials and would be used in HIV vaccine trials (5, 6, 76). For nonvaccine interventions, Phase I could examine issues like feasibility of intervention schedules, Phase II could include larger studies like those evaluations that have been carried out so far, and Phase III trials could be RCTs that use the relevant endpoint of infection (6). Phase II would typically use self-reported behavioral endpoints to provide preliminary rather than definitive evidence for the efficacy of the intervention.

The vaccine trials provide a unique opportunity to circumvent significant impediments usually associated with the use of HIV infection as the endpoint in evaluations of nonvaccine interventions. Since the vaccine cohort would already be assembled with HIV-infection status being measured for vaccine evaluation, the sample size/cost argument against using HIV infection as the endpoint in a RCT would become moot. There would be costs associated with implementing the interventions, but, as long as they do not detract from the evaluation of vaccine efficacy, they may be far outweighed by the value of the definitive results attainable in this setting.

Factorial Designs

One way to incorporate evaluation of nonvaccine interventions into the vaccine trials is through factorial designs, which have previously received limited consideration in the clinical trial setting (16). A factorial design with the factors being vaccine/no vaccine and intervention/no intervention would allow the evaluation of the main effects, i.e. the respective efficacies of the vaccine and nonvaccine intervention, as well as the interaction between the two.

Slud (86) has developed methods for 2 by 2 factorial designs based on the proportional hazards model, where relative risk parameters are defined to represent the main effects of the two interventions and the possible interaction. Slud compares a 2 by 2 factorial design to a 3-group design containing a control group, a group receiving only the vaccine, and a group receiving only the nonvaccine intervention. He concludes that the power for testing the main effects in a factorial design usually is comparable to or better than that of the 3-group design. The exact gain from a factorial study depends on the extent of treatment interactions. Factorial designs are most advantageous if these interactions are nonexistent or modest (16). If the nonvaccine intervention is directed at preventing exposure, whereas the vaccine is directed at preventing infection given exposure, their interaction may be modest. In that situation, factorial designs would allow rigorous evaluation of nonvaccine interventions without significant loss of efficiency for evaluating vaccine efficacy. Larger sample sizes will be needed if each intervention has some positive effect, because the overall number of endpoints is likely to be smaller (78).

CONCLUSION

Several important issues in the design of HIV vaccine trials of remain controversial: the choice of endpoints, the role of blinding, and the type of behavioral interventions to be offered in the trials. Although approaches to vaccine evaluation in other disease areas provide useful guidance in resolving some of these controversies, unique aspects of the HIV-prevention setting will often require new approaches.

Many diseases for which vaccines have been developed have relatively short intervals between infection and disease symptoms. With these diseases, even if an infection occurs, the vaccine's ability or inability to assist in overcoming the infection will be observable during the course of the RCT. By contrast, the median time from infection with HIV until the onset of AIDS is about 10 years (15). In a three- to five-year field trial, this time lag forces at least partial reliance on surrogates such as sterilizing immunity or prevention of transient infection. The latter requires defining some level of infection that is considered to be transient, such as no detectable virus in subsequent viral cultures for a duration of at least three months. However, it may not be known at the end of the trial whether such measures reliably ensure reduction in risks of AIDS-defining events or death. As a result, long-term follow-up of participants will be required in order to validate the use of the surrogates or as a way to observe potential effects of the vaccine on disease progression.

We have discussed the difference between evaluating biological potency and program effectiveness. Traditional vaccine evaluation often has concentrated on evaluating biological potency in controlled trials and has left evaluation of program effectiveness to postmarketing surveillance (8). This approach may not be appropriate when evaluating HIV vaccines. Vaccines for diseases such as mumps, measles, rubella, diphtheria, pertussis, tetanus, smallpox, and polio have resulted in 100- to 1000-fold reduction in occurrence rates (21). Effects of this magnitude can easily be identified, even with the imprecision inherent in postmarketing observational studies. By contrast, HIV vaccines may provide reductions of only twofold or less. Unlike other disease settings, the act of vaccination in HIV-prevention settings may also have the unintended effect of changing the vaccinee's risk behavior owing to a false sense of security, which further reduces or completely eliminates the small potential benefit achieved by vaccine-induced reductions in susceptibility. A blinded trial looking only at biological potency would provide no information about how these increases in risk behavior could impact the HIV-infection rate, and postmarketing surveillance would not provide a sensitive instrument for reliably estimating such small overall effects of the vaccine on the rate of HIV infection. It is therefore important to consider evaluation of program effectiveness, through an unblinded component of a RCT, as part of the evaluation process prior to vaccine approval. Finally, if a vaccine's beneficial effect is anticipated to be substantially through a reduction in infectivity of breakthrough cases, then large-scale premarketing field trials might be required where community would be the unit of randomization, thereby accounting for direct and indirect effects of a vaccine in estimating the program effectiveness.

Another unique aspect of HIV vaccine trials will be the need for care in "matching" the strain(s) of HIV used in the vaccine with the circulating strains in a given area. This will be necessary to provide a fair evaluation of the vaccine system. However, an implication is that results of vaccine evaluation may not be relevant in regions removed from the trial.

Finally, HIV, unlike most other diseases for which vaccines have been developed, can be prevented by behavioral changes. If funding for large-scale interventions to promote these behavioral changes is to be obtained, it will be extremely important to subject interventions to rigorous evaluation. Such evaluations could use HIV infection as endpoints in a randomized controlled setting. The vaccine trials represent an opportunity for such evaluations. Since no vaccines are available for immediate Phase III trials, nonvaccine interventions represent the only way to prevent new infections in the short term. It may therefore be appropriate to use the existing cohorts that have been assembled for vaccine trials to evaluate promising nonvaccine interventions alone.

ACKNOWLEDGMENTS

The authors would like to thank Amy Sheon of the NIAID for help in providing references on nonvaccine interventions.

Literature Cited

1. Aboulker JP, Swart AM. 1993. Preliminary analysis of the Concorde trial. Concorde Coordinating Committee. *Lancet* 341:889–90
2. Abrams DI, Goldman AI, Launer C, Korvick JA, Neaton JD, et al. 1994. A comparative trial of didanosine or zalcitabine after treatment with zidovudine in patients with human immunodeficiency virus infection. The Terry Beirn Community Programs for Clinical Research on AIDS. *New Engl. J. Med.* 330:657–62
3. Allison AC. 1994. Adjuvants and immune enhancement. *Int. J. Technol. Assess. Health Care* 10:107–20
4. Anderson RM, May RM. 1991. *Infectious Diseases of Humans, Dynamics and Control,* pp. 13–23, 70. Oxford: Oxford Univ. Press
5. Aral SO, Peterman TA. 1993. Defining behavioral methods to prevent sexually transmitted diseases through intervention research. *Infect. Dis. Clin. North Am.* 7:861–73
6. Aral SO, Wasserheit JN, Green SB, Judson FN, Sparling PF. 1990. The NIAID Study Group on Integrated Behavioral Research for Prevention and Control of Sexually Transmitted Diseases. Part III: Issues in evaluating behavioral interventions. *Sex. Transm. Dis.* 17:208–10
7. Auerbach JD, Wypijewska C, Brodie HKH, eds. 1994. *AIDS and Behavior: An Integrated Approach,* pp. 98–123. Washington, DC: Natl. Acad. Press
8. Begg N, Miller E. 1990. Role of epidemiology in vaccine policy. *Vaccine* 8: 180–89
9. Berkley S. 1993. AIDS in the developing world: an epidemiologic overview. *Clin. Infect. Dis.* 17:S329–36 (Suppl. 2)
10. Berzofsky JA. 1991. Approaches and issues in the development of vaccines against HIV. *J. Acquir. Immune Defic. Syndr.* 4:451–59
11. Bolognesi DP. 1993. The immune response to HIV: implications for vaccine development. *Semin. Immunol.* 5:203–14
12. Bourinbaiar AS, Krasinski K, Borkowsky W. 1994. Anti-HIV effect of gramicidin in vitro: potential for spermicide use. *Life Sci.* 54:L5–9
13. Bourinbaiar AS, Lee-Huang S. 1994. Comparative in vitro study of contraceptive agents with anti-HIV activity: gramicidin, nonoxynol-9, and gossypol. *Contraception* 49:131–37
14. Breslow NE, Day NE. 1980. *Statistical Methods in Cancer Research. Vol. 1, The Analysis of Case-control Studies,* pp. 84–90. Lyon: IARC
15. Brookmeyer R, Gail MH. 1994. *AIDS Epidemiology: A Quantitative Approach,* pp. 36–50, 109–112. New York: Oxford Univ. Press

16. Byar DP, Piantadosi S. 1985. Factorial designs for randomized clinical trials. *Cancer Treat. Rep.* 69:1055–63

17. Catania JA, Gibson DR, Chitwood DD, Coates TJ. 1990. Methodological problems in AIDS behavioral research: influences on measurement error and participation bias in studies of sexual behavior. *Psychol. Bull.* 108:339–62

18. Centers for Disease Control. 1992. Recommendations for prophylaxis against *Pneumocystis carinii* pneumonia for adults and adolescents infected with human immunodeficiency virus. *Morb. Mortal. Wkly. Rep.* 41(RR-4):1–11

19. Centers for Disease Control. 1993. Recommendations on prophylaxis and therapy for disseminated *Mycobacterium avium* complex for adults and adolescents infected with human immunodeficiency virus. US Public Health Serv. Task Force on Prophylaxis and Therapy for *Mycobacterium avium* Complex. *Morb. Mortal. Wkly. Rep.* 42(RR-9):14–20

20. Centers for Disease Control. 1993. Update: barrier protection against HIV infection and other sexually transmitted diseases. *Morb. Mortal. Wkly. Rep.* 42: 589–91

21. Chen RT, Rastogi SC, Mullen JR, Hayes SW, Cochi SL, et al. 1994. The vaccine adverse event reporting system (VAERS). *Vaccine* 12:542–50

22. Clumeck N. 1993. Current use of anti-HIV drugs in AIDS. *J. Antimicrob. Chemother.* 32:133–38 (Suppl. A)

23. Coates TJ. 1990. Strategies for modifying sexual behavior for primary and secondary prevention of HIV disease. *J. Consult. Clin. Psychol.* 58:57–69

24. Cohen J. 1993. AIDS vaccine research. A new goal: preventing disease, not infection. *Science* 262:1820–21

25. Cohen J. 1993. Jitters jeopardize AIDS vaccine trials. *Science* 262:980–81

26. Cotton P. 1994. Use of antiretroviral drugs in HIV disease declines following preliminary results from Concorde trial. *J. Am. Med. Assoc.* 271:488–89

27. de Gruttola V, Wulfsohn M, Fischl MA, Tsiatis A. 1993. Modeling the relationship between survival and CD4 lymphocytes in patients with AIDS and AIDS-related complex. *AIDS* 6:359–365

28. de Vincenzi I. 1994. A longitudinal study of human immunodeficiency virus transmission by heterosexual partners. European Study Group on Heterosexual Transmission of HIV. *New Engl. J. Med.* 331:341–46

29. Dietz K. 1993. The estimation of the basic reproduction number for infectious diseases. *Stat. Methods Med. Res.* 2:23–41

30. Dixon DO, Rida WN, Fast PE, Hoth DF. 1993. HIV vaccine trials: some design issues including sample size calculation. *J. Acquir. Immune Defic. Syndr.* 6:485–96

31. Ehrhardt AA, Fishbein M, Washington E, Smith W, Holmes KK. 1990. The NIAID Study Group on Integrated Behavioral Research for Prevention and Control of Sexually Transmitted Diseases. Part II: Issues in designing behavioral interventions. *Sex. Transm. Dis.* 17:204–7

32. Ellenberg SS. 1991. Surrogate end points in clinical trials. *Br. Med. J.* 302: 63–4

33. Fast PE, Walker MC. 1993. Human trials of experimental AIDS vaccines. *AIDS* 7:S147–59 (Suppl. 1)

34. Fischl MA. 1994. Combination antiretroviral therapy for HIV infection. *Hosp. Pract. Off. Ed.* 29:43–48

35. Fischl MA, Olson RM, Follansbee SE, Lalezari JP, Henry DH, et al. 1993. Zalcitabine compared with zidovudine in patients with advanced HIV-1 infection who received previous zidovudine therapy. *Ann. Intern. Med.* 118:762–69

36. Fischl MA, Richman DD, Grieco MH, Gottlieb MS, Volberding PA, et al. 1987. The efficacy of azidothymidine (AZT) in the treatment of patients with AIDS and AIDS-related complex. A double-blind, placebo-controlled trial. *New Engl. J. Med.* 317:185–91

37. Fischl MA, Richman DD, Hansen N, Collier AC, Carey JT, et al. 1990. The safety and efficacy of zidovudine (AZT) in the treatment of subjects with mildly symptomatic human immunodeficiency virus type 1 (HIV) infection. A double-blind, placebo-controlled trial. The AIDS Clinical Trials Group. *Ann. Intern. Med.* 112:727–37

38. Fisher JD, Fisher WA. 1992. Changing AIDS-risk behavior. *Psychol. Bull.* 111: 455–74

39. Fleming TR. 1992. Evaluating therapeutic interventions: some issues and experiences. *Statist. Sci.* 7:428–56

40. Fleming TR. 1994. Surrogate markers in AIDS and clinical trials. *Stat. Med.* 13:1423–35

41. Fleming TR, Prentice RL, Pepe MS, Glidden D. 1994. Surrogate and auxiliary endpoints in clinical trials, with potential applications in cancer and AIDS research. *Stat. Med.* 13:955–68

42. Fletcher CV. 1993. Current perspectives on antiretroviral therapy. *Pharmacotherapy* 13:627–33

43. Gazzard BG. 1993. After Concorde. *Br. Med. J.* 306:1016–17
44. Gerber AR, Campbell CH Jr., Dillon BA, Holtgrave DR. 1994. Evaluating behavioral interventions: need for randomized controlled trials. *J. Am. Med. Assoc.* 271:1317–18
45. Girard M. 1993. The needs and hopes for an AIDS vaccine. *Biochimie* 75:583–89
46. Goldschmidt RH, Dong BJ. 1994. Current report—HIV. Treatment of AIDS and HIV-related conditions—1994. *J. Am. Board Fam. Pract.* 7:155–78
47. Graham BS, Karzon DT. 1990. Development of an AIDS vaccine. Biological and ethical challenges. *Infect. Dis. Clin. North Am.* 4:223–43
48. Greenland S, Frerichs RR. 1988. On measures and models for the effectiveness of vaccines and vaccination programmes. *Int. J. Epidemiol.* 17:456–63
49. Greenwood M, Yule UG. 1915. The statistics of anti-typhoid and anti-cholera innoculations and the interpretation of such statistics in general. *Proc. R. Soc. Med.* 8 (Pt. 2):113–94
50. Haber M, Longini IM Jr, Halloran ME. 1991. Measures of the effects of vaccination in a randomly mixing population. *Int. J. Epidemiol.* 20:300–10
51. Halloran ME, Haber M, Longini IM Jr, Struchiner CJ. 1991. Direct and indirect effects in vaccine efficacy and effectiveness. *Am. J. Epidemiol.* 133:323–31
52. Halloran ME, Longini IM Jr, Haber MJ, Struchiner CJ, Brunet RC. 1994. Exposure efficacy and change in contact rates in evaluating prophylactic HIV vaccines in the field. *Stat. Med.* 13:357–77
53. Hamilton JD, Hartigan PM, Simberkoff MS, Day PL, Diamond GR, et al. 1992. A controlled trial of early versus late treatment with zidovudine in symptomatic human immunodeficiency virus infection. Results of the Veterans Affairs Cooperative Study. *New Engl. J. Med.* 326:437–43
54. Haynes BF. 1993. Scientific and social issues of human immunodeficiency virus vaccine development. *Science* 260:1279–86
55. Hellinger FJ. 1991. Forecasting the medical care costs of the HIV epidemic: 1991–1994. *Inquiry* 28:213–25
56. Hellinger FJ. 1993. The lifetime cost of treating a person with HIV. *J. Am. Med. Assoc.* 270:474–78
57. Higgins DL, Galavotti C, O'Reilly KR, Schnell DJ, Moore M, et al. 1991. Evidence for the effects of HIV antibody counseling and testing on risk behaviors. *J. Am. Med. Assoc.* 266:2419–29
58. Hirsch MS, D'Aquila RT. 1993. Therapy for human immunodeficiency virus infection. *New Engl. J. Med.* 328:1686–95
59. Kahn JO, Birx DL. 1993. Vaccines directed against HIV: preventive and therapeutic strategies. *AIDS Clin. Rev.* 94:213–38
60. Kahn JO, Lagakos SW, Richman DD, Cross A, Pettinelli C, et al. 1992. A controlled trial comparing continued zidovudine with didanosine in human immunodeficiency virus infection. The NIAID AIDS Clinical Trials Group. *New Engl. J. Med.* 327:581–87
61. Kelly JA, Murphy DA. 1992. Psychological interventions with AIDS and HIV: prevention and treatment. *J. Consult. Clin. Psychol.* 60:576–85
62. Kelly JA, Murphy DA, Sikkema KJ, Kalichman SC. 1993. Psychological interventions to prevent HIV infection are urgently needed. *Am. Psychol.* 48:1023–34
63. Kelly JA, St-Lawrence JS, Hood HV, Brasfield TL. 1989. Behavioral intervention to reduce AIDS risk activities. *J. Consult. Clin. Psychol.* 57:60–67
64. Koff WC, Hoth DF. 1988. Development and testing of AIDS vaccines. *Science* 241:426–32
65. Kosorok MR, Fleming TR. 1993. Using surrogate failure time to increase cost-effectiveness in clinical trials. *Biometrika* 80:823–33
66. Kreiss J, Ngugi E, Holmes K, Ndinya-Achola J, Waiyaki P, et al. 1992. Efficacy of nonoxynol 9 contraceptive sponge use in preventing heterosexual acquisition of HIV in Nairobi prostitutes. *J. Am. Med. Assoc.* 268:477–82
67. Lin DY, Fischl MA, Schoenfeld DA. 1993. Evaluating the role of CD4-lymphocyte counts as surrogate endpoints in human immunodeficiency virus clinical trials. *Stat. Med.* 12:835–42
68. MacQueen KM, Buchbinder S, Douglas JM, Judson FN, McKirnan DJ, Bartholow B. 1994. The decision to enroll in HIV vaccine efficacy trials: concerns elicited from gay men at increased risk for HIV infection. *AIDS Res. Hum. Retroviruses.* 10:S261–64 (Suppl. 2)
69. Mann J. 1993. Acquired immunodeficiency syndrome in the 1990s: a global analysis. *Am. J. Infect. Control* 21:317–21
70. Mascola JR, Mathieson BJ, Zack PM, Walker MC, Halstead SB, Burke DS. 1993. Summary report: workshop on the potential risks of antibody-dependent enhancement in human HIV vaccine tri-

als. *AIDS Res. Hum. Retroviruses* 9: 1175–84

71. McGhee JR, Kiyono H. 1994. Effective mucosal immunity. Current concepts for vaccine delivery and immune response analysis. *Int. J. Technol. Assess. Health Care* 10:93–106

72. McLean AR, Blower SM. 1993. Imperfect vaccines and herd immunity to HIV. *Proc. R. Soc. Lond. Ser. B Biol. Sci.* 253:9–13

73. Meng TC, Fischl MA, Boota AM, Spector SA, Bennett D, et al. 1992. Combination therapy with zidovudine and dideoxycytidine in patients with advanced human immunodeficiency virus infection. A phase I/II study. *Ann. Intern. Med.* 116:13–20

74. Orenstein WA, Bernier RH, Hinman AR. 1988. Assessing vaccine efficacy in the field. Further observations. *Epidemiol. Rev.* 10:212–41

75. Otten MW Jr, Zaidi AA, Wroten JE, Witte JJ, Peterman TA. 1993. Changes in sexually transmitted disease rates after HIV testing and posttest counseling, Miami, 1988 to 1989. *Am. J. Public Health* 83:529–33

76. Peterman TA, Aral SO. 1993. Evaluating behavioral interventions: need for randomized controlled trials. *J. Am. Med. Assoc.* 269:2845

77. Prentice RL. 1989. Surrogate endpoints in clinical trials: definition and operational criteria. *Stat. Med.* 8:431–40

78. Rida WN, Lawrence DN. 1994. Some statistical issues in HIV vaccine trials. *Stat. Med.* 13:2155–77

79. Saltzman SP, Stoddard AM, McCusker J, Moon MW, Mayer KH. 1987. Reliability of self-reported sexual behavior risk factors for HIV infection in homosexual men. *Public Health Rep.* 102:692–97

80. Sande MA, Carpenter CC, Cobbs CG, Holmes KK, Sanford JP. 1993. Antiretroviral therapy for adult HIV-infected patients. Recommendations from a state-of-the-art conference. NIAID State-of-the-Art Panel on Anti-Retroviral Therapy for Adult HIV-Infected Patients. *J. Am. Med. Assoc.* 270:2583–89

81. Saracco A, Musicco M, Nicolosi A, Angarano G, Arici C, et al. 1993. Man-to-woman sexual transmission of HIV: longitudinal study of 343 steady partners of infected men. *J. Acquir. Immune Defic. Syndr.* 6:497–502

82. Schilling RF, El-Bassel N, Gilbert L, Schinke SP. 1991. Correlates of drug use, sexual behavior, and attitudes towards safer sex among African-American and Hispanic women in methodone maintenance . *J. Drug Issues* 21:685–98

83. Schultz AM, Hu SL. 1993. Primate models for HIV vaccines. *AIDS* 7:S161–70 (Suppl. 1)

84. Sheon AR. 1994. Overview: HIV vaccine feasibility studies. *AIDS Res. Hum. Retroviruses.* 10:S195–96 (Suppl. 2)

85. Sheon AR. 1994. Behavioral Considerations in HIV Vaccine Trials, Presentation to the American Public Health Association Annual Meeting, November 1994. Washington, DC

86. Slud EV. 1994. Analysis of factorial survival experiments. *Biometrics* 50:25–38

87. Smith PG, Hayes RJ, Mulder DW. 1991. Epidemiological and public health considerations in the design of HIV vaccine trials. *AIDS* 5:S105–11 (Suppl. 2)

88. Smith PG, Rodrigues LC, Fine PE. 1984. Assessment of the protective efficacy of vaccines against common diseases using case-control and cohort studies. *Int. J. Epidemiol.* 13:87–93

89. Svensson A. 1991. Analyzing effects of vaccines. *Math. Biosci.* 107:407–12

90. Tsoukas CM, Bernard NF. 1994. Markers predicting progression of human immunodeficiency virus-related disease. *Clin. Microbiol. Rev.* 7:14–28

91. Turner CF, Sheon AR. 1994. Behavioral studies relevant to vaccine trial preparation: an introduction. *AIDS Res. Hum. Retroviruses.* 10:S273–76 (Suppl. 2)

92. Volberding PA, Lagakos SW, Koch MA, Pettinelli C, Myers MW, et al. 1990. Zidovudine in asymptomatic human immunodeficiency virus infection. A controlled trial in persons with fewer than 500 CD4-positive cells per cubic millimeter. The AIDS Clinical Trials Group of the Natl. Inst. Allergy Infect. Dis. *New Engl. J. Med.* 322:941–49

93. Walker MC, Fast PE. 1994. Clinical trials of candidate AIDS vaccines. *AIDS* 8:S213–36 (Suppl. 1)

94. Weller SC. 1993. A meta-analysis of condom effectiveness in reducing sexually transmitted HIV. *Soc. Sci. Med.* 36:1635–44

95. World Health Organization. 1994. The current global situation of the HIV/AIDS pandemic. *Wkly. Epidemiol. Rec.* 69:189–96

96. Zekeng L, Feldblum PJ, Oliver RM, Kaptue L. 1993. Barrier contraceptive use and HIV infection among high-risk women in Cameroon. *AIDS* 7:725–31

Annu. Rev. Public Health. 1995. 16:23–41
Copyright © 1995 by Annual Reviews Inc. All rights reserved

BAYESIAN STATISTICAL METHODS IN PUBLIC HEALTH AND MEDICINE

Ruth D. Etzioni

Fred Hutchinson Cancer Research Center, 1124 Columbia Street, Seattle, Washington 98104

Joseph B. Kadane

Department of Statistics, Carnegie-Mellon University, Pittsburgh, Pennsylvania 15213

KEY WORDS: decision theory, prior distribution, estimation, hypothesis testing, likelihood, posterior distribution

ABSTRACT

This article reviews the Bayesian statistical approach to the design and analysis of research studies in the health sciences. The central idea of the Bayesian method is the use of study data to update the state of knowledge about a quantity of interest. In study design, the Bayesian approach explicitly incorporates expressions for the loss resulting from an incorrect decision at the end of the study. The Bayesian method also provides a flexible framework for the monitoring of sequential clinical trials. We present several examples of Bayesian methods in practice including a study of disease progression in AIDS, a comparison of two therapies in a clinical trial, and a case-control study investigating the link between dietary factors and breast cancer.

INTRODUCTION

Bayesian methods are currently enjoying a renaissance in the statistical world. This is largely due to fairly recent advances in computing hardware and algorithms that have made it possible to implement Bayesian analyses previously considered computationally infeasible. As Bayesian methodology be-

23

comes more developed and accepted within the statistical community, its potential for use in applied studies is being recognized. During the past several years, the statistical literature has witnessed a marked increase in the frequency of Bayesian approaches to practical problems, with a significant number in the public health sciences.

In contrast to the growth of interest in Bayesian methods in the statistical world, these methods remain relatively underutilized in public health and medical research. This is partly due to a lack of communication between Bayesian statisticians and the applied research community, although this communication is not entirely nonexistent [see, for example, (40)]. The goal of this article is to bridge this gap; to explain the essence of the Bayesian approach, and to illustrate its utility in a number of research problems in public health and medicine. The article attempts to supply the reader with the beginnings of answers to two key questions namely, (a) What is the Bayesian approach and (b) What is in it for me as a researcher in the health sciences?

The short answer to the first question is that the Bayesian approach means different things to different people. In its purest form it constitutes an alternative way of statistical thinking. Some find the Bayesian way of thinking more natural, coherent, and scientific, and are compelled to adopt a Bayesian approach in all circumstances. However, others view Bayesian methods as simply providing an additional choice of analysis, to be employed should it appear to be more suitable practically, given the problem at hand. As there is clearly a range of motivations for adopting a Bayesian approach to a problem, the discussion and examples that follow attempt to give the reader some insight into the different ways of thinking.

This article considers separately the problems of data analysis and design of studies. Throughout we use real rather than hypothetical data examples to illustrate the practicality of the Bayesian approach. We begin by presenting several examples of problems in the health sciences that have been analyzed using Bayesian methods. In reviewing the results of these studies, we introduce the basic tools upon which Bayesian inferences are based. In some cases, we compare the Bayesian approach with other statistical approaches, noting the relative demands and returns of each.

Often in data analysis, the Bayesian inference corresponds closely to that based on traditional or classical statistical methods. However, Bayesian study designs tend to be quite different from traditional designs based on significance levels and power considerations. We describe the Bayesian approach to design, together with some examples from the clinical trials literature. The final section of the article reviews some of the controversial issues raised by the Bayesian approach, and predicts possible future developments for Bayesian methods in public health and medicine.

BAYESIAN INFERENCE: SOME EXAMPLES

The central idea in the Bayesian approach is a very intuitive one, namely that of updating knowledge. The state of knowledge about quantities of interest before, or *prior* to a study is updated by the study data to yield the state of knowledge after, or *posterior* to the study. The transformation from *prior* to *posterior* is achieved by Bayes Theorem, an explicit mathematical expression for the updating process. This formal mechanism for incorporating prior information is a defining feature of Bayesian inference. Traditional statistical inferences are typically based only on the current study, and little systematic structure exists to facilitate combination of results with those from previous studies.

We explore the idea of the prior-to-posterior transformation by considering several examples of Bayesian inference in problems in the health sciences. We summarize the goals of each study, the prior information, the available data, and the major conclusions based on the posterior state of knowledge.

Example 1: Biological Markers of AIDS Progression

Our first example is a longitudinal study of the decline in CD4 T-lymphocyte counts, a possible marker for disease progression following infection with the AIDS virus. We consider a Bayesian analysis of data from the San Francisco Men's Health Study. Previous studies had suggested that CD4 counts, measured in cells per cubic millimeter of blood, do indeed decline after infection with HIV, and that the rate of decline together with the absolute CD4 level are associated with progression to AIDS.

The major goal of the analysis by Lange et al (39) was to better understand the natural history of this surrogate marker; specifically, to obtain estimates of the average rate of the decline in infected patients, and to assess whether the decline is more rapid immediately after infection than later in the course of the disease.

Some prior information on the rate of change in CD4 counts could be inferred from previous studies. For example, the average period from infection to AIDS had been estimated by several authors to be roughly ten years. In addition, over this period the CD4 T-cell count had been estimated to drop from an average of 1000/mm^3 to 200/mm^3. Based on this information the average annual rate of change in the square root of the CD4 T-cell count was estimated a priori to be −1.75, with a standard deviation of 1; this rate of change was assumed a priori to be constant from infection onwards.

The data for the study consisted of longitudinal series of up to eight repeated CD4 T-cell measurements for 327 infected subjects in the San Francisco Men's

Health Study. CD4 levels were measured approximately twice yearly, beginning in 1984.

Given the data and the prior information, Bayesian analysis of this dataset estimated the average annual change in square root CD4 count to be −1.59, with a standard deviation of 0.56. The analysis also concluded that the study data did not provide evidence for accelerated decline in CD4 counts immediately after seroconversion.

Example 2: Evaluating Clinical Therapies of Potentially Great Benefit

Our second example concerns the analysis of data from the first phase of a clinical trial comparing extracorporeal membrane oxygenation (ECMO), an external system for oxygenating the blood, with conventional therapy, in newborns with respiratory failure (33). The objective was to determine whether randomization was ethically justifiable in a second phase or, equivalently, to evaluate whether the first phase provided sufficient evidence that ECMO was superior to terminate the trial.

Prior information was available on two previous groups of patients. One group of 13 patients had received conventional medical therapy; 11 subsequently died. A second group of eleven patients had received ECMO; only 1 of this group died. In addition, historical mortality rates of up to 80 percent among infants treated with conventional therapy had been reported. Conversely, survival rates of 80 percent among infants treated with ECMO had been reported by several centers using ECMO after 1977.

The data for the analysis consisted of the results of the first phase of the trial, namely four deaths among ten newborns given conventional medical therapy and no deaths among nine patients given ECMO.

Kass & Greenhouse presented a Bayesian analysis of this study (33). In spite of the apparent a priori superiority of ECMO, they chose to interpret the prior information conservatively, as "cautious reasonable skeptics." As a result, their conclusions were based on the probability that ECMO was superior, under a prior assumption of no preference for either ECMO or the conventional therapy. Their analysis strongly suggested that ECMO was superior even when the prior information was interpreted in the most skeptical light. The evidence in favor of ECMO was so strong that even a pessimistic prior assumption of a 75 percent chance that ECMO would do more harm than good, was updated by the study data to about 50 percent that ECMO would be substantially better.

Example 3: Investigating the Link Between Dietary Factors and Breast Cancer

Our third example is an analysis investigating the link between fat and alcohol intake, and breast cancer risk. Raftery & Richardson (48) analyzed data from a case-control study of 854 women that took place in France between 1983 and 1987. The goal of the study was to determine which factors were predictive of disease risk and how to code them in a statistical model adjusting for classical risk factors like parity and age at menarche.

The authors noted that prior studies of the role of fat and alcohol in breast cancer etiology had led to somewhat conflicting conclusions, with some studies succeeding and others failing to show an association. Raftery & Richardson used a description of the prior state of knowledge that captured the lack of precise information on the relative risk corresponding to each dietary covariate.

Bayesian techniques were used to determine which covariates to include in a logistic regression model for breast cancer risk. The covariates considered were alcohol consumption, an indicator of alcohol use, and dichotomization of total and saturated fat intake.

The results of the Bayesian analysis showed that models including the indicator of alcohol use were preferred, given the data. The five most preferred models all included either this variable or the quantitative alcohol consumption variable. Raftery & Richardson concluded that the evidence for the alcohol link was very strong, given the data. This conclusion concurred with the original analysis of the study by Richardson and co-authors (49). Raftery & Richardson also concluded that the evidence for the part played by fat was somewhat weaker, and that the data could not distinguish between the effects of total fat and saturated fat.

We conclude this section by noting a few other examples of areas in the health sciences where Bayesian methods have been successfully employed.

In multicenter clinical trials, Bayesian methods have been used to assess heterogeneity of treatment effects across centers (28, 53, 58). In health services research, Bayesian methods have been used to study the interstate variability in coronary angiography rates for Medicare beneficiaries recovering from recent acute myocardial infarctions (22). Bayesian methods have also been used to investigate the relationship between county-level covariates, like population size and per capita income, and hospital admissions for nonsurgical treatment of back pain in Washington State (51). In medical forensics, Bayesian measures of evidence have been proposed to determine whether a suspect's DNA matches that found at the scene of a crime (6, 50).

The reader is also referred to Racine et al (46) and the volumes edited by Gatsonis et al (23, 24) and Berry and Stangl (8) for further examples of Bayesian methods in practice.

TOOLS OF BAYESIAN INFERENCE

Clearly the Bayesian framework is intuitive and provides answers that respond directly to the questions of interest. But how is Bayesian updating done? This section explains the basic components of the Bayesian updating process, in an attempt to make precise some of the concepts introduced in the previous section. We describe how prior and posterior knowledge are expressed and used to draw inferences, and we introduce Bayesian tools for testing hypotheses.

Prior and Posterior Distributions

Even if prior information is available from previous studies, there is often substantial uncertainty about the exact value of the quantity of interest. This is true also once the study has been completed. This uncertainty is expressed mathematically as a probability distribution over the possible values of the quantity of interest. The probability distribution before the study is termed the *prior distribution* and that after the study the *posterior distribution*. The prior distribution expresses the investigator's knowledge about the quantity of interest prior to the study. Similarly, the posterior distribution expresses the investigator's updated knowledge about the quantity of interest after the study. For example, Lange et al (39) describe their prior state of knowledge about the average annual decline in square-root CD4 counts as a normal distribution with mean −1.75 and a variance of 1. Bayesian updating, together with some modeling assumptions, leads to a normal posterior distribution on this quantity with mean −1.59 and standard deviation 0.56.

Substantial prior uncertainty is expressed by prior distributions with large variances. The larger the prior variance, or the more diffuse the prior distribution, the less influence it has on the end result. In the extreme case of no prior information, or if it is decided to ignore the prior information, noninformative priors may be employed. Such priors generally regard all possible values of the quantity of interest as equally likely. Rather than ignoring the prior information, Kass & Greenhouse (33) interpret it in their own way. They construct a prior distribution that represents the opinion of a cautious, reasonable skeptic, in the sense that the expected benefit of ECMO is zero and if there is a benefit it is likely to be moderate, with a small chance of a significant benefit.

Thus, even if information from previous studies is available, Bayesian analysis may be performed using noninformative, skeptical, or even several prior distributions to investigate sensitivity of inferences to the chosen description of the prior state of knowledge.

Estimation

The posterior distribution is the basic tool of Bayesian estimation. Indeed, it is often graphed as a summary statistic and used directly for inference. By looking at the posterior distribution, one can get an idea of the expected value of quantities of interest (posterior mean), or the most likely value, given the data (posterior mode) as well as the posterior probability of events of substantive interest. For example, when comparing two treatments, the posterior probability that the difference in response rates is positive may be assessed by examining the plot of the posterior distribution of the difference in response rates. Such a plot would display all possible values of the difference in response rates together with an assessment of how likely each value is, given the data.

Several of the examples listed above base inferences directly on plots of the posterior distribution. In a study of interstate variability in coronary angiography rates, Gatsonis et al (24) use one display to graph the posterior distributions of the log-odds of the procedure across states. The posterior distributions are plotted for different age and gender groups. Younger males are seen to have the highest odds on average and older females the lowest. In addition, substantial interstate variability in the probability of angiography is evident. Kass & Greenhouse (33) plot the posterior distribution of the difference between the log-odds of survival on ECMO and the log-odds of survival on standard therapy. The plots show that most of the posterior probability lies above zero. The posterior distributions corresponding to a range of prior distributions are plotted on the same display, giving a clear idea of the sensitivity of inferences to the prior specification.

Estimates based on the posterior include the posterior mean, mode, and median. Interval estimates are called credible intervals, and may be defined in several ways. For example, a 95% equal-tail credible interval is the interval containing the central 95% of the mass of the posterior distribution. The interpretation of a 95% credible interval (L, U) for the quantity of interest is simply that the probability that the quantity lies in (L, U) is 95%. In their analysis of CD4 counts, Lange et al (39) note that the 95% equal-tail credible interval for the change in rate of decline from immediately after infection to later in the course of the disease includes zero. They infer that the data do not provide evidence for a differential decline. Thus, credible intervals are used in much the same way as their classical analogue, the confidence interval.

Bayesian Hypothesis Tests

Consider the test of a null hypothesis H_0 against an alternate H_A. In comparing two treatments, for example, H_0 may be that there is no difference and H_A is that there is one. In DNA fingerprinting, H_0 may be that the blood from the crime scene matches that of the suspect, and H_A that the samples do not match. When selecting models in logistic regression, H_0 may be that a particular covariate need not be included in the model and H_A that the covariate should be included.

Bayesian hypothesis tests require specification of the prior probability of H_0 and H_A and yield corresponding posterior probabilities. The result of a Bayesian hypothesis test is simply the probability that the null hypothesis is true, an interpretation that is often erroneously placed on the result of a classical hypothesis test. Decisions are based on the relative posterior probabilities of H_0 and H_A, interpreted as the evidence provided by the data (and the prior) in favor of one hypothesis versus the other. The procedure is inherently symmetric in that H_A may potentially be rejected in the same way as H_0, as opposed to traditional hypothesis testing in which evidence may be used only to reject, and not to accept the null hypothesis. This particular feature of traditional testing presents a serious problem in clinical equivalence trials, where the goal is to prove H_0, i.e. equivalence of two therapies.

Since the posterior probability of a hypothesis is heavily dependent on its prior probability, there is a need for a measure of evidence in favor of H_0 that is clearly a function of the data alone. In fact, such a measure does exist. It can be shown that the posterior odds of H_0 are simply a multiplicative transformation of the prior odds. The transforming factor is called the Bayes factor, and may indeed be thought of as a measure of evidence provided by the data in favor of H_0; a large value of the Bayes factor implies that the odds of H_0 relative to H_A are increased by the data. In fact, the Bayes factor is the posterior odds when no prior preference is expressed for H_0 or H_A, that is, the prior probability of each is 1/2.

Cornfield (14) discusses the use of Bayes factors in the analyses of clinical trials data; he refers to the Bayes factor as the Relative Betting Odds. Kass & Raftery (34) describe the Bayes factor as a "summary of the evidence, provided by the data in favor of one scientific theory, represented by a statistical model, as opposed to another." Berry (6) uses the Bayes factor quite literally as a measure of evidence for or against the theory that the blood found at the scene of a crime matches that of a suspect. Just how large the Bayes factor needs to be to make a decision in favor of H_0 may depend on the problem (20, 34); Jeffreys (31) suggested some thresholds for this statistic, to be used in much the same way as standard thresholds for the p-value of a traditional hypothesis test.

In model selection problems, the Bayes factor may be used together with the posterior probability to evaluate the evidence in favor of one statistical model versus another. The steps in computing and interpreting the Bayes factor are the same whether or not one model is a special case of the other (nested models); the comparison of two statistical models that are not nested is a ubiquitous problem that does not have a straightforward traditional solution.

Raftery & Richardson (48) used the Bayes factor to select from among four covariates describing alcohol and fat intake in a logistic regression model for breast cancer. They first used a criterion based on the Bayes factor to exclude models from a set of sixteen candidate models. They then calculated posterior model probabilities to select from among the five remaining candidate models. Models that included an alcohol use indicator had higher posterior probabilities. All five retained models included either the alcohol use indicator or a quantitative alcohol consumption variable; the authors concluded that the evidence for an association between breast cancer and alcohol consumption was very strong. Raftery, Madigan & Volinsky (47) have introduced Bayes factors for a similar purpose in Cox regression analysis. Kass & Raftery (34) have authored an extensive review of Bayes factor methodology, with several practical examples and many important insights. However, Kadane & Dickey (32) have criticized the use of Bayes factors because they purport to decide between two hypotheses without taking into account the magnitude of the error resulting from choosing wrongly.

DESIGN

We now turn from the analysis of studies once completed to the topic of study design. Bayesian contributions in the area of design have been especially plentiful in the field of clinical trials, where the monitoring of trials has received a great deal of attention. Bayesian methods for choosing between alternative designs before the start of a trial have also been developed. We consider the monitoring and pretrial design problems separately. For further information on these and other applications of the Bayesian approach to design, the reader is referred to Chaloner & Verdinelli's (13) comprehensive review of the Bayesian design literature.

Monitoring of Trials

The monitoring of sequential clinical trials has been a focal point for debate about the appropriateness of the Bayesian paradigm in clinical research. This is because Bayesian and classical approaches diverge completely on the question of how to monitor clinical trials, and the reasons for the divergence reach to the very foundations of the two paradigms. In a nutshell, classical monitoring of trials requires adjustment of the inference, given the data, for the sampling plan or stopping rule used. Bayesian inferences, on the other hand, require no such adjustment. This difference leads to two very different philosophies of clinical trial monitoring. The debate shows no sign of subsiding; indeed, Anscombe's comment (1) that these "issues [are] much in the air at the present time" is as applicable today as it was then. We summarize the main issues below. Our remarks are abstracted from several articles on the subject, including (1, 2, 7, 14, 15, 29, 43, 56).

The main difference between the Bayesian and classical approaches to monitoring lies in the dependence of inferences, given the data, on the sampling plan. In short, classical inferences depend on the sampling plan; Bayesian inferences do not.

Since the probability of Type 1 error in classical significance testing increases with each look at the data, the significance level at the end of a classical clinical trial depends not only on the data observed, but also on the sampling plan. The *p*-value exhibits a similar dependence on the sampling plan. The *p*-value is the probability of outcomes as or more extreme than that observed; as the sampling plan changes the set of "more extreme" outcomes changes, and with it the *p*-value. Since inferences depend on the sampling plan, they must be explicitly adjusted for the sampling plan used. Equivalently, if a certain overall significance level is desired, the sampling plan must be adjusted so that this is ultimately achieved. There is a large body of work on how to adjust the individual significance levels of the repeat tests used in monitoring clinical trials.

In contrast to the classical approach, Bayesian inference is based on the posterior distribution and is said to follow the *likelihood principle*. In other words, in a trial enrolling 50 patients, the posterior is the same whether the data were examined 5 times, with a decision to continue after each group of 10 patients except for the last, or whether the data were examined for the first time after all 50 patients had enrolled. In other words, the inference depends only on the observed data and on the prior distribution, but not on the sampling plan. As a result, no adjustment is required for the sampling plan used, and even if the sampling scheme implemented differs from that originally planned, the posterior distribution is still a valid inferential tool within the Bayesian framework. Proponents of the Bayesian approach note that unforeseen events requiring alteration of the sampling plan frequently occur in practice. The flexibility of Bayesian methods therefore makes them far preferable to classical methods which are not easily adapted when the original sampling scheme is changed.

We now consider some examples of Bayesian sequential monitoring schemes. Such plans examine the data as they accumulate, and base decisions to stop on the posterior probability of the event of interest. In the common case of clinical trials comparing two treatments, several authors have recommended basing stopping decisions directly on the posterior probability that the treatment difference, Δ, exceeds some bound, ε. If $P(\Delta > \varepsilon \mid data)$ is greater than a given threshold T, then the trial should be stopped; otherwise the trial may be allowed to continue, at least until some truncation point. Carlin et al (9) and Mehta & Cain (43) also recommend this strategy; Freedman & Spiegelhalter (21) describe a similar idea based on a range of equivalence ($\varepsilon_1 \leq \Delta \leq \varepsilon_2$), stopping when the posterior probability that the true treatment difference lies outside this range is high. The threshold T is generally chosen to reflect a common judgment of what constitutes a "high" probability. Berry (4) uses 0.90 or 0.95 for T; Carlin et al follow suit. Mehta & Cain use 0.97, arguing that this conservative value is appropriate in their pilot toxicity setting due to the small number of patients typically accrued to any such trial.

At this point we note that the conceptual and practical simplicity of Bayesian monitoring is, of course, only half of the design story. Methods are needed for evaluating and comparing alternative designs such as stopping rules with different posterior probability thresholds, differing sample sizes, and alternative group-sequential strategies. Such methods are based on Bayesian measures analogous to significance and power: the classical, non-Bayesian ways of discriminating between alternative designs. We discuss some Bayesian measures in the section below. We note, however, that it is also possible to calculate the significance and power of a Bayesian sampling plan. Etzioni & Pepe show how to do this in a pilot toxicity study with a bivariate adverse outcome. The Bayesian monitoring rule is intuitive and ethical, stopping the trial if the posterior probability of toxicity at any point is excessive. Etzioni & Pepe (19) then show how to choose an overall sample size and a threshold for the posterior probability to achieve prespecified significance and power. Grossman et al (27) and Thall & Simon (59) propose a similar approach.

Pre-Trial Design

In general, Bayesian designs do not attempt to control the Type 1 error probability or the power of the study. Rather, Bayesian designs are based on decision theory. The essence of a decision-theoretic approach is the view that the inference given the data is in fact a decision, with possibly adverse or costly consequences. This leads to specification of the loss that will result from an incorrect decision and, conversely, the gain (or utility) from a correct decision. Consider, for example, a clinical trial comparing a new therapy with a standard treatment. At the end of the trial, a decision must be made—either to adopt the new therapy or to continue treating patients with the standard. A decision-theoretic approach considers the losses should the new therapy be selected when the standard is in fact more effective and vice versa. The benefits (negative losses) should the correct decision be made are also be taken into account. Given the data then, the *optimal* decision is simply the one minimizing the loss.

Anscombe, in a paper that has become a classic (1), developed a decision-theoretic approach for the two treatment problem. Anscombe specified the loss to be a function of the difference in treatment effectiveness, the number of patients receiving the inferior treatment during the trial, and the patient horizon or the number of future patients to receive a treatment assignment based on the trial results. In Anscombe's formulation the loss, due to selecting the inferior treatment, increased with the size of the trial and the patient horizon at a rate proportional to the difference in effectiveness between the two treatments. A similar approach was developed by Berry & Ho (7). In formulating stopping rules for a sequential drug development trial, they specified a zero loss associated with not pursuing drug approval at any point, a fixed positive loss associated with pursuing approval for an ineffective drug, and a gain, proportional to the effectiveness of the drug, associated with pursuing approval for an effective drug.

Bayesian designs in the literature can be divided into those that are implicitly decision-theoretic and those that are explicitly decision-theoretic. In explicitly decision-theoretic procedures a loss function is specified, and it provides a recipe for the optimal Bayesian decision, given the data. The implicitly decision-theoretic approaches tend to be developed without reference to formal decision theory, and may be based on traditional decision rules. However, in general, a given decision rule is optimal with respect to some loss and, therefore, even if one uses a standard decision rule based on hypothesis tests, this behavior may be viewed as acting in accordance with some specification of loss. For example, Spiegelhalter, Freedman & Blackburn's (55) predictive power approach to selecting the size of a trial comparing two treatments is interpretable as a decision-theoretic design procedure even though it is presented as a tool for design based on traditional hypothesis testing.

The key to choosing between alternative designs is to think ahead and to compute the expected value, before seeing the data, of the loss that will be incurred by following the planned decision procedure. This is termed the *predictive expected loss*. The costs of collecting the data may be considered in combination with the predictive expected loss. The design that minimizes the combined predictive expected loss and cost is the optimal design. The predictive power of Spiegelhalter, Freedman & Blackburn (55) and Spiegelhalter & Freedman (54) is, in fact, a predictive expected loss corresponding to an implicit loss function.

The appropriate role for the explicitly decision-theoretic approach is a matter of discussion. One school of thought observes that many clinicians and public health researchers feel uncomfortable specifying utilities or losses when money, loss of human life, and/or patient relief from disease may all be at stake (19, 43, 56). This can lead to the use of loss functions that may have mathematical convenience but rarely express the real losses faced by society or by the experimenter. Alternatively, standard or intuitive decision procedures may be employed. The loss functions implicit in such procedures may directly conflict with the real loss. Heitjan, Houts & Harvey (29) suggest that this is in fact the case when standard group-sequential procedures are used for monitoring clinical trials. The implicit loss function conflicts with the patient horizon viewpoint, which specifies losses in terms of the expected response among future patients, assuming that future treatment assignments will be based on the trial results.

A second school of thought believes that the questions posed in loss function elicitation are very important matters that should be addressed. Every decision or decision procedure implicitly uses some trade-off between various risks;

this school believes that it is critical to confront the value trade-off openly, however uncomfortable this may be. Otherwise the risk is very real that behavior will be in accord with an irrelevant system of consequences and losses, and not with the truly pertinent ones.

In a sense, these schools do not differ about Bayesian philosophy at all. Rather the debate is a pragmatic one having to do with the willingness of medical researchers to address difficult value issues. As health care reform gathers momentum, and the need to quantify the costs and benefits of medical interventions grows, investigators are being forced to come to terms with these issues and to specify at least financial costs and benefits. This points to a possibly expanding role for the explicitly decision-theoretic approach in the future.

In addition to elicitation of losses, probability elicitation is generally an important issue for Bayesian design. While Bayesian analyses can be carried out with noninformative or relatively flat priors, this is not the case with Bayesian design. Different priors may be used for design and for analysis, as explored by Etzioni & Kadane (18). Computational tools have been developed to assist in elicitation of prior distributions (12).

With a full elicited loss function and prior distribution, the computational difficulties in evaluating the predictive expected loss can be formidable. Multistage or group-sequential procedures are particularly complex (42). The development of methods to ease the computational burden of Bayesian design is an area of active research.

CONTROVERSIES RAISED BY THE BAYESIAN APPROACH

The Bayesian paradigm stimulates controversy because it forces one to reexamine one's fundamental notions about the concept of probability and the appropriateness of traditionally accepted statistical practices. We have already touched on two major points of controversy, namely the analysis of data that have been collected in a sequential fashion, and the role of decision theory in statistical inference. Traditional and Bayesian approaches in these cases tend to lead to quite different conclusions on a practical level, and these differences result from major differences between the approaches on a foundational level.

The prior distribution, while basic to the Bayesian system of inference, is also a major source of controversy. The definition of the prior as the investigators' beliefs or state of knowledge before seeing the data, a subjective quantity, seems to contrast sharply with the ethic that statistical analyses should be *objective*, defined as inferences being based only on the data observed. Even if the prior distribution is defined instead as a summary of previous evidence, which is usually the case in practice, there is still concern that the historical results upon which the prior is based may not be relevant to the current investigation, or that the investigators' interpretation of the historical results may involve some subjectivity.

One Bayesian response to these concerns is that while objectivity might be desirable, it is simply unattainable in most, if not all, statistical analyses, even outside of the Bayesian paradigm. In parametric analyses, for instance, the choice of likelihood function is under the control of the investigator, and is usually made based on previous studies, the investigators' opinion, or mathematical convenience. Although nonparametric analyses do not generally specify a likelihood, they too require assumptions that may arguably be subjective in nature. Thus, objectivity is rarely attained in data analyses. This is even more so in study design where performing power calculations essentially requires prediction of the true state of nature.

In fact, the use of the prior distribution may be viewed as a strength, rather than a weakness, of the Bayesian paradigm. The prior provides a mechanism for expressing explicitly some of the possibly subjective assumptions that are present, but not usually acknowledged, in classical statistical analyses. Concerns about the relevance or precision of historical information may be expressed through appropriate setting of prior means and variances. Empirical Bayes methods, on the other hand, essentially estimate the prior from the data before applying Bayes Theorem to obtain the posterior, so it is not entirely clear where they fit in the Bayesian framework. There is some debate among Bayesians on this topic. On the one hand, Empirical Bayes methods are often used in analyses that are clearly not Bayesian (38), where they lead to estimates with favorable properties. However, there is no disputing that Empirical Bayes methods rely on the basic Bayesian machinery, that is the transformation from prior to posterior using Bayes Theorem. Therefore, they would appear to be at least partially Bayesian in nature. Discussion of this issue can be found in Morris (44), Hui & Berger (30) and Deely & Lindley (16). The Empirical Bayes primer by Cassella (10) is a very clear introduction to the topic.

CONCLUSIONS

In this article, we have attempted to provide the reader with an understanding of the essence of the Bayesian approach and a feeling for its usefulness in application to problems in the health sciences. We believe that the Bayesian paradigm has a great deal to offer the public health community on a conceptual, foundational, and practical level.

On a conceptual level, the Bayesian transformation from prior to posterior formalizes the scientific processes of interpreting results in the context of other relevant research, and of updating the current state of knowledge as information accumulates. Probability statements based on the posterior distribution are particularly simple to interpret and generally provide direct quantification of probabilities of interest to the subject matter specialist. The conceptual simplicity of the Bayesian framework can be very appealing in complex practical problems, like modeling longitudinal CD4 counts in HIV-positive patients without exact knowledge of the time of infection with the virus. In addition, the Bayesian approach brings with it a new measure of the evidence in favor of a theory or hypothesis, namely the Bayes factor. Like the posterior distribution, the Bayes factor has a simple and direct interpretation, in contrast to standard classical measures of evidence like p-values and significance levels.

The Bayesian approach is also supported by foundational arguments. Briefly, such arguments essentially prove that a rational individual must behave as if maximizing expected utility with respect to some probability distribution. An oft-quoted line of argument leading to the Bayesian approach is the "Dutch Book" argument of deFinetti (17), Kemeny (37), Shimony (52) and Lehman (40). The idea is that if you are willing to take either side of specified bets, at odds you set, either your odds comport with expected utility theory or you can be made to be a sure loser, regardless of random occurrences.

On the practical front, we have observed that as the hurdle of Bayesian computation crumbles, Bayesian methods are being used more frequently to analyze complex practical problems that arise in public health research. The implementation of Bayesian methods is becoming significantly more straightforward and the number of analyses in which the Bayesian approach is preferred from a practical point of view, is bound to increase with the continued development of new Bayesian computational tools and software (see, for example, Zeger & Karim (61). Bayesian methods are particularly useful in testing model selection, and accounting for model uncertainty (see Raftery, Madigan & Volinsky (47) for a recent example in survival analysis). Bayesian methods also have obvious practical appeal in the monitoring of clinical trials. More work is needed to develop and compute Bayesian analogues of power and significance with which clinicians are comfortable, in order to evaluate alternative clinical trial designs.

The practitioner who decides to take a Bayesian approach has several issues to resolve. First, there is the question of whether an explicit decision-theoretic approach is appropriate and, if so, how to formulate expressions for, and obtain information on, losses and costs. Second, there is the question of what prior information exists, and how it relates to the current investigation. All prior assumptions should be justified. This is true also of the likelihood, which must be specified whether or not the approach is Bayesian. Finally, there is the question of the appropriate computational method. The Appendix reviews some important recent advances in this area for the interested reader. Recent developments lead us to predict that in the future, this step will be largely automated; appropriate noninformative, or reference priors, may also become available in Bayesian software packages for design and analysis. Even with this computational assistance, a good deal of thought will still be required. However, as statisticians, we feel that this is entirely appropriate—and not without its rewards; a more thoughtful study, a more thorough resolution of the problem, and a better understanding of the results and their implications.

APPENDIX

Computational Aspects of the Bayesian Approach

Typical Bayesian analyses require integration. Integration is needed to compute the posterior distribution and the posterior moments. In multiparameter problems, integration is needed to obtain marginal distributions of parameters of interest. In a few cases, the likelihood and the prior go together in a particularly neat form for which the integrals can be found analytically. Such a prior is called conjugate. Conjugate priors may not, however, be available or appropriate for a given problem. This section reviews methods available in such situations.

The simplest strategy for integration is to evaluate the function at a suitable grid of points, and to calculate a weighted sum of the results. This method is useful only if the dimensionality of the parameter space is very small. As the dimension grows, the number of evaluations grows exponentially, and most of the important contributions to the integral occur at a very few points, where the integrand is large.

Because the integrand is largest at its maximum, a reasonable idea is to compute the value of the parameter maximizing the integrand (the posterior mode), and the curvature at the maximum. The integral is then approximately equal to the integral under the normal density with mean equal to the posterior mode and variance equal to the inverse of the curvature at the mode. This approximation is a result of the asymptotic normality of the posterior, thus such an approximation generally suffices when the sample size is large. A more refined large-sample technique, especially useful for computing posterior expectations, is the Laplace method (36, 60). Often reparametrization is useful in conjunction with these methods (35). Surprisingly, although the justification for these approximations is asymptotic, they often work well in small samples. The principal limitation is again the dimensionality of the parameter space. Because second derivatives of the integrand are needed, the difficulty of computation grows with the square of the dimension. However, problems with 25 parameters have been successfully treated this way. Raftery & Richardson (48) use the Laplace method to approximate Bayes factors in their case-control study of fat and alcohol intake and breast cancer.

Monte Carlo methods provide a third approach to Bayesian computation. The idea is to simulate from the appropriate posterior distribution and then to approximate functionals of interest by their empirical counterparts based on the simulated sample. For example, the posterior mean of a parameter of interest may be estimated by generating a sample from the corresponding posterior distribution, and calculating the sample mean. Antithetic variates and importance sampling may be used to reduce the variance of the resulting estimate (26).

Until recently, generating a sample from the appropriate posterior distribution was a nontrivial exercise in many practical problems. Recent significant developments in this area have revolutionized the field of Bayesian computation. The resulting techniques are known as Markov Chain Monte Carlo (MC^2), Gibbs sampling or successive substitution sampling. These methods have greatly enhanced our ability to generate random samples from the posterior distribution. Moments, marginal distributions, and other summaries are now much more easily obtained. Software is available to estimate these quantities in a variety of standard and nonstandard models (57). To date, Markov Chain Monte Carlo methods have been used successfully in problems with as many as hundreds of parameters. Indeed, they are fast becoming the tool of choice in Bayesian analyses. Lange et al (39), Stangl (58) and Gatsonis et al (22) all use Gibbs sampling in their analyses. Markov Chain Monte Carlo is especially useful in random effects or hierarchical models, because these lend themselves easily to the structuring required for the algorithm. Gelfand et al (25) illustrate the application of Gibbs sampling in a range of practical problems including some with hierarchical structure. Cassella & George (11) give a very clear introduction to the Gibbs sampling algorithm and its use in Bayesian analysis.

Bayesian computation has been the subject of intensive research recently. As a consequence, further rapid advances may be expected. Two recent reviews are (3) and (45).

Literature Cited

1. Anscombe FJ. 1963. Sequential medicine trials. *Am. Stat. Assoc. J.* 365–83
2. Berger JO, Berry DA. 1988. Statistical analysis and the illusion of objectivity *Am. Sci.* 76:159–65
3. Bernardo JM, Smith AFM. 1994. In *Bayesian Theory.* New York: Wiley
4. Berry DA. 1985. Interim analyses in clinical trials: classical vs. Bayesian approaches. *Stat. Med.* 4:521–26
5. Berry DA. 1991. Inferences using DNA profiling in forensic identification and paternity cases. *Stat. Sci.* 6:175–205
6. Berry DA. 1993. A case for Bayesianism in clinical trials. *Stat. Med.* 12:1377–93
7. Berry DA, Ho C-H. 1988. One-sided sequential stopping boundaries for clin-

ical trials: a decision-theoretic approach. *Biometrics* 44:219–27

8. Berry D, Stangl D, eds. 1994. *Bayesian Biostatistics.* New York: Marcel-Dekker. In press.

9. Carlin BP, Chaloner KC, Church T, Louis TA, Matts JP. 1993. Bayesian approaches for monitoring clinical trials with an application to toxoplasmic encephalitis prophylaxis. *Statistician* 42: 355–67

10. Cassella G. 1985. An introduction to empirical Bayes data analysis. *Am. Stat.* 39:83–87

11. Cassella G, George EI. 1992. Explaining the Gibbs sampler. *Am. Stat.* 46:167–74

12. Chaloner K, Church T, Lewis T, Matts J. 1993. Graphical elicitation of a prior distribution for a clinical trial. *Statistician* 42:341–53

13. Chaloner K, Verdinelli I. 1994. Bayesian experimental design: a review. *Stat. Sci.* Submitted

14. Cornfield J. 1966. A Bayesian test of some classical hypotheses with applications to sequential clinical trials. *J. Am. Stat. Assoc.* 61:577–94

15. Cornfield J. 1966. Sequential trials, sequential analysis and the likelihood principle. *Am. Stat.* 18–24

16. Deely JJ, Lindley DV. 1981. Bayes empirical Bayes. *J. Am. Stat. Assoc.* 76: 833–41

17. deFinetti B. 1975. *Theory of Probability,* Vols. 1, 2. New York: Wiley

18. Etzioni R, Kadane JB. 1993. Optimal experimental design for another's analysis. *J. Am. Stat. Assoc.* 88:1404–11

19. Etzioni R, Pepe MS. 1994. Monitoring of a pilot toxicity study with two adverse outcomes. *Stat. Med.* 13:2311–22

20. Evett IW. 1991. *Implementing Bayesian methods in forensic science.* Presented at Valencia Int. Meet. Bayesian Stat., 4th, Spain

21. Freedman LS, Spiegelhalter DJ. 1989. Comparison of Bayesian with group sequential methods for monitoring clinical trials. *Control. Clin. Trials* 10:357–67

22. Gatsonis C, Hodges JS, Kass RE, Singpurwalla ND, eds. 1993. Case studies in Bayesian statistics. In *Lecture Notes in Statistics,* Vol. 83. New York: Springer. 437 pp.

23. Gatsonis C, Hodges JS, Kass RE, Singpurwalla ND, eds. 1995. Case studies in Bayesian statistics. In *Lecture Notes in Statistics,* Vol. 2. New York: Springer. In press

24. Gatsonis C, Normand S-L, Liu C, Morris C. 1993. Geographic variation of procedure utilization: a hierarchical model approach. *Med. Care* 31:YS54–59

25. Gelfand AE, Hills SE, Racine-Poon A, Smith FM. 1990. Illustration of Bayesian inference in normal data models using Gibbs sampling. *J. Am. Stat. Assoc.* 85: 972–85

26. Geweke J. 1992. Evaluating the accuracy of sampling-based approaches to the calculation of posterior moments. In *Bayesian Statistics,* 4:169–93. Oxford, UK: Oxford Univ. Press

27. Grossman J, Parmar MKB, Spiegelhalter DJ, Freedman L. 1992. Unified hypothesis testing, point estimation and interval estimation for group sequential clinical trials. *Stat. Med.* Submitted

28. Gustafson P. 1993. A Bayesian analysis of bivariate survival data from a multicentre clinical trial. *Tech. Rep. No. 576,* Dep. Stat., Carnegie Mellon Univ., Pittsburgh

29. Heitjan DF, Houts PS, Harvey HA. 1992. A decision-theoretic evaluation of early stopping rules. *Stat. Med.* 11:673–83

30. Hui SL, Berger JO. 1983. Empirical Bayes estimation of rates in longitudinal studies. *J. Am. Stat. Assoc.* 78:753–60

31. Jeffreys H. 1961. *Theory of Probability.* Oxford: Oxford Univ. Press, 3rd ed.

32. Kadane JB, Dickey, JM. 1980. Bayesian decision theory and the simplification of models. In *Evaluation of Econometric Models,* ed. J. Kementa, JB Ransey. New York: Academic

33. Kass RE, Greenhouse JB. 1989. A Bayesian Perspective. Comment on: investigating therapies of potentially great benefit. *Stat. Sci.* 4:310–17

34. Kass RE, Raftery AE. 1995. Bayes factors. *J. Am. Stat. Assoc.* 90: In press

35. Kass RE, Slate EH. 1992. Reparametrization and diagnostics of non-normality (with discussion). In *Bayesian Statistics,* ed. JM Bernardo, JO Berger, AP Dawid, AFM Smith, 4:289–305. Oxford: Clarendon

36. Kass RE, Tierney L, Kadane JB. 1988. Asymptotics in Bayesian inference. *Bayesian Statistics,* ed. JM Bernardo, MH DeGroot, DV Lindley, AFM Smith, 3:261–71. Oxford: Oxford Univ. Press

37. Kemeny JG. 1955. Fair bets and inductive probabilities. *J. Symb. Logic* 20: 263–73

38. Laird NM, Ware JH. 1982. Random-effects models for longitudinal data. *Biometrics* 38:963–74

39. Lange N, Carlin BP, Gelfand AE. 1992. Hierarchical Bayes models for the progression of HIV infection using longitudinal CD4 T-cell numbers. *J. Am. Stat. Assoc.* 87:615–26

40. Lehman RS. 1955. On confirmation and

rational betting. *J. Symb. Logic* 20:251–62

41. Lewis RJ, Wears RL. 1993. An introduction to the Bayesian analysis of clinical trials. *Ann. Emerg. Med.* 22:115–23

42. Lindley DV. 1982. *Bayesian Statistics: A Review.* Philadelphia: SIAM

43. Mehta CR, Cain KC. 1984. Charts for the early stopping of pilot studies. *J. Clin. Oncol.* 2:676–82

44. Morris CN. 1983. Parametric empirical Bayes inference: theory and applications. *J. Am. Stat. Assoc.* 78:47–65

45. O'Hagan AO. 1994. Kendall's advanced theory of statistics. In *Bayesian Inference*, Vol. 2B. London: Edward Arnold

46. Racine A, Grieve AP, Fluhler H. 1986. Bayesian methods: experiences in the pharmaceutical industry. *Appl. Stat.* 35:93–150

47. Raftery AE, Madigan D, Volinsky CT. 1995. Accounting for model uncertainty in survival analysis improves predictive performance. In *Bayesian Statistics,* JM Bernardo, JO Berger, AP Dawid, AFM Smith, Vol. 5. In press

48. Raftery AE, Richardson S. 1993. Model selection for generalized linear models via GLIB, with application to epidemiology. See Ref. 8

49. Richardson S, de Vicenzi I, Gerber M, Pujol H. 1989. Alcohol consumption in a case-control study of breast cancer in Southern France. *Int. J. Cancer* 44:84–89

50. Roeder K. 1994. DNA fingerprinting: a review of the controversy. *Stat. Sci.* 9:222–78

51. Rosenkranz SL, Raftery AE. 1994. Covariate selection in hierarchical models of hospital admission counts: a Bayes factor approach. *Tech. Rep. No. 268,* Dep. Stat., Univ. Washington, Seattle

52. Shimony A. 1955. Coherence and the axioms of confirmation. *J. Symb. Logic* 20:1–28

53. Skene AM, Wakefield JC. 1990. Hierarchical models for multicentre binary response studies. *Stat. Med.* 9:919–29

54. Spiegelhalter DJ, Freedman LS. 1986. A predictive approach to selecting the size of a clinical trial, based on subjective clinical opinion. *Stat. Med.* 5:1–13

55. Spiegelhalter DJ, Freedman LS, Blackburn PR. 1986. Monitoring clinical trials: conditional or predictive power? *Control. Clin. Trials* 7:8–17

56. Spiegelhalter DJ, Freedman LS, Parmar MKB. 1994. Bayesian approaches to randomized trials. *J. R. Statist. Soc. A* 157:1–31

57. Spiegelhalter D, Thomas A, Gilks W. 1993. BUGS Examples, Version 0.3. *Tech. Rep. Med. Res. Counc.,* MRC Biostat. Unit, Univ. Forvie Site, Cambridge, UK. 45 pp.

58. Stangl DK. 1992. *Modeling heterogeneity in multi-center clinical trials using Bayesian hierarchical survival models,* PhD thesis. Carnegie Mellon Univ., Pittsburgh

59. Thall PF, Simon R. 1994. Practical Bayesian guidelines for Phase IIB clinical trials. *Biometrics* 50:337–49

60. Tierney L, Kadane JB. 1986. Accurate approximation for posterior moments and marginal densities. *J. Am. Stat. Assoc.* 81:82–86

61. Zeger SL, Karim MR. 1991. Generalized linear models with random effects: a Gibbs sampling approach. *J. Am. Stat. Assoc.* 86:79–86

Annu. Rev. Public Health. 1995. 16:43–59

EXPOSURE ASSESSMENT ERROR AND ITS HANDLING IN NUTRITIONAL EPIDEMIOLOGY

Lenore Kohlmeier

Department of Nutrition and Epidemiology, School of Public Health, The University of North Carolina, Chapel Hill, North Carolina 27599-7400

Bärbel Bellach

Department of Health Risks and Prevention, Robert Koch Institute, General Pape Strasse 64, D 12101 Berlin, Germany

KEY WORDS: nutritional epidemiology, exposure assessment, energy adjustment, calibration, measurement error

---

ABSTRACT

Exposure assessment is the weakest element in nutritional epidemiologic studies. In the absence of an adequate arsenal of biomarkers of intake in the United States, food frequency questionnaires are widely used to assess habitual frequency of consumption of foods. These tools need to be designed for the population under study, based on prior information on the eating behavior of the population. The questions to be addressed to insure appropriate application of these tools are presented. The influence of various sources and types of measurement error on various scientific hypotheses is addressed. In assessment of nutrient adequacy, information on intra- to interindividual variation of the nutrient or substance of interest is essential. Risk assessment requires examination of sources and extent of bias and differential and nondifferential measurement error within the study. The theory required for error correction is well developed, but rarely carried out because of lack of software and lack of information needed to calibrate the measures.

43

INTRODUCTION

Research on the etiologic role of food-related exposures (both environmental and nutritional) in humans depends on accurate assessment of the exposure, in any of its dimensions. As we understand more about the influence of various aspects of diet-related exposures on the absorption, transport, metabolism, and excretion of other substances, as well as the ability of nutrients to influence gene transcription, most, if not all, epidemiological studies are interested in assessing some dimension of diet as a primary exposure or covariate. As a result, the nutritional epidemiologist is often asked for advice on a method suitable for the assessment of diet in an epidemiological study. The constraints are then outlined as a limit on the number of questions (5–10 preferably) to be self-administered in a paper-pencil questionnaire, and to take no longer than 10 minutes. Total diet should be assessed by this tool since the exact exposure and covariates of interest have not yet been identified.[1]

The range of food-borne exposures of interest include substances carried incidentally on foods, contaminants such as pesticides or heavy metals, chemicals added intentionally as additives, preservatives or fortification, nutrients and an ever-increasing list of nonnutrients produced by the plant or animal, food temperature upon consumption, preparation prior to consumption, packaging, as well as the sum of energy contributed to the diet by all foodstuffs consumed in a defined time period. The dimensions of interest include amount, frequency, and duration of consumption. The exposure most commonly desired is the dietary intake, as an exposure rate, integrated over many years. Collecting information on habitual dietary intake of individuals has long been recognized as a challenging problem in nutrition and epidemiology (5, 13, 22). Scientists wanting to add information about dietary exposure to their studies have been faced with a choice of applying expensive records, employing experienced dietitians, administering an available food frequency questionnaire, or searching for a suitable biomarker of exposure. Each approach has its strengths and weaknesses.

FOOD-BORNE EXPOSURE ASSESSMENT TODAY

Currently, the selection of methods is driven largely by practicability, with little expectation of major improvements (57). The dissatisfaction with currently available methods was evidenced by the popularity of the First International Meeting on Dietary Assessment Methods, held in Minnesota in 1992.

---

[1]Our advice to nutritional epidemiologists asked to construct such a set of questions is, before they are held responsible two years later when very unusual race-, gender-, or age-specific results are found, to just say no.

The bewildering inconsistencies in the results of studies of diet and diseases, such as those on fat and breast cancer, were attributed to tools that are too imprecise to characterize habitual dietary intake of individuals (47). This paper addresses the weaknesses in exposure assessment underlying the current conduct of nutritional epidemiology, and the degree of measurement error arising from our methods of assessing exposure.

Historical and International Perspective

Historically, in the United States, records of consumption were first applied to assess dietary intakes. As food compositional data became available in the 1930s the importance of individual nutrient intake assessment increased (30). Widdowson & McCance introduced a "precise weighing method" in 1936, which has remained the standard in the United Kingdom. Shortly afterward, Burke's diet history method was introduced as a way to shortcut the hand calculation of nutrient intake then current (12). One outcome was the development of food frequency questionnaires, introduced by Stefanik & Trulson in 1962 (48). This method dominates most of nutritional epidemiology in the United States (24). In Europe the situation is different: Computerized diet histories are used in national surveys and case-control studies in Germany (23); weighed records are used in the United Kingdom; and because of strong national preferences, a potpourri of methods is used in the large cohort on diet and cancer—the EPIC study (37).

Anatomy of a Food Frequency Questionnaire

Epidemiological research in the United States relies heavily on semiquantitative food frequency questionnaires for dietary assessment. There are many reasons why this method is preferred: It is designed to allow ranking of individuals whose habitual dietary behavior is known, at a low cost. The development of up-to-date food frequency questionnaires designed specifically for the population of interest in a particular study is hampered by lack of motivation of scientists to insure that methods valid for their population are being applied and scarce resources for developing and validating new methods. Consequently, existing questionnaires are often borrowed and administered uncritically in study populations whose dietary behavior differs substantially from those of the populations for whom the instruments were designed. They are frequently described as validated, implying thereby that they are valid for the purpose at hand. This practice may be due to ignorance of the anatomy of such questionnaires.

Unlike other methods of dietary assessment, food frequency questionnaires are designed specifically to assess variance in the frequency of intake of particular foods, using a minimal number of closed questions. Design decisions are made about which foods to include, which to group, which consumption-frequency levels to allow, what to set as a usual portion size, and how individual foods should be weighted in the development of the nutrient database.

The nutrient database consists of the foods that have been determined to contribute the most to the variance in intake of the nutrient of interest in the population under study (9). These individual food items are often grouped in a much smaller set of questions such as "Please fill in your average use, during the past year, of beef, pork, lamb as a sandwich or mixed dish, e.g. stew, casserole, lasagna, etc." These grouping of foods elicit changes in responses in various ethnic and gender groups (45). The emphasis remains on the frequency of consumption. The person responding to the questionnaire generally then adds up frequencies of consumption across foods and consumption of individual foods across meals—no mean task (44).

Nutrient calculations are based on specially constructed nutrient databases that apply weighted averages of the proportions of intakes of all foods covered by the questions. Determination of average nutrient values requires up-to-date information on the relative consumption of the individual items as a proportion of the group under question in the population of interest. For example, if middle-aged African-American men eat more pork than Caucasian men of the same age, the values for thiamin for the response of daily consumption of beef, pork, or lamb will be based on a different database that weighs pork more heavily than the amount for a daily response for Caucasians. These assumptions about relative consumption need to be checked regularly and updated if necessary.

Finally, it should be kept in mind that the food frequency questionnaire restricts true variance in intake because it limits the number of foods that subjects can report, and truncates the range of quantitative intakes. Generally, 5 to 9 categories of frequency are allowed, ranging from never to a few times per day, whereas more categories seem to improve the validity of the instrument (17). This restriction is responsible for what Beaton refers to as the loss of real variance with this tool due to reductionism and summation (6).

The epidemiologist should therefore consider the following questions before applying a food frequency questionnaire designed for another population:

1. Does this tool capture 80–90% of the interpersonal variance in consumption of the food-borne exposures under study? To do so, the questionnaire must be based on or compared with a recent survey of total diet assessed independently. This information must be conducted in the age, race, gender, ethnic, or religious group under study. The categories of frequency of consumption also need to be examined for appropriateness for the ethnic group understanding.

2. Do the nutrient values attributed to each response apply in this group of people? Individuals consuming more pumpkin pie will have incorrect carotene intakes if the nutrient data are based primarily on apple pie consumption. The nutrient value assigned to the questions should be a weighed

average of up-to-date nutrient information on all consumed items that the question subsumes, because foods differ in some or all of their dietary constituents.

3. Are there systematic biases in response between groups of people of interest? Is the accuracy of information captured, for example, in 50-year-old African-American men similar to that from 50-year-old Caucasian men? Do 70-year-old men respond with a different degree of errors to the same questions than 20-year-old men do? If so, applying the same food frequency questionnaire to all people in studies spanning such different groups can result in an artifactual effect of diet.

4. Are the assumptions about portion size appropriate for the subjects under study, as well as for this gender, age group, and population? Are a significant number of elderly persons, vegetarians, children, or Asians (for whom the assumptions on portion size are inappropriate) included in the study population? Use of a single set of portion sizes could result in inaccurate over- or underestimation of intakes.

5. If this tool is being used to monitor changes in intake of specific foods or nutrients over time, how will changes in diet over time be accounted for? How will the introduction of new foods into the market, changes in price (which affect consumption through changes in portion sizes or frequency of consumption), changes in the use of specific commodities in the food products (such as the oils used in margarine) be captured? Changes in relative consumption levels will need to be accounted for in the weighed estimates of nutrient averages in the nutrient database underlying the food frequency questionnaire.

6. Should a separate dietary assessment instrument or biomarker be administered in a subsample of the population to calibrate the results from the food frequency questionnaire and adjust for errors in it? This procedure has been recommended (8) and is becoming generally recognized (34, 35).

ERROR IN MEASUREMENT OF EXPOSURE

Sources of Error

Errors in nutritional epidemiological studies are partly attributable to the use of flawed dietary intake assessment tools, based on short time spans for the estimation of habitual diet. They include errors in remembering the foods consumed: Either foods are forgotten or phantom foods injected; the frequency of food consumption is inaccurately reported; and the portions consumed are incorrectly quantified. True intraindividual daily and seasonal fluctuations in intake, both of which are highly variable and based on patterns that differ from individual to individual (52), are also components of "error" in the measurement of habitual diet.

Part of the error derives from inadequate cognitive support on the part of the subject. From what is known about memory retrieval, it is unlikely that foods are stored in memory by themselves. They need to be retrieved from long-term memory into short-term memory by reconstruction of the period of time. The time period serves as a memory cue to what was eaten (4). The essential difference between methods of dietary assessment from a psychological point of view lies in the nature of the cues provided to the respondent to elicit information about usual diet (46). In recall and history methods, the cues are the period of time. Food frequency questionnaires use specific foods as the category of "event" that the subject is asked to recall. The better method is the one that best matches the content and organization of memory and the cognitive processes operating on memory representation and response generation.

Types of Error

Error in measurement is a problem in all observational sciences. Since measurement error potentially affects all statistical analysis, considerable attention has been paid to its effect on the properties of estimates and testing procedures. Fuller (20) and Thomas (53) describe this work in detail. From the special nutritional epidemiological point of view, the problem lies in determining the extent of error (including true intraindividual variability) in measures of dietary intakes and how this error affects estimates of adequacy or risk.

If, as is usually the case, measurement errors cannot be avoided, their effect on the estimated exposure-disease relationship should be taken into account. Measurement error can attenuate the observed compared with the true exposure-disease relationship; it can distort associations and interactions between covariates and outcomes; and variance can also be altered. Quantitative assessment of the effects of measurement error requires the structure and distribution of measurement error be known.

Epidemiological publications usually classify measurement errors into "random" and "systematic." Since systematic errors can be randomly distributed, we avoid this terminology and discriminate between unbiased and biased measurement methods and differential and nondifferential errors.

Let X' be an erroneous measurement of the exposure X, for instance, the average daily fat consumption as approximated by a 7-day-weighed dietary protocol. Measuring the daily dietary intake as a surrogate for usual intake results in an error term ε, which is a mixture of methodological error and true individual variation in intake from day to day.

X' is defined as an unbiased measurement of X if the average measurement (7-day-protocol results for fat intake) approaches the true measure as the number of samples increases (habitual fat intake for the individual). Unbiased measurements result for

$$X' = X + \varepsilon,$$ 1.

where ε is a random error variable with expectation 0. Any tendency to over- or underreport the intake of some foods should be adjusted for in each group in which it exists separately. The occurrence of underreporting of alcohol intake or the overestimation of fruit consumption indicates a biased method.

X' is a biased measurement when the average measurement does not approximate the true intake. The simplest case is when the expectation of the error variable ε from equation 1 does not equal 0.

Both biased and unbiased errors can be either differential or nondifferential. Measurement error is nondifferential as long as the error distribution is identical for all individuals of a study or for each subgroup of a population. This would occur in equation 1, when the distribution of the error variable ε would be the same for every individual under study. Measurement errors are differential if the participants of a study react differently to a measurement method that is used within a study. The distribution of the error term ε in equation 1 in this case differs between population groups under study. Take, for example, the case in which hospitalized subjects report a lower variance in their diets than population controls. This discrepancy may be reflective of their current diet, but not the true variance of their habitual diets, The variance and therefore the errors in this case are differential, even if the measurements are unbiased. Biased differential error occurs when obese individuals underestimate or underreport their fat intakes, whereas lean individuals report accurately or overreport.

The distinction between differential and nondifferential measurement error is important for error assessment, adjustment, and correction strategies. For nondifferential errors, the direction of influence on the estimated exposure-disease relationship is presumed to be biased toward zero. With some further information, often the bias can be corrected. Differential errors influence the estimated exposure-disease relations in ways that can be predicted only if there is information about the error in all subgroups under study. Thus, in situations where there are different (but unknown) exposure variances between cases and controls, for whatever reason, the odds ratios from logistic regression may give the appearance of a quadratic relationship between exposure and disease. Robertson et al (40) show an example in which it is impossible to distinguish between differential error and a true curved relationship. Further illustrations of the devastating effects of differential bias are given later.[1]

In summary, dietary intake is rarely, if ever, measured without error; errors can be biased or unbiased; both kinds can be differential or nondifferential. It is important to know the nature of the errors in order to correct the resulting parameter estimates and assess the confidence levels for study conclusions.

---

[1]Energy Adjustment Does Not Correct for Underreporting, B Bellach, L Kohlmeier, submitted.

Validation and Calibration

Validation of the ability of a method to capture habitual intake accurately is not possible. The gold standard for habitual consumption does not yet exist. Because most studies have no basis in "truth," they are therefore calibration and not validation studies. Calibration studies describe the difference between two methods, and provide information on the covariance structure of the errors between methods to allow correction. Furthermore, they are undertaken in order to adjust results between methods or with a single method used over time to a common baseline analogous to calibration in the clinical laboratory.

Assessment of the extent of measurement error inherent in a method is generally presented in validation papers as correlation coefficients between two methods, although this assessment is disputed as a valuable measure (7). Unadjusted correlation coefficients reported in several validation studies for a number of nutrients under various methods are presented in Table 1. They range from 0.21 to 0.74, when food frequency responses are compared with methods considered to be more reliable. Most of the calculated correlation coefficients are under 0.5 and are remarkably consistent for the same nutrient between studies; this consistency may be due to the extent of correlated errors between methods and the similarities in the methods being applied.

Other indices of "validity" include the kappa statistic, Kendall's Tau, and

Table 1 Correlation coefficients for food frequency questionnaire as compared to reference methods

Nutrients	Rimm[a] 1992	Posner[b] 1992	Pietinen[c] 1988	Longnecker[d] 1993	Willett[e] 1985	Block[f] 1990
Calories	.27	.42	.45	.45	.51	51
Fat	.42	.42	.33	.41	.51	.60
PuFA	.29	.29	.38	.60	.34	.48
MuFA	.46	.29	.30		.50	.59
Vitamin A	.45			.40	.35	.47
Iron	.32				.46	.47
Cholesterol		.30	.35	.35	.39	.55

[a] Unadjusted Pearson correlation coefficients between semiquantitative food frequency questionnaires and two one-week records in 157 men from Boston (39).

[b] Spearman rank correlation coefficients between food frequency questionnaires and three-day records in 77 men and 73 women of the Framingham Offspring (34).

[c] Unadjusted Pearson correlation coefficients between food frequency questionnaires and 24 days of food-consumption records (33) in 190 Finnish men.

[d] Unadjusted Pearson correlation coefficients for food frequency questionnaires and 6 days of diet records in 138 adults (28).

[e] Unadjusted Pearson correlation coefficients comparing food frequency results with the means of four one-week diet record (56).

[f] Unadjusted Pearson correlations of the food frequency responses as compared with means of three four-day records in 277 women (10). In this study the authors transformed the data to reduce skewness, which may explain the higher correlation coefficients.

Spearman's rank correlation coefficient. The combination of these three indices gives a better picture of the method's ability to accurately assess intake and to rank individuals (7).

Correlation coefficients as well as many other indices serve only as good summary measures of the performance within a population, since they depend on the range of intakes observed in these groups. For example, the lower correlation coefficients in women than in men can be interpreted either as a lack of precision in women or the result of their smaller range of intake (16). Correlation coefficients only reflect the degree of linear relationship between two methods. Results of regression analysis (estimated regression coefficients and their standard deviation) reflect much more the quantitative differences between methods (8).

To avoid misinterpretation of correlation coefficients and to enhance comparability of different validation or calibration studies, Delcourt et al (16) propose that the standard deviation of the differences between method measurements and the mean difference be used as an indicator of absolute agreement. They also suggest that standard deviation of the average be presented as an indicator of the range of intakes.

Deattenuation of correlation coefficients and energy adjustment of nutrient values are often undertaken in validation reports. Both of these manipulations tend to increase the strength of the relationship. It has been argued that the crude findings underestimate validity, because the method used as a standard inaccurately represents the truth. Careful studies by Plummer & Clayton (34, 35) reveal the existence of large correlated error between various dietary assessment methods and demonstrate that comparison studies that apply methods with correlated errors (where the subjects under- or overestimate with both methods) actually overestimate the validity of the method under study. These authors warn that subjects under close scrutiny may become rehearsed in their responses; a common component of correlated error can occur and thus affect all attempts to adjust for measurement error.

The evaluation of the validity of methods of dietary exposure assessment remains a problem. Since the methods are imperfect, judgment of the degree of validity that a method offers is flawed. Determination of the degree of validity that the measure applied should have to test specific hypotheses remains uncertain. The relationships between validity, error, efficiency, and study size and the effects on estimates are discussed later.

THE INFLUENCE OF MEASUREMENT ERROR

Questions posed by nutritional epidemiologists generally include some of the following (21):

1. How well nourished is a population? What is the nutritional adequacy of a population or subpopulation with regard to a specific nutrient?
2. Is there a relationship between a food-borne exposure and risk of a specific disease?
3. What is the quantitative relationship between unit of consumption of a food or food component under study, be it a biomarker or reported intake, and the outcome of interest?

From a statistical point of view, each of these questions demands different sets of information, sets different demands on the quality of the information, and requires different approaches to measurement and adjustment. We discuss these three components individually in the following sections.

Assessing Nutrient Adequacy or Toxicity

Many nutritional epidemiologists are primarily concerned with the evaluation of the status of a population, with regard to their dietary intakes and requirements. This evaluation involves (a) comparison of true exposures with some reference values to determine whether the population average is indicative of low risk in general, and (b) examination of the population distribution of exposure to determine the extent and nature of the part of the population at high risk (of either deficiency or excessive exposure). This process is analogous to toxicological risk assessment, and requires stable quantitative information on the true absolute levels of intake. Intraindividual variance is not relevant in the estimation of means or group averages. However, to estimate the prevalence of deficiency, intra- to interindividual variances need to be considered. The ratio of intra- to interindividual variance is not only nutrient or substance specific, but can differ by gender, age, ethnic group, and country. This ratio is also determined by the variety of foods available to the population. These considerations apply not only to dietary assessment methods, but also to biomarkers of exposure. For comparison sake, the extreme differences in intra- to interindividual ratios for different nutrients (21, 29, 55) are shown in Table 2.

These variances, and the level of efficiency that is acceptable (55), determine the number of repeated measures or days of intake to be included in the sampling plan. The desirable number of repeated measures is averaged per person and treated as the best individual estimate of exposure (intake). This estimate is used as the individual value in the population distribution of intakes. This new distribution is then used as a basis to estimate the size of the population at risk of high or low intakes. The probability approach (32) is better for determining the size of a population at risk than is using the percentage of individuals below a cutoff level. This approach uses the probability of deficiency at a given level of intake, and sums up the probabilities across

Table 2 Within- to between-person variance ratios

	24 days of records [a]	3 days of records [b]	7 days of records [c]
Energy	1.5	0.9	1.7
Protein	2.2	1.5	
Total fat	1.9	1.3	2.0
Saturated fat (S)	1.4	1.7	
Monosaturated fat	2.6		
Polyunsaturated fat (P)	1.5	2.6	
P/S quotient	1.0		2.6
Cholesterol	3.2	4.2	4.0
Vitamin A	4.6		
Vitamin C	2.9		
Vitamin E	1.6		
Calcium	1.5	.09	

[a] Ref. (21)   [b] Ref. (55)   [c] Ref. (29)

the population distribution. Knowledge of or assumptions about the risk of deficiency or excess at various levels of intakes are needed.

Assessment of Dietary Contributions to Risk of Disease

Whereas nutritionists are traditionally interested in adequacy, epidemiologists are traditionally interested in determining the presence of risk related to exposure. Accurate information on absolute intake levels is therefore not essential. The overriding need is to categorize individuals into groups of exposure with minimal misclassification. A clear differentiation of individuals exposed to high and low levels of the dietary factor of interest at the relevant time period is critical. It is only when the results of studies are being compared or pooled that the accuracy and quantification of exposure become important.

Measurement error, independently of its type, may lead to misclassification and attenuation in this type of analysis (6). Flegal showed that if the underlying hypothesis of a nutrient effect is true, unbiased, nondifferential measurement error of a metrical dietary exposure can result in differential misclassification of individuals into quintiles of this exposure (18). This misclassification results in an unpredictable attenuation of a corresponding estimation of risk. Brenner & Loomis (11) expand on Flegal's work by assessing the direction and magnitude of the resulting misclassification bias under several assumptions about the underlying nondifferential measurement error. Their simulation studies confirm that unbiased nondifferential measurement error leads to bias toward the null of the estimated exposure-disease relationship. They note further that this bias is less than the expected bias with nondifferential misclassification.

Biased nondifferential and nonrandom error (systematic over- or underestimation of exposure) biases the exposure-disease relationship either toward the null or away from the null. The direction depends on the underlying distribution of exposure, the true exposure-disease relationship, and the cut points used for categorization. These results stress the need for careful evaluation of possible effects of categorizing a continuous exposure variable that is erroneously measured.

Dietary assessment methods employed in epidemiological risk assessment should assess the exposure level or frequency for those foods contributing most to the explanation of variance in the outcome of interest in the population under study. If a method assesses this level well, misclassification of exposure will be minimal. The degrees of misclassification resulting from food frequency questionnaire responses for extreme quintiles have been reported in a few validation papers (38, 58). Misclassification of the extreme quintiles by one quintile ranges from 47 to 59%, depending on the nutrient of interest.

Walker & Blettner evaluated the degree of misclassification associated with various levels of correlation coefficients (54). Under the assumption that M, the method being evaluated, and R, the reference method, follow a bivariate normal distribution with a correlation coefficient ρ, they calculated that when ρ falls below 0.8, half of the population will be misclassified. At ρ equal to 0.5, two thirds of the population are misclassified. The loss of power to detect a difference can be compensated to some degree by increasing the sample size. Compensation for error by increasing size may allow detection of statistical significance, but does reduce the estimate of risk (54). Large increases in sample size are required to compensate in cohort studies for loss of power due to misclassification of disease risk. A 30-fold increase is needed to allow detection of a trend in risk across quintiles with correlation coefficients of 0.2 between M and R (54). If the results for validity of food frequency questionnaires presented in Table 1 are taken into account, the high degree of misclassification potential with these methods becomes obvious.

Quantitative Risk Assessments

Although most nutritional epidemiological analyses are currently based on risk detection, optimal levels or toxic levels need to be determined, and the increase or decrease in risk per unit of food or nutrient consumed needs to be quantified. Absolute intake levels are required to conduct such quantitative analyses of risk, just as with determination of adequacy. For some hypotheses, systematic error may not be relevant. One such example is when risk per increment of dietary substance is considered, e.g. the increase in risk of hypertension per mg of sodium consumed, without concern about the baseline. In other cases, both the intercept and the slope are important, which places the greatest challenge on the instrument of measurement. However, strategies to correct measurement error are available for all types of quantitative epidemiological analyses, provided the requisite information on the nature of the error is available.

In nutritional epidemiology, exposure variables X considered in equation 1 are components of dietary intake. This intake can be the long-term, the average true intake, or the actual intake of some nutrient. The most frequently used mathematical model for the relationship between some disease measure d, exposures **X** and some other factors **Y** (confounders, effect modifiers) is

$$d = a + b\mathbf{X} + c\mathbf{Y}, \text{ (\textbf{X} and \textbf{Y} can be vectors).} \qquad 2.$$

For the sake of simplicity the relationship is assumed to be linear. The expectation d of a continuous variable in the classical linear regression model is related to a linear exposure expression. The logistic regression model assumes a linear relationship between the odds of disease occurrence and exposure for a binary disease indicator. In a Cox regression model the logarithm of the hazard function $h(t)$ is approximated by a linear function of exposure variables. The statistical theory of error correction applicable to each of these models has become highly developed in recent years. Because all these models fit into the theoretical concept of generalized linear models, the corrections for measurement errors based on these models can be applied (3, 14, 15, 26, 27, 31, 51, 50).

Armstrong (2) provides a simple illustration of procedures to correct measurement error in those models: It was assumed that the error in measurement error equation 1 is normally distributed with expectation 0 and variance σ_ε, independently of the true value of **X** (i.e. nondifferential unbiased measurement error). Under the further assumption that the true exposure **X** has a normal distribution in the observed population, he used the statistical result that in equation 2, parameter estimates of b are attenuated toward 0, and that the attenuation factor depends only on the variances σ_x of **X** and σ_ε of ε. Therefore, correcting for attenuation due to measurement error requires knowledge of the variances, which usually must be estimated. σ_ε can be estimated by a validation or calibration study, while the estimation of σ_x comes from the main study.

Unfortunately, the simple model for measurement error described above rarely applies exactly to data arising from epidemiological studies. Nevertheless, generalizations can be used to models with one or more erroneously measured exposure(s). Rosner et al (41) present a correction method for logistic regression when there is error (possibly correlated) in one or more covariates, and data are available from both a main study and a validation substudy. The assumption of multivariate normal distribution of all covariates as well as of the error variable is again needed. Because no gold standard exists for many exposures, these authors also propose (42) correction procedures whereby a reproducibility study instead of a validation study is used to obtain data to estimate the error variable variance. In this case, the average of a large number of individual measurements by one method is considered to be the gold standard for an individual's true mean. The assumption here too is that error has to be nondifferential and unbiased.

A growing number of papers deal with measurement error correction in nutritional epidemiology. Some of the models used assume normal distributed errors (43, 49, 50), and some only the knowledge about the true covariance structure of the errors (26, 31). Each paper proposes a statistical procedure to correct the bias that occurs in estimating the parameter vectors **a, b, c** in equation 2 if nondifferential or known differential measurement errors exist. Unfortunately, these procedures have not yet been implemented into widely available statistical software.

There a few examples of the applications of these methods in the nutritional epidemiological substance area. Armstrong et al (1) studied the risk of colon cancer in relation to calories, protein, and fat intake. Using the same approach as Rosner et al (41), they adjusted for measurement error in the estimation of calories, protein, and fat. Estimation of error structure and distribution of the dietary assessment method came from a validation substudy (19). Adjustment for measurement error in each measure singly did not have a great impact on the estimates. However, the simultaneous corrections for variance in trivariate models resulted in strong enhancement of the estimate of risk induced by fat (odds ratio from 1.07 to 1.20) and the protective effect of protein (odds ratio from 0.80 to 0.47).

Rosner et al corrected risk estimates within the Framingham Heart Study, where the incidence of coronary heart diseases is related to several risk factors (42). Reproducibility data (e.g. blood pressure, serum cholesterol, serum glucose) were obtained from a subgroup of people seen at examination two or three times. After correcting for measurement error, estimated odds ratios comparing extreme quintiles of risk factors increased considerably (serum cholesterol 2.2 vs 2.9, serum glucose 1.3 vs 1.5, systolic blood pressure 2.8 vs 3.8).

Thomas et al (53) used a different approach to study the relationships between body mass index and intakes of total energy and fat in American men; in this study, 24-h recall data were available from all participants, and 7-day records were available from a subgroup. Instead of separately estimating uncorrected risks, estimating covariance structures, and recalculating a corrected risk estimation, they used the structural equation approach, fitting the model in only a single step. This approach requires a normal distribution of all variables and the linear relationship between them (53). The authors show that the model fit was much improved by incorporating the covariance of the measurements from the 24-h recalls and the 7-day records into the multivariate normal likelihood function to be maximized (53, p. 82). The usage of these calibration data changes the maximum likelihood estimations of coefficient for energy intake from 0.518 to 0.267. The slope for the impact of total energy on BMI changes from 0.121 to −0.0120.

RECOMMENDATIONS

Measurement error is important in nutritional epidemiology. The goal of a study will dictate the required accuracy and thus the sample size and other aspects of the design. Since some data are virtually guaranteed to contain errors of measurement, the study design should attend to estimating the error distribution. The increasing number of procedures to correct for these errors means that these estimated error distributions can be used to make the estimated parameters more precise and increase confidence in the conclusions. As a consequence, epidemiological studies of food-borne exposures should incorporate calibration studies. The commission of the Federal Health Office in Germany of Nutritional Epidemiology (8) offers good recommendations for the design and analysis of nutritional epidemiological studies.

Literature Cited

1. Armstrong BG, Whittemore AS, Howe GR. 1989. Analysis of case-control data with covariate measurement error: application to diet and colon cancer. *Stat. Med.* 8:1151–63
2. Armstrong BG. 1990. The effects of measurement errors on relative risk regressions. *Am. J. Epidemiol.* 132:1176–84
3. Armstrong BG. 1985. Measurement error in the generalized linear model. *Community Stat.* 14:529–44
4. Baranowski T, Domel SB. 1994. A cognitive model of children's reporting of food intake. *Am. J. Clin. Nutr.* 59:212S–7S (Suppl.)
5. Barrett-Connor E. 1991. Nutrition epidemiology: how do we know what they ate? *Am. J. Clin. Nutr.* 54:182S–7S
6. Beaton GH. 1994. Approaches to analysis of dietary data: relationship between planned analyses and choice of methodology. *Am. J. Clin. Nutr.* 59:253S–61S (Suppl.)
7. Bellach B. 1993. Remarks on the use of Pearson's correlation coefficient and

other association measures in assessing validity and reliability of dietary assessment methods. *Eur. J. Clin. Nutr.* 47: S42–S45 (Suppl. 2)
8. BGA Commission on Nutritional Epidemiology. 1993. Recommendations for the design and analysis of nutritional epidemiologic studies with measurement errors in the exposure variables. *Eur. J. Clin. Nutr.* 47:S53–S57
9. Block G, Hartman AM, Dresser CM, Carroll MD, Gannon J, Gardner L. 1986. A data-based approach to diet questionnaire design and testing. *Am. J. Epidemiol.* 124:453–69
10. Block G, Woods M, Potosky A, Clifford C. 1990. Validation of a self-administered diet history questionnaire using multiple diet records. *J. Clin. Epidemiol.* 43:1327–35
11. Brown CC, Kipnis V, Freedman LS, Hartman AM, Schatzkin A, Wacholder S. 1994. Energy adjustment methods for nutritional epidemiology: the effect of categorization. *Am. J. Epidemiol.* 139 (3):323–38
12. Burke BS. 1947. The dietary history as

a tool in research. *Can. J. Public Health* 23:1041

13. Cameron ME, van Staveren WA, eds. 1988. *Manual on Methodology for Food Consumption Studies.* New York: Oxford Univ. Press

14. Carroll RJ. 1989. Covariance analysis in generalized linear measurement error models. *Stat. Med.* 8:1075–93

15. Carroll RJ, Wand MP. 1991. Semiparametric estimation in logistic measurement error models. *J. R. Statist. Soc. B* 53:573–85

16. Delcourt C, Cubeau J, Balkau B, Papoz L. 1994. Limitations of the correlation coefficient in the validation of diet assessment methods. *Epidemiology* 5:518–24

17. Feskanich D, Marshall J, Rimm EB, Litin LB, Willett WC. 1994. Simulated validation of a brief food frequency questionnaire. *Ann. Epidemiol.* 4:181–87

18. Flegal KM, Keyl PM, Nieto FJ. 1991. Differential misclassification arising from nondifferential errors in exposure measurement. *Am. J. Epidemiol.* 134:1233–44

19. Friedenreich CM, Howe GR, Miller AB. 1991. An investigation of recall bias in the reporting of past food intake among breast cancer cases and controls. *Ann. Epidemiol.* 1:439–53

20. Fuller WA, ed. 1987. *Measurement Error Models.* New York: Wiley

21. Hartman AM, Brown CC, Palmgren J, Pietinen P, Verkasalo M, Myer D, et al. 1990. Variabiliy in nutrient and food intakes among older middle-aged men: implications for design of epidemiologic and validation studies using food recording. *Am. J. Epidemiol.* 132:999–1012

22. Kohlmeier L. 1988. Analytical problems in nutritional epidemiology. In *Epidemiol. Nutr. Health Proc. Berlin Meet. Nutr. Epidemiol., 1st,* ed. L Kholmeier, E Helsing, pp. 9–18

23. Kohlmeier L. 1994. Gaps in dietary assessment methodology: meal- vs list-based methods. *Am. J. Clin. Nutr.* 59: 175S–9S (Suppl.)

24. Kohlmeier L, ed. 1994. *Dietary Assessment Resource Manual.* J. Nutr. 124: 2245S–317S

25. Kohlmeier L, Mensink GBM, Rehm J, Hermann-Kunz E, Haussler A, Maierhofer B. 1990. Development of a fully automated tool for nutrition surveys: diet history. *Annu. Rep. Fed. Health Off. (Bundesgesundheitsamt), Prog. Rep.,* pp. 226–28. Munich: MMV Med. Publ. (In German)

26. Liang K-Y, Liu XH. 1991. Estimating equations in generalized linear models with measurement error. In *Estimating Functions,* ed. VP Godambe, pp. 47–64. Oxford: Clarendon

27. Liu X, Liang K-Y. 1991. Adjustment for non-differential misclassification error in the generalized linear model. *Stat. Med.* 10:1197–211

28. Longnecker MP, Lissner L, Holden JM, Flack VF, Taylor PR, et al. 1993. The reproducibility and validity of a self-administered semiquantitative food frequency questionnaire in subjects from South Dakota and Wyoming. *Epidemiology* 4:356–65

29. Marr JW, Heady JA. 1986. Within- and between-person variation in dietary surveys: number of days needed to classify individuals. *Hum. Nutr. Appl. Nutr.* 40A: 347–64

30. Medlin C, Skinner JD. 1988. Individual dietary intake methodology: a 50-year review of progress. *J. Am. Diet Assoc.* 88:1250–56

31. Nakamura T. 1990. Corrected score function for errors-in-variables models: methodology and application to generalized linear models. *Biometrics* 77: 127–37

32. National Research Council Subcommittee on Criteria for Dietary Evaluation. 1986. *Nutrient adequacy: assessment using food consumtion surveys.* Washington, DC: Natl. Acad. Press

33. Pietinen P, Hartman AM, Haapa E, Räsänen L, Haapakoski J, et al. 1988. Reproducibility and validity of dietary assessment instruments. II. A qualitative food frequency questionnaire. *Am. J. Epidemiol.* 128:667–76

34. Plummer M, Clayton D. 1993. Measurement error in dietary assessment: an investigation using covariance structure models. Part 1. *Stat. Med.* 12:925–35

35. Plummer M, Clayton D. 1993. Measurement error in dietary assessment: an investigation using covariance structure models. Part 11. *Stat. Med.* 12:937–48

36. Posner BM, Martin-Munley SS, Smigelski C, Cupples LA, Cobb JL, et al. 1992. Comparison of techniques for estimating nutrient intake: the Framingham Study. *Epidemiology* 3:171–77

37. Riboli E. 1992. Nutrition and cancer: background and rationale of the European prospective investigation into cancer and nutrition (EPIC). *Ann. Oncol.* 3:783–91

38. Rimm EB, Giovannucci EL, Stampfer MJ, Colditz GA, Litin LB, Willett WC. 1992. Authors' response to "Invited commentary: some limitations of semi-

quantitative food frequency questionnaires". *Am. J. Epidemiol.* 135:1133–36

39. Rimm EB, Giovannucci EL, Stampfer
    MJ, Colditz GA, Litin LB, Willett WC.
    1992. Reproducibility and validity of an
    expanded self-administered semi-
    quantitative food frequency question-
    naire among male health professionals.
    Am. J. Epidemiol. 135:1114–26

40. Robertson C, Boyle P, Hsieh C-C, Mac-
    farlane GJ, Maisonneuve P. 1994. Some
    statistical considerations in the analysis
    of case-control studies when the expo-
    sure variables are continuous measure-
    ments. *Epidemiology* 5:164–70

41. Rosner B, Spiegelmann D, Willett WC.
    1990. Correction of logistic relative risk
    estimates and confidence intervals for
    random within-person measurement
    error: The case of multiple covariates
    measured with error. *Am. J. Epidemiol.*
    132:734–45

42. Rosner B, Spiegelmann D, Willett WC.
    1992. Correction of logistic relative risk
    estimates and confidence intervals for
    random within-person measurement
    error. *Am. J. Epidemiol.* 136:1400-13

43. Schafer DW. 1987. Covariate measure-
    ment error in generalized linear models.
    Biometrics 74:385–91

44. Sempos CT, Briefel RR, Flegal KM,
    Johnson CL, Murphy RS, Woteki CE.
    1992. Factors involved in selecting a
    dietary survey methodology for national
    nutrition surveys. *Austr. J. Nutr. Diet*
    49:96–104

45. Serdula MK, Byers T, Coates R,
    Mokdad A, Simoes EJ, Eldridge L.
    1992. Assessing consumption of high-
    fat foods: the effect of grouping foods
    into single questions. *Epidemiology* 3:
    503–8

46. Smith AF. 1991. Cognitive processes in
    long-term dietary recall. In *Natl. Cent.
    Health Stat. Vital Health Stat.* Hyatts-
    ville MD: US Dep. Health Hum. Serv.
    6, 4:1–14

47. Stamler J. 1994. Assessing diets to im-
    prove world health: nutritional research
    on disease causation in populations. *Am.
    J. Clin. Nutr. Suppl.* 59:146S–56S

48. Stefanik PA, Trulson MF. 1962. Deter-
    mining the frequency intakes of foods
    in large group studies. *Am. J. Clin. Nutr.*
    11:335

49. Stefanski LA. 1985. The effects of mea-
    surement error on parameter estimation.
    Biometrics 72:583–92

50. Stefanski LA. 1989. Correcting data for
    measurement error in generalized lin-
    ear models. *Comm. Stat.* 18(A):1715–
    34

51. Stefanski LA, Carroll RJ. 1985. Covari-
    ate measurement error in logistic regres-
    sion. *Ann. Stat.* 13:1335–51

52. Tarasuk V, Beaton GH. 1991. Day-to-
    day variation in energy and nutrient
    intake: evidence of individuality in eat-
    ing behaviour. *Appetite* 18:43–54

53. Thomas D, Stram D, Dwyer J. 1993.
    Exposure measurement error: influence
    on exposure-disease—relationships and
    methods of correction. *Annu. Rev. Pub-
    lic Health* 14:69–93

54. Walker AM, Blettner M. 1985. Com-
    paring imperfect measures of exposure.
    Am. J. Epidemiol. 121:783–90

55. Wassertheil-Smoller S, Davis BR,
    Breuer B, Change CJ, Oberman A,
    Blaufox MD. 1993. Differences in pre-
    cision of dietary estimates among dif-
    ferent population subgroups. *Ann. Epi-
    demiol.* 3:619–28

56. Willett WC. 1987. Implications of total
    energy intake for epidemiologic studies
    of breast and large-bowel cancer. *Am.
    J. Clin. Nutr.* 45:354–60

57. Willett WC. 1994. Future directions in
    the development of food-frequency
    questionnaires. *Am. J. Clin. Nutr.* 59:
    171S–74S (Suppl.)

58. Willett WC, Sampson L, Stampfer MJ,
    Rosner B, Bain C, et al. 1985. Repro-
    ducibility and validity of a semiquantita-
    tive food frequency questionnaire. *Am.
    J. Epidemiol.* 122:51–65

Annu. Rev. Public Health 1995. 16:61–81

ECOLOGIC STUDIES IN EPIDEMIOLOGY: Concepts, Principles, and Methods

Hal Morgenstern

Department of Epidemiology and Center for Occupational and Environmental Health, University of California, Los Angeles, School of Public Health, Los Angeles, California 90024–1772

KEY WORDS: epidemiologic methods, study design, sources of bias, causal inference, aggregate studies

ABSTRACT

An ecologic study focuses on the comparison of groups, rather than individuals; thus, individual-level data are missing on the joint distribution of variables within groups. Variables in an ecologic analysis may be aggregate measures, environmental measures, or global measures. The purpose of an ecologic analysis may be to make biologic inferences about effects on individual risks or to make ecologic inferences about effects on group rates. Ecologic study designs may be classified on two dimensions: (*a*) whether the primary group is measured (exploratory vs analytic study); and (*b*) whether subjects are grouped by place (multiple-group study), by time (time-trend study), or by place and time (mixed study). Despite several practical advantages of ecologic studies, there are many methodologic problems that severely limit causal inference, including ecologic and cross-level bias, problems of confounder control, within-group misclassification, lack of adequate data, temporal ambiguity, collinearity, and migration across groups.

INTRODUCTION

An ecologic or aggregate study focuses on the comparison of groups, rather than individuals. The underlying reason for this focus is that individual-level data are missing on the joint distribution of at least two and perhaps all

61

variables within each group; in this sense, an ecologic study is an incomplete design (35). Ecologic studies have been conducted by social scientists for more than a century (14a) and have been used extensively by epidemiologists in many research areas. Nevertheless, the distinction between individual-level and group-level (ecologic) studies and the inferential implications are far more complicated and subtle than they first appear. Before 1980, ecologic studies were usually presented in the first part of epidemiology textbooks as simple descriptive analyses in which disease rates are stratified by place and/or time to generate or test hypotheses; little attention was given to statistical methods or inference (e.g. 41). The purpose of this review is to provide a methodologic overview of ecologic studies that emphasizes study design and causal inference. Although ecologic studies are easily and inexpensively conducted, the results are often difficult to interpret.

CONCEPTS AND RATIONALE

Before discussing the design and interpretation of ecologic studies, we must first define the concepts of ecologic measurement, analysis, and inference.

Levels of Measurement

The sources of data used in epidemiologic studies typically involve direct observations of individuals (e.g. age and sex), sometimes subindividual parts (e.g. intraocular pressure of each eye), and occasionally groups or regions (e.g. air pollution and social disorganization). These direct observations are then organized to measure specific variables in the study population: Individual-level variables are properties of individuals, and ecologic variables are properties of groups. To be more specific, ecologic measures may be classified into three types:

1. *Aggregate measures* are summaries (e.g. means or proportions) of observations derived from individuals in each group (e.g. the proportion of smokers or median family income).
2. *Environmental measures* are physical characteristics of the place in which members of each group live or work (e.g. air-pollution level or hours of sunlight). Note that each environmental measure has an analogue at the individual level, and these individual exposures, or doses, usually vary among members of each group, though they may remain unmeasured.
3. *Global measures* are attributes of groups or places for which there is no distinct analogue at the individual level, unlike aggregate and environmental measures (e.g. population density, level of social disorganization, or the existence of a specific law).

Levels of Analysis

The unit of analysis is the common level for which the data on all variables are reduced and analyzed. In an *individual-level analysis*, a value for each variable is assigned to every subject in the study. It is possible, even common in environmental epidemiology, for one or more variables to be ecologic measures. For example, the average pollution level of each county might be assigned to every resident of that county.

In a *completely ecologic analysis*, all variables (exposure, disease, and covariates) are ecologic measures, so the unit of analysis is the group (e.g. region, worksite, school, demographic stratum, or time interval). Thus, within each group, we do not know the joint distribution of any combination of variables at the individual level (e.g. the frequencies of exposed cases, unexposed cases, exposed noncases, and unexposed noncases); all we know is the marginal distribution of each variable (e.g. the proportion exposed and the disease rate—the T frequencies in Figure 1).

In a *partially ecologic analysis* of three or more variables, we have additional information on certain joint distributions (the M and/or N frequencies in Figure 1 and/or rarely the L frequencies); but we still do not know the full joint distribution of all variables within each group (i.e. the ? cells in Figure 1 are missing). For example, in an ecologic study of cancer incidence by county, the joint distribution of age (a covariate) and disease status within each county (the M frequencies in Figure 1) might be obtained from the census and a population tumor registry.

Multilevel analysis is a special type of modeling technique that combines analyses conducted at two or more levels (6, 71, 72). For example, an individual-level analysis might be conducted in each group, followed by an ecologic analysis of all groups using the results from the individual-level analyses. This approach is described in a later section.

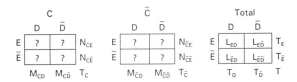

Figure 1 Joint distribution of exposure status (E vs Ē), disease status (D vs D̄), and covariate status (C vs C̄) in each group of a simple ecologic analysis: T frequencies are the only data available in a completely ecologic analysis of all three variables; M frequencies require additional data on the joint distribution of C and D within each group; N frequencies require additional data on the joint distribution of E and C within each group; L frequencies require additional data on the joint distribution of E and D within each group (rarely available); and ? cells are missing in an ecologic analysis.

Levels of Inference

The underlying goal of a given epidemiologic study or analysis may be to make *biologic* (or *biobehavioral*) *inferences* about effects on individual *risks* or to make *ecologic inferences* about effects on group *rates* (45). The target level of causal inference, however, does not always match the level of analysis. For example, the purpose of an ecologic analysis may be to make a biologic inference about the effect of a specific exposure on disease risk. As we see later in this review, such *cross-level inferences* are particularly vulnerable to bias.

If the objective of a study is to estimate the *biologic effect* of wearing a motorcycle helmet on the risk of motorcycle-related mortality among motorcycle riders, the target level of causal inference is biologic. On the other hand, if the objective is to estimate the *ecologic effect* of helmet-use laws on the motorcycle-related mortality rate of riders in different states, the target level of causal inference is ecologic. Note that the magnitude of this ecologic effect depends not only on the biologic effect of helmet use but also on the degree and pattern of compliance with the law in each state. Furthermore, the validity of the ecologic-effect estimate depends on our ability to control for differences among states in the joint distribution of confounders, including individual-level variables such as age and amount of motorcycle riding.

We might also be interested in estimating the *contextual effect* of an ecologic exposure on individual risk, which is also a form of biologic inference (5, 64). If the ecologic exposure is an aggregate measure, we would generally want to separate its effect from the effect of its individual-level analogue. For example, we might estimate the contextual effect of living in a poor area on the risk of disease, controlling for individual poverty level (33). Similarly, in evaluating motorcycle-helmet laws in the U.S., we might want to estimate the contextual effect of living in a state that mandates helmet use on the risk of motorcycle-related mortality in riders, controlling for individual helmet use. Contextual effects are also relevant in infectious-disease epidemiology, where the risk of disease depends on the prevalence of the disease in others with whom the individual has contact (37, 65).

Rationale for Ecologic Studies

There are several reasons for the widespread use of ecologic studies in epidemiology, despite frequent cautions about their methodologic limitations:

1. *Low cost and convenience*   Ecologic studies are inexpensive and take little time because various secondary data sources, each involving different information needed for the analysis, can easily be linked at the aggregate level. For example, data obtained from population registries, vital records,

large surveys, and the census are often linked at the state, county, or census-tract level.

2. *Measurement limitations of individual-level studies*   In environmental epidemiology and other research areas, we often cannot accurately measure relevant exposures or doses at the individual level for large numbers of subjects—at least not with available time and resources. Thus, the only practical way to measure the exposure may be ecologically (45, 46). This advantage is especially true when investigating apparent clusters of disease in small areas (66). Sometimes individual-level exposures, such as dietary factors, cannot be measured accurately because of substantial within-person variability; yet ecologic measures might accurately reflect group averages (31).

3. *Design limitations of individual-level studies*   Individual-level studies may not be practical for estimating exposure effects if the exposure varies little within the study area. However, ecologic studies covering a much wider area might be able to achieve substantial variation in mean exposure across groups (e.g. 50).

4. *Interest in ecologic effects*   As noted above, the stated purpose of a study may be to assess an ecologic effect, i.e. the target level of inference may be ecologic rather than biologic. Ecologic effects are particularly relevant when evaluating the impacts of population interventions such as new programs, policies, or legislation.

5. *Simplicity of analysis and presentation*   In large, complex studies conducted at the individual level, it may be conceptually and statistically simpler to perform ecologic analyses and to present ecologic results than to do individual-level analyses. For example, data from large, periodic surveys, such as the National Health Interview Survey, are often analyzed ecologically by treating some combination of year, region, and demographic group as the unit of analysis.

STUDY DESIGNS

In an ecologic study design, the planned unit of analysis is the group. Ecologic designs may be classified on two dimensions: the method of exposure measurement and the method of grouping (35, 45). Regarding the first dimension, an ecologic design is called *exploratory* if the primary exposure of potential interest is not measured, and *analytic* if the primary exposure variable is measured and included in the analysis. In practice, this dimension is a continuum, since most ecologic studies are not conducted to test a single hypothesis. Regarding the second dimension, the groups of an ecologic study may be identified by place (multiple-group design), by time (time-trend design), or by a combination of place and time (mixed design).

Multiple-Group Study

EXPLORATORY   In this type of exploratory study, we compare the rate of disease among many regions during the same period. The purpose is to search for spatial patterns that might suggest an environmental etiology or more specific etiologic hypotheses. For example, the National Cancer Institute (NCI) mapped the age-adjusted cancer mortality rates in the U.S. by county for the period 1950–69 (42). For oral cancers, they found a striking difference in geographic patterns by sex: Among men, the mortality rates were greatest in the urban Northeast, but among women, the rates were greatest in the Southeast. These findings led to the hypothesis that snuff dipping, which is common among rural southern women, is a risk factor for oral cancers (2). The results of a subsequent case-control study supported this hypothesis (70).

Exploratory ecologic studies may also involve the comparison of rates between migrants and their offspring and residents of their countries of emigration and immigration (31, 41). If the rates differ appreciably between the countries of emigration and immigration, migrant studies often yield results suggesting the influence of certain types of risk factors for the disease under study. For example, if US immigrants from Japan have rates of a disease similar to US whites but much lower than Japanese residents, the difference may be due to environmental or behavioral risk factors operating during adulthood. However, the interpretation of results from these studies is often limited by differences between countries in the classification and detection of disease or cause of death.

In mapping studies, such as the NCI investigation, a simple comparison of rates across regions is often complicated by two statistical problems. First, regions with smaller numbers of observed cases show greater variability in the estimated rate; thus the most extreme rates tend to be observed for those regions with the fewest cases. Second, nearby regions tend to have more similar rates than do distant regions (i.e. autocorrelation) because unmeasured risk factors tend to cluster in space. Statistical methods for dealing with both problems have been developed by fitting the data to an autoregressive spatial model and using empirical Bayes techniques to estimate the smoothed rate for each region (9, 44, 47). The degree of spatial autocorrelation or clustering can be measured to reflect environmental effects on the rate of disease (68, 69). The empirical Bayes approach can also be applied to data from analytic multiple-group studies (described below) by including covariates in the model (e.g. 8, 12).

ANALYTIC   In this type of study, we assess the ecologic association between the average exposure level or prevalence and the rate of disease among many groups. This is the most common ecologic design; typically, the unit of analysis is a geopolitical region. For example, Hatch & Susser (29) examined the association between background gamma radiation and the incidence of child-hood cancers between 1975 and 1985 in the region surrounding a nuclear power plant. Average radiation levels for each of 69 tracts in the region were estimated from a 1976 aerial survey. The authors found positive associations between radiation level and the incidence of leukemia (an expected finding) as well as solid tumors (an unexpected finding).

Data analysis in this type of multiple-group study usually involves fitting the data to a mathematical model. For example, Prentice & Sheppard (51) proposed a linear relative rate model using iteratively reweighted least-squares procedures to estimate the model parameters. Prentice & Thomas (52) also considered an exponential relative rate model, which, they argue, may be more parsimonious than the linear-form model for specifying covariates. These methods can be applied to data aggregated by place and/or time (to be discussed below). Use of ecologic modeling to estimate exposure effects is described in the next section.

Time-Trend Study

EXPLORATORY   An exploratory time-trend or time-series study involves a comparison of the disease rates over time in one geographically defined pop-ulation. In addition to providing graphical displays of temporal trends, time-series data can also be used to forecast future rates and trends. This latter application, which is more common in the social sciences than in epidemiol-ogy, usually involves fitting the outcome data to autoregressive integrated moving average (ARIMA) models (30, 48). The method of ARIMA modeling can also be extended to evaluate the impact of a population intervention (43), to estimate associations betweens two or more time-series variables (7, 48), and to estimate associations in a mixed ecologic design (60; see below).

A special type of exploratory time-trend analysis often used by epidemiol-ogists is age-period-cohort (or cohort) analysis. Through graphical displays or formal modeling techniques, the objective of this approach is to estimate the separate effects of three time-dependent variables on the rate of disease: age, period (calendar time), and birth cohort (year of birth) (32, 35). Because of the linear dependency of these three variables, there is an inherent statistical limitation (identification problem) with the interpretation of age-period-cohort results. The problem is that each data set has alternative explanations with respect to the combination of age, period, and cohort effects; there is no unique set of effect parameters when all three variables are considered simultaneously. The only way to decide which interpretation should be accepted is to consider the findings in light of prior knowledge and, possibly, to constrain the model by ignoring one effect.

Lee et al (40) conducted an age-period-cohort analysis of melanoma mor-tality among white males in the U.S. between 1951 and 1975. They concluded that the apparent increase in the melanoma mortality rate was due primarily to a cohort effect. That is, persons born in more recent years experienced throughout their lives a higher rate than did persons born earlier. In a subsequent paper, Lee (39) speculated that this cohort effect might reflect increases in sunlight exposure or sunburning during youth.

ANALYTIC   In this type of time-trend study, we assess the ecologic association between change in average exposure level or prevalence and change in disease rate in one geographically defined population. As with exploratory designs, this type of assessment can be done by simple graphical displays or by time-series regression modeling (e.g. 48). With either approach, however, the interpretation of findings is often complicated by two problems. First, changes in disease classification and diagnostic criteria can produce very misleading results. Second, the latency of the disease with respect to the primary exposure may be long, variable across cases, or simply unknown. Thus, employing an arbitrary lag between observations—or an empirically defined lag that maximizes the estimated association between the two trends—can also produce misleading results (28).

Darby & Doll (13) examined the associations between average annual absorbed dose of radiation fallout from weapons testing and the incidence rate of childhood leukemia in three European countries between 1945 and 1985. Although the leukemia rate varied over time in each country, they found no convincing evidence that these changes were attributable to changes in fallout radiation.

Mixed Study

EXPLORATORY   The mixed ecologic design combines the basic features of the multiple-group study and the time-trend study. Time-series (ARIMA) modeling or age-period-cohort analysis can be used to describe or predict trends in the disease rate for multiple populations. For example, to test Lee's (39) hypothesis that changes in sunlight exposure during youth can explain the observed increase in melanoma mortality in the U.S., we might conduct an age-period-cohort analysis, stratifying on region according to approximate sunlight exposure (without measuring the exposure). Assuming the amount of sunlight in the regions has not changed differentially over the study period, we might expect the cohort effect described above to be stronger for sunnier regions.

ANALYTIC   In this type of mixed ecologic design, we assess the association between change in average exposure level or prevalence and change in disease rate among many groups. Thus the interpretation of estimated effects is enhanced because two types of comparisons are made simultaneously: change over time within groups and differences among groups. For example, Crawford et al (11) evaluated the hypothesis that hard drinking water (i.e. water with a high concentration of calcium and magnesium) is a protective risk factor for cardiovascular disease (CVD) mortality. They compared the absolute change in CVD mortality rate between 1948 and 1964 in 83 British towns, by water-hardness change, age, and sex. In all sex-age groups, especially for men, the authors found an inverse association between water-hardness change and CVD mortality. In middle-aged men, for example, the increase in CVD mortality was less in towns that made their water harder than in towns that made their water softer.

EFFECT ESTIMATION

A major quantitative objective of most epidemiologic studies is to estimate the effect of one or more exposures on disease occurrence in a well-defined population at risk. A measure of effect in this context is not just any measure of association, such as a correlation coefficient; rather, it reflects a particular causal parameter, i.e. a counterfactual contrast in disease occurrence (21, 24, 27, 46, 58). In studies conducted at the individual level, effects are usually estimated by comparing the rate or risk of disease, in the form of a ratio or difference, for exposed and unexposed populations. In multiple-group ecologic studies, however, we cannot estimate effects directly in this way because of the missing information on the joint distribution within groups. Instead, we regress the group-specific disease rates (Y) on the group-specific exposure prevalences (X). For example, fitting the data to a linear model produces the following prediction equation: $\hat{Y} = B_0 + B_1 X$, where B_0 and B_1 are the estimated intercept and slope, using ordinary least-squares methods. The estimated biologic effect of the exposure (at the individual level) can be derived from the regression results (1, 19). The predicted disease rate $(\hat{Y})$ in a group that is entirely exposed is $B_0 + B_1(1) = B_0 + B_1$, and the predicted rate in a group that is entirely unexposed is $B_0 + B_1(0) = B_0$. Therefore, the estimated rate difference is B_1 and the estimated rate ratio is $1 + B_1/B_0$. Note that this ecologic method of effect estimation requires rate predictions be extrapolated to both extreme values of the exposure variable (i.e. $X = 0$ and 1), which are likely to lie well beyond the observed range of the data. It is not surprising, therefore, that different model forms (e.g. log-linear vs linear) can lead to very different estimates of effect (22). Fitting a linear model, in fact, may lead to negative, and thus meaningless, estimates of the rate ratio.

As an illustration of rate-ratio estimation in an ecologic study, consider Durkheim's (16) examination of religion and suicide in four groups of Prussian provinces between 1883 and 1890 (see Figure 2). The groups were formed by

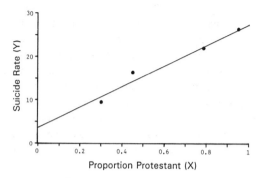

Figure 2 Suicide rate (*Y*, per 10^5/year) by proportion Protestant (*X*) for four groups of Prussian provinces, 1883–90. The four observed points (*X, Y*) are (0.30, 9.56), (0.45, 16.36), (0.785, 22.00), and (0.95, 26.46); the fitted line is based on unweighted least-squares regression [Source: Adapted from Durkheim (16)].

ranking 13 provinces according to the proportion (*X*) of the population that was Protestant. Using ordinary least-squares linear regression, we estimate the suicide rate ($\hat{Y}$, per 10^5/year) in each group to be 3.66 + 24.0(*X*). Therefore, the estimated rate ratio, comparing Protestants with other religions, is 1 + (24.0/3.66) = 7.6. Note in Figure 2 that the fit of the linear model is excellent ($R^2 = 0.97$).

There are two methods used to control for confounders in multiple-group ecologic analyses. The first is to treat ecologic measures of the confounders as covariates (**Z**) in the model, e.g. percent male and percent white in each group. If the individual-level effects of the exposure and covariates are additive (i.e. if the disease rates follow a linear model), then the ecologic regression of *Y* on *X* and **Z** will also be linear with the same coefficients (22, 38). That is, the estimated coefficient for the exposure variable can be interpreted as the rate difference adjusted for other covariates, analogously to the crude estimate discussed above.

The second method used to control for confounders in ecologic analyses is rate standardization for these confounders (57), followed by regression of the standardized rates as the outcome variable. Note that this method requires additional data on the joint distribution of the covariate and disease within each group (i.e. the M frequencies in Figure 1). Nevertheless, it cannot be expected to reduce bias unless all predictors in the model (*X* and **Z**) are mutually standardized for the same confounders (22, 25, 56). Standardization of the exposure prevalences, for example, requires data on the joint distribution of the covariate and exposure within groups (i.e. the N frequencies in Figure 1); however, this information is not often available in ecologic studies.

As in individual-level analyses, product terms (e.g. XZ) are often used in ecologic analyses to model interaction effects, i.e. to assess effect modification. In ecologic analyses, however, the product of X and Z (both group averages) is not, in general, equal to the average product of the exposure (x) and covariate (z) at the individual level within groups. Assuming a linear model, XZ will be equal to the mean xz in each group only if x and z are uncorrelated within groups (22). Thus, as pointed out in the next section, interaction (nonadditive) effects at the individual level complicate the interpretation of ecologic results.

METHODOLOGIC PROBLEMS

Despite the many practical advantages of ecologic studies mentioned previously, there are several methodologic problems that may severely limit causal inference, especially biologic inference.

Ecologic Bias

The major limitation of ecologic analysis for making causal inferences is ecologic bias, which is the failure of expected ecologic effect estimates to reflect the biologic effect at the individual level (18, 19, 25, 45, 54). In addition to the usual sources of bias that threaten individual-level analyses (35, 57), the underlying problem of ecologic analyses for estimating biologic effects is heterogeneity of exposure level and/or covariate levels within groups; as noted earlier, this heterogeneity is not fully captured with ecologic data because of missing information on joint distributions (see Figure 1). Robinson (55) was the first to describe mathematically how ecologic associations could differ from the corresponding associations at the individual level within groups of the same population. He expressed this relationship in terms of correlation coefficients; this relationship was later extended by Duncan et al (15) to regression coefficients in a linear model. The phenomenon became widely known as the *ecologic(al) fallacy* (61), and the magnitude of the ecologic bias may be severe in practice (10, 17, 54, 62, 63).

As an illustration of ecologic bias, consider again Durkheim's data on religion and suicide (Figure 2). The estimated rate ratio of 7.6 in the ecologic analysis may not mean that the suicide rate was nearly eight times greater in Protestants than in non-Protestants. Rather, since none of the regions were entirely Protestant or non-Protestant, it may have been non-Protestants (primarily Catholics) who were committing suicide in predominantly Protestant provinces. It is certainly plausible that members of a religious minority might have been more likely to take their own lives than were members of the majority. The implication of this alternative explanation is that living in a predominantly Protestant area has a contextual effect on suicide risk among non-Protestants, i.e. there is an interaction effect at the individual level between religion and religious composition of one's area of residence.

Interestingly, Durkheim (16) compared the suicide rates (at the individual level) for Protestants, Catholics, and Jews living in Prussia. From his data, we find that the rate was about twice as high in Protestants as in other religious groups. Thus, there appears to be substantial ecologic bias (i.e. comparing rate-ratio estimates of about 2 vs 8). Durkheim, however, failed to notice this quantitative difference because he did not actually estimate the magnitude of the effect in either analysis.

Greenland & Morgenstern (25) showed that ecologic bias can arise from three sources when using simple linear regression to estimate the crude exposure effect: The first may operate in any type of study; the latter two are unique to ecologic studies (i.e. *cross-level bias*), but are defined in terms of individual-level associations.

1. *Within-group bias*   The exposure effect within groups may be biased by confounding, selection methods, or misclassification (35, 57). Thus, for example, if there is positive net bias in every group, we would expect the ecologic estimate to be biased as well.

2. *Confounding by group*   Ecologic bias may result if the background rate of disease in the unexposed population varies across groups, specifically if there is a nonzero ecologic (linear) correlation between mean exposure level and the background rate.

3. *Effect modification by group*   Ecologic bias may also result if the rate difference for the exposure effect at the individual level varies across groups.

Confounding and effect modification by group (the sources of cross-level bias) can arise in three ways: (*a*) Extraneous risk factors (confounders or modifiers) are differentially distributed across groups; (*b*) the ecologic exposure variable has an effect on risk separate from the effect of its corresponding individual-level analogue, e.g. living in a predominantly Protestant area vs being Protestant (in the suicide example); or (*c*) disease risk depends on the prevalence of that disease in other members of the group, which is true of many infectious diseases (37).

Unfortunately, those conditions that produce ecologic bias cannot be observed in ecologic data. Furthermore, the fit of the ecologic regression model, in general, gives no indication of the presence, direction, or magnitude of ecologic bias. Thus, a model with excellent fit may yield substantial bias (e.g. Figure 2), and one model with a better fit than another model may yield more bias.

A potential strategy for reducing ecologic bias is to use smaller units in an ecologic study (e.g. counties instead of states) in order to make the groups more homogeneous with respect to the exposure. On the other hand, this strategy might not be feasible because of the lack of available data aggregated at the same level, and it might lead to two other problems: greater migration between groups (see below) and less precise estimation of disease rates (45, 67).

Problems of Confounder Control

As already indicated, covariates are included in ecologic analyses to control for confounding, but the conditions for a covariate being a confounder are different at the ecologic and individual levels (25, 26). At the individual level, a risk factor must be associated with the exposure to be a confounder. In a multiple-group ecologic study, in contrast, a risk factor may produce ecologic bias (i.e. it may be an ecologic confounder) even if it is unassociated with the exposure in every group, especially if the risk factor is ecologically associated with the exposure across groups (22, 25). Conversely, a risk factor that is a confounder within groups may not produce ecologic bias if it is ecologically unassociated with the exposure across groups.

Control for confounders is more problematic in ecologic analyses than in individual-level analyses (22, 25, 26). Even when all variables are accurately measured for all groups, adjustment for extraneous risk factors may not reduce the ecologic bias produced by these risk factors. In fact, it is possible for such ecologic adjustment to increase bias. It follows from the principles presented in the previous section (25) that there will be no ecologic bias in a multiple-linear-regression analysis if the following conditions are met:

1. There is no residual within-group bias in exposure effect in any group because of confounding by unmeasured risk factors, selection methods, or misclassification.
2. There is no ecologic correlation between the mean value of each predictor and the background rate of disease in the joint reference (unexposed) level of all predictors.
3. The rate difference for each predictor is uniform across levels of the other predictors within groups (i.e. the effects are additive), and each rate difference is uniform across groups (i.e. group does not modify the effect of each predictor at the individual level).

These conditions are sufficient, but not necessary, for the ecologic estimate to be unbiased, i.e. there might be little or no bias even if none of these conditions are met. On the other hand, minor deviations from these conditions can produce substantial ecologic bias (22). Since the sufficient conditions for no ecologic bias cannot be checked with ecologic data alone, the unpredictable and potentially severe nature of such bias makes biologic inference from ecologic analyses particularly problematic. Prentice & Sheppard (51) have suggested that ecologic data be supplemented with individual-level data from each group (or a representative sample) to enhance biologic inference.

Lack of additivity at the individual level (see #3 above) is common in epidemiology, but unmeasured modifiers do not bias results at the individual level if they are unrelated to the exposure (21). Furthermore, interactions may be handled readily at the individual level by including product terms as predictors in the model (e.g. xz). In ecologic analyses, however, lack of additivity within groups is a source of ecologic bias, and this bias cannot be eliminated or reduced by the inclusion of product terms (e.g. XZ) unless the effects are exactly multiplicative and the two variables are uncorrelated within groups (53).

Another source of ecologic bias is misspecification of confounders (26). Although this problem can also arise in individual-level analyses, it is more difficult to avoid in ecologic analyses because the relevant confounder may be the distribution of covariate histories for all individuals within each group. In ecologic studies, therefore, adjustment for covariates derived from available data (e.g. proportion of current smokers) may be inadequate to control confounding. It is preferable, whenever possible, to control for more than a single summary measure of the covariate distribution (e.g. the proportions of the group in each of several smoking categories). In addition, since it is usually necessary to control for several confounders (among which the effects may not be linear and additive), the best approach for reducing ecologic bias is to include covariates for categories of their joint distribution within regions. For example, to control ecologically for race and sex, the investigator might adjust for the proportions of white women, nonwhite men, and nonwhite women (treating white men as the referent), rather than the conventional approach of adjusting for the proportions of men (or women) and whites (or nonwhites).

Within-Group Misclassification

The principles of misclassification bias with which epidemiologists are familiar when interpreting the results of analyses conducted at the individual level do not apply to ecologic analyses. At the individual level, for example, nondifferential misclassification of exposure nearly always leads to bias toward the null. In multiple-group ecologic studies, however, this principle does not hold when the exposure variable is an aggregate measure. Brenner et al (4) have shown that nondifferential misclassification of a binary exposure within groups usually leads to bias away from the null and that the bias may be severe. Greenland & Brenner (23) have provided a simple method to correct for nondifferential misclassification of exposure or disease in ecologic analyses, based on estimates of sensitivity and specificity.

In studies conducted at the individual level, misclassification of a covariate, if nondifferential with respect to both exposure and disease, will usually reduce our ability to control for that confounder (20, 59). That is, adjustment will not completely eliminate the bias due to the confounder. In ecologic studies, however, nondifferential misclassification of a binary confounder within groups does not affect our ability to control for that confounder, provided there is no cross-level bias (3).

If all but one variable (e.g. the exposure or a covariate) in a given analysis is measured at the individual level, this partially ecologic analysis may also be regarded as nonecologic with the ecologic variable misclassified. Thus, the resulting bias may be understood in terms of misclassification bias operating at the individual level.

Other Problems

LACK OF ADEQUATE DATA   Certain types of data, such as medical histories, may not be available in aggregate form; or available data may be too crude, incomplete, or unreliable, such as sales data for measuring behaviors (45, 67). In addition, secondary sources of data from different administrative areas or from different periods may not be comparable. For example, disease rates may vary across countries because of differences in disease classification or case detection. Furthermore, since many ecologic analyses are based on mortality rather than incidence data, causal inference is further limited (35).

TEMPORAL AMBIGUITY   In a well-designed cohort study of disease incidence, we can usually be confident that disease occurrence did not precede the exposure. In ecologic studies, however, use of incidence data provides no such assurance against this temporal ambiguity (45). The problem is most troublesome when the disease can influence exposure status in individuals or when the disease rate can influence the mean exposure in groups (through the impact of population interventions designed to change exposure levels in areas with high disease rates).

The problem of temporal ambiguity in ecologic studies (especially time-trend studies) is further complicated by an unknown or variable latent period between exposure and disease occurrence (28, 67). The investigator can only attempt to deal with this problem in the analysis by examining associations for which there is a specified lag between observations of average exposure and disease rate. Unfortunately, there may be little prior information about latency on which to base the lag, or appropriate data may not be available to accommodate the desired lag.

COLLINEARITY   Another problem with ecologic analyses is that certain predictors, such as sociodemographic and environmental factors, tend to be more highly correlated with each other than they are at the individual level (10, 62).

The implication of such collinearities is that it is very difficult to separate the effects of these variables statistically; analyses yield model coefficients with very large variances, so effect estimates may be severely distorted. In general, collinearity is most problematic in multiple-group ecologic analyses involving a small number of large, heterogeneous regions (15, 64).

MIGRATION ACROSS GROUPS   Migration of individuals into or out of the source population can produce selection bias in a study conducted at the individual level because migrants and nonmigrants may differ on both exposure prevalence and disease risk. Although it is clear that migration can also cause ecologic bias (36, 49), little is known about the magnitude of this bias or how it can be reduced in ecologic studies (46).

CONTEXTUAL AND MULTILEVEL ANALYSES

Knowing the severe methodologic limitations of ecologic analysis for making biologic inferences, many epidemiologists who report ecologic results argue that there can be no cross-level bias because their primary objective is to estimate an ecologic effect. For example, we might want to estimate the ecologic effect (effectiveness) of state laws requiring smoke detectors by comparing the fire-related mortality rate in those states with the law vs other states without the law (45). Although this is a reasonable objective, the interpretation of observed ecologic effects is complicated by two issues:

First, biologic inference may be implicit to the objectives of an ecologic study unless the underlying biologic and contextual effects are already known from previous research. Can smoke detectors placed appropriately in homes reduce the risk of fire-related mortality in those homes by providing an early warning of smoke? Does living in an area where most homes are properly equipped with smoke detectors reduce the risk of fire-related mortality in homes with and without smoke detectors? The first question refers to a possible biologic (biobehavioral) effect; the second question refers to a possible contextual effect. Even if these effects exist, the ecologic effect of smoke-detector laws also depends on other factors, e.g. the level of enforcement, the quality of smoke-detector design and construction, the cost and availability of smoke detectors, and their proper placement, installation, operation, and maintenance. In an ecologic study without additional information, the ecologic effect is completely confounded with biologic and contextual effects.

The second complicating issue in interpreting observed ecologic effects is the need to control for confounders measured at the individual level. Even if the exposure is a global measure, such as a law, groups are seldom completely homogeneous or comparable with respect to confounders. To make a valid comparison between states with and without smoke-detector laws, for example, we would need to control for differences among states in the joint distribution of extraneous risk factors, such as socioeconomic status of residents, firefighter availability and access, building design, and construction (see also *Problems of Confounder Control*).

Perhaps the best solution to these problems is to incorporate both individual-level and ecologic measures in the same analysis. This approach might include different measures of the same factor; e.g. each subject would be characterized by his/her own exposure level as well as the average exposure level for all members of the group to which s/he belongs (aggregate measure). Not only would this approach help to clarify the sources and magnitude of ecologic and cross-level bias, but it would also allow us to separate biologic, contextual, and ecologic effects. It is especially appropriate in social epidemiology, infectious-disease epidemiology, and the evaluation of population interventions.

There are two statistical methods for including both individual-level and ecologic measures in the same analysis. The first method, often called *contextual analysis* in the social sciences, is a simple extension of conventional modeling such as multiple linear regression or logistic regression (5, 34). The model, which is fit to the data at the individual level, includes both individual-level and ecologic predictors. For example, suppose we wanted to estimate the effect of "herd immunity" on the risk of an infectious disease. The risk (y) of disease might be modeled as a function of the following linear component: $b_0 + b_1x + b_2\bar{x} + b_3x\bar{x}$, where x is the individual's immunity status and $\bar{x}$ is the prevalence of immunity in the group to which that individual belongs (65). Therefore, b_2 represents the contextual effect of herd immunity, and b_3 represents the interaction effect, which allows the herd-immunity effect to depend on the individual's immune status. The interaction term is needed in this application, since we would expect no herd-immunity effect among immune individuals. Note, however, that the interpretation of the interaction effect depends on the form of the model (35, 57).

An important limitation of contextual analysis is that observations for individuals within groups are not likely to be independent, which is a basic assumption of conventional modeling. If there are contextual effects, then the outcomes for individuals in the same group are more likely to resemble each other than are the outcomes for individuals in different groups. To handle this problem of within-group clustering, we treat the sampling of individuals from groups as random effects; this approach is called *multilevel modeling, hierarchical regression,* or *random-effects modeling* (6, 71, 72).

Multilevel modeling is a powerful technique with many applications; it can be used to estimate contextual and ecologic effects and to derive improved (empirical Bayes) estimates of biologic effects. At the first level of analysis, we might predict individual risk or health status within each group as a function of several individual-level variables. At the second (ecologic) level, we predict the estimated regression parameters (e.g. the intercept and slopes) from the first level as a function of several ecologic variables. For example, Humphreys & Carr-Hill (33) used multilevel modeling to estimate the contextual effect of living in a poor area on several health outcomes, controlling for the individual's income and other covariates. In a conventional ecologic analysis, the effects of living in a poor area and income would be confounded, and ecologic estimates of effect would be susceptible to cross-level bias.

CONCLUSIONS

Several practical advantages make ecologic studies especially appealing for undertaking various types of epidemiologic research. Despite these advantages, however, ecologic analysis poses major problems of interpretation when making ecologic inferences and especially when making biologic inferences (due to ecologic bias, etc). From a methodologic perspective, it is best to have individual-level data on as many relevant nonglobal measures as possible. Just because the exposure variable is measured ecologically, for example, does not mean that other variables should be as well.

Even when the stated purpose of the study is to estimate an ecologic effect, biologic inference is usually implicit in epidemiology. Thus, to address the underlying research questions, we typically would want to estimate and/or control for biologic and contextual effects, preferably using multilevel analysis. In contemporary epidemiology, the "ecologic fallacy" reflects the failure of the investigator to recognize the need for biologic inference and thus for individual-level data.

ACKNOWLEDGMENTS

The author would like to thank Drs. Sander Greenland and Matthew Longnecker for their helpful comments.

Literature Cited

1. Beral V, Chilvers C, Fraser P. 1979. On the estimation of relative risk from vital statistical data. *J. Epidemiol. Community Health* 33:159–62
2. Blot WJ, Fraumeni JF Jr. 1977. Geographic patterns of oral cancer in the United States: etiologic implications. *J. Chron. Dis.* 30:745–57
3. Brenner H, Greenland S, Savitz DA. 1992. The effects of nondifferential confounder misclassification in ecologic studies. *Epidemiology* 3:456–59
4. Brenner H, Savitz DA, Jöckel K-H, Greenland S. 1992. Effects of nondifferential exposure misclassification in ecologic studies. *Am. J. Epidemiol.* 135: 85–95
5. Boyd LH Jr, Iversen GR. 1979. *Contex-*

tual *Analysis: Concepts and Statistical Techniques.* Belmont, CA: Wadsworth
6. Bryk AS, Raudenbush SW. 1992. *Hierarchical Linear Models: Applications and Data Analysis Methods.* Newbury Park, CA: Sage
7. Catalano R, Serxner S. 1987. Time series designs of potential interest to epidemiologists. *Am. J. Epidemiol.* 126:724–31
8. Clayton DG, Bernardinelli L, Montomoli C. 1993. Spatial correlation in ecological analysis. *Int. J. Epidemiol.* 22:1193–202
9. Clayton D, Kaldor J. 1987. Empirical Bayes estimates of age-standardized relative risks for use in disease mapping. *Biometrics* 43:671–81
10. Connor MJ, Gillings D. 1984. An empiric study of ecological inference. *Am. J. Public Health* 74:555–59
11. Crawford MD, Gardner MJ, Morris JN. 1971. Changes in water hardness and local death-rates. *Lancet* 2:327–29
12. Cressie N. 1993. Regional mapping of incidence rates using spatial Bayesian models. *Med. Care* 31:YS60–65 (Suppl.)
13. Darby SC, Doll R. 1987. Fallout, radiation doses near Dounreay, and childhood leukaemia. *Br. Med. J.* 294:603–7
14. Dogan M, Rokkan S, eds. 1969. *Social Ecology.* Cambridge, MA: MIT Press
14a. Dogan M, Rokkan S. 1969. Introduction. See Ref. 14, pp. 1–15
15. Duncan OD, Cuzzort RP, Duncan B. 1961. *Statistical Geography: Problems in Analyzing Areal Data,* pp. 64–67. Westport, CT: Greenwood Press
16. Durkheim E. 1951. *Suicide: A Study in Sociology,* pp. 153–54. New York: Free Press
17. Feinleib M, Leaverton PE. 1984. Ecological fallacies in epidemiology. In *Health Information Systems,* ed. PE Leaverton, L Massö, pp. 33–61. New York: Praeger
18. Firebaugh G. 1978. A rule for inferring individual-level relationships from aggregate data. *Am. Sociol. Rev.* 43:557–72
19. Goodman LA. 1959. Some alternatives to ecological correlation. *Am. J. Sociol.* 64:610–25
20. Greenland S. 1980. The effect of misclassification in the presence of covariates. *Am. J. Epidemiol.* 112:564–69
21. Greenland S. 1987. Interpretation and choice of effect measures in epidemiologic analysis. *Am. J. Epidemiol.* 125:761–68
22. Greenland S. 1992. Divergent biases in ecologic and individual-level studies. *Stat. Med.* 11:1209–23
23. Greenland S, Brenner H. 1993. Correct-

ing for non-differential misclassification in ecologic analyses. *Appl. Statist.* 42:117–26
24. Greenland S, Maclure M, Schlesselman JJ, Poole C, Morgenstern H. 1991. Standardized regression coefficients: a further critique and review of some alternatives. *Epidemiology* 2:387–92
25. Greenland S, Morgenstern H. 1989. Ecological bias, confounding, and effect modification. *Int. J. Epidemiol.* 18:269–74
26. Greenland S, Robins J. 1994. Invited commentary: ecologic studies—biases, misconceptions, and counterexamples. *Am. J. Epidemiol.* 139:747–60
27. Greenland S, Schlesselman JJ, Criqui MH. 1986. The fallacy of employing standardized regression coefficients and correlations as measures of effect. *Am. J. Epidemiol.* 123:203–8
28. Gruchow HW, Rimm AA, Hoffman RG. 1983. Alcohol consumption and ischemic heart disease mortality: are time-series correlations meaningful? *Am. J. Epidemiol.* 118:641–50
29. Hatch M, Susser M. 1990. Background gamma radiation and childhood cancers within ten miles of a US nuclear plant. *Int. J. Epidemiol.* 19:546–52
30. Helfenstein U. 1991. The use of transfer function models, intervention analysis and related time series methods in epidemiology. *Int. J. Epidemiol.* 20:808–15
31. Hiller JE, McMichael AJ. 1991. Ecological studies. In *Design Concepts in Nutritional Epidemiology,* ed. BM Margetts, M Nelson, pp. 323–53. Oxford: Oxford Univ. Press
32. Holford TR. 1991. Understanding the effects of age, period, and cohort on incidence and mortality rates. *Annu. Rev. Public Health* 12:425–57
33. Humphreys K, Carr-Hill R. 1991. Area variations in health outcomes: artefact or ecology. *Int. J. Epidemiol.* 20:251–58
34. Iversen GR. 1991. *Contextual Analysis.* Newbury Park, CA: Sage
35. Kleinbaum DG, Kupper LL, Morgenstern H. 1982. *Epidemiologic Research: Principles and Quantitative Methods,* pp. 77–81, 130–34, 184–280. New York: Van Nostrand Reinhold
36. Kliewer EV. 1992. Influence of migrants on regional variations of stomach and colon cancer mortality in the western United States. *Int. J. Epidemiol.* 21:442–49
37. Koopman JS, Longini IM Jr. 1994. The ecological effects of individual exposures and nonlinear disease dynamics in populations. *Am. J. Public Health* 84:836–42

38. Langbein LI, Lichtman AJ. 1978. *Ecological Inference.* Beverly Hills, CA: Sage
39. Lee JAH. 1982. Melanoma and exposure to sunlight. *Epidemiol. Rev.* 4:110–36
40. Lee JAH, Petersen GR, Stevens RG, Vesanen K. 1979. The influence of age, year of birth, and date on mortality from malignant melanoma in the populations of England and Wales, Canada, and the white population of the United States. *Am. J. Epidemiol.* 110:734–39
41. MacMahon B, Pugh TF. 1970. *Epidemiology: Principles and Methods,* pp. 137–98, 175–84. Boston: Little, Brown & Co.
42. Mason TJ, McKay FW, Hoover R, Blot WJ, Fraumeni JF Jr. 1975. *Atlas of Cancer Mortality for US Counties: 1950–1969,* pp. 36, 37. DHEW Publ. No. (NIH) 75–780. Washington, DC: US GPO
43. McDowall D, McCleary R, Meidinger EE, Hay RA Jr. 1980. *Interrupted Time Series Analysis.* Beverly Hills, CA: Sage
44. Mollie A, Richardson S. 1991. Empirical Bayes estimation of cancer mortality rates using spatial models. *Stat. Med.* 10:95–112
45. Morgenstern H. 1982. Uses of ecologic analysis in epidemiologic research. *Am. J. Public Health* 72:1336–44
46. Morgenstern H, Thomas D. 1993. Principles of study design in environmental epidemiology. *Environ. Health Perspect.* 101:23–38 (Suppl. 4)
47. Moulton LH, Foxman B, Wolfe RA, Port FK. 1994. Potential pitfalls in interpreting maps of stabilized rates. *Epidemiology* 5:297–301
48. Ostrom CW Jr. 1990. *Time Series Analysis: Regression Techniques.* Newbury Park, CA: Sage. 2nd ed.
49. Polissar L. 1980. The effect of migration on comparison of disease rates in geographic studies in the United States. *Am. J. Epidemiol.* 111:175–82
50. Prentice RL, Kakar F, Hursting S, Sheppart L, Klein R, Kushi LH. 1988. Aspects of the rationale for the Women's Health Trial. *J. Natl. Cancer Inst.* 80: 802–14
51. Prentice RL, Sheppard L. 1989. Validity of international, time trend, and migrant studies of dietary factors and disease risk. *Prev. Med.* 18:167–79
52. Prentice RL, Thomas D. 1993. Methodologic research needs in environmental epidemiology: data analysis. *Environ. Health Perspect.* 101:39–48 (Suppl. 4)
53. Richardson S, Hémon D. 1990. Ecological bias and confounding (letter). *Int. J. Epidemiol.* 19:764–66
54. Richardson S, Stücher I, Hémon D. 1987. Comparison of relative risks obtained in ecological and individual studies: some methodological considerations. *Int. J. Epidemiol.* 16:111–20
55. Robinson WS. 1950. Ecological correlations and the behavior of individuals. *Am. Sociol. Rev.* 15:351–57
56. Rosenbaum PR, Rubin DB. 1984. Difficulties with regression analyses of age-adjusted rates. *Biometrics* 40:437–43
57. Rothman KJ. 1986. *Modern Epidemiology,* pp. 41–49, 82–94. Boston: Little, Brown & Co.
58. Rubin DB. 1978. Bayesian inference for causal effects: the role of randomization. *Ann. Stat.* 6:34–58
59. Savitz DA, Baron AE. 1989. Estimating and correcting for confounder misclassification. *Am. J. Epidemiol.* 129:1062–71
60. Sayrs LW. 1989. *Pooled Time Series Analysis.* Newbury Park, CA: Sage
61. Selvin HC. 1958. Durkheim's "Suicide" and problems of empirical research. *Am. J. Sociol.* 63:607–19
62. Stavraky KM. 1976. The role of ecologic analysis in studies of the etiology of disease: a discussion with reference to large bowel cancer. *J. Chron. Dis.* 29: 435–44
63. Stidley C, Samet JM. 1994. Assessment of ecologic regression in the study of lung cancer and indoor radon. *Am. J. Epidemiol.* 139:312–22
64. Valkonen T. 1969. Individual and structural effects in ecological research. See Ref. 14, pp. 53–68
65. Von Korff M, Koepsell T, Curry S, Diehr P. 1992. Multi-level analysis in epidemiologic research on health behaviors and outcomes. *Am. J. Epidemiol.* 135:1077–82
66. Walter SD. 1991. The ecologic method in the study of environmental health. I. Overview of the method. *Environ. Health Perspect.* 94:61–65
67. Walter SD. 1991. The ecologic method in the study of environmental health. II. Methodologic issues and feasibility. *Environ. Health Perspect.* 94:67–73
68. Walter SD. 1992. The analysis of regional patterns in health data: I. Distributional considerations. *Am. J. Epidemiol.* 136:730–41
69. Walter SD. 1992. The analysis of regional patterns in health data: II. The power to detect environmental effects. *Am. J. Epidemiol.* 136:742–59
70. Winn DM, Blot WJ, Shy CM, Pickle LW, Toledo A, Fraumeni JF Jr. 1981. Snuff dipping and oral cancer among

women in the southern United States. *N. Engl. J. Med.* 304:745–49

71. Wong GY, Mason WM. 1985. The hierarchical logistic regression model for multilevel analysis. *J. Am. Statist. Assoc.* 80:513–24

72. Wong GY, Mason WM. 1991. Contextually specific effects and other generalizations for the hierarchical linear model for comparative analysis. *J. Am. Statist. Assoc.* 86:487–503

Annu. Rev. Public Health. 1995. 16:83–103

BIOMARKERS AND MECHANISTIC APPROACHES IN ENVIRONMENTAL EPIDEMIOLOGY

Jonathan M. Links, Thomas W. Kensler, and John D. Groopman

Department of Environmental Health Sciences, The Johns Hopkins University School of Hygiene and Public Health, Baltimore, Maryland 21205

KEY WORDS: molecular epidemiology, molecular biomarkers, carcinogenesis, exposure assessment

ABSTRACT

Environmental epidemiological research involves the identification of relationships between previous exposures to putative causative agents and subsequent biological effects with study populations. Such relationships are often hard to fully characterize because of difficulties in accurately quantifying exposure, dose, and effect. Biomarkers are indicators, residing in biological systems or samples, of exposure, dose, effect, or susceptibility. Biomarkers of exposure indicate the presence of previous exposure to an environmental agent; a biomarker of dose bears a quantitative relationship to previous exposure or dose; these include exogenous substances, interactive products, or interactions that change the status of the target molecule. Biomarkers of effect indicate the presence and magnitude of a biological response to exposure to an environmental agent; these include endogenous components, or measures of the functional capacity or state of the system. Biomarkers of susceptibility indicate an elevated sensitivity to the effects of an environmental agent; these include the presence or absence of an endogenous component, or abnormal functional responses to an administered challenge. The development of molecular biomarkers for environmental agents is based upon specific knowledge of metabolism, interactive product formation, and general mechanisms of action. The validation of any biomarker-effect link requires parallel experimental animal and human epidemiological studies.

83

0163-7525/95/0510-0083$05.00

INTRODUCTION

Epidemiological research fundamentally involves the identification of relationships between previous exposures to putative causative agents and subsequent biological effects in clusters of individuals within study populations. In the broad field of environmental health, such relationships are often difficult to fully characterize because of impediments to accurately quantifying exposure, dose, and effect. Exposure is any condition that provides an opportunity for an external environmental agent to enter the body. Dose is the amount of agent actually deposited within the body. Typically, the distinction between exposure and dose is blurred, although in reality significantly different doses can result from the same exposure. Effect is the biological response of an individual to the agent. Methods to more accurately and sensitively characterize exposure, dose, and effects are needed in research involving environmental agents. These methods will produce more appropriate risk assessments for populations.

In the course of identifying putative causative agents, and in the context of characterizing relationships between agents and effect, successful elucidation of the underlying mechanisms involved in the continuum between exposure and clinical disease can make the association much more credible. It is helpful to think of a multistage process, often referred to as the toxicological paradigm, which starts with exposure, and progresses through internal dose (e.g. deposited body dose), biologically effective dose (e.g. dose at the site of toxic action), early biological effect (e.g. at the subcellular level), and altered structure or function (e.g. subclinical changes), and ends with clinical disease. Any stage of this process may be modified by host-susceptibility factors, including genetic traits.

In both quantitatively characterizing agent-effect relationships and deriving mechanistic descriptions of the process, it would be useful to distinguish each stage in the process, and to be able to assess or measure directly the conditions at each stage (or the passage of an individual through each stage). Since all of the stages except initial exposure represent processes occurring within the body, in vivo indicators of the condition of each stage are needed. Biological markers (biomarkers) are such indicators, residing in biological systems or samples, that signal the occurrence of specific events or status. Molecular epidemiology focuses on the use of these biomarkers in epidemiologic research.

Molecular biomarkers are typically indicators of exposure, dose, effect, or susceptibility (49, 50–53). As defined below, a biomarker of exposure indicates the presence of previous exposure to an environmental agent; a biomarker of dose bears a quantitative relationship to previous exposure or dose. Such a biomarker may be an exogenous substance, an interactive product (e.g. between a xenobiotic compound and endogenous components), or an interaction that changes the status of the target molecule. A biomarker of effect indicates the presence (and magnitude) of a biological response to exposure to an environmental agent. Such a biomarker may be an endogenous component, a measure of the functional capacity of the system, or an altered state recognized as impairment or disease. A biomarker of susceptibility indicates an elevated sensitivity to the effects of an environmental agent. Such a biomarker may be the presence or absence of an endogenous component, or an abnormal functional response to an administered challenge. Biomarkers thus offer significant potential in clarifying the relationships between environmental agents and disease (81).

The development of molecular biomarkers for environmental agents should be based upon specific knowledge of metabolism, interactive product formation, and general mechanisms of action (37). The validation of any biomarker-effect link requires parallel experimental and human studies. Ideally, an appropriate animal model is used to determine the associative or causal role of the marker in the disease or effect pathway and to establish relationships between dose and response. The putative marker can then be validated in pilot human studies where sensitivity, specificity, accuracy, and reliability parameters are established (36). Data obtained in these studies can be used to assess background levels, relationship of the marker to external dose or to disease status, and intra- or interindividual variability, as well as feasibility of the analytic methods for use in larger population-based studies. Prospective epidemiological studies may be necessary to demonstrate the role that the marker plays in the overall pathogenesis of the disease or effect. In the context of assessing the passage of an individual through the toxicological paradigm, it is important to understand whether the biomarker represents a transient or irreversible event. For transient events, the measurement must be made while the biomarker exists.

ENVIRONMENTAL AGENTS

Environmental agents, whether naturally occurring or man-made, may be broadly classified as chemical, physical, or biological in character. Human exposure to environmental agents occurs as a result of contaminated air, water, soil, or food. This exposure is the result of the proximity between the agent-containing vector and humans. In general, the vector quantities and concentrations of the agents, and the interplay of any modifying factors, determine the actual exposure. Host factors then modify this exposure in leading to internal dose.

Biomarkers of these agents may themselves be chemical, physical, or biological in character. The agent may itself be the biomarker; many metals are measurable directly in body tissues and fluids, for example. Frequently, however, metabolic products of agent-body interactions serve as markers of exposure, dose, or effect. Carcinogen-DNA and carcinogen-protein adducts are good examples. Finally, altered structure or function may serve as the marker, such as the altered expression of a gene, or a decrease in organ function.

BIOMARKERS OF EXPOSURE AND DOSE

In general, epidemiologic research requires knowledge of both dose and response. Ideally, the biologically effective dose would be assessed, and correlated with response. As described above, this dose is the result of exposure and internal dose processes. A mechanistic understanding of the progression from exposure to internal dose to biologically effective dose is necessary for the complete understanding of this relationship. Unfortunately, it is usually difficult to separate exposure, internal dose, and biologically effective dose. Accordingly, we directly monitor either exposure or internal dose, and relate these measurements to effect.

There is potential confusion regarding the distinction between a biomarker of exposure and of dose. In general, the term exposure refers to an assessment of the opportunity for transfer of an environmental agent to the body. Typically, such an assessment would include measurements of the quantity or concentration of the agent present in the environment, and the duration of exposure. Thus, the conventional use of the term exposure deals only with conditions, not results. In the context of biomarkers, exposure must take on a different meaning, because biomarkers, by definition, involve measurements of substances residing within the body. Accordingly, we differentiate biomarkers of exposure from those of dose by considering qualitative indices as markers of exposure, and quantitative indices as markers of deposited body dose. Thus, when no exact quantitative relationship exists between the degree of prior exposure and the amount of biomarker present, the biomarker's presence is only an indicator that previous exposure occurred.

Exposure

In the absence of biomarkers, an assessment of exposure typically requires measurement of toxicant levels in the environment, and characterization of the individual's presence in, and time of interaction with, that environment. The measurement of toxicants in media (e.g. air, water, soil, or food) is accomplished by a wide array of analytical methodologies. Assessments of exposure include questionnaires, personal external monitors, and measurements of chemicals or physical agents in the ambient environment. Questionnaires have been used extensively to estimate broad dietary exposures to chemical compounds and smoking histories, for example. This approach is imprecise for measuring certain kinds of exposures, such as those occurring through diet, since knowledge of specific dietary chemical agents is still limited.

A complexity arising from the use of ambient measurements to determine exposure status of individuals is the heterogeneous nature of most environmental contaminations. It is rare for an agent to be evenly distributed in environmental media. For example, the distribution of aflatoxins in grains is very uneven due to variable patterns of mold growth; the sampling procedure used often results in a greater than 100% coefficient of variation (11). Thus, extrapolation from data on grain contamination to an individual's exposure is imprecise. Given such problems, the goals for the development of specific biomarkers to assess exposure must include an ability to integrate multiple portals of entry, integrate fluctuating exposures over time, relate time of exposure to dose, and examine mechanistically important biological targets. These requirements assume increased relevance when we recognize that safety regulations designed to limit human risk are often set on the basis of ambient exposure determinations.

Human breath analysis has been used to determine specific solvent vapors in exhaled air (64). In this type of analysis, the subject exhales through a carbon-containing tube connected to a respirometer, with subsequent measurement by gas chromatography. This method has been used to determine styrene exposure, particularly in workers in the shipbuilding industry.

Internal Dose

Because of the problems described above for extrapolating ambient measurements to specific individual exposures, measures of internal dose of a specific agent provide a clearer demonstration that a toxicant has been absorbed and distributed in the body. Many direct measurements of toxic chemicals or their metabolites in body fluids and excreta (e.g. blood, urine, feces, milk, amniotic fluid, sweat, hair, nails, saliva, breath) have been done. When a quantitative measurement of body burden is possible, we consider the marker to indicate deposited body dose. For example, fat tissue concentrations of compounds such as polychlorinated biphenyls (PCBs), polybrominated biphenyls (PBBs), organochlorine pesticides, and dioxins (TCDD) can be measured. One recent study reported relationships between previous exposures to PCBs and to DDE [1,1-dichloro-2,2-bis(p-chlorophenyl) ethylene], the major metabolite of DDT [2,2-bis(p-chlorophenyl)-1,1,1-trichloroethane], and breast cancer risk in women (82). These researchers collected sera from over 14,000 participants enrolled between 1985 and 1991. In a nested case-control study, they found that mean levels of DDE and PCBs were higher for breast cancer patients than for control subjects. It is important to note that the serum samples were obtained after (or at most six months before) diagnosis. In the most recent study with prospectively gathered data (41), no differences in DDE or PCB levels between cases and controls were found. The investigators emphasized the importance of prospective study design in the validation of biomarkers, and concluded that "... future investigations must consider the biologic mechanisms involved ...."

Smoking status in people has been extensively examined by using urinary and blood nicotine or cotinine levels (30, 31). Data derived from these studies have shown that cigarette-smoking status can be assessed qualitatively; however, the quantitative level (i.e. the number of cigarettes smoked) is difficult to estimate by these methods. This use of blood nicotine or cotinine presence is thus consistent with our definition of a biomarker of exposure. In a more recent study, specific metabolites of one of the tobacco-specific nitrosamines, 4-(methylnitrosamino)-1-(3-pyridyl)-1-butanone (NNK), a potent chemical carcinogen, were quantified in the urine of smokers (13). These metabolites were not detected in the urine of nonsmokers. This study provides the first evidence for metabolites of tobacco-specific nitrosamines in human urine. This is an important finding because these tobacco-specific nitrosamines may be causally related to both active and passive smoking-induced cancers, and variations in the levels of these markers might thus be related to disease risk in exposed individuals (see below). To the extent that a quantitative relationship between the degree of exposure to cigarette smoke and the amount of these nitrosamines or their metabolites can be demonstrated, their use is consistent with our definition of biomarkers of dose.

An example of the use of the agent as its own biomarker is in bone-seeking radionuclides. These alpha-emitting actinides (isotopes of uranium, plutonium, americium, and curium) are typically inhaled, and concentrate in bone. There they decay to daughters (which can be thought of as metabolites), and in the process emit alpha particles that deposit significant energy in bone. These daughters are themselves radioactive. Some of these daughters emit low-energy photons, which are easier to detect than the alpha particles. While initial attempts to assay the body burden of these radionuclides used excreta or external measurements over the thorax, a more direct measure of bone deposition was desirable. Cohen and colleagues (14) developed a method in which the low-energy photons are measured by scintillation detectors surrounding the skull. This approach, when used with background correction and appropriate calibration, enables an estimation of body burden. Another example of the use of the daughter of a radionuclide is in measurement of Pb-210 as an indicator of cumulative radon exposure (16). In this application, scintillation detectors surround the skull, and a calibrated measurement of the photon emissions from Pb-210 permits estimation of cumulative exposure. Here it is actually the daughters of radon, which are alpha-emitting radionuclides, that are of principal interest. The decay chain includes Pb-210, so a measurement of its concentration directly implies amounts of the alpha-emitting daughters.

The measurement of the body burden of lead is an example of both an agent acting as its own biomarker, and the distinction between internal dose and biologically effective dose (discussed in greater detail below). It is well-established that blood lead levels reflect recent environmental exposure (29). However, some manifestations of lead toxicity, such as renal dysfunction or diminished neuropsychological performance, correlate better with other measures of body burden, such as bone or tooth levels. Furthermore, it is known that bone contains over 90% of the lead body burden (3). Thus, the body burden of lead, as characterized by bone stores, may be the more relevant measure in relating dose to effect.

In an attempt to directly measure bone lead, x-ray fluorescence has been used (35, 73). In this approach, an external radiation source is used to ionize lead atoms in bone. This ionization process leads to a rearrangement of the electrons orbiting the lead nucleus, which in turn results in emission of x-rays. The energies of these so-called fluorescent x-rays are characteristic for lead, and may be externally detected. By careful calibration of the system, the measured x-ray intensity may be converted to bone lead concentration in bone.

Biologically Effective Dose

Internal dose measurements provide unequivocal identification of chemical exposures, although they do not provide evidence that toxicologic damage has occurred; it is this damage that possibly results in cancer or other diseases. Among the various possible biomarkers reflective of these disease endpoints, the measurement of carcinogen-DNA and protein adducts is of significant interest because they are direct products of (or surrogate markers for) damage to critical macromolecular targets. These adducts result from the covalent interactions of chemical carcinogens (or their metabolites) with DNA or other proteins. If pro-mutagenic DNA adducts are not repaired prior to replication, replication errors (e.g. base-pair insertions, deletions, substitutions, or recombination) may occur; these errors represent initiating events in the multistage carcinogenesis process (see below).

CHEMICAL-DNA ADDUCTS   Many different types of analytical techniques have been devised to measure chemical-macromolecular adducts, as reviewed by Kaderlik (38) and Wogan (81). These techniques have been used to measure composite and specific DNA adducts in cellular DNA isolated from peripheral lymphocytes, bladder, and colonic tissues, as well as excreted DNA adducts in the urine of humans exposed to environmental toxicants. In addition, these types of techniques have been applied in a clinical setting to examine DNA adducts of people undergoing chemotherapy with alkylating agents, in an attempt to associate adduct levels with clinical outcome (61, 62).

As discussed above, we consider biomarkers of exposure to have a qualitative relationship to exposure or dose, whereas biomarkers of dose have a quantitative relationship. With these definitions, chemical-DNA adducts can serve as biomarkers of either exposure or dose. For example, Kaderlik and colleagues (39) have documented in a pilot study the occurrence of DNA adducts in exfoliated urothelial cells of a worker exposed to the aromatic amine 4,4′-methylene-bis(2-chloroaniline) (MOCA) by P-32 postlabeling analysis. This analysis revealed the presence of a single, major DNA adduct that co-chromatographed with the major N-hydroxy-MOCA-DNA adduct [N-(deoxyadenosin-8-yl)-4-amino-3-chlorobenzyl alcohol] formed in vitro. Thus examination of DNA from exfoliated urothelial cells may provide an effective, noninvasive means for biomonitoring the formation of carcinogen-DNA adducts resulting from occupational or environmental exposures.

In a manner similar to that described above, DNA adducts have been detected in biopsy samples of human urinary bladder tissue, as reviewed by Bartsch and colleagues (5). Total polycyclic aromatic hydrocarbon (PAH)-carcinogen-DNA adduct levels and the average levels of several specific adducts were significantly elevated in samples of current smokers, as opposed to never-smokers or ex-smokers with at least five years' abstinence from smoking (74). Putative aromatic amine adducts were detected, and one of these displayed chromatographic behavior identical to the predominant adduct induced by the human urinary bladder carcinogen, 4-aminobiphenyl, which is present in cigarette smoke.

An example of exposure to complex mixtures occurs with cigarette smoking, as reviewed by Perera (59, 60). PAH-DNA adduct levels have been detected in smokers, but the data across many different studies have not been consistent. This is especially true if the total cell population found in the white cell buffy-coat is used as a source of DNA. Recently, Santella and colleagues (66) found that only DNA combined from lymphocyte and monocyte fractions of smokers exhibited detectable levels of PAH-DNA adducts, at an approximately fourfold higher rate than in nonsmokers. Only these particular populations of white blood cells seemed to represent a valid, readily accessible tissue for monitoring genotoxicity from cigarette smoke; the lymphocytes can be considered as surrogates for the actual target tissues.

In addition to monitoring carcinogen-DNA adducts in situ in DNA, the eliminated products of these adducts can be determined in urine. These urinary biomarkers have been especially amenable to comprehensive validation studies (68). One example of these studies is the examination of the dose-dependent excretion of urinary aflatoxin biomarkers in rats following a single exposure to aflatoxin B_1 (AFB_1) (21). The relationship between AFB_1 dose and the excretion of the major nucleic acid adduct, aflatoxin B_1-N^7-guanine (AFB-N^7-Gua), over the initial 24 hour period following exposure demonstrated an excellent linear correspondence between oral dose and excretion of a biologically relevant metabolite in urine. In contrast, other oxidative metabolites, such as aflatoxin P_1 (AFP_1), revealed no linear excretion characteristics.

As noted above, it is useful in the development and validation of a biomarker to perform parallel experiments in animal models and systematic evaluation in humans; the development of biomarkers for aflatoxins is a good example (24). A study of the urinary excretion of aflatoxin metabolites in an area of the People's Republic of China with a high incidence of liver cancer has been completed (23). Total 24-hr urine samples were collected and analyzed by an immunoaffinity HPLC analysis to determine individual aflatoxins in the urine samples. $AFB-N^7-Gua$, aflatoxin M_1 (AFM_1), AFP_1, and AFB_1 were the aflatoxins most commonly detected. However, only $AFB-N^7-Gua$ and AFM_1 showed a dose-dependent relationship between aflatoxin intake and urinary levels, indicating that these two metabolites might be useful biomarkers of dose. Of interest, these studies also demonstrated that the kinetics of formation and excretion of $AFB-N^7-Gua$ in human urine were almost identical with those in the F344 rat, thereby enhancing the value of rodent studies for assessing risk to humans.

Oxidative stress is thought to play important roles in xenobiotic-induced chronic degenerative diseases. Immunoaffinity column methods have been described for the analysis of oxidative damage products of nucleic acids excreted in urine (57). A monoclonal antibody that recognizes 8-oxo-7,8-dihydro-2'-deoxyguanosine was isolated and used in the preparation of immunoaffinity columns to facilitate the isolation of these damage products from various biological fluids. Quantitative analysis of these adducts in urine of rats fed a nucleic acid-free diet suggests that this is the principal repair product in DNA of both eukaryotes. In addition, excretion of oxidative DNA-damage products in urine has been correlated inversely with dietary antioxidant consumption in humans (71, 72). Finally, markers of nitric oxide oxidative damage have been identified (54). Thus these markers may eventually be used to assess protection status as well as risk (46).

CHEMICAL-PROTEIN ADDUCTS   A wide variety of aromatic amines and polynuclear aromatic hydrocarbons bind at high levels to hemoglobin following environmental exposures (75). Indeed, knowledge regarding chemical-hemoglobin adducts is much more extensive than for chemical-DNA adducts. These chemical-protein biomarkers have been particularly well characterized for the potent bladder carcinogen, 4-aminobiphenyl (4-ABP). One recent study examined the relationship between exposure to environmental tobacco smoke and levels of 4-ABP-hemoglobin adducts in nonsmoking pregnant women compared to adduct levels in those women who smoked during pregnancy (26). A questionnaire on smoking and exposure to environmental tobacco smoke was administered to pregnant women who smoked cigarettes and those who did not smoke. Samples of maternal blood and cord blood collected during delivery were analyzed for 4-ABP-hemoglobin adducts by gas chromatography with negative ion chemical ionization mass spectrometry. The mean adduct level in smokers was approximately ninefold higher than that in nonsmokers. Among nonsmokers, the levels of 4-ABP adducts increased by a factor of 1.7 with a fourfold increase in environmental tobacco smoke level. This relationship between environmental tobacco smoke exposure and 4-ABP-hemoglobin adduct levels supports the concept that environmental tobacco smoke is a probable hazard during pregnancy.

In addition to hemoglobin adduct analyses, albumin chemical adducts have also been investigated, in particular for AFB_1 exposures. In recent studies conducted in The Gambia, West Africa, a strong dose-response relationship was seen (78), similar to that previously reported in China (19). From a practical perspective pertinent to epidemiologic studies, the measurement and quantification of the aflatoxin-serum albumin adduct offers a rapid, facile approach that can be used to screen very large numbers of people (79, 80). Of importance, chemical-protein markers offer the further advantage of reflecting longer, cumulative exposure periods in people when compared to urinary adduct markers. This advantage results from the longer biological half-life of serum proteins (e.g. three weeks for albumin) compared with excreted DNA adducts (e.g. six hours for $AFB-N^7-Gua$).

ELECTRON PARAMAGNETIC RESONANCE-BASED BONE DOSIMETRY   Although chemical-DNA adducts and chemical-protein adducts represent the most fully developed biomarkers of biologically effective dose, other examples exist. Of these, electron paramagnetic resonance (EPR)-based bone dosimetry is of interest because the biologic tissue of interest (bone) is made to act as a radiation dosimeter (67). Paramagnetic centers are formed in the crystalline matrix (hydroxyapatite) of bone as a result of exposure to ionizing radiation. The radiation-absorbed dose within the bone matrix is proportional to the emitted signal intensity from a small biopsy sample following EPR excitation. By further, stepwise addition of known doses of radiation to the irradiated bone sample, an "internal" calibration approach can be used to directly relate EPR signal intensity to dose.

Relationship Between Exposure and Disease Risk

Rigorous evidence for an association between exposure and disease outcome is found in prospective epidemiological studies, where healthy people are followed until the diagnosis of disease. A nested case-control study, initiated in 1986 in Shanghai, examined the relationship between markers for aflatoxin and hepatitis B virus (HBV) and the development of liver cancer (63, 65). In this study, over 18,000 urine samples were collected from healthy males between the ages of 45 and 64. In the subsequent seven years, fifty of these individuals developed liver cancer. The urine samples for cases were age-matched and residence-matched with controls, and analyzed for both aflatoxin biomarkers and HBV surface antigen status. A significant relative risk of about three was observed for those liver cancer cases where urinary aflatoxins were detected. The relative risk for people who tested positive for the HBV surface antigen was about seven. Individuals with both urinary aflatoxins and positive HBV surface antigen status had a relative risk for developing liver cancer of about 60. These results demonstrate a relationship between the presence of carcinogen-specific biomarkers and cancer risk. Moreover, these findings provide the first demonstration of a multiplicative interaction between two major risk factors for liver cancer, HBV and AFB_1 exposure. When individual aflatoxin metabolites were stratified for liver cancer outcome, the presence of $AFB-N^7$-Gua in urine always resulted in a two- to threefold elevation in risk of developing liver cancer. These findings extend the conclusions from earlier rodent chemoprotection studies that monitoring urinary levels of this biomarker may also be appropriate for assessing individual risk.

BIOMARKERS OF EFFECT

Biomarkers of effect represent health impairment, or an event predictive of subsequent health impairment. Health impairment includes functional changes or the occurrence of frank disease. Events predictive of subsequent health impairment include subcellular changes and subclinical functional changes. The corresponding biomarkers can conceptually be divided into those of altered structure and those of altered function.

Biomarkers of Altered Structure

One recent study has examined a variety of molecular biomarkers to assess human exposure to complex mixtures of environmental pollution in Poland (58). Measurement of genotoxic damage in peripheral blood samples from residents of high-exposure regions indicated that environmental pollution was associated with significant increases in carcinogen-DNA adducts (polynuclear aromatic hydrocarbon-DNA and other aromatic adducts), sister chromatid exchanges, chromosomal aberrations, and frequency of increased *ras* oncogene expression. Perera and colleagues found that the presence of aromatic adducts on DNA were significantly correlated with chromosomal mutation, providing a possible link between environmental exposure and genetic alterations relevant to disease. This particular example highlights the possibility of the coexistence of biomarkers of multiple stages of the toxicological paradigm (i.e. biologically effective dose and effect).

Biomarkers of Altered Function

On an organ system level, functional changes are particularly useful in assessing the effects of inhaled environmental agents such as ozone, acid fog (composed primarily of a sulfuric acid aerosol), and tobacco smoke. Relevant biomarkers focus on changes in lung function, as measured by spirometry, or on other parameters, such as mucociliary clearance. For example, chronic changes in lung function with cigarette smoking can be quantified by measuring the forced expiratory volume in the first second of exhalation (FEV_1). Dockery and colleagues (15) have shown that there is almost a perfectly linear relationship between this parameter and accumulated pack-years of smoking. As another example, Laube and colleagues (43) have shown that acute exposure to acid fog leads to increased mucociliary clearance, as measured with a radiolabeled aerosol.

This last study used noninvasive nuclear medicine imaging in human subjects. Noninvasive imaging is beginning to offer new approaches to the detection of anatomic and functional abnormalities produced by environmental agents. For example, while lipid blood levels can be related to coronary artery disease, angiography, in which the blood vessels are visualized, provides a direct biomarker of disease (namely, visualization of the blockade itself). As another example, direct visualization of the relationship between regional ventilation and perfusion of the lung following acute ozone exposure can be obtained (JM Links, unpublished data). Perhaps the greatest potential for noninvasive imaging is in the setting of neurotoxins, particularly with metals, in which cerebral blood flow and neurotransmitter/neuroreceptor system function can be monitored. For example, emission tomographic techniques (e.g. PET scanning) have the capability of producing quantitative images of the density of available receptors in regions of the brain, before and after blockade with a receptor-binding ligand (18).

BIOMARKERS OF SUSCEPTIBILITY

Host-susceptibility factors can be very important in determining disease outcomes, and specific differences may account for the wide variations in incidence of cancer despite similar exposures (55). Active research is underway to define important determinants of susceptibility and much progress has been made in two areas, biological markers of metabolism and indices of DNA-repair capacity.

Arylamine metabolism is an area where phenotypic polymorphism is of interest, as reviewed by Lang & Kadlubar (42). One of the metabolic processes observed to exhibit a polymorphism in people is the rate of acetylation by the liver enzyme, N-acetyltransferase. Point mutations in one of the N-acetyltransferase genes result in a polymorphism manifested as either rapid or slow metabolizing activity (6). Several methods have been used to assess acetylator phenotype involving the administration of drugs; a method using urinary caffeine metabolites appears to be the most convenient and noninvasive (10, 20).

The interest in acetylation phenotype results from its potential role in susceptibility to aromatic and heterocyclic amine–induced cancers. Acetyltransferases catalyze both N- and O-acetylation. N-acetylation is a detoxification step for arylamines like 2-naphthylamine and 4-aminobiphenyl, but O-acetylation of N-hydroxy arylamines can form reactive esters that are ultimately carcinogenic by inducing DNA damage. Through the use of various markers, such as caffeine metabolites, as indices of acetylator phenotype, several epidemiological studies have found an association between the slow acetylation phenotype and risk for developing bladder cancer. In contrast, there is some evidence suggesting a relationship between the rapid acetylator phenotype and colon cancer (12).

The superfamily of cytochrome P-450 enzymes found throughout the body also generates possible determinants in cancer susceptibility. These enzymes are responsible for activating a wide range of environmental carcinogens to reactive intermediates; in many cases the amounts of these enzymes vary widely among individuals (25). The development of noninvasive, facile methods to determine the expression and activities of various cytochrome P-450s involved in activating environmental carcinogens will permit a fuller assessment of the role of these enzymes in cancer susceptibility.

The use of urinary caffeine metabolites as a molecular biomarker for the activity of the enzyme cytochrome P-450 1A2 has undergone validation and use in epidemiologic studies. Cytochrome P-450 1A2 catalyzes the N-oxidation of several environmentally important aromatic and heterocyclic amines to reactive carcinogens. The initial step in the biotransformation of caffeine is also catalyzed by this enzyme, so caffeine metabolism can be used as an indicator of metabolic phenotype. Caffeine metabolism data from many human populations suggest a trimodal distribution of this enzyme activity (10). In an ongoing case-control study (9) involving patients with a history of colorectal cancer or polyps and controls, a trend toward an increased proportion of rapid acetylators was observed. In addition, a significantly greater percentage of rapid metabolizers for cytochrome P-450 1A2 was found in the cancer and polyp cases than in the controls. A much more striking observation, however, resulted from a comparison of the prevalence of individuals who were both rapid acetylators and rapid metabolizers for cytochrome P-450 1A2. These results showed that 33% of the patients with colorectal cancer or polyps possessed the rapid/rapid phenotype, compared to only 13% of the controls (76). This difference is consistent with a metabolic activation pathway involving food-borne carcinogenic heterocyclic amines.

Results from a recently reported case-control study demonstrated that lung cancer patients who had only recently stopped smoking had significantly higher specific cytochrome P-450 activity in lung parenchyma compared with smoking noncancer patients (4). In these recent smokers, lung aryl hydrocarbon hydroxylase activity was positively correlated with the level of tobacco smoke-derived DNA adducts as determined by P-32 post-labeling. Pulmonary aryl hydrocarbon hydroxylase activity also showed a good correlation with the intensity of immunohistochemical staining for cytochrome P-450 1A1, suggesting that high pulmonary expression of this gene in tobacco smokers could be associated with increased lung cancer risk.

The repair of damage to DNA is an important individual response that may be a host-susceptibility factor. An assay for the proficiency of DNA repair in human lymphocytes has recently been developed and evaluated in epidemiological studies (2). In this assay, a chemically damaged plasmid DNA containing a reporter gene, chloramphenicol acetyltransferase, is transfected into human lymphocyte samples obtained from an individual. After an incubation period to allow for repair and expression of the reporter gene, DNA excision–repair capacity is scored by determining the amount of reactivated chloramphenicol acetyltransferase enzyme activity. Human cells with decreased ability to repair the damaged DNA will have lower expression of the reporter gene and hence lower enzymatic activity.

This technique has been used to compare the DNA-repair capacities of basal cell carcinoma (BCC) skin cancer patients and controls (77). An age-related decline in DNA-repair capacity was detected, and reduced repair capacity was a particularly important risk factor for young individuals with BCC and for those individuals with a family history of skin cancer. Young individuals with BCC repaired DNA damage poorly when compared with controls. With increasing age, however, differences between cases and controls gradually disappeared. The normal decline in DNA repair observed with increasing age may account for the increased risk of skin cancer that begins in middle age, suggesting that the occurrence of skin cancer in the young may represent a biochemical manifestation of decreased repair capacity.

Functional biomarkers may prove useful in identifying individuals who are at particular risk. For example, the measurement of FEV_1, described above, has been used to identify ozone-susceptible individuals (47). The decrease in FEV_1 from the control to the ozone-challenge state can be used to identify three populations of individuals: those with a particularly marked response (susceptible individuals), those with a mild response (normal individuals), and those with no response (resistant individuals). The observed differences in ozone susceptibility may be genetically determined (40).

As another example, functional asthmatics may be identified by their response to the bronchoconstrictor methacholine. The use of such a challenge in combination with noninvasive imaging may provide a means for direct visualization and identification of the affected regions (43). Noninvasive imaging may also help identify those sites within the airways most likely to be affected by inhaled pollutants by virtue of a high deposition concentration (7).

MECHANISTIC APPROACHES

A major endpoint frequently studied in environmental health research is cancer. It is helpful to think of clinical cancers as the final stage of a multistage carcinogenesis process (27, 28). The process starts with exposure to a putative environmental carcinogen (e.g. a biological agent like a virus, a chemical agent like benzene, or a physical agent like ionizing radiation), and progresses through initiation (involving a genetic change that results in an initiated cell), promotion (involving defects in terminal differentiation or growth control that result in a pre-neoplastic lesion), and conversion and progression (involving activation of proto-oncogenes like *ras* or inactivation or loss of tumor suppressor genes like *p53* that result in a malignant tumor), which leads to clinically manifest cancer.

The increasing mechanistic understanding of the genetic alterations that underlie the progression from initiation to clinical cancer in the process of carcinogenesis has permitted initial development of sensitive tests for diagnosis of oncogenes and tumor suppressor gene activities. For example, there have been many recent studies of the tumor suppressor gene, *p53*, the most commonly mutated gene detected in human cancers. The number and type of mutations in this gene are not equally distributed, but occur in specific hotspots that vary with tumor type (32). Different patterns in mutation type between tumors may be consistent with different etiologies for the specific tumor types. For example, several independent studies of *p53* mutations in hepatocellular carcinomas occurring in populations exposed to aflatoxin found high frequencies of guanine to thymine transversions, with clustering at codon 249 (8, 34). On the other hand, studies of *p53* mutations in liver tumors from Japan and other areas where there is little exposure to aflatoxin revealed no mutations at codon 249 (56). These data have been confirmed in follow-up studies (1). Previous data in bacterial mutagenesis test systems had shown that AFB_1 exposure causes almost exclusively guanine to thymine transversions (17). It is intriguing to speculate that there is a linkage between this type of mutation and putative aflatoxin exposure in high-risk regions. In the future, it may be possible that the mutational spectrum in a target gene such as *p53* can serve as a marker of exposure to, and indicate damage from, specific classes of environmental agents.

Screening for mutations in the *p53* tumor suppressor gene has also been used as a possible diagnostic tool for early stage cancers. For example, mutations could be detected in the *p53* gene from bladder epithelial cells shed into urine of bladder cancer patients (69). Further studies remain to determine the temporal relation between these mutations and disease status. Nonetheless, these types of genetic markers of changes represent a rapidly developing field that will progress from the laboratory to the clinic very quickly (48).

Detectable genetic changes in specific oncogenes may also prove useful as an aid in diagnosis. Recent data indicate that the specific mutations in the *K-ras* oncogene in colon tumors of an individual can be detected in the shed colonic cells found in the stool of patients with colorectal tumors (70). In these experiments, *ras* mutations were detected in the stools of eight out of nine patients with tumors exhibiting this mutation, but were found in none of the stools of the patients whose tumor did not express this mutation. The detection of this mutation relies upon a recently developed technique, the polymerase chain reaction (PCR), that allows the amplification of DNA from tumor cells followed by sequencing to detect mutations. These tools have been integral to recent major advances in an understanding of the genetic changes accompanying and causing cancer, and may now have a direct application to the identification of people with early stage disease. A particularly compelling example is that of Hubert H. Humphrey, who died of bladder cancer in 1978. Analysis of urine samples from 1967, when he first presented with hematuria, disclosed the presence of a *p53* mutation in a number of the cells present (33). This mutation, a transversion from adenine to thymine in codon 227 of the *p53* gene, was identical to that found in a fixed tissue-block specimen of Humphrey's infiltrative transitional-cell bladder carcinoma, obtained in 1976. Of major importance, no diagnosis was established in 1967, and Humphrey was followed with cystoscopy every six months. A definitive diagnosis of cancer was not established until 1973, fully six years after *p53* mutations were already present.

It is clear that one marker alone will not be enough. For example, *K-ras* gene mutations are found in only 40% of colon cancers and 60% of bladder cancers. Thus, additional early markers of genetic change are needed to produce a battery of probes for early biological effects. Indeed, the strength of information derived for all applications of biomarkers is greatly enhanced by the convergence of independent markers to a concordant outcome.

THE FUTURE

To date, many studies of individual molecular biomarkers in experimental animals and human populations have been undertaken. These investigations show that many markers serve as indicators of exposure or dose, or as indicators of the development of altered structure, function, or disease, or as indicators of possible susceptibility to disease. The major challenge facing this field is the ability to link these markers to a toxicological effect. Currently, in most cases, it is only through supposition that this linkage is made. Even in those cases where all of the data are consistent with a specific etiological agent and mutagenic event, such as with aflatoxin and *p53* mutations, the specific information required to tie everything together remains to be elucidated. Such information will eventually be gleaned from both experimental studies and molecular epidemiological investigations in human populations.

Molecular biomarkers will find an important application in cancer prevention trials, where they will be used as intermediate endpoints to assess the efficacy of molecular interventions (45). These intermediate markers are particularly valuable when investigating chemoprotective agents that act at relatively early, preclinical stages of carcinogenesis. The key issue in trials that use biomarkers as the outcome of interest is to have a marker that is directly associated with the development or evolution of neoplasia. These biomarkers are typically organ site-specific genomic, proliferation, or differentiation markers that reflect different intermediary stages of the neoplastic process. As an adjunct to these process-dependent markers, it may also be possible to devise markers specific to interventions in selected groups at high risk for carcinogen exposure. These agent-dependent approaches would be based upon knowledge of the etiologic agent(s) in the study population.

The continued rapid development of the technologies used in molecular epidemiology should lead to more accurate exposure assessment as well as to the development of effective intervention strategies. These marker studies will also improve and refine the ability to identify susceptible populations, thereby increasing the power of epidemiologic investigations. Finally, these tools should quickly evolve to be valuable in the policy and regulatory setting by helping to more accurately characterize the relationship between exposure and effects in people.

ACKNOWLEDGMENTS

We wish to acknowledge support from USPHS Grants P01 ES06052, P30 ES03819, and R01 CA39416.

Literature Cited

1. Aguilar F, Harris CC, Sun T, Hollstein M, Cerutti P. 1994. Geographic variation of p53 mutational profile in nonmalignant human liver. *Science* 264:1317–19

2. Athas WF, Hedayati MA, Matanoski GM, Farmer ER, Grossman L. 1991. Development and field-test validation of an assay for DNA repair in circulating

human lymphocytes. *Cancer Res.* 51: 5786–93

3. Barry PSI. 1975. Distribution of lead in the body. *Br. J. Ind. Med.* 32:119–39

4. Bartsch H, Castegnaro M, Rojas M, Camus AM, Alexandrov K, Lang M. 1992. Expression of pulmonary cytochrome P-450 1A1 and carcinogen DNA adduct formation in high risk subjects for tobacco-related lung cancer. *Toxicol. Lett.* 64–65:477–83

5. Bartsch H, Malaveille C, Friesen M, Kadlubar FF, Vineis P. 1993. Black and blond tobacco cancer risk. IV: molecular dosimetry studies implicate aromatic amines as bladder carcinogens. *Eur. J. Cancer* 29A:1199–1207

6. Blum M, Demierre A, Grant DM, Heim M, Meyer UA. 1991. Molecular mechanism of slow acetylation of drugs and carcinogens in humans. *Proc. Natl. Acad. Sci. USA* 88:5237–41

7. Bowes SM, Laube BL, Links JM, Frank R. 1989. Regional deposition of inhaled fog droplets. *Environ. Health Perspect.* 79:151–57

8. Bressac B, Kew M, Wands J, Ozturk M. 1991. Selective G to T mutations of p53 gene in hepatocellular carcinoma from southern Africa. *Nature* 350:429–31

9. Butler MA, Lang NP, Massengill JP, Lawsen M, Kadlubar FF. 1992. CYP1A2 and AT phenotypes in human colo-rectal cancer or polyps. *Proc. Am. Assoc. Cancer Res.* 33:1749

10. Butler MA, Lang NP, Young JF, Caporaso NE, Vineis P, et al. 1992. Determination of CYP1A2 and NAT2 phenotypes in human populations by analysis of caffeine urinary metabolites. *Pharmacogenetics* 2:116–27

11. Campbell AA, Whitaker TB, Pohland AE, Dickens JW, Park DL. 1986. Sampling, sample preparation, and sampling plans for foodstuffs for mycotoxin analysis. *Pure Appl. Chem.* 58:305–14

12. Caporaso N, Landi MT, Vineis P. 1991. Relevance of metabolic polymorphisms to human carcinogenesis: evaluation of epidemiologic evidence. *Pharmacogenetics* 1:4–19

13. Carmella SG, Akerkar S, Hecht SS. 1993. Metabolites of the tobacco-specific nitrosamine 4-(methylnitrosamino)-1-(3-pyridyl)-1-butanone in smokers' urine. *Cancer Res.* 53:721–24

14. Cohen N, Spitz HB, Wrenn ME. 1977. Estimation of skeletal burden of "bone-seeking" radionuclides in man from in vivo scintillation measurements of the head. *Health Phys.* 33:431–41

15. Dockery DW, Speizer FE, Ferris BG,

Ware JH, Louis TA, Spiro A. 1988. Cumulative and reversible effects of lifetime smoking and simple tests of lung function in adults. *Am. Rev. Respir. Dis.* 137:286–92

16. Eisenbud M, Laurer GR, Rosen JC, Cohen N, Thomas J. 1969. In vivo measurement of lead-210 as an indicator of cumulative radon daughter exposure in uranium miners. *Health Phys.* 16:637–46

17. Foster PL, Eisenstadt E, Miller JH. 1983. Base substitution mutations induced by metabolically activated aflatoxin B1. *Proc. Natl. Acad. Sci. USA* 80:2695–98

18. Frost JJ, Wagner HN, eds. 1990. *Quantitative Imaging: Neuroreceptors, Neurotransmitters, and Enzymes.* New York: Raven

19. Gan L-S, Skipper PL, Peng X-C, Groopman JD, Chen J-S, et al. 1988. Serum albumin adducts in the molecular epidemiology of aflatoxin carcinogenesis: correlation with aflatoxin B1 intake and urinary excretion of aflatoxin M1. *Carcinogenesis* 9:1323–25

20. Grant D, Tang BK, Kalow W. 1984. A simple test for acetylator phenotype using caffeine. *Br. J. Clin. Pharmacol.* 17:459–64

21. Groopman JD, Hasler J, Trudel LJ, Pikul A, Donahue PR, Wogan GN. 1992. Molecular dosimetry in rat urine of aflatoxin-N7-guanine and other aflatoxin metabolites by multiple monoclonal antibody affinity chromatography and HPLC. *Cancer Res.* 52:267–74

22. Groopman JD, Skipper PL, eds. 1991. *Molecular Dosimetry and Human Cancer.* Boca Raton: CRC

23. Groopman JD, Wogan GN, Roebuck BD, Kensler TW. 1994. Molecular biomarkers for aflatoxins and their application to human cancer prevention. *Cancer Res.* 54:1907s–11s

24. Groopman JD, Zhu J, Donahue PR, Pikul A, Zhang L-S, et al. 1992. Molecular dosimetry of urinary aflatoxin DNA adducts in people living in Guangxi Autonomous Region, People's Republic of China. *Cancer Res.* 52:45–51

25. Guengerich FP, Shimada T, Raney KD, Yun C-H, Meyer DJ, et al. 1992. Elucidation of catalytic specificities of human cytochrome P-450 and glutathione S-transferase enzymes and relevance to molecular epidemiology studies. *Environ. Health Perspect.* 98:75–80

26. Hammond SK, Coghlin J, Gann PH, Paul M, Taghiza-deh K, et al. 1993. Relationship between environmental to-

bacco smoke exposure and carcinogen-hemoglobin adduct levels in nonsmokers. *J. Natl. Cancer Inst.* 85:474–78

27. Harris CC. 1991. Molecular epidemiology: overview of biochemical and molecular basis. See Ref. 22, pp. 15–26

28. Harris CC. 1993. p53: at the crossroads of molecular carcinogenesis and risk assessment. *Science* 262:1980–81

29. Heard MJ, Chamberlain AC. 1984. Uptake of lead by human skeleton and comparative metabolism of lead and alkaline earth elements. *Health Phys.* 47:857–65

30. Hecht SS, Carmella SG, Foiles PG, Murphy SE. 1994. Biomarkers for human uptake and metabolic activation of tobacco-specific nitrosamines. *Cancer Res.* 54:1912s–17s

31. Hecht SS, Haley NJ, Hoffmann D. 1991. Monitoring exposure to tobacco products by measurement of nicotine metabolites and derived carcinogens. See Ref. 22, pp. 325–62

32. Hollstein M, Sidransky D, Vogelstein B, Harris CC. 1991. p53 mutations in human cancers. *Science* 253:49–53

33. Hruban RH, van der Riet P, Erozan YS, Sidransky D. 1994. Brief report: molecular biology and the early detection of carcinoma of the bladder—the case of Hubert H. Humphrey. *N. Engl. J. Med.* 330:1276–78

34. Hsu IC, Metcalf RA, Sun T, Welsh JA, Wang NJ, Harris CC. 1991. Mutational hotspot in the p53 gene in human hepatocellular carcinomas. *Nature* 350:427–28

35. Hu H, Milder FL, Burger DE. 1989. X-ray fluorescence: issues surrounding the application of a new tool for measuring burden of lead. *Environ. Res.* 49:295–317

36. Hulka B. 1991. Epidemiological studies using biological markers: issues for epidemiologists. *Cancer Epidemiol. Biomarkers Prev.* 1:13–19

37. Joellenbeck L, Kadlubar FF, Groopman JD. 1994. Molecular biomarkers for use in cancer risk assessment and cancer prevention. In *Cancer Dose-Response in Humans. Int. Life Sci. Inst.* In press

38. Kaderlik KR, Talaska G, DeBord DG, Osorio AM, Kadlubar FF. 1993. 4,4'-Methylene-bis(2-chloroaniline)-DNA adduct analysis in human exfoliated urothelial cells by P-32 postlabeling. *Cancer Epidemiol. Biomarkers Prev.* 2:63–69

39. Kaderlik RK, Lin DX, Lang NP, Kadlubar FF. 1992. Advantages and limitations of laboratory methods for measurement of carcinogen-DNA adducts for epidemiological studies. *Toxicol. Lett.* 64–65:469–75

40. Kleeberger SR, Bassett DJP, Jakab GJ, Levitt RC. 1990. A genetic model for evaluation of susceptibility to ozone-induced inflammation. *J. Appl. Physiol.* 258:L313–20

41. Krieger N, Wolff MS, Hiatt RA, Rivera M, Vogelman J, Orentreich N. 1994. Breast cancer and serum organochlorines: a prospective study among white, black, and Asian women. *J. Natl. Cancer Inst.* 86:589–99

42. Lang NP, Kadlubar FF. 1991. Aromatic and heterocyclic amine metabolism and phenotyping in humans. *Prog. Clin. Biol. Res.* 372:33–47

43. Laube BL, Bowes SM, Links JM, Thomas KK, Frank R. 1993. Acute exposure to acid fog: effects on mucociliary clearance. *Am. Rev. Respir. Dis.* 147:1105–11

44. Laube BL, Links JM, Wagner HN, Norman PS, Koller DW, et al. 1988. Simplified assessment of fine aerosol distribution in human airways. *J. Nucl. Med.* 29:1057–65

45. Lippman SM, Lee JS, Lotan R, Hittleman W, Wargovich MJ, Hong WK. 1990. Biomarkers as intermediate end points in chemoprevention trials. *J. Natl. Cancer Inst.* 82:555–62

46. Malins DC, Holmes EH, Polissar NL, Gunselman SJ. 1993. The etiology of breast cancer: characteristic alterations in hydroxyl radical-induced DNA base lesions during oncogenesis with potential for evaluating incidence risk. *Cancer* 71:3036–43

47. McDonnell WF, Horstman DH, Hazucha MJ, Seal E, Haak ED, et al. 1983. Pulmonary effects of ozone exposure during exercise: dose-response characteristics. *J. Appl. Physiol.* 54:1345–52

48. Miki Y, Swensen J, Shattuck-Eidens D, Futreal A, Harshman K, et al. 1994. A strong candidate for the breast and ovarian cancer susceptibility gene BRCA1. *Science* 266:66–71

49. Natl. Res. Counc. Comm. Biol. Markers. 1987. Biological markers in environmental health research. *Environ. Health Perspect.* 74:3–9

50. Natl. Res. Counc. 1989. *Biological Markers in Reproductive Toxicology.* Washington, DC: Natl. Acad. Press. 395 pp.

51. Natl. Res. Counc. 1989. *Biological Markers in Pulmonary Toxicology.* Washington, DC: Natl. Acad. Press. 179 pp.

52. Natl. Res. Counc. 1989. *Biological*

Markers in Neurotoxicology. Washington, DC: Natl. Acad. Press

53. Natl. Res. Counc. 1989. *Biological Markers in Immunotoxicology.* Washington, DC: Natl. Acad. Press. 206 pp.

54. Nunosiba T, deRojas-Walker T, Wishnok JS, Tannenbaum SR, Demple B. 1993. Activation by nitric oxide in an oxidative-stress response that defends *Escherichia coli* against macrophages. *Proc. Natl. Acad. Sci. USA* 90:9993–97

55. Omenn GS, Omiecinski CJ, Easton DL. 1990. Eco-genetics of chemical carcinogens. In *Biotechnology and Human Genetic Predisposition to Disease,* ed. CR Cantor, CT Caskey, LE Hood, D Kamely, GA Omenn, pp. 81–93. New York: Wiley-Liss

56. Ozturk M. 1991. p53 mutation in hepatocellular carcinoma after aflatoxin exposure. *Lancet* 338:1356–59

57. Park EM, Shigenaga MK, Degan P, Korn TS, Kitzler JW, et al. 1992. Assay of excised oxidative DNA lesions: isolation of 8-oxoguanine and its nucleoside derivatives from biological fluids with a monoclonal antibody column. *Proc. Natl. Acad. Sci. USA* 89:3375–79

58. Perera F. 1993. Biomarkers and molecular epidemiology of occupationally related cancer. *J. Toxicol. Environ. Health* 40:203–15

59. Perera FP, Hemminki K, Gryzbowska E, Motykiewicz G, Michalska J, et al. 1992. Molecular and genetic damage in humans from environmental pollution in Poland. *Nature* 360:256–58

60. Perera FP, Tang DL, Grinberg-Funes RA, Blackwood A, Dickey C, et al. 1993. Molecular epidemiology of lung cancer and the modulation of markers of chronic carcinogen exposure by chemopreventive agents. *J. Cell Biochem.* Suppl. 17F:119–28

61. Poirier MC, Reed E, Litterst CL, Katz D, Gupta-Burt S. 1992. Persistence of platinumamine-DNA adducts in gonads and kidneys of rats and multiple tissues from cancer patients. *Cancer Res.* 52:149–53

62. Poirier MC, Shamkhani H, Reed E, Tarone RE, Gupta-Burt S. 1992. DNA adducts induced by platinum drug chemotherapeutic agents in human tissues. *Prog. Clin. Biol. Res.* 374:197–212

63. Qian G-S, Yu MC, Ross R, Yuan J-M, Gao Y-T, et al. 1994. Urinary markers of aflatoxin exposure and liver cancer risk in Shanghai, P.R.C. *Cancer Epidemiol. Biomarkers Prev.* 3:3–11

64. Rappaport SM, Kure E, Petreas M, Ting D, Woodlee J. 1991. A field method for measuring solvent vapors in exhaled air:

application to styrene exposure. *Scand. J. Work Environ. Health* 3:195–204

65. Ross R, Yuan J-M, Yu M, Wogan GN, Qian G-S, et al. 1992. Urinary aflatoxin biomarkers and risk of hepatocellular carcinoma. *Lancet* 339:943–46

66. Santella RM, Grinberg-Funes RA, Young TL, Dickey C, Singh VN, et al. 1992. Cigarette smoking related polycyclic aromatic hydrocarbon-DNA adducts in peripheral mononuclear cells. *Carcinogenesis* 13:2041–45

67. Schauer DA, Desrosiers MF, Le FG, Seltzer SM, Links JM. 1994. EPR dosimetry of cortical bone and tooth enamel irradiated with X and gamma rays: study of energy dependence. *Radiat. Res.* 138:1–8

68. Shuker DE, Farmer PB. 1992. Relevance of urinary DNA adducts as markers of carcinogen exposure. *Chem. Res. Toxicol.* 5:450–60

69. Sidransky D, von Eschenbach A, Tsai Y-C, Jones P, Summerhayes I, et al. 1991. Identification of p53 gene mutations in bladder cancers and urine samples. *Science* 252:706–9

70. Sidransky D, Tokino T, Hamilton SR, Kinzler KW, Levin B, et al. 1992. Identification of ras oncogene mutations in the stool of patients with curable colorectal tumors. *Science* 256:102–5

71. Simic MG. 1992. Urinary biomarkers and the rate of DNA damage in carcinogenesis and anticarcinogenesis. *Mutat. Res.* 267:277–90

72. Simic MG, Bergtold DS. 1991. Dietary modulation of DNA damage in humans. *Mutat. Res.* 250:17–24

73. Somervaille LJ, Chettle DR, Scott MC. 1985. In vivo measurement of lead in bone using x-ray fluorescence. *Phys. Med. Biol.* 30:929–43

74. Talaska G, al-Juburi AZ, Kadlubar FF. 1991. Smoking related carcinogen-DNA adducts in biopsy samples of human urinary bladder: identification of N-(deoxyguanosin-8-yl)-4-aminobiphenyl as a major adduct. *Proc. Natl. Acad. Sci. USA* 88:5350–54

75. Tannenbaum SR. 1990. Hemoglobin-carcinogen adducts as molecular biomarkers in epidemiology. *Princess Takamatsu Symposia,* pp. 351–60. Tokyo: Jpn. Sci. Soc. Press

76. Turesky RJ, Lang NP, Butler MA, Teitel CH, Kadlubar FF. 1991. Metabolic activation of carcinogenic heterocyclic amines by human liver and colon. *Carcinogenesis* 12:1839–45

77. Wei Q, Matanoski GM, Farmer ER, Hedayati MA, Grossman L. 1993. DNA repair and aging in basal cell carcinoma:

a molecular epidemiology study. *Proc. Natl. Acad. Sci. USA* 90:1614–18

78. Wild CP, Hudson G, Sabbioni G, Wogan GN, Whittle H, et al. 1992. Correlation of dietary intake of aflatoxins with the level of albumin bound aflatoxin in peripheral blood in The Gambia, West Africa. *Cancer Epidemiol. Biomarkers Prev.* 1:229–34

79. Wild CP, Jiang YZ, Allen SJ, Jansen LA, Hall AJ, Montesano R. 1990. Aflatoxin-albumin adducts in human sera from different regions of the world. *Carcinogenesis* 11:2271–74

80. Wild CP, Jiang YZ, Sabbioni G, Chapot B, Montesano R. 1990. Evaluation of methods for quantitation of aflatoxin-albumin adducts and their application to human exposure assessment. *Cancer Res.* 50:245–51

81. Wogan GN. 1992. Molecular epidemiology in cancer risk assessment and prevention: recent progress and avenues for future research. *Environ. Health Perspect.* 98:167–78

82. Wolff MS, Toniolo PG, Lee EW, Rivera M, Dubin N. 1993. Blood levels of organochlorine residues and risk of breast cancer. *J. Natl. Cancer Inst.* 85:648–52

Annu. Rev. Public Health. 1995. 16:105–121

THE IMPORTANCE OF HUMAN EXPOSURE INFORMATION: A Need for Exposure-Related Data Bases to Protect and Promote Public Health[1,2]

Diane K. Wagener

Office of Analysis, Epidemiology, and Health Promotion, National Center for Health Statistics, Centers for Disease Control and Prevention, Hyattsville, Maryland 20782

Sherry G. Selevan

Human Health Assessment Group, US Environmental Protection Agency, Washington, D.C. 20460

Ken Sexton

Office of Health Research, US Environmental Protection Agency, Washington, D.C. 20460

KEY WORDS: exposure assessment, risk assessment, risk management, data collection

ABSTRACT

As a subfield of public health, environmental health is concerned with evaluating and ameliorating the effects of people on the environment and the effects of the environment on people. Separating hazards from risks, and characterizing the magnitude, likelihood, and uncertainty of risks is at the heart of environmental health in the 1990s. To this end, a full range of data is needed, including data that characterize the distribution of hazards, the population potentially at risk, and the contact between people and pollution that creates the risk. Several government-sponsored data systems contain information on a range of exposure estimators. The challenge is to develop meaningful, properly validated models to identify public health needs and evaluate public health programs.

INTRODUCTION

Interactions between people and their environment are an important aspect of public health. Safeguarding the health of individuals and populations often depends on knowledge and understanding of people's exposures to potentially harmful environmental agents that occur during daily activities. Exposure-related information—including (*a*) the number of people exposed to the environmental toxicant, at specific concentrations, for the time period of interest; (*b*) the resulting dose that enters the body and reaches the target organ(s); and (*c*) the relative contribution of important sources and pathways to exposure/ dose—is essential to making informed decisions about the seriousness of environmental health risks and about what to do in response to those risks deemed unacceptable.

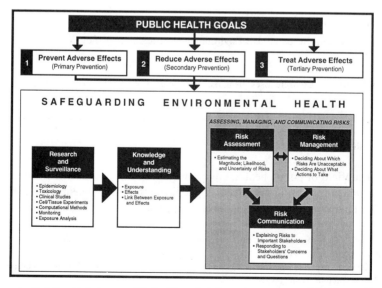

Figure 1   Relationship between public health goals, information sources, and decision-making.

Public health prioritized goals (e.g. prevention, amelioration, and treatment) should drive decisions related to the assessment, management, and communication of health risks associated with exposures to environmental agents, as well as decisions about research needs and priorities to improve and strengthen the underlying scientific knowledge base (Figure 1).

In the context of this discussion, *environmental health* is defined as a subfield of public health that focuses on evaluating and, where necessary, ameliorating the effects of human activity on environmental quality and thus on human health (2). A central function of environmental health is determining the risk associated with a particular environmental agent or mixture of agents. In this context, risk has two essential elements: (*a*) the presence of a biological (e.g. bacteria, virus), chemical (e.g. asbestos, benzene), and/or physical (e.g. radionuclides, noise, heat) agent in the environment that is intrinsically hazardous to human health; and (*b*) contact or interaction between the hazardous agent(s) and people (i.e. exposure). The resulting risk is the chance or probability of adverse health consequences in those who are exposed.

Realistic assessment and prioritization of risks (Figure 2) depend on accurate estimation of both exposure (i.e. contact between people and environmental agents) and toxicity (i.e. the relationship between exposure/dose and adverse health effects). Neither toxicity nor human exposure is well characterized, but there have been more resources devoted to toxicity and so a lack of knowledge about important exposure mechanisms is a major source of uncertainty in many risk assessments (3–9).

The need for exposure-related research is highlighted by the paucity of

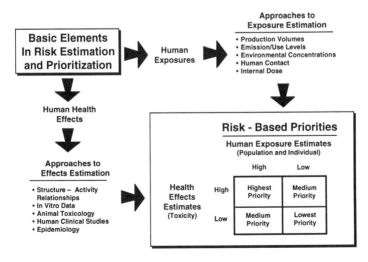

Figure 2   Information needs for prioritization of risks [From Sexton et al (7)].

empirical data available to estimate exposures and associated doses for most environmental agents of public health significance. What information exists tends to be anecdotal, fragmented, or narrowly focused on single pathways and routes of exposure for individual chemicals. For this reason, human exposure analysis is currently an important topic of scientific investigation, complementing such traditional public health disciplines as epidemiology and toxicology (3–9). It is becoming increasingly recognized that exposure information can have value, separate from the traditional epidemiologic studies.

The purpose of this paper is to highlight the importance of human exposure information for protection of public health and to draw attention to the need for more and better exposure-related data bases. In the following discussion, we (a) survey the public health uses of human exposure information; (b) explore the issue of measuring the "right" exposure; (c) review exposure-related data bases that can be used to guide decisions about public health; and (d) discuss the value of exposure-related data bases for decision-making purposes.

USES OF HUMAN EXPOSURE INFORMATION

Every day people are exposed to a multitude of environmental agents, both synthetic and natural, in the air they breathe, the liquids they drink, the food they eat, the surfaces they touch, and the products they use. Sometimes exposures to hazardous agents are sufficient to cause such adverse health consequences as birth defects, cancer, neurobehavioral effects, and respiratory disease. In a few cases, the link between an environmental/occupational agent and a harmful effect is relatively well established; for example, death from carbon monoxide poisoning, pneumonia from *Legionella pneumophila* infection, and mesothelioma and lung cancer from asbestos exposure.

Usually, however, establishing the cause-and-effect relationship is more a matter of scientific inference and expert judgment than of documented fact. Actions to prevent or reduce the harmful consequences of environmental agents are predicated on established or postulated links between emission sources, human exposures, and adverse health effects. Typically, environmentally induced effects on human health are discussed in terms of probabilistic (stochastic) risks. Lifetime risks of developing cancer from a particular exposure (e.g. ambient air pollution or drinking water disinfectants) are commonly described in terms such as one in one million.

An environmental health paradigm that assists in the understanding and evaluation of environmental health risks is depicted in Figure 3. Two primary activities are involved in assessing environmental health risks: exposure assessment and effects assessment. Exposure assessment focuses on the initial portion of the environmental health paradigm: sources of environmental con-

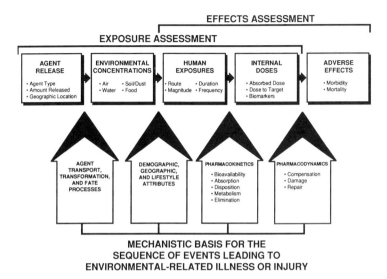

Figure 3   Environmental health paradigm and mechanisms affecting sequence of events leading to environmental-related illness [Adapted from Sexton et al (6)].

taminants, concentrations, exposure, and dose. The goal is to develop a quantitative description of the environmental agent's contact with (exposure) and entry into (dose) the human body. Emphasis is placed on specifying the pathway(s) and route(s) of exposure, estimating the magnitude, duration, and frequency of exposures, and determining the number of people exposed to various concentrations of the agent in question (6–9).

The goals of health effects assessment are twofold: (*a*) to determine the intrinsic hazards associated with the agent (hazard identification); and (*b*) to quantify the relationship between dose and related effects (dose-response assessment). The overlap in exposure and health-effects assessments (see Figure 3) reflects the importance of the exposure-dose relationship to both activities (6).

Risk assessment is, then, a formalized process for estimating the likelihood and magnitude of environmentally related health effects, as well as the uncertainty associated with these estimates. In a step called risk characterization, the results of both exposure and effects assessments are combined to estimate risks for the subject population (e.g. residents of a particular geographic area), important subgroups within the population (e.g. children, residents in an industrial area), and individuals near the center (e.g. median, mean) and at the high-end (e.g. 98th percentile) of the exposure distribution. Currently, due to limited data on humans, risk assessments have emphasized toxicological data.

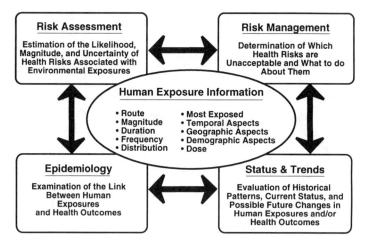

Figure 4   Potential uses of human exposure information in environmental health [From Sexton et al (6)].

In the future, as more human data are developed, risk assessments will reflect these changes.

In addition to risk assessment, human exposure information can be used for: risk management, status and trends analyses, and epidemiologic studies (Figure 4). Risk management is the process of deciding whether risks are unacceptable and, if so, what to do about them. Risk management decisions fall into four basic categories: (*a*) setting priorities; (*b*) determining unacceptable risks; (*c*) selecting the most cost-effective method to prevent or reduce risks; and (*d*) measuring the success of risk management efforts. To make informed decisions, risk managers depend on credible information about exposure and effects as they consider the relevant economic, engineering, legal, social, and political aspects of the issue.

Analysis of current status and historical trends for exposure, an important component of both risk assessment and risk management, requires that exposure data be collected over a period of years, which ensures the identification and understanding of temporal trends. Data on status and trends can be invaluable for identifying new or emerging problems, recognizing the relative importance of sources and exposure pathways, assessing the effectiveness of pollution controls, distinguishing opportunities for epidemiologic research, and predicting future changes in exposures and effects. Because contaminant levels may change over time, as may the sensitivity of the techniques used to measure them, comparison of trends is often a complex undertaking.

Epidemiologic studies can provide unique and powerful information directly relevant to risk assessment and risk-management decisions. In addition to their other uses, these studies can characterize the health status of populations, describe disease occurrence through identification of explanatory factors, and evaluate efforts at disease prevention and reduction. Without reliable exposure data, however, epidemiologic studies are less useful for decision-making. In most cases, the risk associated with environmentally related health effects is relatively small, and failure to correctly classify or quantify exposures can introduce misclassification errors that may artificially reduce or inflate the level of risk observed and thus limit the usefulness of the study.

ESTIMATING THE RIGHT EXPOSURE

Estimating the "right" exposure (i.e. the exposure most directly related to the question being asked) depends on, among other things, the nature of the public health activity, the population exposed, the environmental agent(s) of concern, and the health effect under observation. Efforts to link human exposure with health effects require a thorough understanding of the complexities of both exposure (e.g. route, magnitude, duration, frequency) and effects (e.g. variations in the type and nature of health effect depending on different types of exposures that occur at different times and with different latency periods). For example, exposures that cause cancer might occur many years before the cancer is diagnosed; in contrast, birth defects may result from exposures during early gestation. Thus, risk assessments are frequently complicated by the fact that exposures at the time a health effect is recognized may have little to do with the exposures responsible for causing the effect.

Other key characteristics of exposure may also affect the exposure-effect relationship and often interrelate in a complex manner. For example, in the risk-assessment process, some health effects (e.g. developmental effects) are assumed to have an exposure/dose threshold below which the effect does not occur, whereas others (e.g. cancer) are assumed to have no exposure/dose threshold, which suggests than even one molecule of a carcinogen has a finite probability, albeit low, of causing cancer (7). In addition, each environmental agent has a different residence time in the body. The longer the half-life of the substance in the body, the greater the body burden may become and thus the likelihood increases of receiving a sufficient dose to cause a health effect. Moreover, the intervals between exposures (when exposures are intermittent rather than continuous) can affect the body burden and may have significant ramifications for subsequent health effects. Finally, the body may respond to short-term, acute exposures differently than to long-term, chronic exposures; for example, the body may compensate for chronic exposures (e.g. increased carboxyhemoglobin in smokers), whereas acute exposures may overwhelm the body (e.g. carbon monoxide poisoning with acute exposures). Thus, an investigator looking at hypotheses about a causal relationship between exposure/ dose and effect must consider many exposure-related factors when making decisions about which exposures to measure or to estimate.

Generally, individuals or populations are considered to be at potentially greater risk if (*a*) they are exposed to an environmental agent at concentrations above some health-related benchmark (e.g. occupational or ambient exposure standard) and/or (*b*) they are more susceptible to the effects of exposures (e.g. by reason of age, gender, health status, genetic variability, diet, life-style factors, or access to health care) (8). Often an important aspect of exposure analysis involves addressing questions about (*a*) what individual or population characteristics cause people to be in either or both of these at-risk categories, and (*b*) what are associated levels of exposure for the agents of interest. Realistic answers to these kinds of questions require collection of data on exposures and/or development and application of predictive exposure models.

There are a number of different ways to collect exposure data, some more direct than others (Figure 5). Generally, the further the method is removed from the actual point of contact between people and environmental agents, the less expensive and less accurate the data in terms of estimating specific human exposures. The most accurate and most expensive methods of data collection are personal measurements of exposure concentrations and human tissue monitoring for biomarkers of exposure. As pointed out earlier, however, depending on the agents and health effects of interest, information about current expo-

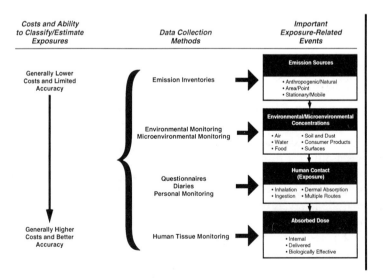

Figure 5 Exposure-related events and their indicators, data collection methods, and the costs associated with estimating exposures [From Sexton et al (6)].

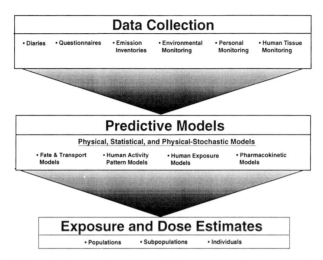

Figure 6 Relationship of data collection, model development, and exposure estimation [From Sexton et al (7)].

sures, no matter how good, may not be very useful in trying to link exposures and effects. Thus, diaries and questionnaires are commonly used to estimate current and past exposures based on factors such as occupation, residential proximity to potential ambient emission sources, smoking history, unvented combustion appliances in the home, and use of consumer products. An increasingly practical approach to historical exposure estimation for some environmental agents is the use of long-lived biological markers of exposure that can be measured in human tissue and other specimens (e.g. blood or urine) (5–7).

Direct measurements are the only way to establish unequivocally whether and to what extent individuals are exposed to specific agents. But it is neither affordable nor technically feasible to measure exposure/dose for everyone in all populations of interest. Models, which are mathematical abstractions of physical reality, may obviate the need for such extensive monitoring programs by providing estimates of population exposures/doses that are based on a smaller number of representative measurements. The challenge is to develop appropriate and robust models that allow for extrapolation from relatively few measurements to estimates of exposure and/or dose for a much larger population. The relationships between data collection, model development, and exposure estimation is summarized in Figure 6.

The path from data collection to modeling to the development of exposure and dose estimates is frequently not as straightforward as depicted in Figure 6. Many people think of complex statistical models when they consider exposure models, but any use of exposure data requires some level of modeling to estimate the exposure of interest. Modeling can span the spectrum from a simple geographic mapping strategy to a complex exposure model that includes detailed information about human activity patterns and physiologically based pharmacokinetics. The suitability of a particular modeling approach depends on factors such as the intended uses, the required certainty of the estimate, and the costs of the information.

The need for realistic estimates of exposure is driving an increasing demand for monitoring data and predictive models. An obvious question is the extent to which existing data and data bases are useful in meeting this demand. The next section surveys exposure-related data bases that might be helpful in estimating exposures to environmental agents.

A SURVEY OF EXPOSURE-RELATED DATA BASES

Concerns about the adequacy of available information to estimate human exposures prompted three Federal agencies, the U.S. Environmental Protection Agency (EPA), the Centers for Disease Control and Prevention—National Center for Health Statistics (CDC-NCHS), and the Agency for Toxic Substances and Disease Registry (ATSDR), to develop an inventory of exposure-related data systems (10). The objectives were to identify existing data bases, examine how and why they were established, briefly describe the contents of each, summarize relevant characteristics, and disseminate that information to interested individuals, groups, and organizations[3]. The inventory contains exposure-related data systems that meet three conditions: Cover a relatively large geographical area (e.g. state or national); provide reasonable access to information; and are supported, at least in part, by Federal funds (6, 9, 10).

Categories

Systems identified through the survey were sorted into four categories: (*a*) those that collect and store exposure-related data (i.e. data collection systems); (*b*) those that provide access, analysis, and displays of data contained in multiple data bases (i.e. data handling systems); (*c*) those that provide tools for generating estimates of exposure or exposure-related parameters; and (*d*) those that characterize other systems that contain information on the physical environment or potential hazards. The major portion of the inventory contains information on 67 systems that fall into category (*a*). These 67 data collection

[3]This may be obtained from the Center for Environmental Research Information, 26 Martin Luther King Drive, Cincinnati, OH 45268 by requesting ORD Publications Document number EPA/600/R-92/078.

systems are managed by 17 different U.S. Federal agencies, the United Nations Environment Program (UNEP), and the World Health Organization (WHO) (9).

Exposure Estimators

Data collection systems contain a wide variety of exposure estimators including production/usage values, discharges estimates, environmental concentrations, microenvironmental concentrations, personal concentrations, and human-tissue concentrations. A comparison of exposure estimators with sample type for the 67 data systems is provided in Table 1.

Five data systems include information on production/usage (e.g. Synthetic Organic Chemicals US Production and Sales—annual information on total output of over 6000 organic chemicals in 15 classes). Eleven data systems provide discharge information (e.g. Air Facility Subsystem of the Aerometric Information Retrieval System—discharge data for air pollution point sources and stack discharges primarily for criteria pollutants). Microenvironmental sampling results are found in ten data systems (e.g. the Study of the Effects of Sulfur Dioxide and Respirable Particles on Human Health, also referred to as the Six-Cities Study). Environmental samples are included in 54 data systems (e.g. National Pesticide Survey—frequency and concentration of pesticide/nitrate occurrence in drinking water wells). Seven data systems include data collected using personal monitors (e.g. carbon monoxide, volatile organic chemical, and particulate measurements from the Total Exposure Assessment Methodology (TEAM) studies). Human-tissue samples are included in 13 data systems (e.g. National Health and Nutrition Examination Survey (NHANES)—blood and urine samples) (9).

Table 1   Comparison of exposure estimators and sample type for 67 federally sponsored data systems[a]

Exposure estimator	Water	Soil	Air	Food	Human tissue	Bulk chemicals
Production/usage volume	—	—	—	—	NA[b]	5
Estimated emissions	5	4	—	9	NA	NA
Environmental concentrations	31	15	27	15	NA	NA
Microenvironmental concentrations	2	—	10	—	NA	NA
Personal monitoring	—	—	7	—	NA	NA
Biological measurements	—	—	—	—	13	NA

[a] Total does not equal 67 because some data bases contain more than one type of estimator or information from more than one type of sample.
[b] NA = not applicable.

Agents/Parameters

Data on a variety of different environmental agents/parameters are collected by the 67 data systems. The most frequently included agents/parameters are inorganic compounds, pesticides, volatile and semivolatile organic compounds, polychlorinated biphenyls (PCBs), dioxins/furans, and radionuclides. Information on acids, bases, and tobacco smoke is included in relatively few systems, and no system includes data on airborne allergens (9).

Geographic Scope

Although most systems report national coverage, this descriptor can be misleading. It is true that the majority contain information from different parts of the country, however, most were not constructed to be population-based, probabilistic samples. Only a few are considered to be representative of the US population (e.g. the NHANES). Because most data systems are not designed to collect a statistically representative sample, there is no assurance that data accurately reflect national, regional, or local conditions. Consequently, substantial uncertainty exists about when and under what conditions reported values can be generalized to different geographical areas or populations (9).

Collection Frequency and Location

Schedules for sample collection vary dramatically among data systems, with 14 obtaining samples annually, 20 on an irregular or mixed schedule, and the rest using other schemes. For 16 data systems, the data are collected either on an as-needed (e.g. for compliance purposes) or a one-time basis. More consistency is exhibited by the location identifiers used in data systems with state (52 systems), latitude/longitude (44 systems), city/municipality/township (30 systems), and county/parish (28 systems) the most common descriptors (9).

Purpose of the Data Base

The lack of uniformity and consistency among data collection systems (e.g. agents/parameters, collection frequency, and location identifiers) results from the disparate purposes for which they were constructed, as well as the different missions of the responsible agencies. Thirty-six systems were established to monitor environmental conditions, 29 to conduct research, 19 to support regulatory programs, and 6 to meet legal requirements. The heterogeneous nature of the data systems, not only in terms of objectives, but also in the quality of the data, suggests that prudence should be exercised when using this information to estimate human exposures (9).

Summary of Findings

Overall, the evidence suggests that existing data systems contain a substantial amount of information that is relevant to exposure estimation. It is clear, however, that the quality of the data is inconsistent and difficult to access and that understanding and accessing the information is often difficult. Furthermore, these systems demonstrate a striking absence of data on actual human exposures, including a lack of information about contact between the agent and the human body (i.e. exposure concentration) and about the amount of the agent or its metabolites that enters the body (i.e. dose) (6).

Recommendations to Improve Exposure-Related Data Systems

Five major recommendations to improve the utility of exposure-related data systems were made, based on a review of the 67 data collection systems (6):

- The inventory reveals that many different data bases have been established by Federal agencies, for a variety of reasons. Standardized procedures for collecting, storing, analyzing, and reporting all information relevant to human-exposure estimation would enhance linkage of data bases and encourage more extensive use by Federal, state and local governments, the private sector, the academic community, and the public. User-friendly software for the submission and retrieval of data would significantly enhance accessibility.
- It is critical that exposure data be compared over time; consequently, bridging studies should be conducted whenever changes are made in general procedures (e.g. data handling and reporting, sampling techniques, or analytical methods). Such studies would generate conversion factors for the comparison of data before and after changes are implemented.
- Formal and informal mechanisms should be established for coordination and cooperation among: Federal agencies; Federal, state, and local governments; and the public and private sectors for design, maintenance, exchange, and review of data bases. Close interactions are essential for the promotion of awareness, accessibility, and cost-effectiveness.
- Very few data bases report actual measurements of either exposure or dose in human populations. There is a critical need to establish and maintain systems that include measurements of concentrations in important micro-environments (e.g. residences, offices, public buildings, commercial buildings, vehicles), time-activity pattern data for individuals and groups, personal exposure information (e.g. use of personal monitors), and biological measurements in human tissues and fluids (e.g. blood and urine). Such systems should also allow for comparison of data over time and for special subgroups (e.g. children or economically disadvantaged persons).
- It is not practical to measure exposures for every person. It follows, therefore, that a crucial use of exposure measurements extends to the construction and validation of models for extrapolation of the data to estimate exposures for specific populations and individuals. Development of predictive models is the ultimate goal of most exposure-measurement pro-

grams, and data bases should be structured to permit easy manipulation of information for both model building and testing.

USING EXPOSURE DATA BASES TO INFORM PUBLIC HEALTH DECISIONS

As described in Figure 1, decisions about safeguarding environmental health should be guided by public health principles. The three hierarchical public health goals of prevention (primary prevention), amelioration (secondary prevention), and treatment (tertiary prevention) successively target more specific/restricted populations. Primary prevention tends to focus on the general population. Therefore, data such as environmental concentrations measured in a geographic area may affect public health decisions. Secondary prevention targets a segment of the general population experiencing either excessive exposures or adverse effects. These public health efforts require more specific exposure data on these targeted groups. Finally, tertiary prevention requires a clinical approach to individuals that existing exposure systems cannot address.

Applying the public health goals to specific environmental agents and situations requires that decision-makers explicitly answer several key questions based on existing scientific knowledge and understanding. As summarized in Table 2, the range of public health questions creates the need for relevant and timely data on (*a*) exposures, (*b*) health status, and (*c*) the link between exposures and health outcomes. Each type of information (i.e. exposure, health, or exposure-health link) is germane to certain kinds of questions.

Many critical public health questions have an exposure component. Decision-makers need reliable exposure data to address questions such as: Are people exposed? If so, to what concentrations over what time period? What are exposures to susceptible populations (e.g. infants)? What is the link, if any, between exposures and adverse health effects (e.g. nature and strength of association based on epidemiologic studies)? How many people are exposed to concentrations that exceed a health-related benchmark (e.g. workplace exposure limit or ambient standard)? How and why do exposures occur (e.g. sources, pathways, and routes)? What is the relative effectiveness and efficiency of viable control options? What are the trends in exposure over time (e.g. are new problems emerging, or are old problems getting better or worse)? Have control measures been successful (e.g. are exposures within acceptable limits)?

As discussed earlier, existing exposure-related data bases are not very helpful in answering many of these critical questions. Moreover, it is often impractical (e.g. not technically feasible and too costly) to conduct exposure measurements to answer these questions directly. Decision-makers must therefore depend heavily on exposure estimates that are derived from combining

Table 2   Data to address important environmental health questions

Key environmental health questions	Information defin- ing exposure[a]	Information defin- ing health effects[b]	Information linking exposure and health[c]
Is an agent a hazard?			X
Are we exposed? (Yes, no)	X		
Who, what, where, when, why are we exposed?	X		
Are we affected now?		X	
Did the exposure cause the health effect?			X
Is there a risk?	X	X	X
What are relative effectiveness and efficacy of viable control strategies?	X		
What are important risk factors and be- haviors to address in public health programs?			X
Is the situation changing over time?	X	X	X

[a] Sources of exposure information include compliance registries, discharge inventories, site investigations, monitoring of ambient concentrations, and exposure registries.

[b] Sources of health information include health registries, vital records, community health studies, descriptive studies, and surveillance activities.

[c] Sources of data on the exposure-health link include toxicology studies, clinical studies, epidemiologic studies, and hazard and community studies.

existing data (e.g. emission inventories, environmental concentrations, residential location, and human time-activity patterns) with critical, and often heroic, assumptions (e.g. lifetime-exposure patterns). The resulting uncertainty seriously hinders realistic assessment of environmental health risks, reduces confidence in the risk-management decisions, and increases the difficulty of risk communication.

Determination of how best to safeguard environmental health in accordance with public health principles depends on accurate information about human exposures. For example, without accurate and timely exposure data it is often not possible to anticipate new or emerging problems, and thus the goal of preventing risks before they occur is difficult or impossible to achieve. Similarly, lack of exposure data can limit our ability to understand the need for stopping or reducing ongoing exposures until some people have already suffered ill-effects. Appropriate information about human exposures to environmental agents, including past, present, and future exposures, is essential to informed and credible public health decisions. Without it, attainment of our two highest priority goals, prevention and reduction of risk, is often out of the question. Consequently, attainment of our third highest goal, treatment of those with environmentally induced illness and injury, is the only achievable objective.

SUMMARY

The field of environmental health focuses on (*a*) the effects of people on the environment, and (*b*) the effects of the environment on people. Consistent with the public health paradigm, decisions about environmental health should be driven by three goals: first, to prevent adverse health effects from exposures to environmental agents from occurring in the first place; second, if that is not possible, then to reduce the magnitude and extent of the adverse effects; and third, if all else fails, to treat the impairments and disabilities of affected individuals. Information about human exposures to environmental agents is a key ingredient in making informed decisions about environmental hazards so as to do the best job possible of protecting public health. Human exposure information is critical to distinguish hazards with little risk to the public from hazards having important risks to the public. Human exposure analysis is pivotal to the major activities related to environmental health, including risk assessment, risk management, status and trends analyses, and epidemiologic studies.

The relationships between environmental exposures and associated health effects are often complex, raising sometimes difficult questions about which exposures and which agents are causally related to observed outcomes. Care must be taken, therefore, in selecting the right exposures to address as part of risk assessment and risk-management activities. At present, many data systems only indicate whether a hazard is present in a geographic area but not the risk for a population. Methods for collecting data on human exposures/doses are limited and there tends to be a direct relationship between costs and data accuracy. Because it is neither desirable nor feasible to measure exposures for everyone, the challenge is to develop robust exposure models that can be used to extrapolate from a few, inexpensive measurements to a much larger population.

A survey of existing exposure-related data bases indicates that data on hand are inadequate and inappropriate for answering many of the important exposure questions confronting decision-makers. Among other things, there is a critical need to establish data bases that are based on direct measurements of exposure and dose. This is the only way to establish the degree to which less-direct and less-costly methods are suitable for estimating exposure.

Information about exposures to environmental agents, environmentally induced health effects, and the link between exposures and effects is needed to answer important environmental health questions realistically. Exposure data and data bases complement and enhance health status information and epidemiologic investigations. All three types of information are necessary for informed decisions about safeguarding public health.

CONCLUSION

The value of collecting and analyzing these data in a comprehensive and systematic manner is substantial, and the costs associated with establishment and maintenance of appropriate data bases are justified. Instead of focusing solely on the costs of implementing the necessary data system, we should be asking whether we can afford not to obtain the relevant human exposure information (6).

Literature Cited

1. Last JM. 1983. *A Dictionary of Epidemiology.* New York: Oxford Univ. Press. 418 pp.
2. Moeller DW. 1992. *Environmental Health.* Cambridge, MA: Harvard Univ. Press. 427 pp.
3. Natl. Res. Counc., Natl. Acad. Sci. 1991. *Frontiers in Assessing Human Exposures to Environmental Toxicants.* Washington, DC: Natl. Acad. Press. 41 pp.
4. Natl. Res. Counc., Natl. Acad. Sci. 1991. *Human Exposure Assessment for Airborne Pollutants, Advances and Opportunities.* Washington, DC: Natl. Acad. Press. 303 pp.
5. Natl. Res. Counc., Natl. Acad. Sci. 1991. *Monitoring Human Tissues for Toxic Substances.* Washington, DC: Natl. Acad. Press. 211 pp.
6. Sexton K, Selevan SG, Wagener DK, Lybarger JA. 1992. Estimating human exposures to environmental pollutants: availability and utility of existing data bases. *Arch. Environ. Health* 47:398–407
7. Sexton K, Callahan MA, Bryan EF. 1995. Estimating exposure and dose to characterize health risks: the role of human tissue monitoring in exposure assessment. *Environ. Health Perspect.* In press
8. Sexton K, Olden K, Johnson BL. 1993. Environmental justice: the role of research in establishing a credible scientific foundation for informed decision making. *Toxicol. Ind. Health* 9:685–727
9. Sexton K, Wagener DK, Selevan SG, Miller TO, Lybarger JA. 1994. An inventory of human exposure-related data bases. *J. Expo. Anal. Environ. Epidemiol.* 4:95–109
10. U.S. Environ. Prot. Agency, Natl. Cent. Health Stat., Agency Toxic Subst. Dis. Regist. 1992. *Inventory of Exposure-Related Data Systems Sponsored by Federal Agencies.* EPA/600/R-92/078. Washington, DC: EPA Publ. 436 pp.

Annu. Rev. Public Health. 1995. 16:123 –40

MICROBIAL CONTAMINATION OF SHELLFISH: Prevalence, Risk to Human Health, and Control Strategies

R. J. Wittman

Virginia Department of Health, Division of Shellfish Sanitation, 1500 East Main Street, Main Street Station, Richmond, Virginia 23219

G. J. Flick

Virginia Polytechnic Institute and State University, Department of Food Science and Technology, Blacksburg, Virginia 24061

KEY WORDS: shellfish-borne disease, naturally occurring bacteria, enteric bacteria, enteric viruses

---

ABSTRACT

There has been significant concern in recent times about the safety of molluscan shellfish for human consumption. Despite extensive efforts to assure a safe supply of molluscan shellfish, the number of cases of disease and death are still great enough to cause concern among the public. The number of cases of illness and death associated with the ingestion of shellfish falls in the lower end of the range of other similar microbial pathogen-related foodborne disease. Disease and deaths due to viruses and naturally occurring bacteria are now of greatest concern because they are the most often cited casusative agents. The greatest risk of disease or death due to shellfish consumption is among the population with underlying health conditions who choose to consume raw shellfish. Control strategies to limit shellfish-borne disease should focus upon disease and death caused by viruses and naturally occurring bacteria among at-risk populations.

123

0163-7525/95/0510-0123$05.00

INTRODUCTION

Molluscan shellfish have held an important place in the diets of Americans since the birth of the United States. During colonial times, shellfish thrived in the estuarine environments and were a staple food. However, as the population grew and transportation systems improved, shellfish-borne disease also increased. Sewage discharges from population centers introduced a variety of human pathogens into coastal waters. Transportation improvements allowed shellfish to be introduced to inland markets, but the lack of adequate control during distribution resulted in reduced quality of shellfish upon arrival at the marketplace. It was not until the late 19th to early 20th century that public health agencies considered controls to reduce shellfish-borne disease (73). In February 1925, the Surgeon General arranged a conference with the Bureau of Chemistry (now the United States Food and Drug Administration) and the Bureau of Commercial Fisheries (now the National Marine Fisheries Service) to establish sanitary controls for the oyster industry. At this conference the agencies resolved to control "the beds on which shellfish are grown" and "the plants in which shellfish are shucked" (73).

Shellfish safety issues continue to revolve around these two categories: the quality of the waters in which shellfish are grown, and the conditions under which shellfish are harvested, processed, and distributed. Significant strides have been made in creating a safer food, but many problems nevertheless remain. We examine first the magnitude of the shellfish-borne disease in terms of its prevalence and the risks associated with shellfish consumption. We next address the issues of water quality, harvesting, processing, and distribution as they relate to shellfish-borne disease, and present strategies to minimize the risk of disease. Sanitary controls have focused upon edible bivalve mollusks, including oysters, clams, mussels, and scallops, of the class Pelecypoda since they are filter feeders and concentrate pathogens from the water (46). We therefore limit our discussion to these edible bivalves.

SHELLFISH-BORNE DISEASE RATES

The most comprehensive inventory of shellfish-related disease has been compiled by Scott Rippey of the Northeast Technical Services Unit (NETSU) of the US Food and Drug Administration (58). The Centers for Disease Control and Prevention (CDC) also maintain surveillance data on outbreaks of shellfish-borne disease (14, 58). While NETSU includes reports of outbreaks (two or more persons who become ill after consumption of a common food during a common time window) and individual cases, the CDC data base includes only outbreaks. Additionally, the CDC data are collected exclusively through submission of outbreak forms from state public health departments, whereas the NETSU report is a compilation of both case and outbreak data reported in written form, most of which are confirmed verbally by the state public health directors. The NETSU data base is therefore more inclusive and precise than the CDC data base for bivalve molluscan shellfish disease and death rates.

The prevalence of shellfish-borne disease over the past ten years, the various disease agents or types of disease involved with disease, the type of shellfish, and the geographic regions from which the shellfish in question originated can all be determined from the NETSU data base. Examination of these data allows risk to be quantified and rates of disease and death to be compared with the rates of other ingestion-related diseases. Additionally, the data can identify areas of focus in formulating control strategies.

Although both the CDC and NETSU have compiled the best available data, only an estimated 5–10% of all cases of seafood-borne disease are actually reported (13). Findings by the Institute of Medicine on seafood safety indicate that it is possible to identify "the source of much of the acute illnesses associated with the consumption of seafood" but that the dimensions of the problem are very difficult to derive from the CDC and NETSU data bases (1). The NETSU data therefore probably reflect only a small percentage of the disease magnitude.

Prevalence

The NETSU data in Table 1 reveal that the largest number of disease cases are of unknown etiology. The greatest percentage of known death (95%) is caused by non-cholera vibrios. Non-cholera vibrios also account for the second highest number of cases of shellfish-borne disease. Norwalk, Norwalk-like viruses, and *Vibrio cholerae* are the second highest causative agents of disease. Of the various diseases caused by shellfish over the past 10 years, 86% were of unknown agents or were caused by non-cholera vibrios, Norwalk, Norwalk-like viruses, and *Vibrio cholerae*.

The next question of interest is what type of shellfish caused the majority of disease and death. Information in Table 2 shows that oysters account for the highest proportion of cases of disease (49%) and death (97%). Clams present the second major health hazard, and account for 38% of the cases of disease and 2% of the deaths. In some instances, illness is associated with the ingestion of more than one type of shellfish. Mixed consumption of shellfish accounts for 12% of the cases of disease and 1% of the deaths. Scallops and mussels account for 2% and 3%, respectively, of recorded cases of disease, although none of these cases resulted in death.

Establishing the geographic source of contaminated shellfish illustrates the distribution of shellfish disease and death. There are three designated coastal regions: East, the Atlantic states except Florida; Gulf, states bordering the Gulf

Table 1 Shellfish-borne disease: cases and deaths

Year	Cases	Deaths		Non-Cholera Vibrio	Hepatitis A	Norwalk and Norwalk-like Viruses	Cholera	Salmonella	Shigella	Plesiomonas	Aeromonas	E. coli	Campylobacter	Unknown
1984	496	6	Cases	36	3	0	34	0	0	16	13	2	0	392
			Deaths	6	0	0	0	0	0	0	0	0	0	0
1985	238	7	Cases	22	0	3	14	0	0	0	0	0	0	199
			Deaths	7	0	0	0	0	0	0	0	0	0	0
1986	359	9	Cases	66	0	0	31	0	71	4	0	0	0	187
			Deaths	9	0	0	0	0	0	0	0	0	0	0
1987	118	12	Cases	47	0	0	11	0	0	2	0	0	0	58
			Deaths	12	0	0	0	0	0	0	0	0	0	0
1988	142	14	Cases	48	69	0	14	0	0	0	0	0	0	11
			Deaths	14	0	0	0	0	0	0	0	0	0	0
1989	858	9	Cases	52	22	270	14	4	1	0	0	0	5	490
			Deaths	7	0	0	1	0	0	0	0	0	0	0
1990	242	11	Cases	58	4	0	9	4	4	0	0	0	6	157
			Deaths	10	0	0	1	0	0	0	0	0	0	0
1991	33	4	Cases	22	0	0	5	0	0	0	0	0	0	6
			Deaths	4	0	0	0	0	0	0	0	0	0	0
1992	99	15	Cases	34	0	4	8	0	0	0	0	0	1	52
			Deaths	13	0	0	2	0	0	0	0	0	0	2
1993	210	9	Cases	21	0	156	0	0	0	1	0	0	0	32
			Deaths	9	0	0	0	0	0	0	0	0	0	0
TOTALS	2795	96	Cases	406	98	333	140	8	76	23	13	2	12	1573
			Deaths	91	0	0	4	0	0	0	0	0	0	1

Table 2 Shellfish-borne disease: types of shellfish and location of harvest

Year		Type of Shellfish						US Coastal region of harvest			
		Clams	Oysters	Scallops	Mussels	Multiple	Unknown	West	East	Gulf	Unknown
1984	Cases	265	206	0	0	25	0	3	239	99	155
	Deaths	0	6	0	0	0	0	0	0	1	5
1985	Cases	164	73	0	0	1	0	0	128	17	93
	Deaths	0	7	0	0	0	0	0	0	0	7
1986	Cases	65	292	0	0	2	0	0	82	100	177
	Deaths	0	9	0	0	0	0	0	0	1	8
1987	Cases	4	113	0	0	1	0	0	0	9	109
	Deaths	0	12	0	0	0	0	0	0	4	8
1988	Cases	1	136	0	0	5	0	5	3	66	68
	Deaths	0	14	0	0	0	0	0	0	9	5
1989	Cases	390	184	2	3	279	0	16	241	115	486
	Deaths	0	9	0	0	0	0	0	0	3	6
1990	Cases	159	70	0	0	3	10	1	1	36	204
	Deaths	0	11	0	0	0	0	0	0	11	0
1991	Cases	3	30	0	0	0	0	0	0	3	30
	Deaths	0	4	0	0	0	0	0	0	0	4
1992	Cases	24	74	0	0	1	0	13	0	32	54
	Deaths	2	12	0	0	1	0	0	0	2	13
1993	Cases	1	184	0	0	25	0	4	4	167	35
	Deaths	0	9	0	0	0	0	0	0	8	1
TOTALS	Cases	1076	1362	2	3	342	10	42	698	644	1411
	Deaths	2	93	0	0	1	0	0	0	39	57

of Mexico including Florida; and West, Pacific states. Shellfish harvested from waters along the Gulf Coast states accounted for 23% of all reported cases of shellfish-borne disease and 41% of resultant deaths during the ten-year period, 1984–1993. Twenty-five percent of all cases of shellfish-related disease originated from East Coast states, but had no associated deaths. Shellfish from West Coast waters yielded 5.5% of cases of disease with no associated deaths. The remaining cases (50%) resulted from shellfish in which the location of harvest could not be identified.

Shellfish from the East and Gulf Coasts are essentially equally likely to cause disease. Most molluscan shellfish illnesses on the East Coast are from outbreaks associated with virally contaminated clams, whereas on the Gulf Coast they are due to individual cases involving oysters with non-cholera vibrios.

In general, the NETSU data indicate that in the late 1800s and early 1900s most outbreaks involved cases of typhoid or hepatitis resulting from sewage contamination of waters where shellfish was grown. From the late 1970s to the present, increased incidence of disease associated with non-cholera vibrios indicates a rapidly emerging problem with naturally occurring environmental pathogens (58). Rippey noted that while nearly 25% of all shellfish-borne disease outbreaks in the NETSU data were cases of typhoid fever, the last such recorded outbreak occurred in 1954 (58). Similarly, cases of hepatitis A associated with the consumption of shellfish have steadily decreased over the same time period, while cholera is sporadically reported. Beginning in the early 1980s, outbreaks associated with Norwalk and Norwalk-like viruses have increased. Many of cases of unknown agents reported during this time are similar in nature to symptoms associated with Norwalk and Norwalk-like viruses.

IDENTIFYING THE POPULATION AT RISK

Both the CDC and NETSU data show that of all the shellfish-borne disease agents, none produces heat-stabile toxins, and that all, except for possible human enteric viral agents in the unknown categories, are deactivated by varying degrees of heat under most conditions (9, 32). Research results suggest that a wider heat range is needed to kill viruses than bacteria (48, 54). Heating molluscan shellfish to an internal temperature of 85–90°C for one minute completely inactivates viruses (48) and thus eliminates risk due to viral or bacterial agents.

However, the preference of many people for raw shellfish poses the greatest risk from bacterial or viral agents. This risk is greatly enhanced in individuals with underlying health conditions and predisposes them to illness and/or prolonged illness and death. For most diseases caused by the consumption of raw shellfish, higher infection rates occur most frequently in immunocompromised hosts—patients who have neoplasia of the immune system, a hematopoietic disorder, liver disease or alcoholism, chronic renal failure, acquired immune deficiency syndrome, or who are receiving pharmacological immunosuppression for neoplasia or transplantation of an organ (6, 34). Additionally, the risk of infection is higher for patients with diabetes mellitus, individuals with naturally low levels of gastric acid, or those taking prescription or over-the-counter medication to reduce stomach acidity (6, 41). Individuals with hepatic disorders and iron metabolism dysfunction are at much higher risk of progressive *Vibrio vulnificus* infection, often resulting in death (64). The elderly, the debilitated, the malnourished, and young children also are more susceptible to disease and death from the ingestion of raw shellfish (6).

Since the risk is highest for consumers of raw or partially cooked shellfish, this specific population should be defined. However, there are no national statistics to provide this information (21, 72). The best estimate of raw shellfish consumption is obtained from surveys performed in Virginia and Florida. A 1992 Commonwealth Poll estimated approximately 850,000 raw shellfish consumers in the State of Virginia [18% of the population aged 18 or older] (37). The 1988 Florida Behavioral Risk Factor Survey estimated that approximately 3 million adults in Florida consume raw oysters [23% of the population aged 18 or older] (23). Large numbers of people are thus at risk of disease and death via raw oyster consumption in both Virginia and Florida. It is not known how these rates of consumption in Virginia and Florida translate to other areas of the country. However, it can be assumed that the consumption of raw molluscan shellfish is more popular in coastal areas of the East Coast than in inland states, based upon an informal survey of local sales of shellstock oysters (74).

Of the estimated 850,000 raw shellfish consumers in Virginia, 93,000 (11%) have at least one high-risk characteristic: liver disease, stomach disorders, diabetes, immune system disorder, or immune suppressant drug therapy. In Florida, 71,000 (2.5%) of these raw oyster eaters have liver disease, a high-risk characteristic (23). The larger number of at-risk raw shellfish consumers in Virginia is likely to be partially due to the more inclusive definition of who is considered to be at risk.

Table 3 indicates that the relative risk for raw oyster eaters with liver disease in Florida of contracting a *Vibrio vulnificus* infection is approximately 92 times greater than for a raw oyster eater without liver disease, and 120 times greater than for a nonraw oyster eater. The relative risk of death for a raw oyster eater with liver disease in Florida is 190 times greater than for a raw oyster eater without liver disease and 345 times greater than for a nonraw oyster eater. In Virginia, the relative risk of contracting a *Vibrio vulnificus* infection is approximately 13 times greater for a raw oyster eater with at least one high-risk condition than for a raw oyster eater without any high-risk conditions, and 60 times greater than for a nonraw oyster eater.

Non-cholera vibrios, Norwalk, Norwalk-like viruses, and *Vibrio cholerae*, are the top three shellfish disease-causing agents, respectively. Non-cholera vibrios and *Vibrio cholerae* occur naturally throughout the marine environment within US coastal waters (28, 38, 50, 68–70). Norwalk virus is associated with human fecal contamination either in the shellfish-growing waters or through postharvesting contamination (27, 55). The remaining diseases identified with the ingestion of molluscan shellfish are associated with fecal pollution of the marine environment or with postharvesting contamination during processing

Table 3 Relative risk data; Florida and Virginia

Florida 1981–1993*	
Nonraw oyster eaters	
.6 illnesses/1 million adults	(95% C.I. .57–.64)
.131 deaths/1 million adults	(95% C.I. .124–.139)
Raw oyster eaters	
.8 illnesses/1 million adults	(95% C.I. .7–1)
.236 deaths/1 million adults	(95% C.I. .196–.297)
Raw oyster eaters with liver disease	
74.1 illnesses/1 million adults	(95% C.I. 37.8–215.9)
45.3 deaths/1 million adults	(95% C.I. 23.1–1320.7)
Virginia 1974–1993	
Nonraw oyster eaters	
.483 illnesses/1 million adults	(95% C.I. .466–.502)
.0402 deaths/1 million adults	(95% C.I. .0380–.043)
Raw oyster eaters	
2.2 illnesses/1 million adults	(95% C.I. 2.03–2.40)
.191 deaths/1 million adults	(5% C.I. .176–.208)
Raw oyster eaters with at least one high-risk characteristic	
28.9 illnesses/1 million adults	(95% C.I. 25.4–133.6)
2.51 deaths/1 million adults	(95% C.I. 2.15–62.86)

Source: GW Hlady (30).

(55, 73). Enteric pathogens account for 80% of reported shellfish-borne disease. Naturally occurring bacteria account for 20% of shellfish-borne disease but 99% of the deaths. Therefore, enteric pathogens pose a greater risk of disease through the ingestion of raw or partially cooked molluscan shellfish, whereas naturally occurring bacteria pose a greater risk of death.

The number of cases of microbial pathogen-related food-borne disease, calculated from CDC data, for all age groups reveals that the rate of disease is ~36 cases per 100,000 per year for the period from 1983 through 1987 (12). The prevalence of microbial pathogen-related shellfish-borne disease, calculated from the NETSU data for the same period, was ~9 cases per 100,000 (58). Prevalence rates for other ingestion-related diseases such as amebiasis, botulism, hepatitis A, salmonellosis, and shigellosis are described in Table 4. The data indicate that shellfish-borne disease is exceptionally low in relation to other similar diseases with the exception of botulism. The death rates for shellfish-borne disease are not significantly different from those for amebiasis

Table 4 Disease and death rates per 100,000 for shellfish-borne and related diseases 1983–1991, 1992.

	Shellfish-borne disease	Amebiasis	Botulism	Hepatitis A	Salmonellosis	Shigellosis
Disease rate per 100,000 1983–92	.127	1.74	.047	11.79	20.91	10.26
Death rate per 100,000 1983–1991	.0043	.0035	.011	.031	.036	.0043

and shigellosis. The death rate for botulism is significantly less, while the rates for hepatitis A and salmonellosis are significantly greater ($p \leq .01$). The death rate for shellfish-borne disease falls in the middle of the range of death rates identified for the diseases.

CONTROL STRATEGIES

Food safety is a value judgment of how much risk an individual or a community is willing to accept (5, 42). Of the food groups implicated in outbreaks of food-borne illness in the U.S. from 1977–84, seafood was most frequently associated with disease (~25%) (2, 15). Of these cases, 28% were related to shellfish, and of these, 22% were associated with a bacterial or viral agent (4). Control strategies to minimize shellfish-borne disease associated with viruses or bacteria could reduce food-borne disease in the U.S. by more than 6%.

Naturally Occurring Pathogens

The naturally occurring pathogens of concern that cause shellfish-borne disease are those of the family *Vibrionaceae*, *Plesiomonas shigelloides* and *Aeromonas hydrophilia*. These organisms vary seasonally (i.e. temperature sensitivity) and geographically (i.e. salinity sensitivity) in the marine environment.

Bacteria from the family *Vibrionaceae* cause the majority of identifiable illness and death from shellfish consumption. Patterns in their environmental distribution may provide a basis upon which to develop an effective disease control strategy. The species of this family associated with shellfish-borne disease are *Vibrio cholerae*, *V. vulnificus*, *V. parahaemolyticus*, *V. mimicus*, *V. hollisae*, and *V. furnissi*.

Toxigenic strains of *V. cholerae* are of public health concern. These strains of *V. cholerae*, identified by two groupings, serotype 01 and non-01, are found in greater concentrations during the warmer months of the year, with significantly higher incidence of disease occurring during this same time period (44).

Both strains of *V. cholerae* are adapted to waters with lower salinities (4 ppt to 17 ppt) (3, 61).

Vibrio parahaemolyticus has been found in marine environments in higher concentrations during warm weather periods (29, 53). This organism exists in the upper-salinity regimes of the marine environment (18).

A number of studies indicate a strong correlation between temperature, salinity, and the presence of *V. vulnificus* in seawater and oysters (36, 39, 51, 52). Although *V. vulnificus* has been isolated from waters with a wide range of temperatures and salinity, the highest concentrations of the organism are more frequently isolated from waters with temperatures of 17° to 31°C and salinities of 15 ppt to 25 ppt (52). Tamplin's study found significant associations ($p \leq 0.0001$) between salinities from 10 ppt to 20 ppt and numbers of *V. vulnificus* organisms (66). Additionally, there were high populations of *V. vulnificus* when water temperatures increased from 20° to 30°C (66).

The influence of temperature on the geographic distribution of *V. vulnificus* in the U.S. can easily be observed. Tamplin's study shows that the lowest concentrations of *V. vulnificus* for all sample sites in the United States (<100 MPN/g) occur in northern East Coast waters and all West Coast waters (66). Concentrations of *V. vulnificus* in oysters increased from Virginia south to Texas, with oysters from Texas sometimes exceeding 1 million MPN/g (66). Tamplin derived a predictive model predicated on the data from this study that estimates concentrations of *V. vulnificus* based upon temperature and salinity levels in specific geographic areas (65).

Tamplin's research examined the concentrations of virulent (opaque) and weakly virulent (translucent) strains of *V. vulnificus* at various sample sites in the Gulf of Mexico throughout a two-year period. The mean concentrations of virulent strains of *V. vulnificus* in oysters were 56.57 MPN/g (S.D. 214.21) during cold weather months (November to March), while during warm weather months (April to October) the concentrations were 7204.76 MPN/g (S.D. 34810.87) (66). Concentrations of weakly virulent strains during cold weather months were .289 MPN/g (S.D. 0.269), and during warm weather months they were 79.81 MPN/g (S.D. 246.10) (66). There is a significant ($p \leq .05$) increase in the number of virulent strains of *V. vulnificus* during periods of warm weather. Furthermore, there is also a significant increase in weakly virulent strains in warm weather. It may be possible to use the concept of seasonal or geographical distribution of strains and variable degrees of pathogenicity as a basis for identifying harvest areas that pose the greatest risk to consumers of infections from *V. vulnificus* (65).

Concentrations of *V. mimicus* vary seasonally, with higher concentrations present during warm weather periods (18). The organism persists in a wide range of salinities, but prefers salinities common to brackish water environments (7, 18).

The seasonal distribution and ecology of *V. hollisae* is not well understood because the organism is difficult to isolate (55). *V. furnissi* is found in greater concentrations during periods of warm weather, as are the other pathogenic members of the family *Vibrionaceae*. This organism has been isolated from a wide variety of salinities, ranging from fresh to brackish water environments (59).

Both *P. shigelloides* and *Aeromonas hydrophilia*, like some *Vibrionaceae*, are found ubiquitously in both fresh and saltwater environments. Both organisms exhibit higher natural concentrations in water during warm weather conditions (75).

Concentrations of naturally occurring pathogenic bacteria are distributed in the shellfish-growing coastal environments based upon temperature and salinity. These pathogens are distributed over a wide range of salinities with different genera and species thriving in relatively narrow ranges. Common to all of these pathogens is their increase in numbers with temperature. Since there is a definite relationship between temperature and the concentrations of these organisms in the environment, a twofold strategy to reduce death and disease is suggested. The first would limit harvesting of molluscan shellfish to cold weather months (November to March) in areas where these pathogens are known to exist in significant concentrations. This restriction would, in turn, necessitate an extensive monitoring program to determine when harvesting could be permitted.

Salinity preferences vary; many pathogens are able to grow throughout a wide range. Furthermore, salinities change constantly in the shellfish-growing environment. Thus a strategy to limit harvest based upon salinity alone, although possible, would be difficult to implement effectively.

The Institute of Medicine Food and Nutrition Board's Committee on Evaluation of the Safety of Fishery Products suggests that shellfish-growing waters be monitored during periods of warm weather for *Vibrio* species and that other means be investigated and implemented to eliminate or reduce the potential for disease from naturally occurring pathogenic bacteria through the ingestion of molluscan shellfish (1). Monitoring shellfish-growing areas for *Vibrio* species would not be a feasible proposition for public health agencies. More promising is a harvest-control strategy supported by a validated geographic model that predicts concentrations of *V. vulnificus* based upon temperature and salinity. If this model could be coupled with data on the identification and ecology of virulent strains, it would be possible to predict when harvesting areas should be closed to minimize risk. Such a model would work well for steady state conditions. However, the typically large fluctuations of salinity and temperature over small periods of time in estuarine environments would limit its usefulness, and alternative strategies would be needed.

The second component of this disease-reduction strategy—consumer education—holds greater potential for success. Individuals who consume raw shellfish, especially those with underlying risk factors, should be adequately apprised of the risks by health care providers and warnings should be posted at establishments where shellfish is purchased and/or consumed (76). In most instances the health care providers are the first to discover that an individual has an underlying risk factor, and should therefore be made aware of the importance of informing these patients that their condition requires abstinence from raw or partially cooked molluscan shellfish in order to avoid serious illness or possible death. If an individual is unaware of the personal risk, a health warning attached to the shellfish package or posted at the establishment where shellfish is sold will not prevent consumption.

Public warning notices should be provided both by health care providers and at the point of sale. Point of sale warnings should alert consumers to the increased risk of infection associated with the consumption of raw molluscan shellfish if they have neoplasia of the immune system, a hematopoietic disorder, liver disease or alcoholism, chronic renal failure, or acquired immune deficiency syndrome (34, 41). Also included are patients receiving pharmacological immunosuppression for neoplasia or transplantation of an organ or diabetes mellitus, individuals with naturally low levels of gastric acid, and those taking prescription or over-the-counter medication to reduce stomach acidity. Any warning system, to be effective, must contain language that clearly conveys potential risk and should be posted at all points of sale of molluscan shellfish if it is to reduce the incidence of disease and death.

Cooking the oyster to an internal temperature of 85–90°C will destroy both viruses and bacteria of public health concern in molluscan shellfish. Control strategy would require that consumers be advised to cook oysters during periods of warm weather.

Enteric Bacteria Associated with Contamination

Enteric bacteria and viruses can also contaminate shellfish either in the growing waters or during harvesting, processing, and distribution. Pathogens of concern that have been associated with disease from consumption of contaminated molluscan shellfish include human enteric viruses; hepatitis A, non-A, non-B enteral hepatitis (hepatitis E), unclassified viruses; and such bacteria as *Salmonella, Shigella, Camplyobacter jejuni*, and pathogenic *Escherichia coli* (14, 55, 58). The group of unclassified viruses includes the Norwalk, Norwalk-like virus, Snow Mountain agent, and small round structured virus. Although human viruses are inert outside of their host and therefore do not multiply in other organisms, they are resilient and persistent in the environment and in molluscan shellfish (22, 24, 47, 54). These viral and bacterial enteric pathogens are of public health concern because of their link with disease caused by fecal contamination of the waters from which molluscan shellfish are harvested and of the environment in which they are processed (12, 14, 17, 31, 54, 56).

Other pathogenic bacteria (*E. coli, Yersinia enterolytica, Listeria mono-cytogenes, Clostridium botulinum*, and *Staphylococcus aureus*) that are not exclusively of enteric origin can also potentially contaminate molluscan shellfish, both in their natural environment and through processing and distribution (45).

Prevention of shellfish-borne disease caused by these enteric related pathogens should focus upon strategies to increase sensitivity in detecting contamination of shellfish, avert the entry of pathogens into areas open to shellfish harvesting, and eliminate pathways by which pathogens could contaminate shellfish through their harvesting, processing, and distribution. A National Indicator Study sponsored by the National Oceanic and Atmospheric Administration is currently under way to identify better indicators of fecal pollution than either total or fecal coliforms (49). This study seeks to identify an organism or series of organisms that will provide a more specific mechanism to detect polluted shellfish-growing areas. Total or fecal coliforms are limited as indicators because they cannot be correlated with the presence of enteric viruses (25, 33). This limitation is especially important in light of the significant 10-year increase in viral enteric shellfish-borne disease (14, 56). Fecal coliforms do not differentiate well between human and nonhuman pollution sources (63). Once the best available indicator(s) is identified, the regulatory community should implement a classification system of shellfish-growing areas based upon such indicator(s).

The United States Food and Drug Administration has proposed to mandate a quality assurance program to regulate molluscan shellfish safety based on the Hazard Analysis Critical Control Point (HACCP) concept (71). Currently, the molluscan shellfish industry is regulated by the National Shellfish Sanitation Program. Although this voluntary framework has been effective, the adoption of a HACCP-based program will provide a system of preventive controls and corrective actions to be implemented by molluscan shellfish processors and handlers and monitored by regulators to insure that conditions under which shellfish are harvested, processed, and distributed minimize the risk from contaminated shellfish reaching the consumer.

A recent outbreak of shellfish-borne disease—oyster-related Norwalk-like virus gastroenteritis—occurred in November 1993, and was associated with fecal contamination from fishing boats (16). This incident suggests that similar sporadic cases of pollution, which are very difficult if not impossible to trace, could potentially have been responsible for some of the many unidentifiable cases of shellfish-borne disease. Comprehensive education for users of the waterways on the importance of proper sewage disposal and imposition of stiff penalties for improper disposal of fecal material could reduce such sporadic discharges into approved shellfish harvest waters.

Likewise, harvest areas adjacent to sewage treatment facilities with point source discharges should be more closely evaluated, especially for the presence of viruses. Conventional sewage treatment facilities do not reduce numbers of enteric viruses in their discharges to low concentrations (40, 43). Outbreaks of disease associated with Norwalk virus have increased, and many cases where the agent is unknown are similar to those associated with this virus (58). Areas that receive discharges from a sewage treatment facility and that also support resources of molluscan shellfish that have been approved for harvesting must be carefully evaluated for the presence of viruses. Improvement in the technology of sewage treatment is needed to eliminate viruses in these areas.

Oysters have a persistent microbial flora in the gut region. Controlled purification involves the supervised processes of depuration and relaying. Depuration requires placing of molluscan shellfish in recirculating seawater tanks where the water is continuously disinfected. The circulation of water in these tanks stimulates molluscan shellfish to feed, which thus facilitates defecation of the bacteria and viruses populating the gut into the tank water, where they are inactivated by disinfection. Under most holding conditions, this depuration process does not successfully remove *V. vulnificus* or lower concentrations of enteroviruses in shellfish (26, 43, 57, 67). Depuration will not produce oysters free of *V. vulnificus* or viruses and therefore will not predictably reduce the risk of disease or death.

Relaying is the transfer of molluscan shellfish from contaminated growing areas to approved areas (i.e. with no contamination) so that the gut will be naturally purged of pathogenic organisms. This strategy has been shown to be effective in reducing total numbers of organisms in shellfish (10, 11, 62). *V. vulnificius* as part of the natural microflora of the gut of oysters does not depurate in an artifical environment. Since relaying can be thought of as depuration in the natural environment, the elimination of *V. vulnificius* through this process has not been considered to be effective. However, recent research suggests that in the natural environment, if the waters to which the shellfish are to be relayed are free of *Vibrio vulnificus*, the numbers of these organisms will be reduced over time in cold water conditions (35).

Irradiation has been proposed as a means of killing or inactivating the *V. vulnificus* organism without killing the oyster. The United States Food and Drug Administration and the United Nation's World Health Organization have determined that there is no health risk associated with foods irradiated by approved commercial procedures (20). However, the FDA has yet to approve commercial irradiation procedures for shellfish. The potential for such approval appears encouraging; Dr. George Hoskin, associate director of FDA's Office of Seafood, described the process as "promising for control of pathogens including vibrios" (60).

Processes such as rapid chilling and mild heat treatment of oysters can limit the growth of *V. vulnificus*—and actually reduce its concentration over time—in oysters that are not shucked (8, 19). The National Shellfish Sanitation Program has taken the first step toward implementation of strict time-temperature controls, which are technologically feasible and attainable. However, these measures fall short of what will reduce or limit the growth of the organism. Intensive rapid chilling, cold storage, and heat treatment (which does not change the protein nature of the shellfish) can significantly reduce *V. vulnificus*. Thermal processing is also lethal to several other pathogens. Both processes are not an inclusive control strategy for all pathogens of concern.

The most effective control strategy would be to ban the sale of raw molluscan shellfish either totally or at food service facilities, although this proscription would not eliminate consumption resulting from the recreational harvest or from illegal sales. However, such an extreme measure is unlikely for political reasons, and it would be virtually impossible to adequately enforce. To estimate the risk reduction, it would be necessary to calculate the magnitude of the illegal market and recreational catch and the risk factors of those who would consume such product.

Strategies to control shellfish-borne disease should focus upon illness caused by bacteria of the family *Vibrionaceae* and upon viral illness since the majority of cases and deaths (86%) are a result of these agents. The strategies that have been outlined focus upon minimizing all types of shellfish-borne disease with an emphasis upon maximizing the reduction of risk from *Vibrionaceae* and viral disease and death. If these strategies are fully implemented, the risk of shellfish-borne disease and death can be significantly reduced.

The disease and death rates from eating raw shellfish are small in relation to other similar risks and consumers appear willing to bear this risk in order to enjoy the food. However, steps can be taken to increase the safety of raw shellfish, and consumers should be warned of the risks. The control strategies presented here provide various levels of potential risk reduction. A determination of which strategies to use should be based upon the level of risk that is considered acceptable, the costs to the shellfish industry, and the costs to the consuming public (in deaths and disease). Risk can be eliminated by prohibiting the consumption of raw or partially cooked shellfish. If lesser reductions of risk are desired, consumer education, seasonal harvest restrictions, strict time-temperature controls, changes in indicator organisms, and the inclusion of viruses in evaluation of shellfish growing areas can be selected.

Literature Cited

1. Ahmed FE. 1991. *Seafood Safety.* Washington, DC: Natl. Acad. Press
2. Archer DL, Kvenberg JE. 1985. Incidence and cost of foodborne diarrheal disease in the United States. *J. Food Prot.* 48:887–94
3. Baumann P, Furniss AL, Lee JV. 1984. Genus 1. *Vibrio pacini* 1854. In *Bergey's Manual of Systematic Bacteriology,* ed. NR Kreig, 1:518–38. Baltimore, MD: Williams & Wilkins
4. Bean NH, Griffin PM. 1990. Foodborne disease outbreaks in the United States, 1973–1987: pathogens, vehicles, and trends. *J. Food Prot.* 53:804–17
5. Benarde MA. 1989. *Our Precarious Habitat.* New York: Wiley
6. Benenson AS, ed. 1990. *Control of Communicable Diseases in Man.* Washington, DC: Am. Public Health Assoc.
7. Bockemuhl J, Roch K, Wohler B, Aleksia S, Wokatsch R. 1986. Seasonal distribution of facultative enteropathogenic vibrios (*Vibrio choleras, Vibrio mimicus, Vibrio parahaemolyticus*) in the freshwater of the Elbe river at Hamburg. *J. Appl. Bacteriol.* 60:435–39
8. Boutin BK, Reyes AL, Peeler JT, Twedt RM. 1985. Effect of temperature and suspending vehicle on survival of *Vibrio parahaemolyticus* and *V. vulnificus. J. Food Prot.* 48:875–78
9. Brown MRW, Melling J. 1971. Inhibition and destruction of microorganisms by heat. In *Inhibition and Destruction of the Microbial Cell,* ed. WB Hugo, pp. 180–212. New York: Academic
10. Cabellia VJ, Hefferman WP. 1970. Elimination of bacteria by the soft shell clam, *Mya drendria. J. Fish. Res. Board Can.* 27:1579–87
11. Canzonier WJ. 1971. Accumulation and elimination of coliphage S-13 by the hard clam *Mercenaria mercenaria. Appl. Microbiol.* 21:1024–31
12. Centers for Disease Control Prevention. 1983–92. Annual summary, 1983, 1984, 1985, 1986, 1987, 1988, 1989, 1990, 1991, 1992. CDC Surveillance Summaries. *Morbid. Mortal. Wkly. Rep.*
13. Centers for Disease Control and Prevention. 1988. *Foodborne Disease Outbreaks. Annual Summaries 1973–1987.* USDHHS Publ. Cent. Dis. Control
14. Centers for Disease Control and Prevention. 1989. *Foodborne Surveillance Data for all Pathogens in Fish/Shellfish for years 1973–1987.* Dec.
15. Centers for Disease Control and Prevention. 1990. Foodborne disease outbreaks, 5-year summary, 1983–87. CDC Surveillance Summaries. *Morbid. Mortal. Wkly. Rep.* 39(No. SS-1):15–57
16. Centers for Disease Control and Prevention. 1993. Multistate outbreak of viral gastroenteritis related to the consumption of oysters—Louisiana, Maryland, Mississippi, and North Carolina. *Morbid. Mortal. Wkly. Rep.* 42:945–48
17. Cliver DO. 1988. Virus transmission via foods. A scientific status summary by the Institute of Food Technologists' Expert Panel on Food Safety and Nutrition. *Food Technol.* 42:241–47
18. Colwell R. 1984. *Vibrios in the Environment.* New York: Wiley
19. Cook DW, Ruple AD. 1992. Cold storage and mild heat treatment as processing aids to reduce the numbers of *Vibrio vulnificus* in raw oysters. *J. Food Prot.* 12:985–89
20. Cowen RC. 1991. Beware scares about irradiated food risks. *Christian Sci. Monitor,* July 17
21. Dayal HH, Trieff NM, Dayal VD. 1993. Preventing *Vibrio vulnificus* infections: who should bear responsibility? *Am. J. Prev. Med.* 9:191–93
22. DeLeon R, Gerba CP. 1990. Viral disease transmission by seafood. In *Food Contamination from Environmental Sources,* ed. JO Nraigu, MS Simmons, pp. 639–62. New York: Wiley
23. Desenclos JC, Klontz KC, Wolfe LE, Hoecherl S. 1991. The risk of Vibrio illness in the Florida raw oyster eating population, 1981–1988. *Am. J. Epidemiol.* 134:290–97
24. DiGirolamo R, Liston J, Matches JR. 1970. Survival of virus in chilled, frozen and processed oysters. *Appl. Microbiol.* 20:58–63
25. Ellender RD, Mapp JB, Middlebrooks BL, Cake EW. 1980. Natural enterovirus and fecal coliform contamination of Gulf Coast oysters. *J. Food Prot.* 43:105–10
26. Eyles MJ, Davey GR. 1984. Microbiology of commercial depuration of the Sydney Rock Oyster, *Crassostrea commercialis. J. Food Prot.* 47:703–6
27. Gerba CP. 1988. Viral disease transmission by seafoods. *Food Technol.* 42:99–103
28. Hackney CR, Kilgen MB, Kator H. 1992. Public health aspects of transferring mollusks. *J. Shellfish Res.* 11:521–33
29. Hackney CR, Ray B, Speck ML. 1980. Incidence of *Vibrio parahaemolyticus*

and the microbiological quality of sea-foods in North Carolina. *J. Food Prot.* 43:769–72

30. Hlady GW. 1994. *Summary of* Vibrio vulnificus *infections in Florida, 1981–1993.* Dep. Health Rehabil. Serv., Fla.

31. Hood MA, Ness GE, Blake NJ. 1983. Relationship among fecal coliform, *Escherichia coli* and *Salmonella* spp. in shellfish. *Appl. Environ. Microbiol.* 45:122–26

32. Int. Comm. Microbiol. Specific. Foods. 1980. *Microbial Ecology of Foods.* Vol. 1. *Factors Affecting the Life and Death of Microorganisms.* New York: Academic

33. Jehl-Pehtri C, Hugues B, Deloince R. 1990. Viral and bacterial contamination of mussels exposed in an unpolluted marine environment. *Lett. Appl. Microbiol.* 11:126–29

34. Johnston JM, Becker SF, McFarland LM. 1985. *Vibrio vulnificus:* man and sea. *J. Am. Med. Assoc.* 253:2850–52

35. Jones S. 1994. *The effects of relaying upon concentrations of* Vibrio vulnificus *in oysters in Maine waters.* Presented at FDA/NMFS/ISSC *Vibrio vulnificus* Workshop, June 15, 16

36. Kaysner CA, Abeyta C Jr, Wekell MM, DePaola A, Stott RF, Leitch JM. 1987. Virulent strains of *Vibrio vulnificus* isolated from estuaries of the United States west coast. *Appl. Environ. Microbiol.* 53:1349–51

37. Keeter S. 1992. *The Commonwealth Survey—1992.* Commissioned by the Virginia Dep. Health. Performed by Virginia Commonwealth Univ. Sur. Res. Lab.

38. Kelly MT. 1982. Effect of temperature and salinity on *Vibrio vulnificus* occurrence in Gulf Coast estuaries. *Appl. Environ. Microbiol.* 44:820–24

39. Kelly MT, Stroh EM. 1988. Occurrence of Vibrionaceae in natural and cultivated oyster populations in the Pacific Northwest. *Diagn. Microbiol. Infect. Dis.* 9:1–5

40. Keswick BH, Satterwhite TK, Johnson PC, DuPont HL, Secor SL, et al. 1985. Inactivation of Norwalk virus in drinking water by chlorine. *Appl. Environ. Microbiol.* 50:261–64

41. Klontz KC, Spencer L, Schreiber M, Janowski HT, Baldy LM, Gunn RA. 1988. Syndromes of *Vibrio vulnificus* infections: clinical and epidemiologic features in Florida cases, 1981–1987. *Ann. Intern. Med.* 109:318–23

42. Lechowich RV. 1992. Current concerns in food safety. In *Food Safety Assessment,* ed. JW Finley, SF Robinson, DJ Armstrong. Washington, DC: Am. Chem. Soc.

43. Lewis GD, Austin FJ, Loutit MW. 1986. Enterovirus of human origin and fecal coliforms in river water and sediments downstream from a sewage outfall in the Tieri River, Otago. *NZ J. Mar. Fresh Res.* 20:153–62

44. Madden JM, McCardell BA, Read RB. 1982. Vibrio cholera in shellfish from U.S. coastal waters. *Food Technol.* 36:93–96

45. Martinez-Manzanares E, Morinigo MA, Cornax R, Egea F, Borrego JJ. 1991. Relationship between classical indicators and several pathogenic microorganisms involved in shellfish-borne diseases. *J. Food Prot.* 54:711–17

46. Metcalf TG. 1975. *Evaluation of Shellfish Sanitary Quality by Indicators of Sewage Pollution.* Oxford, UK: Pergamon

47. Metcalf TG, Stiles WC. 1965. The accumulation of enteric viruses by the oyster *Crassostrea virginica. J. Infect. Dis.* 115:68–76

48. Millard JH, Appleton H, Parry JV. 1987. Studies on heat inactivation of Hepatitis A virus with special reference to shellfish. *Epidemiol. Infect.* 98:397–414

49. Natl. Oceanic Atmos. Admin. 1993. *Interstate Shellfish Sanit. Conf. The National Indicator Study*

50. Oliver JD, Warner RA, Cleland DR. 1982. Distribution and ecology of *Vibrio vulnificus* and other lactose-fermenting marine vibrios in coastal waters of the Southeastern United States. *Appl. Environ. Microbiol.* 44:1404–14

51. Oliver JD, Warner RA, Cleland DR. 1983. Distribution and ecology of *Vibrio vulnificus* and other lactose-fermenting marine vibrios in the marine environment. *Appl. Environ. Microbiol.* 45:985–98

52. O'Neill KR, Jones SH, Grimes DJ. 1992. Seasonal incidence of *Vibrio vulnificus* in the Great Bay estuary of New Hampshire and Maine. *Appl. Environ. Microbiol.* 58:3257–62

53. Paille D, Hackney C, Reily L, Cole M, Kilgen M. 1987. Seasonal variation in the fecal coliform population of Louisiana oysters and its relationship to microbiological quality. *J. Food Prot.* 50:545–49

54. Peterson DA, Wolfe LG, Larkin EP, Deinhardt FW. 1978. Thermal treatment and infectivity of Hepatitis A virus in human feces. *J. Med. Virol.* 2:201–6

55. Regan PM, Margolin AB, Watkins WD. 1993. Evaluation of microbial indicators for the determination of the sanitary

quality and safety of shellfish. *J. Shellfish Res.* 12:95–100

56. Richards GP. 1985. Outbreaks of shellfish associated enteric virus illness in the United States: requisite for development of viral guidelines. *J. Food Prot.* 48:815–23

57. Richards GP. 1988. Microbial purification of shellfish: a review of depuration and relaying. *J. Food Prot.* 51:218–51

58. Rippey SR. 1994. *Seafood borne disease outbreaks.* Kingstown, RI: DHHSS Public Health Serv., FDA, NE Seafood Lab. Branch

59. Roberts NC, Bradford HB, Barbay JR. 1984. Ecology of Vibrio choleras in Louisiana coastal waters. See Ref. 18

60. Seafood irradiation called safe but misunderstood. 1992. *Food Chem. News,* June 22

61. Singleton FL, Attwell RW, Jangi MS, Colwell RR. 1982. Influence of salinity and organic nutrient concentration on survival and growth of *Vibrio choleras* in aquatic microcosms. *Appl. Environ. Microbiol.* 43:1080–85

62. Son NT, Fleet GH. 1980. Behavior of pathogenic bacteria in the oyster, *Crassostrea commercialis,* during depuration, relaying and storage. *Appl. Environ. Microbiol.* 80:994–1002

63. Stelma GN, McCabe LJ. 1992. Nonpoint pollution from animal sources and shellfish sanitation. *J. Food Prot.* 55:649–56

64. Tacket CO, Brenner F, Blake PA. 1984. Clinical features and an epidemiological study of *Vibrio vulnificus* infections. *J. Infect. Dis.* 149:558–61

65. Tamplin ML. 1994. *The distribution of concentrations of* Vibrio vulnificus *in oysters in United States.* Presented at FDA/NMFS/ISSC *Vibrio vulnificus* Workshop, June 15, 16

66. Tamplin ML. 1994. *The seasonal occurrence of* Vibrio vulnificus *in shellfish, seawater and sediment of the United States coastal waters and the influence of environmental factors on survival and virulence.* Final res. rep. to Salstonstall-Kennedy program

67. Tamplin ML, Capers GM. 1992. Persis-

tence of *Vibrio vulnificus* in tissues of Gulf Coast oysters, *Crassostrea virginica,* exposed to seawater disinfected with UV light. *Appl. Environ. Microbiol.* 58:1506–10

68. Tamplin M, Roderick GE, Blake NJ, Cuba T. 1982. Isolation and characterization of *Vibrio vulnificus* from two Florida estuaries. *Appl. Environ. Microbiol.* 44:1466–70

69. Tilton RC, Ryan RW. 1987. Clinical and ecological characteristics of *Vibrio vulnificus* in Northeastern United States. *Diagn. Microbiol. Infect. Dis.* 2:109–17

70. Tison DL, Kelly MT. 1986. Virulence of *Vibrio vulnificus* strains from marine environments. *Appl. Environ. Microbiol.* 51:1004–6

71. US Dep. Health Hum. Serv. 1994. FDA, 21 FCR, parts 123, 1240 [Doc. No. 9ON-0199, 93N-0195] Proposal to establish procedures for the safe processing and importing of fish and fishery products. *Fed. Regist.* 4192–214

72. US Dep. Health Hum. Serv. 1992. *Health United States and Healthy People 2000 Review.* Washington, DC: Natl. Cent. Health Stat.

73. US Dep. Health Hum. Serv. 1993. *National Shellfish Sanitation Program, Manual of Operations, Part II. Sanitation of the Harvesting, Processing and Distribution of Shellfish. Revision.* Washington, DC: Public Health Serv., FDA

74. VA Dep. Health. Div. Shellfish Sanit. 1993. *Informal survey conducted of the major molluscan shellfish dealers in Virginia, Louisiana and Florida*

75. Wadstrom T. 1987. *Aeromonas* and *Plesiomonas*-enteric infections and fecal carriage in research on *Aeromonas* and *Plesiomonas.* I. Taxonomy, ecology, isolation and identification. *Experientia* 43:362–64

76. Wittman RJ, Croonenberghs RC. 1992. Vibrio vulnificus *in shellfish: an examination of public health risks and public health policy recommendations.* VA Dep. Health. Policy Anal. Comm. Health

Annu. Rev. Public Health. 1995. 16:141–64

INFECTIOUS RISKS FOR HEALTH CARE WORKERS

Linda Hawes Clever and Yannick LeGuyader

Department of Occupational Health, California Pacific Medical Center, San Francisco, California 94120

KEY WORDS: infectious, risks, health care workers

ABSTRACT

Although health care has been practiced for eons and although hundreds of thousands of workers are engaged in it, we know distressingly little about ways to prevent work-related infectious illnesses in this important group. Assumptions may be dangerous and expensive: Are "universal precautions" effective; when are respirators necessary? These kinds of questions have taken on particular urgency in the face of multiple-drug resistant tuberculosis and the spread of human immunodeficiency virus and other blood-borne pathogens. Furthermore, health care has moved from the traditional hospital setting into ambulatory, home, and other noninstitutional settings, thus increasing the complexity of worker protection measures. Steps to ensure the safety and health of health care workers must therefore include research and action that lead to identifying workers at risk; planning; education; providing necessary equipment and assuring adequate staffing; using appropriate techniques and precautions; immunizing workers; appropriately isolating patients; record-keeping; and evaluation. Curricula in schools for health professionals should include material on ways to achieve good health for health care workers. Public health officials and regulators should pay more attention to this arena.

INTRODUCTION

Health care workers through the ages have been plagued by infectious diseases. During the eras of greatest risk, the most prevalent and serious infections such

141

as syphilis, hepatitis, human immunodeficiency virus (HIV), tuberculosis (TB), and influenza have been incurable. Although these diseases pale in importance by comparison with occupational injuries in terms of numbers, cost, and suffering, they deserve attention because of their effects on people, policies, and the professions.

In 1700, the astute Bernadino Ramazzini, noting the frequency of syphilis among midwives, said, "How, then, shall the medical profession safeguard ... [midwives], how to assist them to follow their calling with all possible impunity? The only way is for them to wash the hands and arms in water or wine when they have a breathing spell; when their work is done they should wash the face and rinse the throat with vinegar and water, put on clean clothes when they go home, in short be very careful to keep themselves clean. I was told by an aged midwife that, whenever she attended a woman who was either suspected of suffering from French disease or was in any way sickly, she used to wait till the patient was in the very last throes before she placed on the [birthing] chair; this was to shorten the time in which her own hands would be wetted by the contaminated lochia" (104, p. 167). Characteristically, Ramazzini urged prevention, since there was no cure. And prevention needed to be technological, since there was no vaccine. A century ago, recognition of the problem, rigorous antisepsis, hand washing, avoidance of breaks in skin, and, finally, use of rubber gloves, essentially eliminated work-related syphilis for health professionals (89).

That tuberculosis is contagious has been known since Aristotle. After years of conflicting data and debate, opinion coalesced in the 1960s that tuberculosis can be a work-related disease (110). Somewhat earlier, recommendations for tuberculin skin testing, chest X-rays, isolation of patients, asepsis, and, finally, effective treatment and prophylaxis of tuberculosis, decreased the risk for health care workers, at least temporarily.

HIV was recognized as a threat to health care workers early in its course (12), and a stream of recommendations followed (13, 14, 16–18). Regulations were later developed (95). The effectiveness of these measures remains to be seen, although instituting techniques to isolate body fluids reliably can decrease spread of at least some organisms (83), and universal precautions can decrease incidents of exposure (120). As is so often the case, more good occupational research is urgently needed to assure the health of health care workers. The focus should be on benefit-cost. That is, if applied as directed, do universal precautions or body substance isolation techniques decrease or prevent transmission of infectious diseases from patients to health care workers and beyond? If so, what is the cost in money, time, and effort? Some analysts have estimated millions of dollars and billions of gloves (53). Immediate attention must be given to these questions, because therapeutic approaches are wanting (91, 116).

RISKS

What risks of HIV infection do health care workers face? The consensus is that, after a needle stick or sharps cut from an HIV antibody-positive patient, a health care worker has a chance of about 1 in 250 of being infected (19, 64, 87, 105). That amounts to a loss of life expectancy of 39 days for a 30 year-old female health care worker (97). Factors other than the incident itself affect the outcome. The frequency of needle sticks varies by specialty, experience, and job title (65, 71, 85, 98, 102). The HIV titer seems to be higher in patients with more severe illness, so the chance of infecting a health care worker is correspondingly greater with sicker patients (97). The picture with hepatitis B (HBV) is more alarming, given its higher prevalence. About 1 in 20 health care workers will be infected after a percutaneous injury if the patient is hepatitis Be antigen (HBe Ag) negative; more than 1 in 4 will be infected if the patient is HBe Ag positive (97).

The consequences of exposures go beyond mere microbiology. Whether or not a health professional is actually infected by an injury, there is a period of anxiety, guilt, worry, fear, anger, sadness, and perhaps depression. Relationships may founder; pregnancy may be deferred. If infection is transmitted, sickness or death may ensue. Infection can also be passed along to patients, family members, and others. Professional lives may be threatened or ended by breaches of privacy and by the need for sick leave, restrictions of practice (10, 35, 49, 93), disability, or death. Thus, these incidents have poignant human dimensions that have meaning beyond numbers and models. As Sir Richard Doll has been quoted, "Statistics are people with the tears wiped away."

DEFINITION OF HEALTH CARE WORKER

Before discussing selected infections and proposed risk modifications, we need to define "health care workers." The Centers for Disease Control and Prevention (CDC) definition is inclusive: "any persons, including students or trainees, whose activities involve contact with patients or with blood or other body fluids from patients in a health-care setting" (17, p. 3S). Thus, clinical clerks in medical schools, geriatric workers, aides, and psychiatric and drug rehabilitation technicians may be included in the definition. Some of these workers may be considered more social service than health care workers, but the exposure potential is real. The exposure is real, too, for emergency workers and public safety workers, and protection guidelines have been published for them as well (21). The CDC does not refer to volunteers, but volunteers should be included if they are at risk. Family members should be of concern as well, because they provide an enormous amount of care, and because in-home transmission of tuberculosis, hepatitis B, influenza, HIV (15, 44, 59), and cytomegalovirus (CMV) (99) is well recognized.

Counting only persons who touch patients for whom they are paid to care, 8.5 million people in the United States are health care workers (8). This number is expected to rise; indeed, four of the top six fastest-growing occupations are in health: home health aides, personal and home-care aides, medical assistants, and radiologic technologists and technicians (9).

High costs of in-patient services, increasing numbers of older persons who require chronic care, and the desire of many patients with acquired immunodeficiency syndrome (AIDS) and cancer to die in noninstitutional surroundings are forces expanding and dispersing health care work and sites. Hospices, day care and rehabilitation centers, and private homes are joining the ranks of hospitals, clinics, and nursing homes as "health care facilities." More than one half of health care workers are employed outside of hospitals (8). Physicians' offices, also possible sites for worker exposure, are covered by occupational safety and health administration (OSHA) regulations and CDC recommendations (95, 121). Assuring safe and healthy workplaces for tens of millions of paid and unpaid workers providing an array of services in countless sites is daunting but doable.

RISK MODIFICATION

In medicine, health care, and life, *decreasing* risk to a practical minimum is desirable, necessary, and feasible. As Murray noted, "Epidemics of nosocomial diseases in health care settings can be costly and tragic." Epidemics are even more unfortunate since diseases can be prevented with vaccines (92, p. 5), respiratory isolation, and placing susceptible hospital personnel on leave (39).

The question is how to achieve the ideal under conditions that occasionally include worker indifference or resistance and always include relentlessly tightening resources. First, an employer must know formal and informal local, state, and national standards and practices. Official guidelines (20, 24, 32, 41, 43) have almost the same force as formal rules and regulations (95) since following them lessens liability, enhances recruitment and satisfaction of employees, and helps mitigate the harsh glare of media attention in case of nosocomial transmission of disease (i.e. in the health care setting). Second, a robust alliance between workers and employer is essential. Acknowledging and working toward shared goals, beginning with a healthy, productive workforce, is essential. A good foundation is needed for the structure requisite to lessen risk and adverse events, and to deal with them when they happen. Creating this structure involves crafting a beneficent philosophy and assembling a coalition to develop and approve guidelines for handling serious incidents such as needle sticks (68). A straightforward checklist of steps includes (84, 95):

- Identifying workers at risk
- Planning
- Educating—now and forever

- Providing necessary *equipment*, such as respirators; barrier *supplies*, such as gloves; and assuring *adequate staffing*
- Using appropriate precautions, including hand-washing and disposal methods
- Immunizing workers against work-related illness without charge to the workers
- Appropriately isolating patients
- Keeping records of training and of workers' health (for 30 years after exposure)
- Evaluating the program

Although this checklist seems clear, each item can be fraught with frustration. Differing priorities, cultures and languages; low morale secondary to uncertainty or layoffs; insufficient time, money, storage space, or computer experience and equipment can complicate the establishment of a sound program. Underestimates or denial of risk, fear of adverse reactions, or inconvenience can interfere even with *free* immunizations. Resistance, disagreements, and disputes can delay progress. Leadership (61) and conflict resolution skills (58) as well as profound knowledge of occupational health, public health, and individual and organizational behavior are necessary to move ahead. Progress would be more certain if schools for health professionals set the tone with inspired, leading-edge curricula on infection control, and requirements for immunizations of students (10).

REVIEW OF REGULATIONS

Information regarding infectious diseases designated as "reportable" must be sent to local health departments and eventually to the Centers for Disease Control and Prevention (CDC). The CDC collects weekly, monthly, and yearly statistics on many infectious disease and makes recommendations about disease control. Because of the recognized risk and the negative consequences to health care workers, some infectious diseases are now considered reportable to the Occupational Safety Health Administration (OSHA), as work-related conditions. For example, the bloodborne pathogen standard, 29CFR 1910.30, in effect since 1992, mainly encompassing hepatitis B and HIV, mandates that the hepatitis and HIV status of the source patient be discoverable in case of a health care worker's exposure. Some states require an authorization from the source patient before studies are done. In October, 1993, OSHA issued mandatory guidelines for protecting exposed workers against tuberculosis (24). All persons with positive TB skin tests (except pre-placement tests) and all employees with clinical TB are presumed to have employment-related conditions to be recorded on the OSHA 200 Log (24).

The purpose of the Occupational Safety and Health Act of 1970 is to "ensure safe and healthful working conditions for every working man and woman" (94, p. 1). The Act also protects workers who exercise their rights under the Act from being fired or discriminated against by their employer. OSHA, an agency of the Department of Labor, is responsible for promulgating and enforcing standards in most workplaces, whereas the primary role of the National Institute for Occupational Safety and Health in the Department of Health and Human Services is to support education and research in occupational health and recommend new standards for OSHA. NIOSH has no enforcement authority.

INFECTIONS SELECTED FOR DISCUSSION

We selected infectious agents for this review based on their frequency in patients, likelihood for health care worker exposure, seriousness of effects, and new information. We focus on hepatitis, HIV, influenza, measles, meningococcal disease, mumps, rubella, tuberculosis, and varicella. For a variety of reasons, herpes simplex, hantavirus, *Coxiella burnetii,* cytomegalovirus, diphtheria, tetanus, Legionellosis, rabies, and zoonoses have been excluded.

HEPATITIS

Hepatitis A and Other Fecal-Oral Infections

Hepatitis A (HAV) can be transmitted by the fecal-oral route to health care workers (81). Good hand-washing practices and glove use discourage transmission. A report of an outbreak of acute gastroenteritis in a geriatric convalescent facility highlighted the pervasiveness of the fecal-oral transmission. Since 25% of 57 affected employees had no routine stool or patient contact, the question of airborne or multiple viruses was raised, especially since both stool and vomitus have plentiful organisms and can be projectile (81). Face shields may therefore be advisable in some settings. Although most researchers have found similar prevalence of hepatitis A antibodies in health care workers and in the general public, Germanaud recently suggested that breaks in technique could account for the significantly higher prevalence of hepatitis A IgG antibodies among nursing staff over 30 years of age compared to hospital office workers and technicians (67), but job analysis, history of immunization, and length of service were not described, so firm conclusions are not possible. When postvaccination immunity lasting 5 to 10 years is established, inactivated hepatitis A vaccine will be a boon for health care workers who work in long-term care facilities and in areas where the disease is highly endemic (75). But eternal vigilance and precautions will remain necessary against other agents transmitted by the fecal-oral route.

Hepatitis B

Hepatitis B is a bloodborne pathogen that, via a variety of injections and inseminations, infects about 300,000 new people in the United States per year (62). Three injections of the yeast-based, genetically engineered vaccine now in use, available since 1986, prevents infection in about 90% of healthy young people. Boosters are customarily given to health care workers every five to seven years, or if testing after exposure shows an inadequate antibody titer. Attention to these details is important. One study recently showed that only 35% of employees who reported parenteral exposures had completed hepatitis B vaccination (82). Another reported that 23% of health care workers were unvaccinated altogether (113). The consequences of this lack of immunity and failed universal precautions are immense: 10,000 to 12,000 health care workers are infected with hepatitis B every year, and 200 to 300 die of it. The most recent report available, which does not reflect use of liver transplantation, cites fulminant liver necrosis, chronic liver disease (cirrhosis), and hepatocellular carcinoma as the primary causes of death (21).

Hepatitis B vaccine must be given to all health care workers, using every legal persuasion. If health care workers cannot or prefer not to have the vaccine, they should not be assigned to patient contact responsibilities. Protection against disease is important for careers as well as health purposes. For example, because of the low but measurable risk of health care workers transmitting hepatitis B *to* patients, applicants to medical school in the United Kingdom are now being rejected if they are HBeAg positive (79). This new recommendation is being protested and has no counterpart in the U.S. (28).

Hepatitis C

Some studies have found the risk of health care workers developing hepatitis or becoming hepatitis C antibody (HCVAb) positive after percutaneous exposure to HCVAb-positive patients is low, but worrisome (73). One study found the prevalence of HCVAb in hospital workers with patient care responsibilities to be 0.9%, compared to 1.7% in hospital office workers (66). On the higher side, another population study found that 0.7% of health care workers were HCVAb positive compared to 0.4% of local blood donors ($P = 0.10$) (113). Prospective evaluation found that 4 of 110 (4%) hospital workers with percutaneous injuries from HCVAb-positive patients developed hepatitis with alanine aminotransferase (ALT) levels over ten times the upper limit of normal; three of these four workers became HCVAb positive, and two had elevated ALT for at least one year (80). Even more striking is the report by Mistui et al, which showed seven of 68 (10%) medical personnel who had needle sticks from HCV RNA- and antibody-positive patients developed evidence of hepatitis and/or a positive HCV core antibody test; ALT levels ranged from two to 50 times normal; all seven became HCV RNA positive, and one had persistently abnormal liver function tests and positive antibody for two years (90). The relatively low, but real, risk of seroconversion may be secondary to a low circulating virus titer in patients. Strict precautions are reasonable because of the propensity of hepatitis C infection to become chronic and because of its link to hepatocellular cancer. Unlike hepatitis A and B, no good prophylaxis is available. Administering immunoglobulin immediately after exposure receives only an ambiguous endorsement by the Advisory Committee for Immunization Practices (27). HBIG has no place in prophylaxis. Safety, efficacy, and cost of after-exposure interferon need evaluation (109).

Hepatitis D

Hepatitis D (HDV) causes havoc in the form of chronic active hepatitis only in the presence of hepatitis B infection (32). It is most devastating when superinfection occurs in a HBV carrier, but fulminant hepatitis D can also occur with hepatitis B coinfection (32). Although the virus is uncommon, risk after exposure is high. HDV has by far the highest infectivity titer of any bloodborne hepatitis: 10^2 chimpanzee-infection units for human non A–non B hepatitis-positive sera; 10^8 for HBeAg-positive sera, and 10^{11} for hepatitis D virus-positive sera (80).

HUMAN IMMUNODEFICIENCY VIRUS

As the human immunodeficiency virus (HIV) epidemic relentlessly disperses beyond high-incidence urban areas (42), as heterosexual spread increases and women and young people are affected at an alarming rate (42, 46), and as health care is given more often in ambulatory, hospice, and home settings, work-related exposures of health care workers to HIV increase. Untamed by vaccine or behavior change, the prevalence of HIV infection is rising in the United States (about one in 250 persons) (42) and around the world. In 1991, the World Health Organization (WHO) estimated that 8 to 10 million adults worldwide were infected (31, 42); in mid-1994, it estimated that over 16 million adults were infected (WHO Global Programme on AIDS, July 1994). Coupled with the lack of certain means to prevent progression of infection to AIDS, this pattern leads to the inexorable conclusion that the health of health care workers is threatened by the imperative to care for an ever-growing number of patients with HIV-related illness. According to information available to the CDC, nearly 50 health care workers in the United States already have clear-cut documentation of HIV infection from work (42a). Almost 100 others are HIV Ab positive after work-related accidents and have no other known risk factors but did not have baseline HIV titers done, so the time of seroconversion cannot be established. More laboratory workers and nurses have occupational HIV than any other health care workers, but physicians, therapists, technicians, and environmental services workers have also been infected on the job. Most of the incidents involved punctures or cuts, but a few were mucocutaneous splashes or spills (42a). Creative new equipment may decrease the number of accidents secondary to manipulating intravenous lines. Injunctions against recapping used needles may also decrease needle sticks. Nevertheless, using and disposing of needles and other sharps can present a special problem in homes, for example. Complacency, born of denial or outdated information about prevalence and risk groups, may lull employers into providing inadequate supplies and equipment and may lull workers into inappropriate work habits. Time constraints and inexperienced house officers (and students) unfamiliar with the procedures and risks may lead to tragic injuries (74). Furthermore, it is not possible always to know if a sample (70) or a patient is infected with any bloodborne pathogen, including HIV (76, 77). A recent study involving urban and suburban emergency rooms of teaching hospitals found that the HIV status of 69% of HIV antibody-positive patients was not known to the staff (86). Another study from the emergency department of an urban university hospital showed that about 30% of patients who were bleeding or who had procedures done were positive for HBV, HCV, and/or HIV antibodies. Screening for HIV alone would have detected only 13% of HBsAg positive patients and 20% of HCV antibody-positive patients (78). These kinds of data reinforce worker health and safety dicta: *Think* and *be prepared* at all times because we will never know all of the hazards that a patient may present. As already noted, despite fears raised by the specter of occupational HIV infection, health care workers are far more likely to be infected with and die of hepatitis B. Compared to HIV, many more patients have occult hepatitis B viremia and are far more likely to be infectious (19, 64, 80, 87, 97, 105). It has been estimated, for example, that the annual cumulative risk for dentists to become infected at work is 50 times greater with HBV than with HIV, and they are 1.7 times more likely to die from HBV than from HIV (11).

One of the knottiest problems for a health care worker after exposure to HIV concerns prophylaxis. Unfortunately, despite hopes to the contrary, there is no encouragement that zidovudine (AZT) is effective in preventing occupational infection (29, 72, 103). Proof of efficacy is wanting because controlled studies have been impossible to complete and the risk of infection is low. Furthermore, despite immediate, intensive, and prolonged administration of zidovudine, health care workers have become infected with HIV after punctures from needles, lancets, and intravenous cannulas (115). At this time, most experienced programs continue to offer zidovudine after exposure, but not with enthusiasm. Workers who have injuries involving more than a needle prick and/or those who are particularly anxious tend to start the drug, but most do not complete a full course because of side effects, including "nausea, malaise, fatigue, and headache" (115, p. 915). Insomnia can also be a problem for professionals already short on sleep and hematocrits can drop substantially (115). In contrast, psychological prophylaxis is essential. In our experience, counseling for injured workers should be done as soon as possible and should be available during the entire medical surveillance period, since fear and anger may flare with each HIV antibody test. Material to cover includes estimates of risks, methods of safer sex, coping with guilt and fear, and discussions of safer work practices. Formal psychotherapy is rarely needed but should be undertaken without hesitation, if necessary, while protecting the worker's confidentiality within the workers' compensation system. Families may need to be involved.

The resurgence of tuberculosis has led to heightened concerns and recommendations about the interactions of HIV and tuberculosis (24, 45, 50). As HIV and tuberculosis spread on intersecting paths, and multiple drug-resistant tuberculosis (MDR) becomes more prevalent (7, 54), risks to health care workers increase (5, 57). Nearly 12,000 health care workers are HIV positive (8) for life-style reasons. They are at special risk for developing MDR tuberculosis, because of prolonged exposure to infectious patients and infection-control challenges (41). For the protection of these and other workers and patients, TB infection-control practices must be mandatory, vigorous, and rigorous. The efficacy of using respirators and environmental ultraviolet (UV) radiation to control tuberculosis spread remains to be established; studies of efficacy, costs and interference with patient care are urgently needed.

RUBELLA

Significant numbers of hospital personnel are susceptible to rubella; rates vary from 14% to 20% (96). Because a history of rubella alone does not indicate immunity, health care workers need to show serologic testing for rubella-specific antibodies (6, 107). Ten to 20 percent of young adults in the U.S. are at risk for contracting rubella (69). About 98% to 99% of susceptible persons will show antibody response following attenuated rubella vaccine (6).

Reporting of all cases of rubella to local health authorities is mandatory. Medical personnel should be excluded from work for seven days after onset of rash. The benefit of immunization with immunoglobulin has not been proved.

Health departments in the U.S. reported an all-time low of 225 cases of rubella in 1988, but there were 1093 cases reported to the National Notifiable Disease Surveillance System (NNDSS) for 1990 (33), plus 10 confirmed cases of congenital rubella syndrome reported to CDC's National Congenital Rubella Syndrome Registry (33). Of the 26 rubella outbreaks in 1990, some occurred in the workplace (33). The goal of rubella vaccination is to prevent intrauterine rubella infection that can result in miscarriage, stillbirth, or congenital rubella syndrome. The sudden increase in the congenital rubella syndrome (CRS) emphasizes the need for proof of immunity of susceptible health care workers. The immunity provided by the vaccine may persist for a long time.

MUMPS

Transmission of mumps from patient to health care workers has occurred (39). In Tennessee between 1986 to 1987, six health care workers in three different hospitals contracted mumps after nosocomial exposure (119). Most adults, however, particularly those born before 1957, may be considered to be immune. Preventive vaccination is administered as a live attenuated vaccine as single vaccine or in combination with rubella and measles live virus vaccine (MMR), and provides long-lasting immunity in 95% of persons vaccinated. Vaccine is contraindicated if a person is immunosuppressed or pregnant (6). Relative contraindications include sensitivity to egg or neomycin.

Reporting to local health authority is selective (6). Susceptible medical personnel should be excluded from the workplace from the 12th through the 25th day of exposure.

MEASLES

Measles can be a serious public health and work place problem. More than 18,000 cases were reported in 1989, whereas there were only 1497 cases in 1983 (25, 33). The cost of controlling a single outbreak ranges from $26,000 to more than $100,000 (33). Between 1985 and 1989, 3.5% of all reported cases of measles were acquired in a medical setting, including 28 cases in health care workers (2). A group of four health care workers who contracted measles represented secondary measles vaccine failure. Three of the health care workers had proof of having received one live measles vaccine, and one had received a second dose; furthermore, their pre-illness sera had shown immunity to measles (1).

The Centers for Disease Control and Prevention recommend verification of two live measles vaccinations, documentation of physician-diagnosed measles, or laboratory evidence of measles immunity to prove health care worker immunity to measles (22). Persons born in or after 1957 who have no documentation of vaccination or other evidence of measles immunity should be vaccinated. Contraindications to the use of live vaccine include pregnancy and suppressed immune responses. HIV-infected individuals and AIDS patients may develop severe complications from measles and therefore should be vaccinated. It should not be given to people with known allergies to eggs, and it should be given 14 days before blood transfusion or immunoglobulin or deferred. Recommendations for the immunization of health care personnel are summarized in Table 1 and work restrictions in Table 2.

Table 1 Vaccines used in adults

Vaccine	Type	Schedule	Indications	Precautions and contraindications	Side effects
Attenuated, live-bacteria vaccine					
Bacille Calmette-Géurin	—	Primary: 1 dose i.d. or s.c.	Debatable benefits for selected adult groups	Immunocompromised host	Local progression; disseminated infection
Attenuated, live-virus vaccines					
Measles	—	Primary: 2 doses s.c.	For adults born after 1956 without measles (diagnosed by a physician or immunologic test) or live virus immunization; for revaccination of persons given killed measles vaccine, 1963 to 1967	Pregnancy; immunocompromised host; history of anaphylaxis to eggs or neomycin	Temperature of $\geq 39.4°C$, 5 to 21 days after vaccination in 5 to 15%; transient rash in 5%; local reaction in 4 to 55% of persons previously immunized with killed vaccine 1963 to 1967
Mumps	—	Primary: 1 dose s.c.	For susceptible adults	Pregnancy; immunocompromised host; history of anaphylaxis to eggs or neomycin	Mild allergic reactions uncommon; rare parotitis
Rubella	—	Primary: 1 dose s.c.	For adults, particularly women of childbearing age, without documented illness or live vaccine on or after first birthday	Pregnancy; immunocompromised host; history of anaphylaxis in response to neomycin	Joint pains, transient arthralgias in up to 40%, beginning 3 to 5 days after vaccination, persisting 1 to 11 days; frank arthritis in <2%

Inactivated-virus vaccines

Hepatitis B	Recombinant hepatitis B surface antigen	Primary dose: 2 doses (10 g/dose) i.m. in deltoid, 1 month apart; third dose 5 months after second	For health workers in contact with blood; persons residing 6 months in areas of high endemicity of hepatitis B surface antigen; others at risk	Safety to fetus unknown; pregnancy not a contraindication in high-risk persons	Mild local reaction in 10 to 20%; occasional systemic symptoms of fever, headache, fatigue, and nausea
Influenza	Inactivated whole and split	Annual vaccination with current vaccine	For adults with high-risk conditions; healthy persons more than 65 years old; medical care personnel	First trimester of pregnancy a relative contraindication; anaphylaxis in response to eggs	Mild local reaction in less than one third; occasional systemic reaction of malaise, myalgia, beginning 6 to 12 h after vaccination and lasting 1 to 2 days; rare allergic reaction

Data are from the Centers for Disease Control and Prevention and the American College of Physicians Task Force on Adult Immunization

Table 2   Work restrictions for hospital personnel exposed to or infected with certain vaccine-preventable diseases

Disease	Relieve from direct patient contact	Duration
Mumps		
Active	Yes	Until 9 days after onset of parotitis
Postexposure*	Yes	From day 12 through 26 after exposure, or until 9 days after onset of parotitis
Measles		
Active	Yes	Until 7 days after rash appears
Postexposure*	Yes	From day 5 through 21 after exposure and/or 7 days after rash appears
Rubella		
Active	Yes	Until 5 days after rash appears
Postexposure*	Yes	From day 7 through 21 after exposure and/or 5 days after rash appears

*Susceptible personnel
Modified from Williams WW. Preblud SR, Reichelderfer PS, Hadler SC. *Infect. Dis. Clin. North Am.* 3:701–21 (with permission).

Most states require case reporting and cases should be reported to the local health authority (6). In hospitals, respiratory isolation during the most infectious period reduces the exposure to susceptible patients and health care workers (6). Protection after contact may be achieved by live vaccine, which must be given within 72 hours of exposure. Passive immunization with immunoglobulin (IG) can be used for susceptible contacts when measles vaccine is contraindicated or to avoid risk of complications. When given, it must be used within six days of exposure (6).

INFLUENZA

Unfortunately, health care workers generally do not comply with the recommendations from the US Public Health Services for "physician, nurse, and other personnel in both hospital and out patient care settings who have contact with high risk persons among all age groups including infants" to receive annual influenza vaccination (34). Among the reasons for poor compliance in health care and the general public are doubts about the efficacy and safety of vaccine and inadequate reimbursement (52). In addition, there seems to be more emphasis even from the US Public Health Service to immunize high-risk patients rather than health care workers. Stress on vaccination of health care workers appears to be more to protect patients than the health care workers themselves. For health care workers to comply to the recommendations, educational efforts about the benefits of the vaccine should be emphasized, and access to vaccination should be easy.

The use of inactivated influenza virus vaccine, which may protect up to 80% of the population, depending on the strain, is considered to be safe. Worldwide surveillance and current antigenic characterization of strains provide the basis for selecting the two strains of influenza A and one strain of influenza B in each year's vaccine. Chemoprophylaxis is not a substitute for vaccination (34), but unvaccinated health care workers may be protected by administering amantadine hydrochloride, which is effective in the chemoprophylaxis of influenza A but not B (6, 56). Central nervous system side effects occur in 5% to 10% of those who receive amantadine. The side effects are more severe in older persons and in those with chronic renal disease.

VARICELLA-HERPES ZOSTER

Varicella is transmitted mainly via airborne spread or direct contact. When varicella is prevalent, only personnel with known immunity should be assigned to varicella patients to avoid transmission. The incubation period is usually from two to three weeks. Communicability occurs one to two days before the onset of rash and up to five days afterwards. Infectiousness occurs for 10 to 20 days after exposure. Varicella zoster immunoglobulin (VZIG), if given within 96 hours of exposure, may prevent or modify disease in susceptible close contacts of cases.

Herpes zoster (shingles) is the skin manifestation of reactivated varicella virus. Susceptible contacts will develop varicella. Because the immune status of health care workers is reported to vary from 50% to 97% (88), varicella zoster virus is an infectious risk for hospital health care workers, especially pregnant workers. Varicella infection during pregnancy may be associated with complications as well as risk, albeit low, of congenital varicella syndrome (88). Employees who are seronegative are considered infectious from 10 to 21 days after exposure, and need to be removed from work if they have no proof of immunity. Many states do not require that the disease be reported to the local authorities (6).

MENINGOCOCCAL DISEASE

Although the transmission of *Neisseria meningitidis* to health care workers is rare, it has occurred following mouth-to-mouth resuscitation (117). Meningococcal pneumonia is also dangerous to health care workers, especially if the patient has a productive cough (106).

Use of proper precautions is important, and in health care personnel who have had significant unprotected exposure, prophylaxis is indicated (117).

SCABIES

Scabies is a pruritic disease of the skin caused by a mite, *Sarcoptes scabiei*. It is transmitted primarily by skin-to-skin contact and, less commonly, by infected fomites (3). It presents as papules, vesicles, or tiny linear burrows, and causes intense itching at night. In immunosuppressed patients, it presents as generalized dermatitis and is highly infectious (3). It is also known as Norwegian scabies, disseminated scabies, crusted scabies, or hyperkeratotic scabies. An outbreak has been described (3) that involved six nursing staff and one medical resident who developed scabies after being exposed to a patient whose scabies was not initially recognized because of its unusual presentation. Another similar hospital outbreak occurred from a patient with AIDS involving eleven nurses, two radiology technicians, and one resident (108). Isolation precautions should be instituted until 24 hours after the start of effective treatment. Official reporting to local health authorities is not required (6).

TUBERCULOSIS

After a steady decline from 84,000 cases reported to CDC in 1953 to 22,000 in 1984, there were 39,000 cases of tuberculosis above the expected downward trend from 1985 through 1991 (37). Contributory factors to the increase in tuberculosis include immigration of persons from TB-prevalent countries, drug abuse, overcrowding and homelessness (60, 114). An even more important factor is the HIV epidemic, since HIV-infected individuals are more likely to develop active disease (114). HIV-infected patients often present with normal chest X-rays and are more likely to develop extra-pulmonary disease (37).

Tuberculosis is spread by airborne transmission. Primary infection is usually acquired through inhaled droplet nuclei containing the acid fast bacilli (AFB) during "coughing, singing, or sneezing," (6, p. 459), as well as during prolonged exposure to an infected case. Anyone inhaling the bacteria may become infected. The infection can remain latent in persons with a healthy immune system, and causes disease when the immune system declines (37, 114). A positive TB skin test may be the only evidence of infection.

Communicability of the disease depends on the number and viability of bacilli in the air and their virulence, as well as the adequacy of ventilation (6, 24). Communicability is rapidly decreased with effective antimicrobial chemotherapy. HIV infection and immunosuppression increase the risk of developing the disease (6). Methods of control are mainly preventive measures and are summarized in Table 3 (24, 30).

Table 3 Summary of recommendations for preventing the transmission of tuberculosis in health-care settings*

1. Early identification and treatment of persons with active tuberculosis (TB)
   - Maintain a high index of suspicion for TB to identify cases rapidly.
   - Promptly initiate effective multidrug anti-TB therapy based on clinical and drug-resistance surveillance data.
2. Prevention of spread of infectious droplet nuclei by source control methods and by reduction of microbial contamination of indoor air
   - Initiate acid-fast bacilli (AFB) isolation precautions immediately for all patients who are suspected or confirmed to have active TB and who may be infectious. AFB isolation precautions include use of a private room with negative pressure in relation to surrounding areas and a minimum of six air exchanges per hour. Air from the room should be exhausted directly to the outside. Use of ultraviolet lamps and/or high-efficiency particulate air filters to supplement ventilation may be considered.
   - Persons entering the AFB isolation room should use disposable particulate respirators that fit snugly around the face.
   - Continue AFB isolation precautions until there is clinical evidence of reduced infectiousness (i.e., cough has substantially decreased, and the number of organisms on sequential sputum smears is decreasing). If drug resistance is suspected or confirmed, continue AFB precautions until the sputum smear is negative for AFB.
   - Use special precautions during cough-inducing procedures.
3. Surveillance for TB transmission
   - Maintain surveillance for TB infection among health-care workers (HCWs) by routine, periodic tuberculin skin testing. Recommend appropriate preventive therapy for HCWs when indicated.
   - Maintain surveillance for TB cases among patients and HCWs.
   - Promptly initiate contact investigation procedures among HCWs, patients, and visitors exposed to an untreated, or ineffectively treated, infectious TB patient for whom appropriate AFB procedures are not in place. Recommend appropriate therapy or preventive therapy for contacts with disease or TB infection without current disease. Therapeutic regimens should be chosen based on the clinical history and local drug-resistance surveillance data.

*Reproduced from *Morbid. Mortal. Wkly. Rep.* Aug. 30, 1991, p. 586

Patients with active pulmonary tuberculosis and with sputum positive for pulmonary tuberculosis need to be placed in a private room with air pressure negative to adjacent areas. Hand washing and universal precautions should always be observed. Routine PPDs are administered to health care personnel at risk every 6 to 12 months. In addition, if unprotected exposure to a potentially infectious patient occurs, the CDC recommends, "Unless a negative skin test has been documented within the preceding 3 months, each exposed health care facility worker (except those already known to be positive reactors) should receive a Mantoux tuberculin test as soon as possible after exposure and should be managed in the same way as other contacts. If the initial skin test is negative, the test should be repeated 12 weeks after the exposure ended. Exposed persons with skin test reaction more than 5 millimeters or with symptoms suggestive of tuberculosis should receive chest radiographs. Persons with previously known positive skin test reactions who have been exposed to an infectious patient do not require repeat skin test or chest radiograph unless they have symptoms suggestive of tuberculosis" (24, pp. 18–19).

In addition to the upsurge of tuberculosis cases, there also has been an increase in drug-resistant tuberculosis (30). In the past, drug resistance was the result of intermittent compliance or noncompliance, but now drug resistance can be the result of primary infection with a multiply drug-resistant strain. In a recent survey carried out in New York City, 33% of cases had organisms resistant to at least one drug and 19% had organisms resistant to two (37). Drug resistance is not limited to New York City; it occurs nationwide. From 1982 to 1986, only .5% of new cases were resistant to both isoniazid and rifampin. By 1991, this resistance had increased to 3.1% (37). In addition, there have been outbreaks of multi-drug-resistant TB (mDRTB) in institutional settings (30a, 37, 101). Seven outbreaks were investigated in Florida and New York City. Although nosocomial transmission of *Mycobacterium tuberculosis* to health care workers has been recognized, the outbreak in a large Florida hospital was the first documentation of transmission of drug-resistant tuberculosis in a hospital setting (30a). Eight health care workers had tuberculin skin test conversion from January through April 1990 (30a). There has been further documentation of work-related MDR TB in at least nine health care workers and prison guards. Of nine affected, five have died (37, 55, 101). In these outbreaks, more than 200 multiple drug-resistant cases occurred. Most were resistant to isoniazid and rifampin, and some were resistant to seven anti-tuberculosis drugs. Most patients were also infected with HIV. Mortality was high, ranging from 72% to 89%; the median time from diagnosis to death ranged from 4 to 16 weeks (37). Despite tripling the length of the course of treatment, effectiveness has declined from 100% to 70% in immunocompetent hosts (114). These outbreaks are thought to be caused mainly by delay in diagnosis of TB in HIV-infected patients because of unusual clinical and radiographic appearance, as well as by delayed recognition of drug resistance attributable to the lengthy time required for laboratory identification, confirmation, and reporting. As a result, AFB isolation procedures were sometimes delayed (5, 30). Control measures that were carried out were believed to have decreased the number of MDR TB cases substantially. Recommendations for preventing the transmission of tuberculosis in health care settings are summarized in Table 3. In addition to the CDC guidelines for preventing the transmission of tuberculosis in health care settings (24), in October, 1993, the Occupational Safety and Health Administration issued an enforcement policy and procedures for occupational exposure to tuberculosis which are based upon the CDC 1990 guidelines (51). OSHA has the authority under the General Duty Clause of the OSHA Act of 1970 to enforce compliance with existing industrial standards such as CDC guidelines, even if a final standard has not been established.

BCG Vaccine

Although the BCG vaccine has been in use since 1921, its efficacy, duration of protective immunity, and the effect of age of vaccination are still debated. A meta-analysis based on data from 14 prospective trials and 12 case control studies concluded that BCG vaccination significantly reduces the risk of active TB cases and death with an overall protective effect of 50% (48). Vaccination with BCG is still controversial, but may be considered where there is unprotected and prolonged exposure to patients who are sputum positive for TB (48).

SUMMARY

Infectious risks for health care workers continue. As the population ages, and as HIV and TB spread and amplify each other, health care workers will come into contact with sicker patients in unusual settings. Challenges mount as more and more persons become "health care workers"; the definition should include students, volunteers, and family members. Care of patients is no longer centered in hospitals, where safe equipment may easy to find and dispose of. Although hepatitis B, influenza, measles, mumps, and rubella vaccines usually prevent infection, a substantial number of health care workers remain unvaccinated. HIV transmission at work can only be prevented by behavior change and safer equipment; no prevention or cure is available or in sight. Scabies is far from life-threatening but can spread like wildfire, especially in immunosuppressed individuals, and has become resistant to lindane. Health care itself is undergoing revolutionary changes, and health professionals may be distracted, discouraged, exhausted, and undertrained. Human factors in preventing occupational infection are little understood. Data are lacking in crucial areas: use of zidovudine to prevent HIV infection; use of specific types of masks and respirators, plus UV light, to decrease the spread of tuberculosis. Schools where health professionals train, public health officials, researchers, and practitioners themselves will need to lead the way to a healthier future for health care workers.

Literature Cited

1. Ammari LK, Bell LM, Hodinka RL. 1993. Secondary measles vaccine failure in health care workers exposed to infected patients. *Infect. Control Hosp. Epidemiol.* 14:81
2. Atkinson WL, Markowitz LE, Adams NC, Seastrom GR. 1991. Transmission of measles in medical settings—United States, 1985–1989. *Am. J. Med.* 91 (Suppl. 3B):S320–24
3. Bannatyne RM, Patterson T, Wells B, MacMillan SA, Cunningham GA, Tellier R. 1992. Hospital outbreak traced to a case of Norwegian scabies. *Can. J. Infect. Control* 7:111–13
4. Bassett DCJ, Ho AKC, Cheng AFB.

1993. Susceptibility of hospital staff to varicella zoster virus infection in Hong Kong. *J. Hosp. Infect.* 223:161–62

5. Beck-Sagué C, Dooley SW, Hutton MD, Otten J, Breeden A, et al. 1992. Hospital outbreak of multidrug-resistant mycobacterium tuberculosis: factors in transmission to staff and HIV-infected patients. *J. Am. Med. Assoc.* 268:1280–86

6. Benenson AS, ed. 1990. *Control of Communicable Diseases in Man.* Washington, DC: Am. Public Health Assoc. 15th ed.

7. Bloch AB, Cauthen GM, Onorato IM, Dansbury KG, Kelly GD, et al. 1994. Nationwide survey of drug-resistant tuberculosis in the United States. *J. Am. Med. Assoc.* 271:665–71

8. Bur. Census. 1993. *Statistical Abstract of the United States*, p. 117. 113th ed.

9. See Ref. 8, p. 408

10. Calif. Dep. Health Serv. 1993. *Guidelines for Preventing the Transmission of Blood-borne Pathogens in Health Care Settings*, pp. 1–6

11. Capilouto EI, Weinstein MC, Hemenway D, Cotton D. 1992. What is the dentist's occupational risk of becoming infected with hepatitis B or the human immunodeficiency virus? *Am. J. Public Health.* 82:587–589

12. Cent. Dis. Control Prev. 1982. Acquired immune deficiency syndrome (AIDS): precautions for clinical and laboratory staffs. *Morbid. Mortal. Wkly. Rep.* 31:577–80

13. Cent. Dis. Control Prev. 1983. Acquired immunodeficiency syndrome (AIDS): precautions for health care workers and allied professionals. *Morbid. Mortal. Wkly. Rep.* 32:450–51

14. Cent. Dis. Control Prev. 1985. Recommendations for preventing transmission of infection with human T-lymphotropic virus type III/lymphadenopathy-associated virus in the workplace. *Morbid. Mortal. Wkly. Rep.* 34:681–86, 691–95

15. Cent. Dis. Control Prev. 1986. Apparent transmission of human T-lymphotropic virus type III/lymphadenopathy-associated virus from a child to a mother providing health care. *Morbid. Mortal. Wkly. Rep.* 35:76–79

16. Cent. Dis. Control Prev. 1986. Recommendations for preventing transmission of infection with human T-lymphocyte virus type III/lymphadenopathy-associated virus during invasive procedures. *Morbid. Mortal. Wkly. Rep.* 35:221–23

17. Cent. Dis. Control Prev. 1987. Recommendations for prevention of HIV transmission in health-care settings. *Morbid. Mortal. Wkly. Rep.* 36(Suppl. 2S):S3–18

18. Cent. Dis. Control Prev. 1987. Update: human immunodeficiency virus infection in health-care workers exposed to blood of infected patients. *Morbid. Mortal. Wkly. Rep.* 36:285–89

19. Cent. Dis. Control Prev. 1988. Update: acquired immunodeficiency syndrome and human immunodeficiency virus infection among health-careworkers. *Morbid. Mortal. Wkly. Rep.* 37:229–39

20. Cent. Dis. Control Prev. 1988. Update: universal precautions for prevention of the transmission of human immunodeficiency, hepatitis B virus, and other blood-borne pathogens in health-care settings. *Morbid. Mortal. Wkly. Rep.* 37:377–82, 387–88

21. Cent. Dis. Control Prev. 1989. Guidelines for prevention of transmission of human immunodeficiency virus and hepatitis B virus to health-care and public-safety workers. *Morbid. Mortal. Wkly. Rep.* 38(S-6):1–36

22. Cent. Dis. Control Prev. 1989. Measles prevention recommendations of the Immunization Practice Advisory Committee (ACIP). *Morbid. Mortal. Wkly. Rep.* 38(S-9):1–18

23. Cent. Dis. Control Prev. 1989. Summary of notifiable diseases, United States, 1989. *Morbid. Mortal. Wkly. Rep.* 38:1–59

24. Cent. Dis. Control Prev. 1990. Guidelines for preventing the transmission of tuberculosis in health-care settings, with special focus on HIV-related issues. *Morbid. Mortal. Wkly. Rep.* 39(RR-17):1–29

25. Cent. Dis. Control Prev. 1990. Measles, Washington 1990. *Morbid. Mortal. Wkly. Rep.* 39:473–76

26. Cent. Dis. Control Prev. 1990. Nosocomial transmission of multi-drug resistant tuberculosis to health care workers and HIV infected patients in an urban hospital—Florida. *Morbid. Mortal. Wkly. Rep.* 39:718–22

27. Cent. Dis. Control Prev. 1990. Protection against viral hepatitis: non-A, non-B hepatitis. *Morbid. Mortal. Wkly. Rep.* 39(RR-2):23–29

28. Cent. Dis. Control Prev. 1990. Protection against viral hepatitis: recommendations of the Immunization Practices Advisory Committee (ACIP). *Morbid. Mortal. Wkly. Rep.* 39(RR-2):1–26

29. Cent. Dis. Control Prev. 1990. Public health service statement on management of occupational exposure to human immunodeficiency virus, including considerations regarding zidovudine exposure

use. *Morbid. Mortal. Wkly. Rep.* 39(RR-1):1–14
30. Cent. Dis. Control Prev. 1991. Nosocomial transmission of multi-drug tuberculosis resistant among HIV infected persons—Florida and New York, 1988–1991. *Morbid. Mortal. Wkly. Rep.* 40: 585–91
30a. Cent. Dis. Control Prev. 1991. Nosocomial transmission of multi-drug resistant tuberculosis to health care workers and HIV infected patients in an urban hospital—Florida. *Morbid. Mortal. Wkly. Rep.* 39:718–22
31. Cent. Dis. Control Prev. 1991. The HIV/AIDS epidemic: the first 10 years. *Morbid. Mortal. Wkly. Rep.* 40:357–63, 369
32. Cent. Dis. Control Prev. 1991. Hepatitis B virus: a comprehensive strategy for eliminating transmission in the United States through universal childhood vaccination: recommendations of the Immunization Practices Advisory Committee (ACIP). *Morbid. Mortal. Wkly. Rep.* 40(RR-13):1–25
33. Cent. Dis. Control Prev. 1991. Increase in rubella and congenital rubella syndrome, United States 1988–1990. *Morbid. Mortal. Wkly. Rep.* 40:93–99
34. Cent. Dis. Control Prev. 1991. Prevention and control of influenza: recommendation of Immunization Practices Advisory Committee (ACIP). *Morbid. Mortal. Wkly. Rep.* 40(RR-6):1–15
35. Cent. Dis. Control Prev. 1991. Recommendations for preventing transmission of human immunodeficiency virus and hepatitis B virus to patients during exposure-prone invasive procedures. *Morbid. Mortal. Wkly. Rep.* 40(RR 8):1–9
36. Deleted in proof
37. Cent. Dis. Control Prev. 1992. National action plan to combat multiple drug-resistant tuberculosis; meeting the challenge of multi-drug resistant tuberculosis; summary of conference; management of persons exposed to multidrug tuberculosis. *Morbid. Mortal. Wkly. Rep.* 41:5, 51, 261
38. Cent. Dis. Control Prev. 1992. Prevention and control of tuberculosis in U.S. communities with at risk minority populations. *Morbid. Mortal. Wkly. Rep.* 41(RR-5):1–11
39. Cent. Dis. Control Prev. 1992. Tuberculosis mortality, United States 1992. *Morbid. Mortal. Wkly. Rep.* 42:696–97, 703–4
40. Cent. Dis. Control Prev. 1993. *AIDS information: reported Cases of AIDS and HIV infection in health care workers.* Doc. 320230:1
41. Cent. Dis. Control Prev. 1993. National

action plan regarding multiple-drug resistant TB. *Morbid. Mortal. Wkly. Rep.* 41:1–45
42. Cent. Dis. Control Prev. 1993. *AIDS information: statistical projections/trends.* Doc. 320210:1
42a. Cent. Dis. Control Prev. 1993. *AIDS information: reported cases of AIDS and HIV infection in health care workers.* Doc. 320230:1
43. Cent. Dis. Control Prev. 1993. Prevention and control of influenza: part I, vaccines. Recommendations of the Advisory Committee on Immunization Practices (ACIP). *Morbid. Mortal. Wkly. Rep.* 42(RR-6):1–14
44. Cent. Dis. Control Prev. 1993. HIV transmission between two adolescent brothers with hemophilia. *Morbid. Mortal. Wkly. Rep.* 42:948–51
45. Cent. Dis. Control Prev. 1994. Expanded tuberculosis surveillance and tuberculosis morbidity—United States, 1993. *Morbid. Mortal. Wkly. Rep.* 43:361–66
46. Cent. Dis. Control Prev. 1994. Heterosexually acquired AIDS—United States, 1993. *Morbid. Mortal. Wkly. Rep.* 43: 155–60
47. Cent. Dis. Control Prev. 1994. Human immunodeficiency virus transmission in household settings—United States. *Morbid. Mortal. Wkly. Rep.* 43:347–56
48. Colditz GA, Brewer TF, Berkey CS, Wilson ME, Burdick E, Fineberg HV. 1994. Efficacy of BCG vaccine in the prevention of tuberculosis. Meta analysis of the published literature. *J. Am. Med. Assoc.* 271:698–702
49. Conn. Dep. Health Serv. 1992. Recommendations: HIV\BV infected health care workers. *Conn. Med.* 56:213–16
50. Curtis JR, Hooton TM, Nolan CM. 1994. New developments in tuberculosis and HIV infection: an opportunity for prevention. *J. Gen. Int. Med.* 9:286–94
51. Decker MD. 1993. OSHA enforcement for occupational exposure to tuberculosis. *Infect. Control. Hosp. Epidemiol.* 14:689–93
52. DiPerri G, Cadeo GP, Castelli F, Micciolo R, Bassetti S, Rubini F. 1993. Transmission of HIV associated tuberculosis to health care workers. *Infect. Control Hosp. Epidemiol.* 14:67–72
53. Doebbeling BN, Wenzel RP. 1990. The direct costs of universal precautions in a teaching hospital. *J. Am. Med. Assoc.* 264:2083–87
54. Dooley SW, Jarvis WR, Martone WJ, Snyder DE. 1992. Multidrug-resistent tuberculosis. *Ann. Intern. Med.* 117: 257–58
55. Dooley SW, Villarino ME, Lawrence

M, Salinas L, Amil S, et al. 1992. Nosocomial transmission of tuberculosis in
a hospital unit for HIV infected patients.
J. Am. Med. Assoc. 267:2632–34

56. Douglas RG. 1988. Influenza. In *Cecil
Textbook of Medicine*, Chapter 333, pp.
1762–67. Philadelphia: WB Saunders

57. Fischel MA, Uttamchandani RB, Daikos
GE, Poblete RB, Moreno JN, et al. 1992.
An outbreak of tuberculosis caused by
multiple-drug-resistant tubercle bacilli
among patients with HIV infection. *Ann.
Intern. Med.* 117:177–83

58. Fisher R, Ury W, Patton B. 1991. *Get-
ting to Yes: Negotiating Agreement
Without Giving In.* New York: Penguin
Books. 200 pp. 2nd ed.

59. Fitzgibbon JE, Gaurs S, Frenkel LD,
Laraque F, Edlin BR, Dubin DT. 1993.
Transmission from one child to another
of human immunodeficiency virus type
1 with a zidovudine-resistance mutation.
N. Engl. J. Med. 329:1835–41

60. Frieden TR, Sterling MD, Pablos-Mendez A, Kilburn JO, Cauthen GM, Dooley
SW. 1993. The emergence of drug re-
sistent tuberculosis in New York City.
N. Engl. J. Med. 328:521–26

61. Gardner JW. 1990. *On Leadership.* New
York: Free Press. 220 pp.

62. Gardner P, Schaffner W. 1993. Immunization of adults. *N. Engl. J. Med.*
328:1252–58

63. Gellert GA, Waterman SH, Ewert D,
Ohiro L, Giles MP, et al. 1990. An
outbreak of acute gastroenteritis caused
by a small round structured virus in a
geriatric convalescent facility. *Infect.
Control Hosp. Epidemiol.* 11:459–64

64. Gerberding JL, Bryant-LeBlanc CE,
Nelson K, Moss AR, Osmond D, et al.
1987. Risk of transmitting the human
immunodeficiency virus, cytomegalovirus, and hepatitis B virus to health careworkers exposed to patients with AIDS
and AIDS-related conditions. *J. Infect.
Dis.* 156:1–8

65. Gerberding JL, Littell C, Tarkington A,
Brown A, Schecter WP. 1990. Risk of
exposure of surgical personnel to
patients' blood during surgery at San
Francisco General Hospital. *N. Engl. J.
Med.* 322:1788–93

66. Germanaud J. 1994. Hepatitis A and
health care personnel. *Arch. Intern. Med.*
154:820–22

67. Germanaud J, Barthez J-P, Causse X.
1994. The occupational risk of hepatitis
C infection among hospital employees.
Am. J. Public Health 84:122

68. Go GW, Baraff LJ, Schriger DL.
1991. Management guidelines for
health care workers exposed to blood

and body fluids. *Ann. Emerg. Med.*
20:1341–50

69. Greaves WL, Orenstein WA, Steter HC,
Preblud SR, Hinman AR, Bart KJ. 1982.
Prevention of rubella transmission in
medical facilities. *J. Am. Med. Assoc.*
248:861–64

70. Handsfield HH, Cummings MJ, Swensen PD. 1987. Prevalence of antibody
to human immunodeficiency virus and
hepatitis B surface antigen in blood samples submitted to a hospital laboratory:
implications for handling specimens. *J.
Am. Med. Assoc.* 258:3395–97

71. Heald AE, Ransohoff DF. 1990.
Needlestick injuries among resident
physicians. *J. Gen. Intern. Med.* 5:389–
93

72. Henderson DK, Gerberding JL. 1989.
Prophylactic zidovudine after occupational exposure to human immunodeficiency virus: an interim analysis. *J. Infect.
Dis.* 160:321–27

73. Hernandez ME, Bruguera M, Puyuelo
T, Barrera JM, Tapias JMS, Rodés J.
1992. Risk of needlestick injuries in the
transmission of hepatitis C virus in hospital personnel. *J. Hepatol.* 16:56–58

74. Hoffman-Terry M, Rhodes LV, Reed
JF. 1992. Impact of human immunodeficiency virus on medical and surgical
residence. *Arch. Intern. Med.* 152:1788–
96

75. Innis BL, Snitbhan R, Kunasol P, Lao-
rakpongse T, Poopatanakool W, et al.
1994. Protection against hepatitis A by
an inactivated vaccine. *J. Am. Med.
Assoc.* 271:1328–34

76. Kelen GD, DiGiovanna T, Bisson L,
Kalainov D, Sivertson KT, Quinn TC.
1989. Human immunodeficiency virus
infection in emergency department patients: epidemiology, clinical presentations, and risk to health care workers:
The Johns Hopkins experience. *J. Am.
Med. Assoc.* 262:516–22

77. Kelen GD, Fritz S, Qaqish B,
Brookmeyer R, Baker JL, et al. 1988.
Unrecognized human immunodeficiency virus infection in emergency department patients. *N. Engl. J. Med.* 318:
1645–50

78. Kelen GD, Green GB, Purcell RH, Chan
DW, Qaqish BF, Siverton KT, et al.
1992. Hepatitis B and hepatitis C in
emergency department patients. *N. Engl.
J. Med.* 326:1399–404

79. Kingman S. 1994. Hepatitis B status
must be known for medical school. *Br.
Med. J.* 308:876

80. Kiyosawa K, Sodeyama T, Tanaka E,
Nakano Y, Furuta S, et al. 1991. Hepatitis C in hospital employees with nee-

dle stick injuries. *Ann. Intern. Med.* 115: 367–69

81. Lettau LA. 1992. The A, B, C, D, and E of viral hepatitis: spelling out the risks for health careworkers. *Inf. Control Hosp. Epidemiol.* 13:77–81

82. Longbottom HM, Cox K, Sokas RK. 1993. Body fluid exposure in an urban tertiary care medical center. *Am. J. Indus. Med.* 23:703–10

83. Lynch P, Cummings MJ, Roberts PL, Herriott MJ, Yates B, Stamm WE. 1990. Implementing and evaluating a system of generic infection precautions: body substance isolation. *Am. J. Infect. Control* 18:1–12

84. Lynch P, Jackson MM, Cummings MJ, Stamm WE. 1987. Rethinking the role of isolation practices in the prevention of nosocomial infections. *Ann. Intern. Med.* 107:243–46

85. Mangione CM, Gerberding JL, Cummings SR. 1991. Occupational exposure to HIV: frequency and rates of underreporting of percutaneous and mucocutaneous exposures by medical housestaff. *Am. J. Med.* 90:85–90

86. Marcus R. 1988. Surveillance of health care workers exposed to blood from patients infected with the human immunodeficiency virus. *N. Engl. J. Med.* 319:1118–23

87. Marcus R, Culver DH, Bell DM, Srivastava PU, Mendelson MH, et al. 1993. Risk of human immunodeficiency virus infection among emergency department workers. *Am. J. Med.* 94:363–70

88. McKinney WP, Horowitz MM, Battiola RJ. 1989. Susceptibility of hospital based health care personnelto varicella-zoster virus infections. *Am. J. Infect. Control.* 17:26–30

89. Meyer GS. 1993. Occupational infection in health care: the century-old lessons from syphilis. *Arch. Intern. Med.* 153: 2439–47

90. Mitsui T, Iwano K, Masuko K, Yamazaki C, Okamoto H, et al. 1992. Hepatitis C infection in medical personnel after needle stick accident. *Hepatology* 16:1109–14

91. Murray BE. 1994. Can antibiotic resistance be controlled? *N. Engl. J. Med.* 330:1229–30

92. Murray DL. 1990. Vaccine preventable diseases and medical personnel. *Arch. Intern. Med.* 150:25–26

93. Natl. Comm. AIDS. 1992. *Preventing HIV Transmission in Health Care Settings,* pp. 1–48. Washington, DC

94. *Occupational Safety and Health Act of 1970.* Public Law 91–596 91st Congr., S. 2193, Dec. 29

95. Occup. Saf. Health Admin. 1991. Occupational exposure to bloodborne pathogens; final rule. 29 CFR 1910.103.*Fed. Regist.* 56:64003–182

96. Orenstein WA, Haseltine PNR, LeGagnoux SJ, Portnoy B. 1981. Rubella vaccine and susceptible hospital employees: poor physician participation. *J. Am. Med. Assoc.* 245:711–13

97. Owens DK, Nease RF Jr. 1992. Occupational exposure to human immunodeficiency virus and hepatitis B virus: a comparative analysis of risk. *Am. J. Med.* 92:503–12

98. Panlilio AL, Foy DR, Edwards JR, Bell DM, Welch BA, et al. 1991. Blood contacts during surgical procedures. *J. Am. Med. Assoc.* 265:1533–37

99. Pass RF, Little AE, Stagno S, Britt WJ, Alford CA. 1987. Young children as a probable source of maternal and congenital cytomegalovirus infection. *N. Engl. J. Med.* 316:1366–70

100. Paterson WB, Craven DE, Schwartz DA, Nardell EA, Kasmer J, Noble J. 1985. Occupational hazards to hospital personnel (Review). *Ann. Intern. Med.* 102: 658–80

101. Pearson ML, Gereb JA, Friedan TR, Crawford JT, Davis BJ, Dooley SW. 1992. Nosocomial transmission of multidrug resistant mycobacterium tuberculosis. *Ann. Intern. Med.* 117:191–96

102. Popejoy SL, Fry DE. 1991. Blood contact and exposure in the operating room. *Surg. Gynecol. Obstet.* 172:480–83

103. Puro V, Ippolito G, Guzzanti E, Serafin I, Pagano G, et al. 1992. Zidovudine prophylaxis after accidental exposure to HIV. The Italian Study Group on Occupational Risk of HIV Infection. *AIDS* 6:693–99

104. Ramazzini B. 1713. *Diseases of Workers.* New York/London: Hafner. Reprinted 1964. 549 pp.

105. Rogers PL, Lane HC, Henderson DK, Parillo J, Masur H. 1989. Admission of AIDS patients to a medical intensive care unit: causes and outcome. *Crit. Care Med.* 17:113–17

106. Rose HD, Lenz IE, Sheth NK. 1981. Meningococcal pneumonia: a source of nosocomial infection. *Arch. Intern. Med.* 141:575–78

107. Rosenberg J, Clever HL. 1990. Medical surveillance of infectious disease end points. *Occupation Medicine: State of the Art Reviews,* 5:583–605. Philadelphia: Hanley & Belfus

108. Rostami G, Sorg TB. 1990. Nosocomial outbreak ofscabies associated with Norwegian scabies in an AIDS patient. *Int. J. STD AIDS* 1:209–10

109. Schiff ER. 1992. Hepatitis C among health care providers: risk factors and possible prophylaxis. *Hepatology* 16: 1300–1

110. Sepkowitz KA. 1994. Tuberculosis and the health careworker: a historical perspective. *Ann. Intern. Med.* 120:71–79

111. Snider DE, Dooley SW. 1993. Nosocomial tuberculosis in the AIDs era with an emphasis on multi-drug resistant disease. *Heart Lung* 22:365–69

112. Deleted in proof

113. Thomas DL, Factor SH, Kelen GD, Washington AS, Taylor E, Quinn TC. 1993. The seroprevalence of and risk factors for hepatitis B virus and hepatitis C virus infection. *Arch. Intern. Med.* 153:1705–12

114. Tlzak EE. 1993. Eight questions on resurgence of tuberculosis. *Hudson Monit.* 1:40–43

115. Tokars JI, Marcus R, Culver DH, Schable CA, McKibben PS, et al. 1993. Surveillance of HIV and zidovudine use among health care workers after occupational exposure to HIV-infected blood. *Ann. Intern. Med.* 118:913–19

116. Tomasz A. 1994. Multiple-antibiotic-resistent pathogenic bacteria: a report on the Rockefeller University Workshop. *N. Engl. J. Med.* 330:1247–51

117. US Dep. Health Hum. Serv. Public Health Serv. Cent. Dis. Control. Natl. Inst. Occup. Saf. Health. Div. Stand. Dev. Technol. Transfer. 1988. *Guidelines for Protecting the Safety and Health of Health Care Workers*

118. Weber DJ, Rutala WA, Orenstein WA. 1991. Prevention of mumps, measles and rubella among hospital personnel. *J. Pediatr.* 119:322–29

119. Wharton M, Cochi SL, Hutchenson RH, Schaffner W. 1990. Mumps transmission in hospitals. *Arch. Intern. Med.* 150:47–49

120. Wong ES, Stotka JL, Chinchilli VM, Williams DS, Stuart CG, Markowitz SM. 1991. Are universal precautions effective in reducing the number of occupational exposures among health care workers? A prospective study of physicians on a medical service. *J. Am. Med. Assoc.* 265:1123–28

121. Zuber TJ, Geddie JE. 1993. Occupational Safety and Health Administration regulations for the physician's office. *J. Fam. Pract.* 36:540–47

Annu. Rev. Public Health. 1995. 16:165–88

SAFETY AND HEALTH IN THE CONSTRUCTION INDUSTRY

K. Ringen and J. Seegal

Center to Protect Workers' Rights, 111 Massachusetts Avenue, NW, Washington, D.C. 20001

A. Englund

Arbetarskyddsstyrelsen, Ekelundsvägen 16, 17184 Solna, Sweden

KEY WORDS: construction, ergonomics, occupational disease, surveillance, traumatic injury

ABSTRACT

Workers in the building, renovation, and demolition of roads and commercial structures in the U.S. suffer a disproportionate share of occupational fatalities and lost-time injuries. Nearly all of the injuries and deaths are preventable. The fatality rate from work-related ailments, such as cancers and silicosis, is believed to be excessive, but is not generally computed. The safety and health problems are tied largely to the construction industry's organization and how the work is performed. Many hazardous exposures result from inadequacies in access to information, measurement technology, and personal protective equipment. Potential solutions are in labor-management site safety and health planning and management, education and training of workers and supervisors, new technologies, federal regulation, workers' compensation law, medical monitoring, and occupational health delivery. Public health opportunities involve health care delivery systems, improved preventive medicine, disability determination and rehabilitation programs, and research, beginning with the standardization of data to monitor these problems.

INTRODUCTION

Construction workers in many industrialized countries suffer a disproportionate share of work-related injuries and illnesses. In the U.S., the industry employs 5

165

to 6% of the labor force, but has 15% of the fatal injuries (37) and well over 9% of all workdays lost to injuries (J Barnhardt, personal communication). Construction workers disabled or killed each year by work-related illness are believed to number in the tens of thousands, but the numbers are anyone's guess.

The workforce faces some predictable dangers, such as trauma from falls experienced by the roofer, steel worker, or laborer. Predictable occupational ailments include pneumoconiosis of the tunnel builder and the welder; the white finger of the jackhammer operator; low-back pain of the bricklayer; skin allergies of the mason; carpal tunnel syndrome of the iron worker or the electrician; kidney ailments of the painter and the roofer from exposure to solvents; lead poisoning of the bridge rehabilitation worker; asbestosis of the building demolition worker; and heat stress of the hazardous waste cleanup worker (from wearing moon suits) (see 3).

The causes of work-related injuries are well-defined, which means they could relatively easily be prevented. But chronic occupational health risks are poorly defined, in terms of the relations between toxic exposures and health outcomes. In any case, the costs of injuries and illnesses are substantial, not only in workers' poor quality of life and lives cut short, but in financial terms.

Estimates for the total cost of injuries in construction in the U.S. range from $10 billion to $40 billion annually (see 24); at $20 billion, the cost per construction worker would be $3500 yearly. The workers' compensation premiums for three trades—carpenters, masons, and structural iron workers—averaged $28 per $100 of payroll nationally in mid-1993 (25); these rates vary enormously, depending on the trade and jurisdiction. In addition to workers' compensation, there are liability insurance premiums and other indirect costs—reduced work-crew efficiency, cleanup (from a cave-in, for instance), overtime necessitated by the injury, etc. These indirect costs can exceed the workers' compensation claim for an injury by several multiples (21). In the United Kingdom, one study found that accidents—including injuries—cost an average of 8.5% of the contract price. The ratio of uninsured losses to recoverable losses from construction accidents in that country is 11 to 1 (J Hinksman, personal communication).

This review of construction worker safety and health first outlines some of the difficulties, pinpointing the extent and causes of the problems, and then lists health policy and health care issues identified by researchers.

HOW CONSTRUCTION IS ORGANIZED

Several factors contribute to the grim picture for safety and health in construction. Many are related to how the industry operates or how the work is performed.

Construction rarely provides steady employment; construction workers are always working themselves out of their jobs. Although some projects may last several years, many last only a few months. And some assignments—such as roofing or painting—on a project may last only a few days. Thus, a construction worker may have four, five, or more employers in a year. Because of bad weather and layoffs between assignments, in most countries an individual worker may clock only 1500 hours of work or less yearly in construction, compared with 2000 hours in other industries. (There are about 7 million people in construction in the U.S., which equals 4 million to 5 million full-time equivalents or FTEs.)

On a construction project, not only do the work assignments change, but so do the topography of the worksite and, sometimes, the cast of employers. Several trades may work on a site simultaneously, with each trade working for a different contractor. The universe of contractors is marked by high turnover. The U.S. Department of Commerce found 1.9 million employer establishments in 1987. Many contractors are self-employed individuals or mom-and-pop operations; 80 to 90% of construction firms have ten or fewer employees. Less than 20% of all firms belong to a construction organization. These features all create problems from the point of view of public health. With so many job changes and small and short-lived firms, it is difficult to monitor an individual's work history. It is even more difficult to monitor injuries or exposures to hazards.

The constantly changing worksite has another marked effect on safety and health. Unlike in an industrial setting, where the tasks are often repetitive and controlled by the location of machinery, the construction site allows, and requires, extensive movement by the worker from place to place. The worker is therefore much more responsible for his or her own protection.

In addition to potential injuries and exposures to hazardous substances, construction workers face long-term risk from the stress of on- and off-again employment—the fear of not having a paycheck. And because construction jobs can be few and far apart, construction workers may have to travel very long distances to work. This travel, too, takes its toll. For these reasons, it is increasingly difficult to recruit career-oriented workers into construction, and in many states there is a significant decline in the proportion of experienced workers (1).

The lack of comprehensive employer organizations to work with and the huge number of small firms make it difficult to implement preventive programs, including training. In Germany, the Netherlands, Sweden, and Ontario, Canada, the successful safety and health programs were implemented by labor-management organizations. An estimated 25% of the blue-collar construction workforce in the U.S. is unionized; the percentages are much higher for certain trades, nonresidential construction, large projects, the public sector, and certain localities.

MORBIDITY AND MORTALITY DATA FOR CONSTRUCTION

What the U.S. Data Show

With the death rate from injuries for 1980–89 estimated at 25.6 per 100,000 FTEs (18), four or more workers, on average, are killed by injuries sustained on the job each workday. In the U.S., lost-time injuries—requiring restricted activity or time off to recover—affect 5.7 per 100 FTEs yearly, according to the U.S. Bureau of Labor Statistics (BLS) (J Barnhardt, personal communication). That rate and the average time taken off to recover remain essentially unchanged since 1975 (J Weeks, personal communication; 39).

Experience is a factor in such injuries, with the rate of injuries "decreas[ing] substantially as length of service increases" (8). Familiarity with a job site is also a consideration. For laborers, who may suffer the highest injury rates, 12% of lost-time injuries occur during the first day on a job site (2); this pattern appears to hold for most of the trades. Self-employment (37) and small worksite size (23)—both widespread—also appear to correlate with increased risk of injury. Although some researchers maintain that construction workers make matters worse by being risk takers, one study questions that contention (18a).

For a mix of reasons—work-related and not, many still poorly understood— the average age at death for many construction trade workers is lower by 8 to 12 years than those of low-risk groups such as teachers or physicians (5).

Problems with the Data

In addition to the predictable impediments to isolating occupational causes of any illness or chronic injury, other factors hamper efforts to obtain reliable and comparable health statistics about construction workers. These include the way the industry is organized and a lack of data standardization.

Although statistics on deaths from injuries might seem to be the most clear-cut and the easiest to compile, there is wide divergence. FTEs provide the best mode of comparison, particularly in construction where many workers do not work 2000 hours yearly. Nonetheless, the BLS reports a U.S. rate in 1992 of 14 per 100,000 workers, rather than FTEs (J Windau, personal communication). For 100,000 FTEs of 2000 hours yearly, the rate would range from about 18.7 to 23.4, depending, say, on whether the average worker is believed to be employed 1500 or 1200 hours in construction each year. The National Institute for Occupational Safety and Health (NIOSH) reports a rate of 25.6 per 100,000 FTEs, using the National Traumatic Occupational Fatalities data base. The yearly estimated *number* of deaths in construction in the

1980s ranges from 778 (BLS) to 958 (OSHA, for 1985 to 1989), and even higher (18).

A researcher comparing death rates from injuries thus needs to know whether they cover FTEs; whether full-time is considered 2000 hours yearly or, say, 1875; and how many hours the average worker is employed in construction annually. Other key factors in death-rate determination are the industry parameters (what trades are included), the data source and the likelihood of accuracy in listing cause of death, whether the data include self-employed workers and very small sites, whether there is an age cutoff, whether there is a time limit for considering a death following an injury as work-related, and whether motor vehicle accidents are included—on site and to and from work.

When comparing numbers of serious nonfatal injuries, other information is needed, beginning with the definition of *lost-time injury*. For instance, some states or countries count injuries only after a worker has missed three or five days of work; some may not count injuries that result in reduced hours of work (rather than absence from work). Another consideration is whether the reporting system encourages underreporting, even of serious injuries, possibly to avoid higher insurance costs. In the U.S., the recording of injuries (except those that can be handled with first aid) in a log—as required by the U.S. Occupational Safety and Health Administration (OSHA)—has proved virtually unenforceable. A 1987 study commissioned by the National Academy of Sciences noted the difficulties in obtaining injury and illness data for construction. Among other things, the study cited poorly defined responsibility for reporting injuries and illnesses (28).

Comparisons across Countries

The death rate for construction workers in the U.S. appears to be substantially higher than the rates elsewhere, including Germany (FRG in 1991), the Netherlands, Sweden, and Ontario (6). Since 1970, the rate of deaths from worksite injuries has been reduced by 75% in Sweden while the rate has declined by 83% in Ontario since 1965 (A Lindblad & D McVittie, personal communications).

Unfortunately, a lack of uniform parameters bars useful comparisons across countries. For instance, official estimates of the number of hours are unavailable in many cases; none has been available from government or industry in Canada or the U.S. Some U.S. studies include hazardous waste cleanup and the abatement of lead or asbestos in construction, but European studies generally do not. German death rates for construction exclude structural steel erection, electric installation, joinery, and installation of heating systems. In the Netherlands, a death 49 hours after a worksite injury is not considered work related.

The Swedish Longitudinal Study

Despite the problems with health data for construction, one landmark longitudinal study in Sweden has provided insights (10). In the late 1960s, the construction unions and employers in Sweden established Bygghälsan, the Swedish Construction Industry's Organization for Working Environment, Occupational Safety, and Health. Its aim was to identify safety and health risks and develop strategies to reduce them. Physicians, nurses, physical therapists, safety engineers, and industrial hygienists provided an integrated program focusing on safety and health from the perspectives of exposures on the worksite and medical problems of the worker.

TWO COHORTS   In 1969, Bygghälsan began offering preventive and occupational medical examinations to all construction workers. Participation has been voluntary. Starting in 1971, Bygghälsan established a cohort of all participating construction workers. By 1979, 226,704 workers were registered in the cohort. Bygghälsan's longitudinal study has used the results of the medical examination of the cohort and its listings in the national cancer incidence registry and the national mortality registry (11).

Bygghälsan has simultaneously followed a separate, smaller cohort, which included all 48,754 male union painters and certified plumbers and insulators. This cohort was divided into those who participated in the voluntary medical examinations (n = 25,761) and those who did not (n = 22,993). Both cohorts have been followed through 1988 for mortality and through 1987 for cancer incidence.

For the larger cohort, Bygghälsan has reported 18,659 deaths and 9940 cancer cases diagnosed after the first medical examination. As was true for the overall male Swedish population, cardiovascular disease was the main cause of death, but the rate of such deaths was lower in the cohort. Cancer incidence was at 90 to 95% of the rate for the overall population. Bygghälsan attributes the differences partly to selection mechanisms, but also to preventive programs on hypertension, smoking, diet, and exercise.

THE NONPARTICIPANT FACTOR   One striking finding involved the smaller cohort. Nonparticipants showed mortality rates 72% greater than those of participants (Table 1). Similar results were obtained for cancer incidence.

The differences between nonparticipants and participants were especially noteworthy for features associated with poor health behaviors. Differences between the two groups in alcohol and tobacco consumption likely can explain a disparity in mortality rates from cancer of the larynx. But for cancer of the pleura, there is little difference between the two groups, which reflects the strong causal relationship between asbestos and this disease. Only prostate

Table 1 Standardized mortality ratios for nonparticipants and participants, Swedish construction industry preventive health program

Cause of death	Standardized mortality ratios			Confidence intervals (95%)
	Nonparticipants	Participants	Nonparticipants/ participants	
All causes	1.29	0.75	1.71	1.62, 1.80
Alcoholism	2.24	0.38	5.92	3.41, 10.8
Liver cirrhosis	2.17	0.70	3.08	2.16, 4.45
Violent death	1.49	0.71	2.11	1.78, 2.51
All cancers	1.24	0.93	1.34	1.21, 1.48
Laryngeal	3.12	1.11	2.81	0.92, 10.2
Pleural	2.6	2.34	1.11	0.46, 2.63
Esophageal	1.29	0.94	1.37	0.68, 2.78
Liver	1.28	0.78	1.62	0.76, 3.57

Note: Standardized mortality ratios are based on comparison with the white male Swedish population. The cohort was established 1971 to 1979; mortality was followed through the end of 1988. Nonparticipant deaths totaled 3506 and participant deaths 2299. (Source: G Engholm, Bygghälsan.)

cancer diagnosis showed a significant excess incidence for participants compared with nonparticipants. The researchers speculate that this disparity might be attributable to better diagnosis resulting from the regular use of preventive services.

These findings point up the need for caution in interpreting results of screening programs, where participation may be subject to bias. Although screenings can suggest whether a problem exists, other inferences would require a long-term population-based follow-up. In the study described here, the findings paint much too rosy a picture of the health status of construction workers generally.

EXPOSURE-RELATED PROBLEMS

Access to Information

U.S. law requires that material safety data sheets (MSDSs) be readily available on all worksites for all hazardous products introduced to the worksite. Similar provisions apply in Canada. Each MSDS must describe the chemical components, how the substance should be handled, recommended controls such as ventilation or protective equipment, and what to do in an emergency, among other instructions. Unfortunately, many MSDSs are incomplete or are written in language too complicated for a lay reader to understand.

There is also a shortage of industrial hygiene expertise on construction sites to assist with assessments and to advise on protections. Only 16 of 100 large

U.S. construction companies surveyed in 1993 employed an industrial hygien-
ist (31).

Measurement Technology

Industrial hygienists and other researchers have been stymied in their efforts
to develop a reliable system for measuring potential exposures in construction.
In addition to the common difficulties of identifying substances on a site, such
as knowing their condition, there are problems tied to the logistics of worksites
and to available technology. Because each construction worker moves about
a site, the worker's position in relation to exposure sources may change
constantly. At some moments, a worker may be directly exposed while using
a hazardous substance, but at other times the worker may be exposed to another
substance as a bystander 10 feet downwind. It is thus difficult to anticipate all
the substances and degrees of exposure that someone will encounter on a given
day.

To measure exposures in manufacturing, integrated samples are collected
to determine 8-hr time-weighted averages. Such an approach may not tell the
whole story about health effects in construction, however. Brief, high-level
exposures may have different and significant health effects compared with
longer-term low-level exposures. In addition, construction work is marked by
types of exposures that time-weighted averages do not account for: through
the skin and, to a lesser extent, ingestion.

Personal Protection

Workers may not know when they need to use specific personal protective
equipment, and if they do know, they may lack the equipment or needed
training. In addition, the use of some controls can create problems. For instance, while construction workers often perform as teams, respirators may
prevent coworkers from communicating with each other. And full-body protective clothing can contribute to heat stress.

Having protective gear without knowing its limitations can do more harm
than good, because it gives the worker or employer the illusion that the worker
is protected. For instance, there are no gloves that can protect for more than
two hours against methylene chloride, which is in paint strippers. Solvent
mixtures—such as those containing both acetone and toluene or both methanol
and xylene—seep through gloves in less than one work shift.

A lack of eating and sanitary facilities may also lead to increased exposures.
Often, workers cannot wash before meals and must eat in the work zone, which
means they may inadvertently swallow toxic substances transferred from their
hands to cigarettes or food. A lack of changing facilities may result in transport
of contaminants from the workplace to a worker's home.

MAJOR HEALTH OUTCOMES

Traumatic injuries

Construction workers are at great risk of injury partly because of where they work—from scaffolding hundreds of feet up to trenches underground (Table 2). Specific hazards and overall risk vary by trade. Based on what is known in the U.S., iron workers appear to have the highest risk of work-related deaths from injuries; in other countries, roofing may be the most dangerous trade because of the danger of falls and exposures to hot tar (15, 36, 37).

The rankings of causes of fatal and nonfatal injuries appear to differ, however. For instance, falls from elevations tend to be so serious that they are responsible for most traumatic deaths on site. But they are not the main reported overall cause of nonfatal injuries; most studies list being struck by an object first and overexertion second.[1] The leading causes of lost-time injuries vary by trade. In regions where a large proportion of the construction labor force

Table 2 Lost-time injuries, fatal and nonfatal, among roofers and laborers

Cause of injury	Roofers	Laborers
	(percentage)	
Falls from elevations	23	11
Overexertion	23	22
Struck by an object	14	25
Contact with temperature extremes	9	2
Struck against	7	10
Falls from same level	6	7
Bodily reaction[a]	5	3
Caught in/under/between (including cave-ins)	3	8
Rubbed/abraded	3	7
Contact with radiation, caustics, etc	2	3
Other[b]	5	2

[a] Includes, e.g., slipping and twisting body to catch oneself or twisting an ankle while climbing a ladder.
[b] Includes transport injuries and nonclassifiable.
Note: Numbers are rounded.
Source: For laborer injuries, Ref. 3, Table 3, p. 8; for roofer injuries, ME Personick, BLS, based on workers' compensation data, selected states.

[1]Two slightly different conclusions were found in published reports. A study of data compiled by the Army Corps of Engineers showed that being struck by an object was the major cause of fatalities (33%), while falls from an elevation were second (21%) (26). An OSHA study of construction found that overexertion was the leading cause of all lost-time injuries, including fatalities (24%), and being struck by an object was the second-highest cause (22%) (8).

consists of immigrants, such as Southern California, the worker's inability to understand English may increase the risk of injury (Table 3).

Musculoskeletal Disorders

Some musculoskeletal disorders result from traumatic injuries, but many others develop incrementally. These stem from repetitive tasks and awkward body positions. The bricklayer lifts an estimated 3 to 4 tons daily, with 1000 trunk-twist flexions. The iron worker tying intersections of the perpendicular rods used to reinforce concrete may bend over more than half the workday, repeatedly twisting the wrist under pressure. In building construction, much of the finishing work involves areas either above shoulder height or below knee level (33).

Although musculoskeletal disorders are not fatal, they are significant, and little progress has been made in controlling them. According to data for construction in Ontario, about 66% of all workers' compensation claims and 90% of all days lost are the result of soft-tissue injuries (G Atherley, personal communication). In the U.S., these disorders are believed to use 40 to 65% of workers' compensation costs in construction. In Finland, the disorders are responsible for half the early retirements in construction (H Riihimäki, personal communication). A three-year study in Washington State found that certain trades are more at risk generally for musculoskeletal disorders: laborers, carpenters, roofers, and electricians (B Silverstein, personal communication).

The problems of each trade have received little detailed analysis. And what has been done has relied largely on subjective judgments or surveys using

Table 3 The main safety and health hazards for the construction worker

Musculoskeletal disorders, all trades	
Cause of injury	Organs most affected
Lifting	Lower back, shoulders
Awkward postures	Knee, hip, shoulders
Repetitive motion	Wrists
Hand-tool vibration	Fingers, wrists
Chronic health hazards, all trades	
Hazard	Organ/system most affected
Noise	Hearing
Silica; asbestos, other manmade fibers	Lungs
Lead and other metals	Kidneys, nervous and reproductive systems
Solvents	Kidneys, liver, nervous system
Hazardous wastes	All systems
Heat and extreme cold	Circulatory system

questionnaires or interviews. A Bygghälsan questionnaire, conducted since 1989 and completed by more than 83,000 construction workers about work postures and about the location of the most prevalent musculoskeletal complaints, suggests a correlation. For instance, 20% reported working with hands above shoulders "often," and 22% reported shoulder problems "often" or "very often;" in both cases, these were the top items on five-point scales (G Engholm, personal communication). Although whole-body vibration, such as that experienced by operators of heavy construction machinery, is commonly believed to be correlated with lower-back or disk degeneration problems, no studies to date have established this connection (for example, see 30).

THE HOLMSTRÖM STUDY   One of the most detailed scientific reports on musculoskeletal disorders in construction workers is by Holmström, who produced a series of studies—one of them on a randomized, cross-sectional sample of 1773 construction workers in Malmö, Sweden, using questionnaires and some clinical examinations (16). Holmström found that low-back pain correlated with increasing age, trade, personal habits, and psychosocial factors.

Only 8% of the workers studied reported no musculoskeletal problems in the preceding year. For the preceding year, low-back pain was reported by 72%, knee problems by 52%, and neck-shoulder pains by 37%. By contrast, a Bygghälsan survey of foremen and office workers found the following percentages answered "often" or "very often" when asked if they had experienced pain in the preceding year: lower back, 19%; knee, 13%; shoulder, 15%; and neck, 13%.

In Holmström's study, the prevalence of most musculoskeletal symptoms increased with age. Low-back pain correlated with frequent handling of hand-held machines, handling of bricks and roofing materials, and awkward postures—such as stooping or kneeling for more than an hour a day. The prevalence and type of disorder varied by trade. Roofers, carpet and tile layers, and scaffolding erectors had the highest prevalence of low-back pain, compared with the other construction trades. Reported low-back pain was 2.7 times more prevalent for smokers than for nonsmokers. Psychosocial factors also contributed significantly to explain low-back pain, when other factors were kept constant. Workers who reported no low-back problems were generally in better physical condition, were more involved in recreational activities, smoked less, and had a more positive outlook. They reported fewer psychosomatic symptoms and were more active participants in worksite decision-making. The average length of employment in construction for this group was 15 years. Both groups of workers were found to have the same maximum abdominal and back muscle strength. Workers reporting severe low-back problems had significantly reduced back muscle endurance.

Chronic and Fatal Illnesses

Some work-related illnesses appear to be correlated with specific construction trades (Table 4), although there are often many difficulties, including long latencies, in tying a disease to an individual's employment history. In New York State, for instance, a study from the Mount Sinai School of Medicine estimates that 3700 people died yearly in 1979 through 1982 of occupational cancers. The deaths in 1979 included 80 caused by mesothelioma. Mesothelioma is believed to be almost always caused by occupational or family-contact exposures to asbestos, although there may occasionally be other explanations (for example, see 13). Yet the workers' compensation board accepted just three cancer deaths as work-related for each of the four years (19). Similarly, in Finland, many asbestos-induced cancers are still not diagnosed as occupational diseases, although more of the other asbestos-caused diseases are being so labeled (17).

PULMONARY DISEASES, INCLUDING LUNG CANCERS   Construction sites are generally dusty—as powdered bags of cement are emptied for mixing, as wood

Table 4   Common toxic hazards on the construction site

Substance	Key source of exposure
Dusts	
Asbestos*	Demolition, maintenance, insulation
Cement	Foundations, sidewalks, floors
Fiberglass, other insulation	Insulation on pipes, air conditioning
Silica	Sandblasting, tunneling
Wood dust*	Remodeling, demolition, sawing
Metals (dusts and fumes)	
Cadmium*	Welding, cutting pipe
Hexavalent chromium*	Welding, cutting pipe
Copper	Welding, cutting pipe
Lead	Demolition, lead-paint surfaces
Magnesium	Welding, cutting pipe
Zinc	Welding, cutting pipe
Solvents	
Benzene*	Hazardous waste cleanup, petrochemical plant sites
Methylene chloride	Paint strippers
Toluene	Varnishes, paints, adhesives, cleaners
Trichloroethylene	Varnishes, paints, adhesives, cleaners
Other chemicals	
Epoxy resins	Impermeable paints, wood floor primers
Polyurethanes (isocyanates)	Seam sealers, insulation, electrical wire coating
Coal tar pitch*	Roofings, road work

*Human carcinogen
Source: Based on Ref. 41

is sawed, as heavy machinery lumbers across uneven terrain, and as pneumatic tools are used on concrete, drywall, and rock containing quartz. There are also fumes from such activities as welding, roofing, and paving. Construction workers' lungs are thus multiply exposed to potential toxic hazards.

Asbestos and silica are the two best-documented hazards. Recent research by NIOSH has found that the highest proportionate mortality ratios (PMRs) for white male construction workers under age 65 are for asbestosis [393] and silicosis [327] (32). These findings, from underlying cause-of-death codes on death certificates for 1984-86, compare with a PMR for falls of 177.

In 1964, Selikoff et al laid out a clear pattern of pulmonary carcinoma among insulation (asbestos) workers, the risk for other neoplasms, and the likelihood that other workers besides those producing or handling asbestos were at risk (35). The researchers found a 6.8 times greater risk of death from bronchogenic carcinoma and mesothelioma compared with the general U.S. white male population. Circumstantial evidence suggested that smoking habits alone, which the researchers did not document, would not account for so large an increased risk. The authors discussed what has come to be known as bystander exposure. They noted that "the floating fibers do not respect job classifications" on a worksite.

Although the spray application of asbestos insulation has in effect been banned in the U.S. since 1973 and most uses of asbestos are controlled, construction workers continue to be exposed to asbestos installed years ago. Levin has reported lung abnormalities consistent with exposure to asbestos among building demolition workers in New York City who have no other known exposure to the mineral (20). Results of screenings in Finland "seem ... to indicate that all construction workers experience direct or indirect exposure to asbestos" (27).

Similarly, although OSHA has set permissible exposure limits for respirable silica and although personal protective measures such as local exhaust are known, new cases of silicosis are still reported. Those at risk include tunnel workers, sandblasters, trades working with concrete and mortar—laborers, masons, concrete finishers, tile setters, and plasterers—and bystanders (22). Depending partly on the percentage of silica in the materials used, a wide range of tasks can prove hazardous; these include drilling holes, grinding concrete surfaces, power-cleaning concrete forms, or cutting through concrete block, walls, or pipe. The risks are not limited to new construction. For instance, powered grinders may be used to remove mortar for restoration.

OTHER CANCERS   Potential exposures to carcinogens are common in all types of construction. Some sources are well-known, such as hydrocarbons in roofing tar. Welding can produce carcinogenic fumes, such as nickel and hexavalent chromium from stainless steel welds, and cadmium. Many new products have

potential carcinogenic effects. For instance, the use of plastics has been mul-
tiplying, and the health effects of their use remains unknown. Many specialty
paints include metals and dangerous solvents, such as mercury and benzene.
Among resins, acrylontirile in acrylics, epichlorhydrin in epoxies, and isocy-
anates in polyurethanes all pose potential, but poorly documented, risks. Benzene and vinyl chloride are among the substances commonly found at Super-
fund sites (12).

CENTRAL NERVOUS SYSTEM DISORDERS   Lead poisoning continues to be a
particular concern for construction workers. Although lead is restricted to trace
amounts in residential paints in the U.S., it is still allowed in many states for
boats, bridges, and other nonresidential uses. The California Occupational Lead
Registry found that construction workers accounted for 18% of the workers
who had peak blood-lead levels of 80μ/dL [i.e. well above the level at which
OSHA requires removal. (See below; 38)]. Exposures to lead occur during
rehabilitation or demolition of lead-painted structures, for instance, scraping,
cutting with torches, sandblasting, and during welding. Welders may be exposed to fumes containing lead, but also epoxy resins, manganese, nickel,
polyurethane, and vinyl chloride.

Threats to the nervous system commonly encountered by hazardous waste
cleanup workers include toluene, trichloroethylene, tetrachloroethylene, arse-
nic, benzene, lead, and mercury (12).

On a lesser scale, painters and laborers are at risk of mercury exposure from
latex paints, through skin contact, ingestion, or inhaled vapor or dust. Two
voluntary agreements between the U.S. Environmental Protection Agency and
the paint industry should reduce the problem. Mercury compounds were no
longer added to latex paints used for interiors after August 1990 and manufacturers agreed to stop selling phenylmercuric acetate to paint companies for
use in exterior latex paints as of September 1991 (14), but existing stock could
still be used.

SKIN DISORDERS   Laborers, bricklayers, masons, and others who handle concrete or cement are prone to allergic and toxic dermatitis on the hands and
other exposed areas. The symptoms can be severe enough to necessitate early
retirement. The allergic dermatitis is believed to be caused by water-soluble
hexavalent chromium.

NOISE-INDUCED HEARING LOSS   Noise levels on construction sites commonly
exceed 95 dB around heavy machinery, such as bulldozers or front-end loaders.
Noise levels of 95 to 105 dB have been measured around power tools, such
as saws. Bygghälsan found that bilateral normal hearing among construction
workers decreased gradually with age, so that in 1974 only about 26% of those

examined at ages 38 to 40 had hearing in the normal range. At the same time, about 3.6% of construction workers aged 38 to 40 suffered bilateral severe high-frequency hearing loss (4000 Hz or above). This problem hampers team-work; it also endangers workers who cannot be warned of immediate dangers or hear approaching vehicles.

FAMILY CONTACT DISEASE   In some cases, asbestos fibers may be transported in asbestos products carried home to show to family members, as well as inadvertently carried on clothing, in hair, etc (34). A similar risk may exist for lead poisoning among construction workers' families, particularly children, whose systems are more vulnerable than adults'. No epidemiologic studies directly link parental occupation with childhood lead poisoning, but there appears to be a correlation. In one case documented at Mt. Sinai School of Medicine, the elevated blood-lead level of a child of a construction worker was believed to result from lead dust on the parent's clothing (PJ Landrigan, personal communication).

WHAT IS BEING DONE

In recent years construction safety and health in the U.S. has received increased attention. Several changes under way could prove critical in site safety and health planning and management, worker and supervisor training, safer con-struction technologies, health care delivery, and health monitoring. Some changes are being spurred by federal and state regulation or legislation. In-creasingly the belief is taking hold that improved safety and health can produce greater productivity, and several large contracting companies are acting on that assumption (see 4).

Site Safety and Health Planning and Management

There is widespread agreement that planning is a key to better safety and health on the worksite (6, 7, 21). Planning involves all details of logistics and begins well before the first shovelful of earth is turned. A critical element is assigning responsibility for safety and health, while at the same time improving coordi-nation among subcontractors and the trades. Some large contractors have begun to stress planning in cooperation with labor, plus accountability for safety, and have set goals of zero accidents (21, 24).

Education and Training

Safety training and worker and manager education have long been provided by some companies and the trade unions in the U.S. The training programs include site orientation and skills; they cover such topics as rigging, trenching, stretching exercises, and substance abuse recovery. Many training programs also include instruction about dangerous substances that is now mandated under OSHA's Hazard Communication Standard.

The same concern in Germany has led to development of a program entitled Gefahrstoff-Informationssystem der Berufsgenossenschaften der Bauwirt-schaft, or GISBAU. GISBAU works with manufacturers to determine the content of all substances used on construction sites. Equally important, it provides the information in a form suitable to the differing needs of health staff, managers, and workers. The information is available through training programs, in print, and on computer terminals at worksites. GISBAU gives advice about how to substitute for some risky substances and tells how to safely handle others. The program may be made available in English.

New Technologies

Technological improvements are reducing the risks of musculoskeletal and other health problems. Many of the changes are straightforward. One example is a two-handed screwdriver with a longer handle that is used in Sweden, which increases torque and reduces stress on the wrist(s). Another example is the redesign of tower crane cabins in Germany and Sweden. One change extends the window to the cabin floor, enabling the operators to see below without having to lean forward constantly. As a result, they report less chronic neck pain.

To make lifting easier for the bricklayer, bricks in Germany are now de-signed with holes or handles. Regulations require that bricks weighing more than 25 kg (55 pounds) be lifted only by machine. In the Netherlands, brick manufacturers, unions, and management have developed a different system in which bricks are packaged in sets that are easily moved about the worksite on dollies and lifted by levers to a convenient height.

Many countries have stopped the manufacture, sale, importation, and use of asbestos products. In the U.S. and many other countries, for instance, the dismantling of material containing asbestos requires a license, although this requirement is often not enforced.

To reduce the risk of silicosis from sandblasting by about 90%, researchers in Germany have turned to wet blasting, using water to dampen the sand as it is being sprayed and thus minimize dust. Nevertheless, throughout Europe, silica sandblasting is being banned, except where essential.

Beginning in the mid-1980s researchers in Denmark, Sweden, Finland, and more recently Germany, have found that adding small amounts of ferrous sulfate to cement changes water-soluble hexavalent chromium to trivalent chromium. This change appears to explain the substantial decline in allergic dermatitis in the Nordic countries. The change costs about $1 per ton.

Some efforts to improve worker health combine technologies and training. The Swedish construction industry has been reducing noise on site and em-phasizing instructing workers in hearing conservation. By 1986–90, 42% of workers at age 38 to 40 had normal bilateral hearing, compared with 26% in 1974. Severe high-frequency loss had been reduced to 2.2% for the same age level, compared with 3.6% previously.

Federal Regulation

Since 1989, OSHA has issued three regulations that are giving new direction to the construction industry.

- *Hazardous Waste Operations and Emergency Response Standard* (29CFR1926.65) This standard took effect in 1990 and governs all work where hazardous wastes exist. It was the first regulation to require site safety and health plans, extensive specialized training of workers and supervisors, and health monitoring, record-keeping, and reporting. It is gradually becoming a model for general construction.
- *Process Safety Management of Highly Hazardous Chemicals Standard* (29CFR1926.64) This standard, passed in 1992, was adopted to prevent catastrophic explosions, especially when construction and maintenance are performed at such places as refineries and chemical plants. Like the hazardous operations standard, this regulation focuses on site safety and health planning and worker training. Contractors at industrial facilities are required to identify the hazards associated with construction tasks and provide training. The standard also requires that a facility owner evaluate a contracting firm's safety record before hiring it.
- *Lead Exposure in Construction; Interim Final Rule* (29CFR1926) Patterned on the existing standard for general industry, this rule, established in 1993, sets allowable limits for lead. The standard also provides requirements for reducing excessive exposures and providing medical care and job security for lead-poisoned workers, in certain circumstances. Permissible airborne concentrations at the worksite are $50\mu g/m^3$, averaged over 8 hours. Initial medical surveillance is triggered when air monitoring shows exposures above 30 $\mu g/m^3$ for one day and a blood-lead level of $50\mu g/dL$ (measured twice, over 2 weeks) is enough to trigger medical removal. It is generally agreed, however, that the levels are not stringent enough. A consortium of representatives from public health, labor, government, and industry has taken this move a step further, drafting model specifications for a lead-protection program that could be included in bid documents.[2]

Workers' Compensation Law

A 1991 reform of the Massachusetts workers' compensation law permitted collective bargaining for workers' compensation agreements, benefits higher

---

[2]The consortium was organized by the Center to Protect Workers' Rights and the Steel Structures Painting Council.

than those required by the state, managed care arrangements, and alternative dispute resolution. This change, which has been replicated in California and Florida, allows employers and workers to find ways to cut costs while reducing injuries and improving health care delivery.

In 1993, an agreement between Bechtel Construction Co. and the building trades unions, based on the Massachusetts legislation, reportedly cut claims and litigation, provided access to better medical care, and better disability benefits, where needed, while cutting costs by more than half, from $2.21 to $0.98 per hour (T Manley & J Dart, personal communications).

Other Health Care Delivery

For 40 years the unionized sector has provided health insurance through health and welfare funds that are jointly trusteed with employers. There are about 750 such funds of varying size in the U.S., most of them local. To address the episodic employment question, the health and welfare funds have established hour banks in which workers can accumulate hours worked to qualify for coverage for themselves and their families. Workers can thus maintain group coverage through as much as three to six months of unemployment by drawing on their bank reserves. But this system has its limitations. With erratic employment, some workers still are not able to build up reserve hours. And, even with health care coverage, medical care usage has been poor, and hospitalization rates for preventable disorders like substance abuse and perinatal problems are excessive in comparison with rates for the general population (29).

One experiment in preventive medicine is being conducted with a health and welfare fund in the Pacific Northwest. A protocol was designed comprising procedures, history forms, data reporting, and frequency for periodic examinations. It was based on the experience of Bygghälsan, recommendations of the U.S. Preventive Services Task Force, and patterns of local medical practice. An outpatient preferred provider organization (PPO) network serving this health and welfare fund identified providers best suited to provide the examinations. Selection criteria included special medical expertise, interest in workers, and a willingness to submit data. The health and welfare office verifies worker eligibility for the examination. The PPO clinical director's office performs quality control, collects and enters data, and assures continuity between examinations. This program is exceptional, however.

Medical Monitoring

Germany has long specified and required medical monitoring in any work setting for biological (hepatitis), chemical, and physical hazards (noise, vibration). Checkups are required before work is begun, at specified intervals, and, when there has been known exposure to carcinogens (for a given length of time, depending on the carcinogen), at regular intervals for the rest of the worker's life. Information from the checkups that can be used to improve workplace conditions is given to employers. Employers are responsible for continuing medical monitoring according to a schedule begun with a different employer. If a worker is unemployed for longer than the scheduled interval for routine checkups, however, the examination schedule usually begins again with a baseline examination at the time of next employment (G Linke-Kaiser, personal communication).

RECOMMENDATIONS: OPPORTUNITIES IN PUBLIC HEALTH

Construction is a field in which the occupational health professions can play major roles. To be effective, however, health professionals must first understand the organizational and sociological aspects of construction work, so that effective medical delivery systems can be put into place. Second, the risks that workers face on the job must be understood by health professionals. Third, they must develop protocols and programs that are appropriate to the needs of construction workers and their families.

Delivery Systems

There are numerous opportunities to provide improved health programs for construction workers by working with health and welfare plans, workers' compensation carriers, employers, and unions. Structured care systems are needed that are based on close cooperation among clinicians and experts in physical therapy, occupational hygiene, and safety engineering.

Few employers provide their own medical staff. Existing community or academic occupational health clinics generally have a large volume of building trades activities; they see individual workers who have been referred or self-referred and also investigate special problems in the worker population. This pattern, however, does not reflect industry-wide health care use. Because of the episodic nature of their employment and the high cost of health care, most construction workers have not had continuous medical care and a long-term relationship with a medical provider who knows his or her case. (This may change if universal health care is established.)

Preventive Medicine, In General

Targeted preventive services are needed in most health insurance plans that cover construction workers and their families. These services should include discussions with patients about the precautions to take around the hazardous substances that their trades are most likely to encounter.

• *Development of Protocols* Few occupational medicine protocols have been developed and validated for use for construction groups, even for preventive medicine generally. Issues include whether there is a role for chest x-rays in periodic preventive medical examinations. Another is whether liver enzyme tests have a useful role in predicting fitness for work in hazardous waste cleanup.

- *Targeted Medical Monitoring* Because of the difficulties of reliably establishing work histories and exposures, medical monitoring is especially important, particularly in hazardous waste cleanup and lead and asbestos abatement.
- *Screening for Disease* Despite a long history of screening programs for asbestos-related diseases, little is known about the prevalence or incidence of hearing loss, most musculoskeletal disorders, dermatitis, or other chronic diseases. Although questionnaires and interviews should be used at first to identify potential cases of musculoskeletal disorders, in part because such approaches are cost-effective, an objective measure needs to be developed for follow-up. One approach may be to use functional capacity—mobility, muscle strength, etc (H Riihimäki, personal communication). As the first and second waves of asbestos disease reach their conclusion, it will be useful to study whether overall incidence is in decline.

Determination of Disability and Support for Rehabilitation

MEDICAL PANELS   Better medical support is needed to determine disability under workers' compensation and help workers return to work as early as possible. Newly forming closed medical panels for disability determination can help make the system more responsive to the needs of disabled workers. The occupational physician can also help identify light-duty tasks that match a worker's level of disability.

STANDARDS SETTING   Occupational physicians can help with the setting and implementation of health-related standards. In the U.S., most OSHA standards are inadequate in terms of medical monitoring requirements for construction workers. The medical monitoring requirements of the OSHA Hazardous Waste Operations Standard, for instance, are vague. The recently issued OSHA interim final rule for lead in construction has clear medical requirements for monitoring and actions, but is impractical for implementation in the construction sector. For example, a worker with a high blood-lead level is supposed to be provided with another job that is removed from the lead exposure and at the same pay, but if a project is completed, the contractor no longer is required to provide a job. The worker then may have difficulty finding another job until the blood-lead level goes down.

Research

Issues such as the measurement of and consequences of exposures to toxic substances and musculoskeletal overload are poorly understood, largely because of inadequate past research on work-related safety and health in construction. The problems have partly been tied to funding. As recently as 1988, federally funded safety research averaged $2.16 per manufacturing worker and $0.08 per construction worker. The investment in construction research, however, has been increasing.

For health researchers, construction is largely unexplored terrain. Areas that have not been addressed are exposure characterization, epidemiology, health services, interventions, and policy.

EXPOSURE CHARACTERIZATION   An exposure assessment model is needed that addresses the unique nature of construction work. The model should efficiently collect descriptive and quantitative data on exposures so they can be predicted before each job starts. The model should be in a form that construction workers can use easily on site. And it should be part of a system that permits storage of data for reference years later.

Given the limits of existing technology, the best approach may be to develop estimates of the range of exposures for given tasks—such as rod tying, riveting, and welding—taking into account such factors as the substances used, duration, and ventilation. For welding, for instance, an estimate would consider the welding method, the welding rod used, and materials welded, including any coatings. These estimates will need to include ingestion and dermal exposures (for example, see 40). Exposures worth special attention include noise, dusts, vibration, manual lifting, and work postures. For instance, back belts are in widespread use, but no study has determined whether they are effective.

EPIDEMIOLOGY   Good epidemiological surveillance systems and descriptive studies are needed. There is a shortage of reliable data on the morbidity patterns by trade. Virtually no research has been conducted on patterns of disability for the trades.

HEALTH SERVICES   No research has been published in recent years on the delivery of occupational or general medical services for construction workers in the United States. Thirty years ago, the Tennessee Valley Authority developed mobile health centers to provide occupational and preventive medicine to construction workers building its major power plants, dams, etc, but the papers published to describe these programs did not include any evaluation of process or outcome (7a, 7b). In addition, little is known about patterns of health care use among construction workers. If one accepts that continuity of care is a key determinant of the effectiveness of medical care, the episodic nature of construction employment appears to be a major barrier.

INTERVENTIONS   Studies are needed in four types of intervention. First, different approaches to the delivery of preventive services should be tested. Information is also needed on preventive measures such as training (see 9), certification of workers and contractors, use of personal protective equipment, and technologies that may reduce exposures. To date no studies have been performed on the best systems for monitoring the health of construction workers, including exposure monitoring, medical monitoring, and the tracking of workers in a transient industry. Last, experiments should be performed to reduce the sequelae of disability and to return injured workers promptly to gainful employment.

POLICY   Little consideration has been given to the economics of improved safety and health in construction. There have been no geographically defined projects to characterize the construction industry and to intervene in its basic characteristics of small employers, transient work, temporary worksites, and multi-employer worksites. Nor have there been valid studies to examine the effects of disability on workers and their families.

INFORMATION EXCHANGES   To facilitate useful comparisons among programs and across countries, data on work-related injuries and their outcomes need to be standardized. Guidelines for the reporting of occupational illness also need standardization.

Literature Cited

1. Azari-Rad H, Yeagle A, Philips P. 1994. The effects of the repeal of Utah's prevailing wage law on the labor market in construction. In *Restoring the Promise of American Labor Law*, ed. S Friedman, R Hurd, R Oswald, R Seeber, pp. 207–22. Ithaca, NY: ILR Press

2. Bureau of Labor Statistics. 1986. *Injuries to Construction Laborers. Bull.* 2252:7. Washington, DC

3. Burkhart G, Schulte PA, Robinson C, Sieber WK, Vossenas P, Ringen K. 1993. Job tasks, potential exposures, and health risks of laborers employed in the construction industry. *Am. J. Ind. Med.* 24:413–25

4. Business Roundtable. 1982. *Improving construction safety performance: a construction industry cost effectiveness project report*. Rpt A-3

5. Calif. Dep. Health Services. 1987. *California Occupational Mortality 1979–81*. Sacramento

6. Cent. Protect Workers' Rights. 1993. *Agenda for change*. Rep. Natl. Conf. Ergonom. Saf. Health Constr. Washington, DC: Cent. Protect Workers' Rights

7. Construction Industry Institute. 1993. *Zero Injury Techniques*. Austin, Texas. Publ. 32–1

7a. Craig JL. 1968. Mobilized occupational

health services: the TVA experience. *J. Occup. Med.* 10:179–84
7b. Craig JL. 1974. A practical approach to cost analysis of an occupational health program. *J. Occup. Med.* 16:445–48
8. Culver C, Marshall M, Connolly C. 1992. *Construction Accidents: The Workers' Compensation Data Base, 1985–1988.* Washington, DC: Off. Constr. Eng., OSHA
9. Dedobbeleer N, German P. 1987. Safety practices in the construction industry. *J. Occup. Med.* 29:863–68
10. Engholm G. 1992. *Prospective Follow-up of a Medical Surveillance Programme.* Danderyd, Sweden: Bygghälsan
11. Englund A, Engholm G, Michaels D, Ringen K. 1992. Twenty years of follow-up of mortality and cancer incidence in Swedish construction workers. In *Uniting for Healthy Communities: Abstracts,* 1105:57. Washington, DC: Am. Public Health Assoc.
12. Freshwater Foundation. 1993. *Special report: health effects of hazardous waste,* p.4. Health Environ. Digest. Wayzata, MN
13. Glickman LT, Domanksi LM, Maguire TG, Dubielzig RR, Churg A. 1983. Mesothelioma in pet dogs associated with exposure of their owners to asbestos. *Environ. Res.* 32:305–13
14. Hefflin BJ, Etzel RA, Agoos MM, Stratton JW, Ikawa GK, et al. 1993. Mercury exposure from exterior latex paint. *J. Appl. Occup. Environ. Hyg.* 8:866–70
15. Helander MG. 1991. Safety hazards and motivation for safe work in the construction industry. *Int. J. Ind. Econ.* 8:205–23
16. Holmström E. 1992. *Musculoskeletal Disorders in Construction Workers.* Lund, Sweden: Lund Univ. Dep. Phys. Ther.
17. Huuskonen MS, Karjalainen A, Koskinen K, Rinne J-P, Tossavainen A, Rantanen J. 1993. *Asbestos program 1987–92: final report.* Helsinki: Inst. Occup. Health
18. Kisner SM, Fosbroke DA. 1994. Injury hazards in the construction industry. *J. Occup. Med.* 36:137–43
18a. Landeweerd JA, Urlings IJM, DeJong AHJ, Nijhuis FJN, Bouter LM. 1990. Risk taking tendency among construction workers. *J. Occup. Accidents* 11:183–96
19. Landrigan P, Markowitz SB. 1987. *Occupational Disease in New York State.* New York: Mt. Sinai Sch.Med.
20. Levin S. 1994. *Abnormalities Consistent with Asbestos Exposure in Demolition Workers.* Washington: Cent. Prot. Workers' Rights
21. Levitt RE, Samelson NM. 1993. *Construction Safety Management.* New York: Wiley. 2nd ed.
22. Lofgren, DJ. 1993. Silica exposure for concrete workers and masons. *J. Appl. Occup. Environ. Hyg.* 8:832–36
23. Marsh B. 1994. Chance of getting hurt is generally far higher at smaller companies. *Wall St. J.* Feb. 3, A-1 (original research)
24. Meridian Research. 1994. *Worker Protection Programs in Construction.* Silver Spring, Md. OSHA Contract J-9-F-1–0019
25. Powers MB. 1994. Cost fever breaks. *ENR.* Sept. 26, 233:40–41, based on figures from Marsh & McLennan Inc.
26. Off. Constr. Eng., OSHA. 1992. *Construction Lost-Time Injuries: The U.S. Army Corps of Engineers Data Base 1984–1988.* pp. xii & 73
27. Oksa P, Koskinen H, Rinne J-P, Zitting A, Roto P, Huuskonen MS. 1992. Parenchymal and pleural fibrosis in construction workers. *Am. J. Ind. Med.* 21:561–67
28. Pollack ES, Keimig DG, eds. 1987. *Counting Injuries and Illnesses in the Workplace: Proposals for a Better System.* Washington, DC: Natl. Acad. Press
29. Pollack ES, Ringen K. 1993. Risk of hospitalization for specific non-work-related conditions among laborers and their families. *Am. J. Ind. Med.* 23:417–25
30. Pope MH, Hansson TH. 1992. Vibration of the spine and low back pain. *Clin. Orthop. Rel. Res.* 279:49–59
31. Rekus JF. 1994. Chronic risks in construction. *Occup. Health Saf.* May, pp. 102–28
32. Robinson C, Stern F, Halperin W, Venable H, Petersen M, et al. 1995. Assessment of mortality in the construction industry in the United States. 1984–1986. *Am. J. Ind. Med.* In press
33. Schneider S, Susie P. 1993. *Ergonomics and Construction: A Review of Potential Hazards in New Building Construction.* Washington, DC: Cent. Prot. Workers' Rights. Rpt E1–93
34. Selikoff IJ. 1977. Cancer risk of asbestos exposure. In *Origins of Human Cancer,* ed. HH Hiatt, JD Watson, JA Winsten, Book C:1778. Cold Spring Harbor, NY: Cold Spring Harbor Lab.
35. Selikoff IJ, Churg J, Hammond EC. 1964. Asbestos exposure and neoplasia. *J. Am. Med. Assoc.* 188:22–26

36. Sorock GS, Smith EO, Goldoft M. 1993. Fatal occupational injuries in the New Jersey construction industry, 1983 to 1989. *J. Occup. Med.* 35:916–21

37. Toscano G, Windau J. 1994. The changing character of fatal work injuries. *Mon. Labor Rev.* October:17–28. Washington, DC: US Dep. Labor

38. Waller K, Osorio AM, Maizlish N, Royce S. 1992. Lead exposure in the construction industry: results from the California occupational lead registry, 1987 through 1989. *Am. J. Public Health* 82:1669–71

39. Weeks JL. 1993. *Lost-Time Injury Rates in Construction, 1975–90.* Washington, DC: Cent. Prot. Workers' Rights. Rpt D1–93

40. Wolff MS, Herbert R, Marcus M, Rivera M, Landrigan PJ, Andrews LR. 1989. Polycyclic aromatic hydrocarbon (PAH) residues on skin in relation to air levels among roofers. *Arch. Env. Health* 44: 157–63

41. Workplace Hazard and Tobacco Education Project. 1993. *Construction Workers' Guide to Toxics on the Job.* Berkeley: Calif. Public Health Found.

Annu. Rev. Public Health. 1995. 16:189–218

WORKERS' COMPENSATION IN THE UNITED STATES: High Costs, Low Benefits

L. I. Boden

Department of Environmental Health, Boston University School of Public Health, Boston, Massachusetts 02118

KEY WORDS: workers' compensation, occupational safety, occupational health, medical costs, litigation

ABSTRACT

Studies suggest that income replacement is low for many workers with serious occupational injuries and illnesses. This review discusses three areas that hold promise for raising benefits to workers while reducing workers' compensation costs to employers: improving safety, containing medical costs, and reducing litigation.

In theory, workers' compensation increases the costs to employers of injuries and so provides incentives to improve safety. Yet, taken as a whole, research does not provide convincing evidence that workers' compensation reduces injury rates. Moreover, unlike safety and health regulation, workers' compensation focuses the attention of employers on individual workers. High costs may lead employers to discourage claims and litigate when claims are filed.

Controlling medical costs can reduce workers' compensation costs. Most studies, however, have focused on costs and have not addressed the effectiveness of medical care or patient satisfaction. Research also has shown that workers' compensation systems can reduce the need for litigation. Without litigation, benefits can be delivered more quickly and at lower costs.

INTRODUCTION

Over the past 25 years, workers' compensation has moved from an issue unknown to governors and legislators to a central focus of public debate in

189

many states. In the 1970s, legislative changes focused on improving coverage of workers and conditions, the adequacy of benefits, and the effective delivery of these benefits. A prime mover was the report of the National Commission on State Workmen's Compensation Laws (57), created by the Occupational Safety and Health Act of 1970. The National Commission's report described deficiencies in and made recommendations for improving workers' compensation systems (57). In the decade that followed, many states changed their statutes, increasing coverage and raising benefits. In 1972, the 50 states complied, on average, with 6.8 of the 19 essential recommendations of the National Commission. By 1980, they had moved to complying with an average of 12.0 of these recommendations (23).

During the past decade, the public policy discussion has changed from delivering benefits to containing costs. Between 1972 and 1992, the costs of workers' compensation rose from $6 billion to $62 billion (24), an annual rate of growth of 12.5 percent, with workers' compensation costs going from 1.1 percent to 2.6 percent of payroll.

As employers became aware of the substantial growth in costs, they increasingly looked for ways to reduce them. One obvious way is to lobby for limits on benefits or on compensable conditions, and some states have recently legislated such cutbacks (69). But there are other methods of reducing costs, more consistent with the goals established by Congress in the Occupational Safety and Health Act of 1970 for "an adequate, prompt, and equitable system of compensation." This review explores some of these other options.

First, prevention of occupational injuries and illnesses reduces the need for workers' compensation benefits, lowering costs without reducing benefit levels. This article reviews evidence about the impact of workers' compensation on safety. Unfortunately, we find little evidence that workers' compensation provides employers with incentives to improve safety. This suggests that government officials look elsewhere for policies to reduce injury and illness rates.

Second, if workers' compensation systems provide benefits at lower cost, expenditures can be reduced without cutting benefits. Over the past 20 years, medical costs in workers' compensation have been rising rapidly. Workers' compensation systems can look for ways to reduce these costs without sacrificing the quality of care. We find evidence that managed care may reduce costs in workers' compensation, but mixed evidence about the success of fee schedules. Overall, research does not support the contention that employer choice of medical providers reduces medical costs, and virtually no research addresses how cost-control affects the quality of care and patient satisfaction.

Litigation also can generate unnecessary costs. Workers' compensation systems were designed to replace common-law liability suits with systems that rendered attorney representation superfluous. However, data suggest that litigation is a substantial and growing aspect of workers' compensation. We review evidence about the causes of litigation in workers' compensation.

Finally, even in a cost-conscious environment, the adequacy and equity of workers' compensation systems remain important issues. We examine how benefits vary among states, among injuries of different severity, and among types of injuries and illnesses. We should find adequate replacement of lost earnings in these categories. Yet, the picture is far from ideal. Benefits vary greatly among states, and the most serious injuries and illnesses are the least well compensated. This finding supports the search for reforms that provide a better match between income losses and benefits.

INCOME BENEFITS: A BRIEF OVERVIEW

Workers' compensation provides income benefits, medical payments, and rehabilitation payments to workers injured on the job and their families. In the United States, each state has its own system with its own statute, regulations, and administration. Federal systems cover federal employees, longshoremen and harbor workers, and workers employed in the District of Columbia.

Besides benefits to families of fatally injured workers, workers' compensation pays four types of income benefits, distinguished by whether the worker's loss is temporary or permanent and whether the loss is partial or total. Temporary total disability benefits cover income losses when injured workers are off work during their healing period. Temporary partial disability benefits cover income losses during the healing period when workers take lower-paying jobs or work part-time.

Most injured workers fully recover from their injuries and return to their preinjury jobs. But some injured workers never completely recover: They remain permanently impaired. The American Medical Association defines impairment as "the loss of, loss of use of, or derangement of any body part, system, or function" (1, p. 236). One possible consequence of impairment is disability, that is a reduction in the ability to earn wages.

If a worker is deemed permanently unable to work, states pay permanent total disability benefits. State workers' compensation programs treat other injuries with permanent effects in different ways. Some states base benefits on impairment, providing permanent partial benefits based on an *impairment* rating, a measure of functional losses, between one to 100 percent. Other states use a *disability* rating, estimating loss of earning capacity, again as a percentage. Still other states use the difference between current earnings and preinjury earnings to calculate benefits; these are called *wage-loss* systems.

INJURY AND ILLNESS PREVENTION

A principal stated goal of workers' compensation is influencing employers to provide safer working conditions. Given the limitations of regulatory enforcement by the Occupational Safety and Health Administration (OSHA) (67), workers' compensation has been suggested as an alternative to regulation. On the other hand, if both programs are very limited in their impacts, we should look to other approaches to provide the desired improvement in workplace safety (4, 14).

In theory, workers' compensation provides safety incentives to employers because it requires them to pay substantial benefits to injured workers. Because injuries and illnesses are more expensive with workers' compensation than without, employers benefit more from safety activities and, in theory, invest more in hazard reduction, decreasing the number of occupational injuries and illnesses. The extent of these impacts depends on several factors.

Factors Affecting Safety Incentives

SELF-INSURANCE AND EXPERIENCE RATING   Russell (67) pointed out that insurance arrangements can attenuate the relationship between benefit payments and the employer's costs, diluting safety incentives. The premiums of very large employers closely reflect recent injury costs through self-insurance (where the employer directly pays benefits) or, when they purchase insurance, experience rating or retrospective rating[1] (33, 73). Yet, the sensitivity of premiums to injury costs varies inversely with size, and the smallest employers pay a fixed premium that depends on their industry, but not on their own injury experience. If they improve safety, their premiums do not fall; and if they become less safe, their premiums do not rise. Because their costs are insensitive to benefit payments, workers' compensation provides minimal safety incentives to smaller employers (67)—where most workers and most injuries occur.

HAZARD WAGES   Economists have suggested that without workers' compensation employers still would pay at least part of the costs of occupational injuries, in the form of hazard wages. If workers are well informed and have choices between safer and less-safe jobs, they will demand hazard pay to work in less-safe jobs. Hazard wages reflect the risk of lost wages and medical expenses and in part cover the "pain and suffering" that accompany injuries and illnesses.

Controlling for education, experience, and other labor-market characteristics, research finds that workers receive hazard wages for safety risks

---

[1]For the rest of this review, "experience rating" will refer to any method of determining premiums based on past expereince.

(44, 75). Yet this is not so for risks of chronic occupational diseases (7). And it is unlikely that hazard wages fully reflect the costs of injuries or illnesses.

Where they are present, hazard wages provide incentives to employers to improve workplace safety. If employers improve safety, they can pay lower hazard wages, offsetting safety costs.

But in some situations, the interaction of hazard wages and workers' compensation coverage could *reduce* workplace safety (68). Without workers' compensation insurance, employers in dangerous industries might pay substantial hazard wages, providing incentives to improve safety. Workers' compensation covers much of workers' out-of-pocket injury costs, reducing their demand for hazard wages, and making the employer's wage costs less responsive to injury rates (73, 76). Workers' compensation premiums of smaller employers are insensitive to injury rates, so their overall incentive to invest in safety declines.

PROBABILITY OF COMPENSATION   If workers' compensation is to provide financial incentives to eliminate hazards, employers must pay benefits when workers become sick or injured. This is a reasonable assumption for most workplace injuries. However, few cases of chronic occupational diseases are compensated (19, 36). When compensation is paid, it is long after exposure, and the responsible managers are unlikely to be held accountable (40). In this case, safety incentives cannot be substantial.

Evidence about Safety Impacts of Workers' Compensation

INCOME BENEFITS AND SAFETY   Table 1 summarizes sixteen studies of the impact of workers' compensation on safety.[2] These studies generally focus on income benefit levels. As benefit levels rise, workers' compensation payments per injury rise. Employers' costs become more responsive to injury rates, providing an additional incentive to improve safety conditions. Most studies find that reported injuries increase or remain unchanged when benefit levels rise.

The studies use diverse data sources and methods. Nine of the sixteen studies in Table 1 rely on injury data collected by or reportable to the Bureau of Labor Statistics (BLS) of the US Department of Labor. Employers report annually the total number of injuries and the number of injuries involving one or more days lost from work. Four of the studies use workers' compensation claim data to measure safety. Two rely on self-reported workers' compensation claim information, one from the Current Population Survey and one from the Panel

---

[2]This review focuses on injury rates, not days lost from work, as the measure of safety.

Table 1 Studies of the impact of workers' compensation on injuries

Study	Injury measure	Source of data	Unit of observation	Measure of workers' compensation benefits	Association of higher benefits to injury rates	How employer size affects the impact of benefits on injury rates
Chelius (a) (29) (b) (30)	Injuries per 100 full-time workers	Injuries: BLS,[a] all injuries and injuries with lost workdays per 100 full-time workers	Two-digit SIC[a] manufacturing industries (a) in 36 states, 1972–75, 1482 observations (b) in 28 states, 1972–78, 1967 observations	Estimate of average proportion of wages replaced in industry and state by temporary total disability benefits	(a) Frequency of injuries rose, and lost-workday rate did not change (b) both rates increased	Not tested
Butler (26)	Workers' compensation claim rates in South Carolina	South Carolina labor department and workers' compensation agency	South Carolina: 15 industries, 1940–71, 468 observations	Average real annual indemnity payments per worker: temporary total, permanent partial, permanent total, and fatality claims	Using a principal-components benefit measure, all injury rates but temporary total increased	Not tested
Butler & Worrall (27)	Rates of workers' compensation claims	National Council on Compensation Insurance, temporary total, minor and major permanent partial claims	35 States, 1972–78	Average benefit per claim within each state for each type of claim	Injury rates generally increased or did not change	
Chelius & Smith (32)	Difference between large and small firms in injuries per 100 full-time workers, by industry	BLS, injuries with lost workdays	15 Two-digit manufacturing industries in 37 states, 1979, 305 observations	Temporary total disability statutory payment at industry average wage	5 of 60 estimates show significant reductions at p < .05; 32 of 60 show reductions	Little or no impact detected

Study	Dependent variable	Data	Benefit measure	Result	Firm size effect
Robertson & Keeve (62)	Number of injuries reportable to BLS, number of sprains and strains, and number of "objective" injuries	Three metal fabrication plants in three states	Worker-years of exposure, by individual and department, 2700 workers, 1973–80	State maximum temporary total disability rate	Injuries grew; effect stronger for sprains and strains than for "objective" injuries	Not tested
Bartel & Thomas (6)	Injuries per 100 full-time workers	Injuries: BLS, injuries with lost workdays Industries: OSHA[a], BLS Employment and Earnings, Bureau of the Census	Three-digit SIC manufacturing, averaged over 22 states, 1972–78	Expected benefit per claim for each three-digit industry	Injury rate increased, but change not significant	Not tested
Leigh (53)	Individual's receipt of workers' compensation benefits	Panel Study of Income Dynamics, 1977–79	11,889 person-years, interviewed in 1977–79	State's temporary total disability formula applied to worker's wage	Probability of receiving benefits increased, but impact not significant	Not tested
Ruser (63)	Injuries per 100 full-time workers	Injuries: BLS, nonfatal injuries with lost workdays, all reported injuries Size: County Business Patterns	25 three-digit industries by state, 1972–79, 3243 observations	Measure of average real temporary total disability benefit paid, using state wage distribution and benefit formula	Both total injuries and lost-workday injury rates increased	Increase in injury rates smaller in larger firms

Table 1 (Continued)

	Injury measure	Source of data	Unit of observation	Measure of workers' compensation benefits	Association of higher benefits to injury rates	How employer size affects the impact of benefits on injury rates
Chelius & Kavanaugh (31)	Frequency of workers' compensation claims with lost time and of claims with more than seven days' lost time	Workers' compensation claim files of two community colleges in New Jersey	24 quarters at each of two colleges, 1978–84	Temporary disability benefit levels	Rates for both types of injuries were higher before benefits cut by 30%	Self-insurance associated with fewer accepted workers' compensation claims
Worrall & Butler (79)	Workers' compensation claim rates in South Carolina: temporary total, permanent partial, and all claims with income benefits	South Carolina labor department and workers' compensation agency	South Carolina: 15 industries, 1940–71, 468 observations	Expected workers' compensation benefits for the average worker	Permanent partial rates rose; other rates rose, but not significantly	Impact on permanent partial rates lower in industries with larger average employment; impact on other rates lower, but not significantly
Moore & Viscusi (55)	Fatalities per 100,000 workers	Injuries: NIOSH National Traumatic Occupational Fatality surveillance system Individuals: Panel Study of Income Dynamics	Injuries: 7 one-digit industries by state, 1980–84 Firm size: Census, one-digit industries by state, 1982 Other data: 1173 individuals, 1982	State maximum temporary total disability rate	Fatality rates fell	Reduction in fatality rates greater in larger firms (significant in three of four specifications)
Krueger (52)	Probability of filing a workers' compensation claim	Current Population Survey	19,082 individuals, 1984–85	State maximum temporary total disability rate	Probability of filing increased	Not tested

Study						
Ruser (a) 64 (b) 65	Injuries per 100 full-time workers	(a) BLS, injuries with lost workdays (b) BLS, injuries at four levels of severity (a) and (b) BLS Current Employment Survey, other data	(a) 2788 (b) 2798 manufacturing establishments, 1979–84, (a) 16,728 (b) 16,788 observations	(a) State maximum temporary total disability rate (b) Estimate of average proportion of wages replaced by temporary total disability benefits	(a) Rates generally increased (b) Rates declined for fatal injuries, but increased for others	(a) Greatest increase in smallest workplaces, no increase in largest (b) For injuries with and without lost workdays, larger increase in smaller workplaces; no size impact for fatal injuries
Chelius & Smith (34)	Injuries per 100 full-time workers	BLS, injuries with lost workdays	Washington vs. other states, 1979–81, by three-digit SIC and 7 size classes	Not used	Not tested	Experience-rating of small firms in Washington did not reduce their injury rates relative to large firms

[a] BLS: US Department of Labor, Bureau of Labor Statistics, SIC: Standard Industrial Classification, OSHA: US Occupational Safety and Health Administration

Study of Income Dynamics. Another study uses data from the National Traumatic Occupational Fatality surveillance system (50), which is based on death certificates.

Most of the studies are ecological, relying on average injury rates by state (27), by industry (6), by industry within a state (26, 79), or by industry and state (29, 30, 32, 34, 63). Three examined injury rates by workplace (31, 64, 65), one used injury data by state and industry, attributing these risks to individuals (55), while three others used data on individuals (52, 53, 62). Most of the studies use least squares regression to fit the data, although one (52) uses probit estimates. One author, Ruser (63–65), uses methods designed for count data (number of injuries).

Only one of the nine studies using BLS injury rates (64) found an inverse relationship between injury rates and benefit levels. The six studies in Table 1 using workers' compensation claim rates all failed to show a safety impact of benefit levels. Two studies, using data on individuals, also could not find a safety impact (52, 53). In fact, these studies generally found that injury rates rose when benefits increased.

Because these studies rely on reported injuries, we cannot draw the firm conclusion that higher benefits lead to less-safe working conditions. This is because benefit levels affect injury reporting. When benefit levels rise and paying benefits becomes more expensive, we expect employers to discourage the filing of workers' compensation claims more frequently and to encourage earlier return to work (31, 68). At the same time, workers lose less income if they miss work, so they may report more injuries and stay off work longer (45, 46). Even if injury rates fell as benefits rose, reported injury rates might rise.

EXPERIENCE RATING, SELF-INSURANCE, AND SAFETY   Recognizing this ambiguity, some researchers have looked for ways to minimize the impact of reporting on measures of the safety impact of workers' compensation. One method compares the effect of benefits on injuries among employer-size groups, looking for an "experience-rating" effect.

The impact of benefit changes on workers' incentives to report injuries should be similar in smaller and larger firms. Small firms are not experience rated, and thus lack incentives to improve safety when benefits arise. Differences in the response of small and large firms to benefit changes thus should reflect the impact of benefits on injury rates for large firms. As benefits rise, we expect to find that injury rates in large firms decline relative to those in small firms.

Two studies by Chelius & Smith did not find an experience-rating effect (32, 34). On the other hand, studies by Worrall & Butler (79), Moore & Viscusi (55), and Ruser (63, 64) found experience-ratings effects. As benefits rose, injury rates in large firms fell relative to those in small firms. Ruser's most recent study (65) had similar findings for nonfatal injuries with lost workdays and for injuries without lost workdays. However, he did not find an employment-size relationship for fatal injury rates.

A related study suggests that the measured impact of experience-rating on safety could reflect reporting changes by employers and not real changes in injury rates (31). Two community colleges more aggressively challenged the compensability of claims after switching to self-insurance. Self-insurance tied workers' compensation costs more closely to injury costs, leading employers to report fewer injuries. Similarly, when benefits rise, experience-rated employers may discourage claim-filing and reject more workers' compensation claims. Spieler (69) notes that, if employers initiate aggressive loss-control programs, injured workers may fear retaliation and avoid filing injury claims. Rising costs also may cause employers to institute safety contests with group rewards for injury-free periods. Pressure from fellow workers may then decrease reporting by injured workers. Other studies also have found that financial incentives affect employer reporting of injuries (66) and hazardous conditions (16). Employers who deny workers' compensation claims also are unlikely to report the injuries to the BLS.

EVIDENCE FROM "OBJECTIVE" INJURIES   To control for reporting bias, some studies focus on injury types that are less likely to be subject to systematic reporting bias. Robertson & Keeve (62) compared the impact of benefit levels on sprains and strains to the impact on more "objective" injuries, like lacerations and fractures. They found, in both cases, that reported injuries increased with increasing benefits, although the effect was stronger for sprains and strains.

Other researchers have used a similar approach, focusing on fatalities— clear-cut events, and injured workers are unlikely to overreport them. Still, Butler (26) estimated benefit impacts on fatal injury rates and found that benefit increases were associated with higher fatality rates. On the other hand, Moore & Viscusi (55) and Ruser (65) concluded that increases in workers' compensation benefits reduced fatality rates. Moore & Viscusi used a measure of injury rates only at a very aggregated (one-digit) industry level. Also, in Ruser's 1993 study, the estimated impact on fatalities did not decline with employment size (65). This is inconsistent with experience-rating and self-insurance as mechanisms that presumably generate safety incentives. If these function as expected, the sensitivity of premiums to injury experience should increase with size.

Few studies have found evidence for a safety effect, and, where such evidence exists, it can be explained by incentives for employers to discourage and contest expensive injuries. In all the studies to date, the investigators did not control the collection of injury data and thus could not distinguish safety effects from reporting effects. Attempts to control statistically for reporting bias have had only limited success.

Despite many studies addressing this question, we cannot be confident that workers' compensation reduces injury rates, even for large experience-rated or self-insured firms. This is puzzling, since workers' compensation has become a significant and growing business cost. Several studies provide evidence that organizational and managerial shortcomings block employers from taking action that would be in their self-interest. A survey of employers suggests that they rarely know the size of their workers' compensation premiums (49). Another study showed that risk managers and engineering departments communicated poorly (40). Sometimes, large companies may treat workers' compensation costs as fixed overhead. Employers may assume that "accident-prone" workers cause injuries or that many reported injuries are fraudulent (69). Still, ignorance and inefficient behavior are less than satisfactory explanations of the limited impact of workers' compensation on safety behavior. Perhaps further study will conclude that the net financial incentives of workers' compensation costs are smaller than we believe them to be.

MEDICAL CARE AND MEDICAL COSTS

Despite the widespread interest in the cost and quality of medical care, researchers only recently have begun to study this issue in the workers' compensation setting. Studies of medical care in other settings have relevance to workers' compensation, but some distinctive features suggest that behavior in workers' compensation may be quite different. In workers' compensation:

- Medical care is fully covered; deductibles and copayments cannot be used to control utilization.
- The employer or insurer pays both income and medical benefits.
- Physicians often provide information that determines income benefits, including whether an injury is compensable when a worker is ready to return to work, and assessments of permanent impairment.
- Because of the physician's role in determining income benefits, patient-physician communication may be impaired, affecting the quality of care.
- Some injuries are litigated, which can interfere with medical treatment.

Workers' Compensation Medical Costs

From 1980 to 1985, workers' compensation medical costs rose at an average annual rate of 14.7 percent, compared to an annual increase of 9.8 percent outside workers' compensation (15, 17). Between 1985 and 1990, this trend continued (70).

A study of medical costs in Minnesota provides additional evidence that workers' compensation medical costs are higher than nonworkers' compensation costs. It analyzed a matched sample of claims from Minnesota's largest workers' compensation insurer and major nonworkers' compensation insurer (71). Workers' compensation treatment averaged 2.4 times as expensive as nonworkers' compensation treatment. Using regression analysis to control for the quantity of medical services used, workers' compensation charges remained over twice those outside workers' compensation. A reanalysis of these data came to the same conclusion and found charges for specific services to be higher in workers' compensation (5). This suggests that prices, not utilization, caused most of the disparities in costs between the two systems.

Another study reported substantially higher medical costs in workers' compensation claims than in group health claims (37). This study of claims from Florida, Illinois, Oregon, and Pennsylvania analyzed treatment costs, using regression analysis to control for state, year, diagnosis, and cost-containment controls used in workers' compensation. It found workers' compensation costs between 1.65 and 2.3 times group health costs. Controlling further for provider mix, number of outpatient service dates, and length of hospital stays, the difference between workers' compensation and group health disappeared. From this, the authors concluded that the differences between workers' compensation and group health costs were caused by greater utilization of medical services and not by higher prices.

Controlling for gender, age, utilization measures, case mix, and severity, another study estimated that workers' compensation prices in California were 25 percent *below* nonworkers' compensation prices (59). Nevertheless, workers' compensation medical costs per episode averaged 21 percent higher than group medical costs after adjusting for case mix, which suggests that higher utilization caused the difference in overall costs. The stringent workers' compensation fee schedule in effect in California may in part explain why workers' compensation prices there are lower than group health prices.

While the three studies disagree about the relative importance of prices and utilization, they agree that workers' compensation medical care is much more expensive.

Workers' Compensation Medical Cost Control

Over the past several years, many states have adopted one or more methods of containing medical costs. In the year before July 1, 1991, 15 states added one or more new cost-containment initiatives or were developing them (18). In the next 15 months, 19 states had added or were developing additional cost-containment activities (70).

CHOICE OF PROVIDER   Employers and insurers support employer choice of medical provider and managed care to achieve control over medical-care costs.

Organized labor, on the other hand, supports control over medical care by the injured worker. Each side has argued that its preferred option is more effective in producing high-quality care and low costs.

A 1989 report of preliminary results (35) found higher medical costs among states that allowed workers to choose their own medical providers. In another (74), Victor & Fleischman reported that changes to employee choice in Illinois and Texas led to increased medical costs.

Several studies, however, have come to the opposite conclusion. One (17) looked at eight states that changed their laws about provider choice during the 1965–1985 period. Except for one state, Illinois, no major changes in medical cost growth occurred when states changed their laws regarding provider choice. Pozzebon (60, 61) found that, controlling for other factors, states limiting employee choice of provider had average medical payments 10 to 15 percent higher than other states. A study by Appel & Durbin found analogous results. In states with employee choice of provider, claims tended to be considerably shorter and thus less costly (2).

The debate about this issue transcends interest in containing medical costs (42, 43). When they choose the medical provider, employers and insurers have a greater say about the provider's behavior in litigated cases. In many workers' compensation systems, treating providers furnish information about when a worker is ready to return to work (and temporary disability benefits may be terminated) or the worker's level of impairment (affecting permanent disability benefits). Because provider choice can affect income benefits, it would be in contention even if everybody agreed it had no impact on medical costs.

MEDICAL FEE SCHEDULES   The use of medical fee schedules in workers' compensation has engendered less controversy. Yet evidence of effectiveness is also in dispute. Preliminary results cited above (35), Borba (21), and Levy & Miller (54) all found lower medical costs among states with fee schedules. However, another study showed that, in 1980–1985, there was no correlation between the growth of medical costs and the use of medical fee schedules (17). Controlling for other factors, Pozzebon did not find that average growth rates of medical costs in fee-schedule states were lower than in other states during 1979–1987 (60, 61).

Another study of workers' compensation fee schedules helps to explain these seemingly inconsistent results. This study (41) found substantial variability among states in the stringency and coverage of medical fee schedules, suggesting that we should not expect similar effects from all fee schedules. In the four most restrictive states, fee-schedule limits averaged between 54 and 64 percent of nonworkers' compensation medical charges in 1992. In the four least restrictive states, they averaged 103 to 112 percent of nonworkers' compensation charges. If a fee schedule allows fees above typical charges, it does not constrain medical costs. In fact, providers billing below the fee schedule may use it as a signal to raise fees. The study also found that the percentage of workers' compensation charges covered by fee schedules varied from a low of 57.5 percent to a high of 100 percent (41).

MANAGED CARE   In recent years, states have begun to look to managed care to reduce workers' compensation medical costs. Oregon undertook the earliest and most extensive move in this direction in 1991. If an employer in Oregon has designated an approved managed-care organization, Oregon requires injured workers to receive medical care from the managed-care organization in most circumstances. In 1992, Minnesota established a similar program, and the legislature in North Dakota required its exclusive state fund to establish a managed-care program. The legislatures in Montana and Ohio enacted laws in 1993 to require copayments from workers who elect to receive treatment outside designated managed-care organizations. These states previously allowed injured workers the initial choice of medical provider.

Despite this growing activity, little research has assessed the impact of managed care on workers' compensation costs. A 1991 study compared the workers' compensation experience of postal employees in Massachusetts enrolled in a health maintenance organization (HMO) with those in a fee-for-service plan (80). It found lower medical payments and somewhat lower income benefits among the HMO enrollees. Using analysis of variance to control for age, job category, and injury type, the reduction in medical costs was significant (p.<05).

The HMO was paid on a fee-for-service basis for workers' compensation injuries. Still, providers at the HMO continued to give lower-cost care than their fee-for-service counterparts. This suggests that the more cost-conscious practice style of the HMO carried over to the fee-for-service workers' compensation services. Additional fees for workers' compensation services increased the income of the HMO, so this arrangement provided incentives to maximize the number of conditions classified as work related (39). Yet workers' compensation claim rates were slightly lower among the fee-for-service enrollees. Organizational financial incentives did not affect the behavior of the HMO's providers.

A pilot program providing workers' compensation managed care to state government employees in south Florida also appears to have reduced medical costs. Beginning in 1991, the State of Florida paid a fixed monthly premium per enrolled worker to an HMO providing workers' compensation medical care. Costs were tracked, and the state and the HMO shared equally in any surplus or deficit, providing the HMO an incentive to reduce costs.

An evaluation (3) compared payments to the HMO with those to fee-for-service providers[3]. Medical payments were almost 60 percent lower in the HMO group. Accounting for HMO administrative fees and controlling for differences in demographic and injury characteristics, savings remained close to 50 percent. Payments of income benefits also were reduced substantially. Consistent with other research on HMOs, hospital costs were reduced more than physician costs.

The authors caution against generalizing from their findings. The pilot nature of this study may have induced a "Hawthorne effect," leading the HMO to watch costs more carefully than it might if providing ongoing care. Also, south Florida is an area of high medical costs, possibly with more leeway to generate savings than other areas.

We draw the tentative conclusion that managed care in workers' compensation can achieve substantial cost-savings. More research in different settings and over longer periods will clarify the size of these savings.

Medical Care Quality and Patient Satisfaction

Few studies address the public health and labor union concerns about the noncost implications of medical cost controls. Two exceptions highlight the importance of these issues. The Florida pilot study included a survey of workers' satisfaction with their medical care. The respondents in the HMO program were less satisfied than the fee-for-service control group with their doctor's treatment, the medical tests they were given, and the appointment scheduling (3). The response rate to this survey was only 23 per cent.

Another study shows that reducing medical care for injured workers delays return to work and increases income losses (38). This implies that single-minded attention to medical costs is misplaced. How cost-control methods affect outcomes remains an important question.

National Health Reform and Workers' Compensation

The discussion about reform of the US health care system has engendered a debate over the relationship of workers' compensation to general health care. Much of this debate centers on whether integration of workers' compensation medical care into the general health care delivery system would increase or decrease costs. Baker & Krueger (5) reanalyzed the Minnesota data described above (71), and they come to the same conclusion—that workers' compensation medical prices are more than twice prices outside workers' compensation. The authors suggest that shifting to an integrated system would eliminate price differences between the currently separate systems and thus reduce workers' compensation costs by half or more. They also suggest other, more speculative,

---

[3]Florida also developed a second pilot using a preferred provider organization (PPO). This pilot used less-comparable groups, which made differences hard to interpret (3).

sources of savings, including easier use of managed care and utilization review, reduced administrative and legal costs, and less medical testing for legal purposes.

Even in an integrated system, many important differences will remain. For example, litigation in workers' compensation will continue to complicate patient-physician communication, making treatment less effective and possibly more costly. Providers will still spend more time on workers' compensation claims because of special reporting requirements, and they will test more often to provide information needed to determine compensability or the level of income benefits. And, finally, it is very unlikely that copayments and deductibles will be introduced into workers' compensation. We cannot therefore expect the entire difference in costs to evaporate in an integrated system.

Grannemann & Victor (48) have pointed out that integrated systems would separate responsibility for paying income and medical benefits. They note that medical providers in health plans, chosen by workers, may lean toward allowing workers more time off than would providers chosen by employers or insurers. Of course, this would only be relevant in the states that now restrict the worker's choice of provider. Another concern is that capitated medical-care plans, intent on holding down medical costs, might forgo medical treatment that would accelerate return to work. This might harm both the worker and the employer. Of course, it is also possible that capitated plans or standardized treatment protocols might eliminate unnecessary and expensive procedures that both increase medical costs and delay return to work.

Integration would affect the choice of provider, now governed by state workers' compensation laws. In employer-choice states, employers would lose some control over providers, while in employee-choice states the reverse would occur. Both sides understand that choosing the provider may give them added say in medical decisions that affect nonmedical outcomes—in particular, income benefits to injured workers. The AFL-CIO has supported integration, viewing it as more like employee choice than employer choice (42, 43). Also, integration might block the move in some "employee-choice" states to workers' compensation managed-care organizations chosen by employers and insurers.

Finally, integration of workers' compensation medical care into a national health care system offers unique opportunities to provide improved surveillance of occupational injury and illness and data for research on medical care in workers' compensation. Currently, there is little standardization of medical data in workers' compensation. A national, integrated system could require standard billing forms, including uniformly coded information on occupation, industry, employer, diagnosis, and procedure. To the extent possible, these could be stored electronically, rather than on paper. Analyses of these data could identify industries where workers face excess risks. They also could provide data to compare prices and utilization in and outside workers' compensation.

LITIGATION

Before workers' compensation, injured workers and their families generally bore the costs of their work-related injuries. To get compensation, workers had the difficult task of proving in a court of law that employer negligence caused their injuries. If workers won negligence suits, payments were made long after they were injured, and a large amount of each settlement was diverted for legal fees. Today, workers with minor injuries covered by workers' compensation generally can expect to receive payments promptly and without contest. Less than 10 percent of claims for occupational injuries are contested.

Causes and Effects of Litigation

Employers and insurers can contest workers' compensation claims because they do not consider the injury to be work-related, for example, or because the workers want greater benefits than the employers or insurers are willing to pay. In most injury cases the employer or insurance carrier has little incentive to contest because proof of eligibility is easy, and the potential gain to the insurer of postponing or eliminating small payments is not enough to offset the legal costs of pursuing a claim.

For expensive injury claims like permanent disability and death claims, insurance companies are much more likely to deny claims or contest benefits. Workers, through their attorneys, more frequently maintain that they deserve additional benefits. In most states, claims for permanent disability and death are litigated more than half the time, compared to less than 5 percent of claims for temporary disability (56). Employers and insurers also contest claims for chronic occupational disease and cumulative trauma much more frequently than claims for injuries (8, 12, 19).

Studies of litigation of permanent partial disability low-back injuries have shown that states vary considerably in how frequently these claims are litigated. In Maryland and New Jersey, workers retain attorneys in more than 90 percent of these claims. However, attorney representation in Oregon and Wisconsin is much less common (20). Information from workers' compensation insurers shows considerable variation among states in attorney involvement, and also suggests that litigation became more frequent during the 1980s (Table 2) (56).

Litigation imposes substantial costs on injured workers, employers, and insurers, and administrative costs on workers' compensation systems. In litigated permanent disability claims, these added costs absorb about one third of income benefits (13). Savings from reducing litigation could be used to improve benefits for injured workers or to reduce insurance premiums paid by

Table 2 Litigation rate, claims with income benefits, insured employers

State	Percent of claims with attorney involvement		
	1980	1985	1989
Florida	6.9	8.2	16.0
Georgia	9.5	14.9	27.6
Illinois	23.1	23.8	29.5
Kentucky	11.9	10.7	12.0
Maine	14.1	17.1	12.7
Massachusetts	11.3	14.4	20.5
Michigan	23.8	15.0	8.8
Minnesota	4.5	7.6	7.3
Pennsylvania	3.1	4.3	5.2
Average	12.1	13.0	17.1

Source: National Council on Compensation Insurance (56)

employers. Litigation also delays the delivery of benefits, often by more than a year.

System and Insurer Factors Affecting Litigation

Studies of permanently disabling back injuries in two litigious states and two less-litigious states identified features that can cause high litigation rates (20). Laws and regulations in the litigious states do not provide clear guidance about benefits owed to injured workers. Workers' compensation agencies in these states do not provide injured workers with information about the benefits they are entitled to, and they do not ensure that insurers and employers pay permanent partial disability benefits in a timely manner. Also, if claims are litigated, adjudicators tend to "split the difference" between disparate medical assessments by defense and claimant experts. In these states, attorneys provide workers with valuable information and services. Without opinions from physicians chosen by their attorneys, injured workers must rely only on the assessments of partisan defense physicians, accepting a lower payment—or none at all.

Less-litigious systems provide employers and insurers with reasonable certainty about what they owe and provide injured workers with information about the benefits they should receive. Practices and rules encourage the use of nonpartisan experts, typically treating physicians, in the evaluation process. With more than one physician opinion, adjudicators do not split the difference, typically relying on the treating physician's opinion. Also, the workers' compensation agency provides information to injured workers and ensures that insurers and employers pay permanent partial disability benefits on time. When insurers and employers make timely payments of amounts that workers expect, workers feel well treated and their cases are resolved promptly and without litigation.

Another study, based on surveys of workers with permanent disabilities in California, provides complementary information about how insurance company behavior can affect the propensity of workers to hire attorneys (22). Using probit regression, this study estimated the impact of injury characteristics, worker characteristics, benefits, and perceptions of insurer behavior on attorney representation. It found that when workers believed that the insurer kept them well informed or were satisfied with the insurers' overall handling of the claim, they were much less likely than otherwise to hire an attorney. Still, from these data, we cannot tell to what extent workers' satisfaction reflected insurer behavior or workers' attitudes.

These studies suggest that states can design workers' compensation systems to provide an environment that reduces litigation without jeopardizing the protection that attorneys afford injured workers.

INCOME BENEFITS UNDER WORKERS' COMPENSATION

Separate workers' compensation systems in fifty states, the District of Columbia, and two federal jurisdictions have established their own benefit structures. Injured workers should face similar benefits wherever they are injured. Yet statutory income benefits vary considerably, suggesting that identical workers with identical injuries can expect to receive different benefits in different jurisdictions.

After comparing overall benefits among jurisdictions, we turn to measures of benefit adequacy for the two most common types of injuries involving lost earnings: temporary total and permanent partial disabilities. For each, we review knowledge about the proportion of lost income replaced by workers' compensation benefits. For temporary disabilities, some states are more generous than others, but workers receiving workers' compensation income benefits typically recover between 80 and 100 percent of after-tax lost earnings. We use after-tax earnings because neither state nor federal income taxes apply to workers' compensation income benefits. Studies of replacement rates for permanently disabling injuries show that, on average, workers' compensation replaces a small proportion of earnings losses of permanently disabled workers. Some also raise the possibility that, among workers with permanent earnings losses, permanent disability benefits are distributed inequitably.

Table 3 Maximum weekly benefits for total disability: selected states (on January 1, 1994)

Jurisdiction	Fraction of workers' wage	Maximum weekly benefit
Arizona	2/3	328
Arkansas	2/3	267 (70% of SAWW)
California	2/3	366
Connecticut	3/4 of after-tax income	638 (SAWW)
Florida	2/3	444 (SAWW)
Georgia	2/3	250
Indiana	2/3	394
Iowa	4/5 of spendable earnings	797 (200% of SAWW)
Kentucky	2/3	394 (SAWW)
Louisiana	2/3	319 (75% of SAWW)
Michigan	4/5 of spendable earnings	441 (90% of SAWW)
Minnesota	2/3	508 (105% of SAWW)
Mississippi	2/3	244 (2/3 of SAWW)
North Carolina	2/3	466 (110% of SAWW)
Ohio	72% first 12 weeks, then 2/3	482 (SAWW)
Oklahoma	7/10	307 (3/4 of SAWW)
Oregon	2/3	479 (SAWW)
Pennsylvania	2/3	493 (SAWW)
Tennessee	2/3	356 (82% of SAWW)
Texas	7/10	466 (SAWW)
Washington	6/10 to 3/4[a]	517 (105% of SAWW)
West Virginia	7/10	420 (SAWW)

[a] Lower proportion if no dependents.
Key: SAWW = State's average weekly wage; NAWW = national average weekly wage.
Source: US Chamber of Commerce. (72).

Interstate Variation in Benefit Payments

Workers' compensation is a state program, and benefits differ substantially from state to state. One commonly used measure of benefit levels is the maximum weekly rate for temporary total disability (Table 3). Temporary disability benefits are calculated as a proportion (usually two thirds) of the worker's preinjury wage, up to a maximum weekly amount. By this measure, states exhibit considerable variation. In 1994, the lowest maximum weekly temporary disability benefits ($244 in Mississippi) were less than one third those in the most generous state ($797 in Iowa) (72). Statutory benefits for permanent disability exhibit similar variation.

Column 1 of Table 4 shows a broad measure of benefit levels, average workers' compensation benefits paid per worker annually (25). Benefits per worker range from a low of $177 in Indiana to a high of $712 in West Virginia. This measure captures variation in benefit levels, wage levels and injury frequency, and injury severity. Column 3 shows workers' compensation ben-

Table 4 Workers' compensation benefits paid in 1990, insured employers

| State | Average benefits paid per covered worker: 1990 | | Benefits as a percentage of wages | | | Ratio of benefits paid to lost wages[b] |
	Dollar amount 1.	As a per-cent of median state 2.	As a per-cent in state 3.	As a per-cent of median state 4.	Lost-workday rate[a] 5.	As a percent of median state 6.
Arizona	314	89	1.50	87	68.0	107
Arkansas	311	88	1.75	102	88.7	96
California	494	140	1.92	112	90.7	103
Connecticut	502	142	1.72	100	83.8	100
Florida	468	133	2.29	133	66.7	167
Indiana	177	50	0.82	48	76.0	53
Iowa	214	61	1.13	66	94.2	58
Kentucky	340	96	1.72	100	98.8	85
Louisiana	530	150	2.54	148	92.9	133
Michigan	353	100	1.38	80	109.9	61
Minnesota	318	90	1.39	81	79.9	85
North Carolina	179	51	0.91	53	62.5	71
Oklahoma	436	124	2.17	126	91.0	116
Oregon	515	146	2.46	143	98.5	122
Tennessee	304	86	1.51	88	76.4	96
Texas	645	183	2.84	165	115.5	120
West Virginia	712	202	3.45	201	105.4	159
Median state	353	100	1.72	100	90.7	100

Data in columns 1–4 from Burton & Schmidle (25).

[a] Calculated from data in columns 1 and 3 and lost workdays per 100 full-time equivalent workers; lost-workday data supplied to the author by Bureau of Labor Statistics, US Department of Labor.

[b] This rough approximation is calculated by the author, under the assumption of a 200-day work year as: (benefits/wages)/(annual lost workdays per worker/200).

efits as a proportion of covered wages. To facilitate comparison, this measure is presented as a proportion of the value for the median state in Column 4. Finally, Column 6 shows an estimate of benefits paid per dollar of lost wages—also as a proportion of the value for the median state. This measure is closest to a replacement rate, although it includes both medical and income benefits. It probably overestimates generosity in states with a greater proportion of severe injuries, because the lost-workday rate underestimates losses for severe injuries. Still, by this measure, the highest-benefit state is three times as generous as the lowest-benefit state.

Rankings of states vary for the different measures in Table 4, but they are quite different from those in Table 3. The two states with the highest maximum temporary disability rate are Iowa and Connecticut, but Iowa is very low and Connecticut is the median state based on the ratio of benefits paid to lost wages. Florida and Louisiana, the median states by temporary disability rate, are two of the highest using the ratio of benefits to lost wages.

Statutory benefit rates are not the only factors affecting the level of income replacement. States can vary in the probability that injured workers will be compensated, the typical duration of temporary disability benefits for similar injuries, or the probability that workers with similar injuries will receive permanent disability benefits, or the degree of permanent disability assigned to similar injuries.

We know that states vary widely in their propensity to pay permanent disability benefits. In recent years, 43 percent of compensated workers in California and 52 percent in Oklahoma received these benefits. In Alabama and Wisconsin, this proportion was 16 and 15 percent, respectively (57). If these states, all of which had three-day waiting periods, had similar distributions of injury severity, disparities would reflect the relative difficulty of qualifying for permanent disability benefits in Alabama and Wisconsin[4].

This considerable variation raises questions about the adequacy of benefits in different jurisdictions. None of the statistics presented above directly addresses this question, and only a few studies have done so. These studies have attempted to measure the replacement rate, the ratio of income benefits received by workers to their economic losses. Some have examined replacement rates for injuries involving only temporary total disability. Others have estimated replacement rates for the largest group of severe injuries, those involving permanent partial disability benefits.

Ideally, each study should address several important substantive aspects of the replacement rate. First, because workers' compensation income benefits are not taxed, the replacement rate should compare after-tax income losses with workers' compensation benefits. Second, lost income should include the value of fringe benefits foregone. For injuries involving permanent partial disability, estimates of lifetime earnings should be compared with estimates of lifetime benefits. Where possible, income benefits should be calculated net of litigation costs paid by the worker.

Studies have met these criteria to varying degrees, although none has accounted for loss of fringe benefits. All the statistical studies suffer from another limitation: Their samples do not include workers with permanent earnings losses who received no permanent disability benefits. For this reason, they overestimate average replacement rates.

---

[4]If time lost from work does not extend past a state's waiting period, workers' compensation does not reimburse lost wages. States with longer waiting periods pay income benefits for fewer minor injuries, so lost-time injuries are more severe, on average.

Studies in this area indicate workers' compensation replaces a reasonable proportion of lost wages for most workers with minor, temporarily disabling injuries. But permanently disabled workers fare much less well. Average replacement rates for chronic occupational diseases are even lower than those for severe injuries.

Replacement Rates for Temporary Total Disability

In a series of studies of temporary total disability, the Workers' Compensation Research Institute (WCRI) has used a computer model to develop a distribution of after-tax replacement rates based on the applicable workers' compensation statute, the wage distribution of covered workers, and the applicable state and federal tax laws (9, 76). Calculated replacement rates assume that all injured workers receive the appropriate workers' compensation payments and that only work-related injuries are compensated. They do not consider the impact of the waiting period, which would reduce the average replacement rate.

These studies conclude that temporary total disability benefits typically replaced between 80 and 100 percent of preinjury after-tax earnings. Most states provided this level of benefits to between 70 and 85 percent of injured workers. Of 21 states listed in recent comparisons, the WCRI model estimates that only Pennsylvania had a replacement rate over 100 percent for more than 25 percent of injured workers. Six of these 21 states (Arkansas, Georgia, Indiana, Louisiana, Mississippi, and Washington) had replacement rates below 80 percent for more than 25 percent of injured workers.

Replacement Rates for Permanent Partial Disability

A primary goal of workers' compensation is providing adequate benefits to seriously injured workers. However, the most recent published studies of replacement rates for severely injured workers cover injuries that occurred more than 20 years ago. Despite the lack of recent data, the qualitative conclusions of this research probably remain true today.

In a study of California workplace injuries during the 1950s, Cheit found considerable variation in replacement rates (28). He estimated that more than half of these workers received permanent disability benefits without any permanent earnings losses. For workers who experienced permanent income losses, however, permanent partial disability benefits typically replaced only a small fraction. For workers with ratings under 70 percent, benefits typically replaced less than 10 percent of losses. Benefits covered 36 percent of losses for workers with the highest disability ratings.

Berkowitz(10) calculated permanent partial disability benefits on the assumption that workers declared 50 percent disabled actually lost half their post-injury lifetime earnings. Using statutory benefits in effect for 1972, Berkowitz calculated the proportion of income losses replaced by permanent partial disability benefits for a 35-year-old worker with average wages. For 29 jurisdictions, the pretax replacement rate ranged between 12.9 percent and 25.9 percent.

Ginnold (47) studied workers in Wisconsin who had an occupational injury in 1968 resulting in permanent disability benefit payments. Permanent disability benefits averaged 16.4 percent or 24.6 percent of lifetime earnings losses, using five percent and ten percent discount rates, respectively.

In a study of people injured at work during 1968 in Florida, California, or Wisconsin, Berkowitz & Burton (11) calculated income benefits net of legal fees for 1968 through 1973. Pretax replacement rates in Wisconsin averaged 75 percent. In Florida they averaged 59 percent, whereas in California they were only 46 percent.

Replacement rates estimated by Berkowitz & Burton for permanently disabling injuries for 1968 in Wisconsin are much higher than those derived by Ginnold. Average benefits paid in the two studies were similar, but Ginnold calculated much higher future earnings, and thus higher earnings losses. The primary difference between the two estimates appears to be that Berkowitz & Burton focused only on the six years after the injury, whereas Ginnold projected earnings losses (but not benefits, which are nearly all paid by six years after injury) to the expected working life of the injured workers. In this light, the Berkowitz & Burton approach appears to overstate the replacement rate substantially.

Johnson et al (50) measured income replacement among workers with permanent impairment ratings of at least 10 percent. These workers were injured between 1968 and 1970 in California, Florida, New York, Washington, or Wisconsin. The authors calculated after-tax replacement rates, focusing on workers whose earnings losses were at least $500[5]. About one third of the injured workers in this study suffered earnings losses less than $500, averaging a $45 loss. This group received average benefits of $163.

Overall, studies show that workers suffering large income losses have had little of their income losses replaced by workers' compensation. Still, two studies (28, 51) showed that some injured workers with little or no permanent income loss received permanent disability benefits.

Workers' compensation almost certainly replaces an even smaller proportion of income losses for occupational diseases than for injuries. Occupational disease claims tend to be litigated more frequently, so legal costs (which the worker usually pays) are higher. This reduces the net benefit to the injured worker. Also, workers file claims for only a small proportion of occupational diseases.

---

[5]The authors expressed concern that losses less than $500 "may have been an artifact of the estimation methods" (51, p.109). One third of the sample had losses less than $500. In this group, losses averaged $45 and benefits averaged $163.

Many victims do not even suspect that their disease is job related. For those who do and wish to make a claim, the causal relationship between disease and workplace exposures may be very difficult to establish. A study of asbestos insulators who died of asbestos-related causes (19) showed that fewer than half of asbestos-related fatalities among insulation workers led to workers' compensation claims. Of those who filed claims, the pretax replacement rate was only 22 percent. Overall, the pretax replacement rate was 10 percent. Because asbestos is the best-known cause of occupational disease and these workers were members of an active and well-informed union, we can be sure that other occupational diseases enter the workers' compensation system much less frequently. A study of occupational disease in Washington and California revealed that workers' compensation claims were filed for only three percent of identified cases of occupational disease (36).

CONCLUSION

Although workers' compensation costs have risen dramatically in the past 20 years, research has not found income benefits to be excessive. Despite considerable variation among states, studies suggest that replacement of lost income is low for many workers with serious occupational injuries and illnesses. This suggests that benefits for these injuries and illnesses should be improved, although additional research must verify the extent and nature of this problem. Current knowledge generally does not support a strategy of reducing workers' compensation costs by cutting benefits or limiting conditions eligible for compensation.

This review has discussed three potential areas for reducing workers' compensation costs to employers while raising benefits to workers: improving safety, containing medical costs, and reducing litigation.

In theory, workers' compensation increases the costs to employers of injuries and so provides incentives for improving safety. Taken as a whole, however, research does not provide convincing evidence that workers' compensation reduces injury rates. Few studies found evidence for a safety effect, and, where such evidence exists, it can be explained by incentives for employers to discourage and contest expensive injuries. Perhaps workers' compensation does affect safety, but, if so, its impacts are blurred, if not overwhelmed, by reporting bias.

Moreover, unlike safety and health regulation, workers' compensation focuses the attention of employers on specific workers and their injuries. Employers and insurers typically see "loss control," not just injury control, as their objective. This can lead to employers discouraging workers' compensation claims, increased conflict between workers and employers over when workers should return to work, and discrimination against workers perceived to be "injury prone" (despite the strictures of the Americans with Disabilities Act).

This does not imply that we cannot reduce workers' compensation costs through better safety performance. It only suggests that workers' compensation premiums have limited value as weapons in the safety arsenal.

Perhaps in response to these limitations, we have seen an expansion of novel efforts to improve safety through workers' compensation. More than a dozen states mandate premium discounts for employers with safety programs. In some, the safety programs must meet defined criteria or must be certified by the state. A growing number of states mandate safety committees through workers' compensation statutes and regulations and through state safety codes. Oregon and Washington, for example, require all employers with more than 10 employees to maintain safety committees. Twenty states require insurers to provide safety services. For instance, in California, insurers must submit to the workers' compensation agency safety plans targeting high-hazard employers and must provide certified safety services to all employers. Other states, including Connecticut, Michigan, and New York, have assessed surcharges on workers' compensation premiums to fund occupational safety and health education. Still, we know virtually nothing about the effectiveness of any of these methods.

Controlling medical costs holds promise as a method of reducing workers' compensation costs without reducing benefits. As in nonworkers' compensation settings, managed care appears to reduce costs. Well-designed fee schedules also may reduce costs. However, research to date has focused on impacts on costs and not on the quality of care. The only information currently available suggests that injured workers are less satisfied with the care provided in an HMO setting than in a fee-for-service setting. Taken as a whole, the evidence does not support the hypothesis that employer choice of medical provider reduces medical costs. But the choice of treating provider may affect how quickly workers return to work and the level of benefits they receive. Although these issues are at the periphery of research, they are central concerns of both employers and labor unions.

Reducing litigation also can improve the functioning of workers' compensation systems. Without litigation, benefits can be delivered more quickly and at lower costs. In states where litigation is common, injured workers need attorneys to give them information and to ensure they receive all the benefits to which they are entitled. To protect workers' rights, attempts to reduce litigation must include provisions for the workers' compensation agency to provide information to workers about benefits due and to ensure that employers and insurers pay these benefits.

Workers' compensation systems are very inefficient, providing limited benefits to injured workers at excessive costs. Additional research, evaluating options for more effective delivery of benefits, could be of great value.

AKNOWLEDGMENTS

I would like to thank Charles Levenstein, David Ozonoff, and Emily Spieler for reading early drafts. Their helpful comments significantly improved this review.

Literature Cited

1. American Medical Association. 1988. *Guides to the Evaluation of Permanent Impairment.* Chicago. 3d ed.
2. Appel D, Durbin D. 1986. Long duration workers' compensation claims. *NCCI Dig.* 1:59–70
3. Appel D, Durbin D, Fung M. 1994. *Workers' Compensation Managed Care Pilot Program: Final Report to the Florida Legislature.* New York: Milliman & Robertson
4. Bacow LS. 1980. *Bargaining for Job Safety and Health.* Cambridge, MA: MIT Press
5. Baker LC, Krueger AB. 1993. Twenty-four-hour-coverage and workers' compensation insurance. *Health Aff.* 12: 271–81 (Suppl.)
6. Bartel AP, Thomas LG. 1985. Direct and indirect effects of regulation: a new look at OSHA's impact. *J. Law Econ.* 28:1–25
7. Barth PS. 1982. Wage premiums for risk of asbestos workers. In *Disability Compensation for Asbestos-Associated Disease in the United States.* New York: Mt. Sinai Sch. Med.
8. Barth PS, Hunt HA. 1980. *Workers' Compensation and Work-Related Illnesses.* Cambridge, MA: MIT Press
9. Beck M. 1993. Income replacement in Pennsylvania. *WCRI Research Brief* 9(3S). Cambridge, MA: Workers Compens. Res. Inst. (WCRI)
10. Berkowitz M. 1973. Workmen's compensation income benefits: their adequacy and equity. In *Supplemental Studies for the National Commision on State Workmen's Compensation Laws.* Washington, DC: US GPO
11. Berkowitz M, Burton JF Jr. 1987. *Permanent Disability Benefits in Workers' Compensation.* Kalamazoo: WE Upjohn Inst. Employ. Res.
12. Blessman JE. 1991. Differential treat-
ment of occupational disease v occupational injury by workers' compensation in Washington State. *J. Occup. Med.* 32:121–126
13. Boden LI. 1988. *Reducing Litigation: Evidence from Wisconsin.* Cambridge, Mass: WCRI
14. Boden LI. 1989. Unlocking OSHA's potential: an inspection strategy for the 1990's. In *Occupational Health in the 1990's: Developing a Platform for Disease Prevention,* ed. PJ Landrigan, IJ Selikoff, pp. 228–34. New York: NY Acad. Sci.
15. Boden LI. 1992. Workers' compensation medical costs: a special case. In *Workers' Compensation Health Care Cost-Containment,* ed. J Greenwood, A Taricco, pp. 27–54. Horsham, Pa: LRP Publ.
16. Boden LI, Gold M. 1984. The accuracy of self-reported regulatory data: the case of coal mine dust. *Am. J. Ind. Med.* 6:427–40
17. Boden LI, Fleischman C. 1989. *Medical Costs in Workers' Compensation: Trends and Interstate Comparisons.* Cambridge, Mass: WCRI
18. Boden LI, Johnson SM, Smith JCH. 1992. *Medical Cost Containment in Workers' Compensation: A National Inventory 1992.* Cambridge, Mass: WCRI
19. Boden LI, Jones CA. 1987. Occupational disease remedies: The asbestos experience. In *Regulation Today: New Perspectives on Institutions and Policy,* ed. E Bailey, pp. 321–46. Cambridge, MA: MIT Press
20. Boden LI, Victor RA. 1994. Models for reducing workers' compensation litigation. *J. Risk Insur.* 61: 457–75
21. Borba PS. 1986. Can medical fee schedules control medical care expenditures? *NCCI Digest* 1:1–13
22. Borba PS, Appel D. 1987. The propen-

sity of permanently disabled workers to hire lawyers. *Ind. Labor Rel. Rev.* 40: 418–29

23. Burton JF Jr. 1992. The twentieth anniversary of the National Commission on State workmen's Compensation Laws: observations by John F. Burton, Jr. *John Burton's Work. Compens. Monit.* 5(6): 1–10

24. Burton JF Jr. 1993. Workers' compensation costs, 1960–1992: The increases, the causes, and the consequences. *John Burton's Work. Compens. Monit.* 6(2): 1–23

25. Burton JF Jr, Schmidle TP. 1993. Workers' compensation: Comparing the states. *John Burton's Work. Compens. Monit.* 6(5):1–11

26. Butler RJ. 1983. Wage and injury rate response to shifting levels of workers' compensation. See Ref. 78, pp. 61–86

27. Butler RJ, Worrall JD. 1983. Workers' compensation: benefit and injury claims rates in the seventies. *Rev. Econ. Stat.* 65:580–89

28. Cheit E. 1961. *Injury and Recovery in the Course of Employment.* New York: Wiley

29. Chelius JR. 1982. The influence of workers' compensation on safety incentives. *Ind. Labor Rel. Rev.* 35:235–42

30. Chelius JR. 1983. The incentive to prevent injuries. See Ref. 78, pp. 154–160

31. Chelius JR, Kavanaugh K. 1988. Workers' compensation and the level of occupational injuries. *J. Risk Insur.* 55:315–23

32. Chelius JR, Smith RS. 1983. Experience-rating and injury prevention. See Ref. 78, pp. 128–137

33. Chelius JR, Smith RS. 1987. Firm size and regulatory compliance costs: The case of workers' compensation. *J. Policy Anal. Manage.* 6:193–206

34. Chelius JR, Smith RS. 1993. The impact of experience-rating on employer behavior: The case of Washington State. In *Workers' Compensation Insurance: Claim Costs, Prices, and Regulation,* ed. D Durbin, PS Borba, pp. 293–306. Boston: Kluwer

35. Cost Containment Committee, Workers Compens. Congr. 1989. Cost containment. *NCCI Dig.* 4:25–49

36. Discher DP, Kleinman GD, Foster FJ. 1975. *Pilot Study for Development of an Occupational Disease Surveillance Method.* Rockville, MD: NIOSH

37. Durbin DL, Corro D, Helvacian NM. 1993. *Workers' compensation medical expenditures, price v. quantity: Implications for a medical price index.* Presented at the Annu. Econ. Issues

Work. Compens. Semin., 12th. Philadelphia, PA

38. Durbin DL, Helvacian HM, Worral JD. 1994. Synergy in workers compensation insurance: is there a tradeoff between indemnity and medical? Manuscript in preparation. Hoboken, NJ: Natl. Counc. Compens. Ins.

39. Ducatman AM. 1986. Workers' compensation cost-shifting: a unique concern of providers and purchasers of prepaid health care. *J. Occup. Med.* 28: 1174–76

40. Eads G, Reuter P. 1983. *Designing Safer Products.* Santa Monica: Rand Corp.

41. Eccleston SM, Grannemann TW, Dunleavy JF. 1993. *Benchmarks for Designing Workers' Compensation Medical Fee Schedules.* Cambridge, Mass: WCRI

42. Ellenberger, JN. 1992. Medical cost containment in workers' compensation. In *Workers' Compensation Desk Book,* ed. JF Burton Jr, TP Schmidle. Horsham, PA: LRP Publ.

43. Ellenberger, JN. 1994. Workers' compensation and national health reform. *New Solut.* 5:72–75

44. Fisher A, Chestnut LG, Violette DM. 1989. The value of reducing risks of death: a note on new evidence. *J. Policy Anal. Manage.* 8:88–100

45. Fortin B, Lanoie P. 1992. Substitution between unemployment insurance and workers' compensation: an analysis applied to the risk of workplace accidents. *J. Public Econ.* 49:287–312

46. Gardner J. 1989. *Return-to-Work Incentives: Lessons for Policymakers from Economic Studies.* Cambridge, Mass: WCRI

47. Ginnold R. 1979. A follow-up study of permanent disability cases under Wisconsin workers' compensation. In *Research Report of the Interdepartmental Workers' Compensation Task Force,* Vol. 6. Washington, DC: US GPO

48. Grannemann TW, Victor RA. 1993. *The Clinton Health Security Act: Implications for Workers' Compensation Costs.* Cambridge, Mass: WCRI

49. Habeck RV, Leahy MJ, Hunt HA. 1988. *Disability Prevention and Management and Workers' Compensation Claims.* Kalamazoo: WE Upjohn Inst. Employ.Res.

50. Jenkins EL, Kisner SM, Fosbroke DE, Layne LA, Stout NA, et al. 1993. *Fatal Injuries to Workers in the United States, 1980–1989: A Decade of Surveillance.* Cincinnati: NIOSH

51. Johnson WC, Cullinan PR, Curington WP. 1978. The adequacy of workers'

compensation benefits. In *Research Report of the Interdepartmental Workers' Compensation Task Force,* 6:95–121

52. Krueger AB. 1990. Incentive effects of workers' compensation insurance. *J. Public Econ.* 41:73–99

53. Leigh JP. 1985. Analysis of workers' compensation using data on individuals. *Ind. Rel.* 24:247–56

54. Miller TR, Levy DT. 1994. The growth in workers' compensation medical payments and the effect of rate regulations. *J. Risk. Insur.* 62: Submitted

55. Moore MJ, Viscusi WK. 1990. *Compensation Mechanisms for Job Risks.* Princeton: Princeton Univ. Press

56. Natl. Counc. Compens. Insur. (NCCI). 1991. *Workers Compensation Claim Characteristics.* New York: NCCI

57. NCCI. 1993. *Annual Statistical Bulletin.* Boca Raton: NCCI

58. Natl. Comm. State Workmen's Compensation Laws. 1972. *Report.* Washington, DC: US GPO

59. Parry T. 1994. *Does Disability Matter?* San Francisco: Calif. Workers' Compens. Inst.

60. Pozzebon S. 1993. Do traditional health care cost containment practices really work? *John Burton's Workers' Compens. Monit.* 6:17–22

61. Pozzebon S. 1994. *Job related health insurance: Cost containment under workers' compensation. Ind. Labor Rel. Rev.* 48:153–67

62. Robertson LS, Keeve AP. 1983. Worker injuries: The effects of workers' compensation and OSHA inspections. *J. Health Polit. Policy Law* 8:581–97

63. Ruser JW. 1985. Workers' compensation insurance, experience-rating, and occupational injuries. *Rand J. Econ.* 16:487–503

64. Ruser JW. 1991. Workers' compensation and occupational injuries and illnesses. *J. Labor Econ.* 9:325–50

65. Ruser JW. 1993. Workers' compensation and the distribution of occupational injuries. *J. Hum. Resourc.* 28:593–617

66. Ruser JW, Smith RS. 1988. The effect of OSHA records-check inspections on reported occupational injuries in manufacturing establishments. *J. Risk Uncertain.* 1:415–35

67. Russell LB. 1974. Safety incentives in workmens' compensation. *J. Hum. Resourc.* 9:361–75

68. Smith RS. 1993. Have OSHA and workers' compensation made the workplace safer? In *Research Frontiers in Industrial Relations and Human Resources,* ed. D Lewin, OS Mitchell, PD Sheer, pp. 557–86. Madison: Ind. Rel. Res. Assoc.

69. Spieler, EA. 1994. Perpetuating risk? Workers' compensation and the persistence of occupational injuries. *Houston Law Rev.* 31:119–264

70. Telles C. 1993. *Medical Cost Containment in Workers' Compensation: A National Inventory, 1992–1993.* Cambridge, Mass: WCRI

71. Thornquist L. 1990. Health care costs and cost containment in Minnesota's Workers' Compensation Program. *John Burton's Workers' Compens. Monit.* 3: 3–26

72. US Chamber of Commerce. 1994. *1994 Analysis of Workers' Compensation Laws.* Washington DC: US Chamb. Commer.

73. Victor R. 1972. *Workers' Compensation and Workplace Safety: The Nature of Employer Financial Incentives.* Santa Monica: Rand Corp.

74. Victor R, Fleischman C. 1990. *How Choice of Provider and Recessions Affect Medical Costs in Workers' Compensation.* Cambridge, Mass: WCRI

75. Viscusi WK. 1993. The value of risks to life and health. *J. Econ. Lit.* 31:1912–46

76. Viscusi WK, Moore MJ. 1987. Workers' compensation: wage effects, benefit inadequacies, and the value of health losses. *Rev. Econ. Stat.* 69:249–61

77. WCRI. 1993. Income replacement in Minnesota. *WCRI Research Brief* 9(5S). Cambridge, Mass: WCRI

78. Worrall JD, ed. 1983. *Safety and the Workforce.* Ithaca, NY: ILR Press

79. Worrall JD, Butler RJ. 1988. Experience rating matters. In *Workers' Compensation Insurance Pricing: Current Programs and Proposed Reforms,* ed. PS Borba, D Appel, pp. 81–94. Boston: Kluwer

80. Zwerling C, Ryan J, Orav J. 1991. Workers' compensation cost shifting: an empirical study. *Am. J. Ind. Med.* 19: 317–25

Annu. Rev. Public Health. 1995. 16:219–38

ADVANCES IN PUBLIC HEALTH COMMUNICATION[1]

E. Maibach
Emory School of Public Health, Atlanta, Georgia 30329

D. R. Holtgrave
Centers for Disease Control and Prevention, Atlanta, Georgia 30333

KEY WORDS: social marketing, risk communication, behavioral decision-making, media advocacy, entertainment education

ABSTRACT

There have been tremendous advances in recent years in the innovative use of communication to address public health problems. This article outlines the use of communication techniques and technologies to (positively) influence individuals, populations, and organizations for the purpose of promoting conditions conducive to human and environmental health. The approaches described include social marketing, risk communication, and behavioral decision theory, entertainment education, media advocacy, and interactive decision support systems. We also address criticism of these approaches among public health professionals because of perceived discrepanices in their inherent goals and objectives. In conclusion, we call for the rapid diffusion of state-of-the-art public health communication practices into public health service agencies and organizations.

INTRODUCTION

Recent years have seen tremendous advances in the innovative use of communication to address public health problems. Some of these advances have been reviewed in recent volumes of this series. Those reviews include mass media use at different levels of health promotion intervention, social marketing, and risk communication (20, 22, 48). To date, however, there has not been a review of the field as a whole, a field that we call public health communication.

We define public health communication as the use of communication techniques and technologies to (positively) influence individuals, populations, and organizations for the purpose of promoting conditions conducive to human

---

[1]The US Government has the right to retain a nonexclusive, royalty-free license in and to any copyright covering this paper.

and environmental health. This definition is intentionally broad and inclusive. The diverse and multifaceted challenges faced in public health require an equally diverse set of intervention strategies. An inclusive definition encourages consideration of diverse approaches.

In this chapter we do not attempt to provide a comprehensive review of all relevant advances in public health communication, but rather we attempt to define the scope of the field. To this end, we overview five unique communication approaches within the field of public health. We do so with two objectives: to demonstrate the diversity among the approaches; and to highlight the recent advances within each approach. In some cases, these advances are the approaches themselves, and in other cases, the advances are extensions of an existing approach. Some of these advances have been evaluated and shown to be effective; others have not yet been rigorously evaluated but appear to have value for public health practice. The approaches include social marketing, risk communication, behavioral decision theory, entertainment education, media advocacy, and interactive decision support systems. Each is overviewed in a section below.

SOCIAL MARKETING

Social marketing is perhaps the most developed approach to public health communication, although it has resisted simple definition. Ling and colleagues (48) defined social marketing most broadly as "a social change management strategy that translates scientific findings into action programs." They clarify by stating that social marketing attempts to persuade specific target audiences to adopt an idea, practice, and/or product through a variety of approaches and channels of communication combined in "an integrated, planned framework." Lefebvre & Flora (46) specify eight essential aspects of social marketing. It is an approach to intervention that: (a) is based on a consumer orientation, i.e. the perceived wants and needs of the target audience; (b) emphasizes voluntary exchange between providers and consumers; (c) uses audience research to define specific audience segments and provide in-depth profiles of those segments; and (d) uses formative research to design and pretest; (e) adopts a range of appropriately priced products and messages (price referring to monetary and nonmonetary costs of adoption); (f) distributes these products and communicates these messages in locations and through channels that match the target audience's life paths and communication patterns. Moreover, (g) implementation of the process is tracked to assess delivery of, and consumer response to, products and messages; and (h) the process is actively managed using mid-course corrections to ensure accomplishment of stated objectives. Chapman Walsh and colleagues (11) incorporated these essential aspects in a redefinition of social marketing: (a) a disciplined approach to public health intervention whereby research and management strategies are used to pursue clearly stated objectives in ways that often include mass media; that is (b) aimed at well-defined (i.e. segmented) audiences who have been carefully profiled (demographically, behaviorally, psychographically, and media-graphically); and (c) offers a set of products and messages that are responsive to consumers' wants and needs, and refined as needed.

Social marketing has received a warm welcome within most public health circles. Some of this acceptance is undoubtedly linked to its progress toward replacing traditional, paternalistic approaches to public health with consumer-driven approaches. Further contributing to its acceptance are the many notable social marketing successes in public health. Historically, these include the Stanford Three Community Project (50), and a series of contraceptive social marketing projects conducted in developing countries (2). More recently, numerous social marketing successes have been demonstrated in the context of the HEALTHCOM Project, which promoted a variety of child health measures including the promotion of immunization, diarrhea control practices, and breast feeding (13, 40), and a variety of condom social marketing projects staged in developing countries worldwide (70).

Social marketing has its critics in public health as well. Wallack and his colleagues (87, 90) note that social marketing, in its commonly used forms, focuses attention inappropriately on individuals and their behavior, rather than on the upstream causes of poor health, which are typically rooted in social problems and public policies (discussed further in the section on media advocacy, below). Other critics have suggested several factors that may limit the utility of traditional marketing methods in changing social ideas and health practices. These include the complexity of the issues involved; the lack of relevant secondary data sources to support marketing decisions; problems in collecting valid and reliable primary data; and difficulty in segmenting audiences (54). Some of these concerns have been supported empirically, but others have not been confirmed (54). Moreover, a number of recent advances in social marketing have addressed precisely these limitations, increasing the promise of this approach. These advances concern sources of data, audience segmentation strategies, and behavioral theories, each of which support tailored message design efforts. Each of these advances is briefly reviewed.

Social marketing is a consumer-driven process that requires considerable information on members of the target audience (63). Primary data collection with randomly selected members of the target audience, although preferable in terms of specificity, can be prohibitively costly for public health programs. Moreover, until recently, there has been a lack of secondary (and therefore relatively inexpensive) data on health behaviors and psychographics. Lefebvre and colleagues (47) have proposed that existing marketing databases can be used creatively and inexpensively to support social marketing programs. For example, in planning the National Cancer Institute's "5 A Day for Better Health" campaign (a nationwide effort to encourage Americans to eat at least five servings of fruits and vegetables per day), Lefebvre and colleagues requested a customized analysis of fruit and vegetable consumption from the Nutritional Marketing Information Services data set, an existing commercial data set that contains detailed information on the dietary habits of a representative sample of US households. The analysis helped them to better understand the differences between persons already eating five servings per day and the target audience, persons eating 2.5 to 3.5 servings but who were trying to increase this level. To obtain more specific information about the target audience, they added a single question to an on-going omnibus consumer survey, and recontacted select participants in the Nutritional Marketing Information study. Use of these databases supported consumer-driven definitions of the target audience as well as creation of a detailed demographic, psychographic, mediagraphic, and behavioral profile of the target audience in a highly efficient manner.

In social marketing, the audience is not one monolithic group for which all messages are intended. Rather, specific messages must be tailored to specific, *relatively* homogeneous audiences. The process of studying and thereby defining relatively homogeneous audiences out of a larger group is called audience segmentation. Audiences can be segmented on the basis of demographic, geographic, psychographic, and behavioral variables. Slater and colleagues (77, 78) are developing innovative ways to analyze public health audience segmentation under a variety of high- and low-resource situations. One related approach involves the use of the stage of behavior change (SBC) models (8, 68, 69, 99) to segment an audience (38, 52). People usually do not change their health behaviors suddenly, completely, and permanently. Rather, the process of, say, quitting smoking involves several sequential stages and may include multiple relapses from one stage to previous ones. To maximize the chances of moving audience members from one stage of change to the next, through the point of long-term behavior change, the audience must be profiled according to its members' current stage of behavior change, and the health communication messages must be tailored and stage specific (8, 52, 68, 99).

The related processes of audience segmentation and audience profiling establish the starting point for social marketing by defining who is being asked to change, and from what baseline. With the starting point defined, an action plan capable of motivating and enabling the target audience to adopt the recommended changes can be devised. Therein lies the integral role of behavioral theory in social marketing. Behavioral theory allows program planners to understand complex human behavior and to develop effective social marketing strategies that address those behaviors. One such example, the Transtheoretical Model (17, 68), posits that persons cycle and relapse through five distinct stages: (a) precontemplation, no intention to change behavior; (b) contemplation, making a decision about whether or not to change; (c) preparation, intending to change behavior in the near future and have experimented with behavior change in the past; (d) action, successfully changing behavior over a relatively short time; and (e) maintenance, successfully changing behavior over a lengthy time period. Prochaska and colleagues go beyond defining these stages; they also posit ten factors believed to be important for moving persons from one stage to the next (17, 68). The Transtheoretical Model has been used to inform the construction of numerous health communication efforts; these include smoking cessation, dietary habits, mammography, pregnancy prevention, and HIV prevention efforts (7, 15, 17, 25–27, 64, 68, 69, 76, 83). Other behavioral theories, such as Bandura's Social Cognitive Theory (3, 5, 52), and the Theory of Reasoned Action (5, 64), can also be used to explain how people may be guided from one stage to the next.

Compelling evidence for using a stage-based approach to audience segmentation and message tailoring is found in two recent randomized controlled trials (one on mammography and the other focusing on dietary habits) that compared a stage-based intervention to a more generic, nonstage-based intervention (7, 76). In both trials, the stage-based approach was superior to the nonstage-based intervention. The dietary intervention, which featured highly tailored direct mail messages (tailored by stage of change as well as other individual psychographic characteristics including self-efficacy and motives for behavior change), was particularly effective (7). Total fat consumption at four-month follow-up decreased by 23% in the tailored message group, 9% in the nontailored message group, and 3% in a no-message control group (p < .05). In summary, recent developments in social marketing involve the use of marketing data and stage-of-behavior change models to define specific, relatively homogeneous audiences and use of behavioral theories to tailor health messages to their specific needs.

RISK COMMUNICATION AND BEHAVIORAL DECISION-MAKING

Risk communication is another well developed, yet not entirely integrated, area of the public health communication field. The National Research Council (61) defines risk communication as " ... an interactive process of exchange of information, and opinion among individuals, groups and institutions. It involves multiple messages about the nature of risk and other messages, not strictly about risk, that express concerns, opinions, or reactions to risk messages or to legal and institutional arrangements for risk management." Ideally, risk communication involves truly interactive communication and shared decision-making about risk-management strategies. For example, if decisions have to be made about the siting of a commercial landfill and the local citizenry wishes not to have the facility in their neighborhood, then individual citizens, advocacy groups, governmental agencies, and industry would share decision-making power about the best resolution to the risk-management problem. This strategy is to be distinguished from purely persuasive campaigns that might be used to convince citizens to accept the local landfill siting.

In their message design efforts, risk communicators have utilized important lessons from the behavioral decision-making (BDM) literature about how people make choices under conditions of risk, how they perceive risks, and how they cognitively process information about probabilities (especially, probabilities of harmful events occurring to them) (16, 20, 34, 35, 61, 86, 91, 100, 101). Other public health communication specialists, too, increasingly are recognizing cognitive factors involved in audience members' decision-making about health behaviors, and are becoming more sophisticated in addressing them. Here we review several advances from the field of BDM that relate broadly to risk communication and other approaches to public health communication. For more complete overviews of risk communication, see recent publications by the National Research Council (61) and Fischhoff et al (20).

Optimistic Bias

People routinely employ heuristics (i.e. shortcuts or rules-of-thumb) and biases (systematic leanings toward a particular outcome or judgment) when they consider their options (42). One such bias, the optimistic bias [for review of other biases see (20, 42)], refers to the unrealistic perception that one is not at risk, or is at a greatly reduced risk, for a particular threat (39, 43, 85, 95–99). For example, people often perceive themselves to be at less risk than similar others for a variety of health threats, such as radon-induced lung cancer. Some research suggests that the optimistic bias may be due more to a false illusion of control over certain events than to unwarranted optimism itself (56).

Knowledge of such biases can provide direction for subsequent public health communication efforts. For example, Holtgrave & Tinsley (36, 39) developed a recycling education campaign for grade- and high-school students who were, at baseline, shown to possess optimistic biases regarding their family's production of garbage. The campaign emphasized, among other things, the need to take personal responsibility for the garbage one produces and the environmental harm that it might cause. Pre- and posttest evaluation of the campaign indicated significant improvements in certain outcome variables related to recycling knowledge, attitudes, and behaviors; however, the extent to which this success can be specifically attributed to reduction in optimistic bias is unknown.

Qualitative and Quantitative Statements of Probabilities and Other Values

Probabilities are expressions of uncertainty that range from zero through one, and are sometimes expressed as percentages on a scale from zero through 100. Lay people, however, rarely communicate using quantitative probabilities; rather, qualitative expressions are used. For instance, a person might say that it is "very likely" that (s)he will buy a new sofa this year, but it would be unusual to say that there is a .90 probability that (s)he will do so.

Words that people use to describe various probabilities have been studied systematically (38, 59, 80). Any given qualitative term may be associated with a wide range of probabilities (with error bars often spanning .5). Nevertheless, use of qualitative probabilistic statements can improve the comprehension of quantitative probability statements in health communication messages. Moreover, communication addressed to people with low numeracy skills may be more effective if only qualitative terms are employed.

For example, Kassler et al (44) used this literature to inform a novel intervention on HIV-prevention counseling. They were faced with the challenge of modifying the traditional approach to HIV-prevention counseling, which accompanies HIV-antibody testing, to accommodate a new, rapid HIV test that provides results within a few minutes. Negative results are definitive but positive results must be confirmed with a Western Blot test, which can take several days to provide results. The positive predictive value (PPV) for the rapid test at one study site was calculated to be .88. Rather than attempt to communicate a .88 PPV to clients, they employed recommendations from the literature on qualitative probabilities. Probabilities near .88 are related to terms like "probably infected," "very likely infected," "highly likely to be infected," and "very good chance of being infected." As a result, these qualitative probability terms are being employed in the modified counseling protocol for use with the rapid test, which continues to be evaluated.

Although unrelated to probabilities as such, the US Food and Drug Administration has mandated another important linkage between qualitative and quantitative terms (14). Food manufacturers' claims that their products have particular characteristics have now been strictly regulated; included are terms such as "light," "low," "reduced," "good source," and "% fat free." Each term has a clearly defined, quantitative, regulatory meaning to ensure that claims are not falsely made.

The growing literature on qualitative terms can be used to help communicate quantitative values, such as probability levels. Clearly, quantitative values are more precise; however, they may not always be readily understood by audience members. If not, then the qualitative term that is closest in meaning, for the audience, should be used instead of or in combination with the quantitative term.

Cumulative and One-Shot Probabilities

The difference between a probability density function and a cumulative probability density function is not generally understood by members of the lay public. Moreover, even when the difference is appreciated, making *intuitive* cumulative probability estimations (without formal calculations) is challenging.

Linville and colleagues (19, 20) found that college students tended to overestimate the probability of infection with HIV from a single exposure, and (assuming as true their own estimates of infection from one exposure) to underestimate the cumulative probabilities. Thus, if designers of HIV-prevention messages only convey the probability of infection from a single unprotected sexual encounter, they risk miscommunicating by leaving the calculation of cumulative probability to the audience they are trying to reach. Emphasizing the cumulative probability of infection over extended periods of time conveys the higher probability associated with that cumulative, long-term risk, and may be more likely to motivate correct and consistent condom use (38).

Risk Perception

As discussed in Fischhoff et al's (20) review of risk perception and communication, people tend to categorize risks according to a number of dimensions. A recent, empirically supported model posits that in forming their perceptions of various financial and health risks, people consider at least the following dimensions: the probabilities of gain, loss, and status quo associated with an activity (e.g. flying an airplane) or situation (e.g. living in a high-crime area), as well as the magnitude of the expected benefits and harm that might result (37, 49, 65, 66, 92–94).

This empirically validated model differs from other widely discussed models (45, 79) by including dimensions related to expected benefits and to the probability of harm. Given this model, perhaps public health communicators should consider using a balance-sheet approach to help audience members consider both the advantages and disadvantages of their health-related behaviors. The model also suggests that when comparing risks, the probability of harm be taken into account; comparisons of risks that have different probabilities of harm might be rejected by audience members as incommensurate (37).

In summary, BDM constructs have been utilized extensively in risk-communication efforts and increasingly in other approaches to public health communication. These constructs are helping to clarify the pervasive role of cognitive factors in people's understanding of and reaction to information about health risks.

MEDIA ADVOCACY

Media advocacy is a relatively new approach to public health communication, although its origins are found in the time-honored public health strategies of community advocacy, coalition building, and leadership development (88). Media advocacy is defined as the strategic use of mass media to advance a social or public policy initiative (82). As such, the philosophy and praxis of media advocacy reside at the societal level of analysis (22). This fundamentally social/environmental approach to public health promotion is often described in contrast to social marketing and other approaches to public health communication that operate primarily at the individual level (87). For example, Wallack (88) characterizes individual level mass media interventions as addressing the information gap (or more accurately, the behavior gap), while media advocacy addresses the power gap.

Wallack and colleagues (90) state "(m)edia advocacy is a part of a strategy to exert pressure on those whose decisions influence the environment, a strategy that uses the mass media appropriately, aggressively, and effectively to support the development of health public policies." Specifically, media advocacy is a process with a twofold aim: to gain access to the media, and with that access, to advance specific social or public policy initiatives. Gaining access to the media allows media advocates to accomplish three key functions

(90). The first function is to place the public health issue on the public's agenda. Although the media may not tell people what to think, it is clearly understood that they do tell people what to think about (55). The second function is the ability to frame (or reframe) the issue properly, by focusing on upstream or societal level causes. The manner in which the media frames social issues is associated with who, or what, is seen as being responsible for the problem (41). The third function is the ability to propose specific social or public policy initiatives as a primary means of addressing the problem.

By successfully setting the agenda, properly framing the issue, and advancing specific solution-oriented initiatives, public health communicators can effect two important outcomes: They can catalyze public opinion and bolster the public's willingness to support the proposed solution(s); and they can gain access to key opinion leaders and community decision makers who have the ability to further advance the suggested initiatives (90).

Much of the work required for effective media advocacy is conducted before ever attempting to gain access to the media (90). This work includes specifying the social or policy initiatives to be advanced, identifying the media goals and objectives, determining the target audience (which may include policy makers, opinion leaders, the general public or certain segments of the public who are likely to influence the policy-adoption process), developing the proper social/environmental frames for the issue (and for the organizations and key players on both supporting and opposing sides of the issue), drafting specific messages to communicate those frames, and establishing the best channels through which to convey the messages.

Media advocacy strategies include both paid and unpaid access to the media. Paid placement of media messages has many advantages including control of the content, placement, and timing of the message (90). Innovative use of paid placement can also generate substantial amounts of free media coverage to the extent that the advertisement is itself newsworthy. The disadvantages of paid placement include the cost, which need not be prohibitive, and the likelihood of provoking the organizations and individuals identified in the ad as contributing to the problem.

Unpaid or earned access to the media is the bread and butter of the media advocacy approach (90). Access can be earned by staging of newsworthy events that promote the advocate's perspective, conducting and publicizing research that supports the advocate's contentions, piggybacking the advocate's perspective on breaking news, writing letters to newspaper editors and contributing op-ed pieces, appearing on radio and television talk shows, and by other related approaches. A more sustainable approach is accomplished by cultivating effective working relationships with journalists. An effective working relationship is one that supports the journalist to perform his or her basic journalistic functions: collecting and interpreting information, and reporting developments that are newsworthy in a balanced and objective manner. Cultivating such relationships may influence not only the frequency of reporting on the issue, but more importantly, the frame provided by the media for the issue.

For a number of reasons including the recency of the approach, and the community unit of analysis, evaluations of public health media advocacy efforts are limited to case studies methodologies. Nevertheless, case studies presented by Adams & Jennings (1) and by Wallack and colleagues (89, 90) present compelling evidence for the efficacy of the approach. For example, the National Heart Savers Association conducted a media advocacy campaign (the "Poisoning of America" campaign) against the food industry to force the removal of tropical oils from the formulation of food products (1). Several major American food suppliers including Kellogg's, General Mills, McDonalds, and Wendys reformulated a number of their products to exclude tropical oils shortly after being targeted by the advocacy campaign (1).

ENTERTAINMENT EDUCATION

Entertainment education is another relatively new approach to public health communication. Entertainment education has been defined by Singhal (73) as "a performance which captures the interest or attention of an individual, giving them pleasure, amusement, or gratification while simultaneously helping the individual to develop a skill to achieve a particular end ...". These approaches begin with a related set of premises: (*a*) entertainment-oriented communication attracts a larger (voluntary) audience than education-oriented communication; (*b*) people understand and are receptive to educational messages presented in the context of entertainment experiences; and (*c*) because of heightened audience size, attention, and receptivity, entertainment education messages are capable of influencing cognitive, affective, and behavioral outcomes that underlie many public health problems. Singhal & Rogers (75) have summarized the promise of the methods by stating that "the entertainment component of such messages helps break down audience barriers and resistance to the educational content (such as the perception that educational messages are usually dull)."

Depending on the medium and format selected for entertainment education efforts, audience sizes can be substantial. For example, Ven Conmigo, a televised soap opera promoting adult literacy in Mexico, attracted a 32.6 audience share rating (i.e. nearly a third of all Mexican households with television sets were tuned into the show) (60). Similarly, Hum Log, an Indian televised soap opera promoting a variety of pro-development issues (e.g. enhanced status for women, family planning), attracted the largest audience of any show on Indian television during 1984–85 (50 million people watched the average broadcast) (75). A Spanish language pop music song promoting sexual abstinence for teens generated an estimated one million hours of free radio and television time throughout Latin America (75).

Entertainment education programming may attempt to influence audience members cognitively, affectively, and or behaviorally (typically through the use of behavioral modeling). Intended cognitive influences may include increased knowledge about a health problem and various possible solutions, enhanced appreciation of the personal relevance of the problem, increased belief that a proposed behavior change is an acceptable solution to the problem, and an increased sense of confidence in one's capability to successfully implement the proposed behavior change (4). Intended affective influences include encouraging or discouraging specific attitudes that contribute to a public health problem. For example, a number of televised soap operas have attempted to encourage women's equality (60, 75), while other soap operas have attempted to discourage attitudes that inhibit illiterate adults from learning to read (60).

The ultimate goal of entertainment education communication is typically defined behaviorally. To date, entertainment education programming has been developed to promote adult literacy, family planning, responsible parenting, condom use and use of other contraceptives, the designated-driver concept, and substance abuse prevention (58, 60, 75). Unfortunately, existing evaluation data include only case studies, historical analyses, and cross-sectional population/viewer surveys. Given obvious limitations, the evaluation data look promising. During the 13 months that Ven Conmigo aired, enrollment in a government-sponsored adult literacy program increased 63 percent over the previous year (as compared to 7 percent in the prior year, and 2 percent in the year following the program) (60). Similarly, during the nine months in which "Accompaname" (a Mexican pro-family planning soap opera) aired, attendance at family planning clinics increased 33 percent (as compared to an increase of less than 1 percent in the previous year), while condom sales increased 23 percent (compared to a 7 percent increase in the previous time period) (60).

The entertainment education concept is not restricted to a specific medium or form of entertainment, although its public health uses to date have tended to feature primarily television and radio. Within the media of television and radio, two distinct approaches to entertainment education have been attempted: the pro-development soap opera, and incorporation of health messages into existing programming. Other media that have been used or that show promise for entertainment education include popular music, theatrical performances, interactive computer software systems, and print materials such as comic books and magazines. Each is reviewed briefly.

Pro-Development Soap Operas

Singhal & Rogers (74) define pro-development soap opera as "a melodramatic television serial that is broadcast in order to convey subtly an educational or development theme." These are also referred to as telenovellas or radio-novellas. The soap operas referred to above (Ven Conmigo, Accompaname, and Hum Log) are examples of pro-development soap operas. The genre of pro-development soap opera was created by Miguel Sabido, a senior executive at Televisa (Mexico's commercial television network). In response to a Peruvian soap opera that inspired masses of women to learn to use sewing machines, Sabido launched a multiyear investigation of the soap opera format as a vehicle for promoting social change (60, 75). Drawing heavily from communication and psychological theories, most notably Bandura's Social Learning Theory (3), Sabido created a script writing formula whereby the audience will predictably identify with certain key characters in a particular cast (60). Over the course of many episodes, the key characters develop a desire to change their behavior (along the advocated lines) in response to positive modeling provided by other characters. These characters are shown to struggle but eventually succeed with their behavior changes, and in the long run, they are rewarded with positive outcomes.

The genre has been both very popular and commercially successful in developing countries. Televisa (Mexico) has developed and aired six such soap operas between the years 1975 and 1981, most of which were commercially successful in the Mexican television market. These six soap operas were also licensed for rebroadcast in numerous other (ranging from 4 to 15) American countries. The approach has been used with commercial success in Jamaica, India, Kenya, Indonesia, and other countries (60, 75).

The point that pro-development soap operas can be very profitable is important. Many social marketers argue that social programs that operate within market forces are generally more successful and longer-lived. Given the commercial viability of pro-development soap operas (as well as pro-development popular music), a strategic technical assistance program whereby television producers and writers are instructed on how to apply Sabido's approach may stimulate the dissemination of this promising public health communication strategy. Population Communication International, a nonprofit organization headquartered in New York City, has taken the lead in this effort.

Messages Incorporated into Existing Programs

A related approach to televised entertainment education calls for the inclusion of specific health messages into existing commercial programming. This approach, rather than developing original television programming, seeks to work with writers, producers, and other executives in the television industry to encourage them to incorporate public health messages into programming that they are already creating.

Although advocacy groups have a long history of lobbying the television industry (57), few such efforts have been made by the public health community. Breed & De Foe (6) used content analytic research (which demonstrated frequent and dysfunctional depictions of alcohol use on entertainment television) in a series of workshops with the television production community. They appealed, with some success, for consumption of alcoholic beverages to be portrayed in "an appropriate context so that a realistic picture of alcohol use and abuse could be shown" (Breed & De Foe as quoted in 58).

The Harvard Alcohol Project, an activity conducted by the Center for Health Communication at Harvard's School of Public Health, worked with representatives of the television industry to promote specific mentions of the risk of drinking and driving, including the designated-driver concept. Their efforts resulted in prominent inclusions of that message in over 25 television programs (58).

Recently, the Centers for Disease Control and Prevention (CDC) convened a working group of television industry and health communication professionals to discuss how CDC can work with the television industry to promote positive portrayals of sexual abstinence and other means of HIV prevention, and to promote destigmatization of people with HIV infection (9). The group encouraged CDC to work proactively with the media industry in a number of ways including: (*a*) to serve as a liaison with and a scientific resource for the entertainment industry; (*b*) reinforce media industry efforts by convening regular meetings with industry groups and presenting awards for outstanding contributions to programming; and (*c*) fund research to assess specific themes and audiences, and to evaluate the effectiveness of entertainment-education strategies.

Alerting viewers to the health content in entertainment media may, for a variety of reasons, amplify its positive effects. Engelberg (18) evaluated this hypothesis using a randomized experiment whereby participants were or were not prompted to attend specifically to health information featured in entertainment television shows. Forewarned participants perceived the health issue to be more personally relevant, and they were more interested in seeking additional information on the topic.

Other Approaches to Entertainment Education

The oldest application of the entertainment education concept can be found in traditional or folk media (84). For millennia, the function of folk media (e.g. story-telling, shadow puppetry) has been to entertain audiences while transmitting important lessons about the values, practices, or ideologies of a cultural group, and to provide current information about events in other places. Innovative environmental education campaigns have featured folk troupes whose performances were taped and aggressively aired on national television (51).

Theatrical arts are the developed world's equivalent to folk media. Inventive public health communicators have used the theatrical arts to entertain audiences while educating them about important health issues. For example, teen theater performances are an effective way to enhance adolescents' willingness to speak with parents and friends about contraception, and to increase sexually active adolescents' intentions to use contraception (33).

CD-ROM technology offers great potential for entertainment education applications. It offers interactive access to vast amounts of multimedia information (text, audio, graphics, animation, and historical and original video footage) nearly instantaneously. Moreover, the quality of the educational experience can be superior to that offered by traditional linear forms of communication because users customize the educational experience as a result of the way in which they interact with the system (including pace, content accessed, order of access, etc). Unfortunately, few of the 2500 CD-ROM titles in print focus on health, and none do so in a manner that takes full advantage of the educational potential of the medium. (71). Pioneering work in this area by Hawkins and colleagues (32) remains one of the few health examples of this approach.

Entertainment-oriented print media such as comic books offer another avenue to reach specific populations including children and adolescents (67). For example, in several recent issues of *The Amazing Spiderman*, the main character directly communicated about abstinence from drug use and encouraged the use of bicycle helmets (67). Another example is *Karate Kids*, an animated video and comic book that promotes HIV-preventive behaviors to street children (81).

INTERACTIVE DECISION SUPPORT SYSTEMS

Telecommunications and computer technology now allow vast amounts of custom-tailored information to be provided rapidly to persons all over the country and the globe. Witness the proliferation of computer bulletin boards, on-line information databases, electronic mail systems, and distance-learning technologies. Such information is available interactively so that the information obtained can be highly customized to meet the user's needs. For this reason, we refer to such information sources collectively as interactive decision support systems (IDSSs). As the information superhighway evolves, IDSSs are being developed for use in public health (62). Currently, IDSSs function primarily to enhance the capacity of the public health workforce, although probably they will increasingly be used as a channel of health information for the general public.

IDSSs can provide important functions to support public health communication and other public health efforts: greatly enhanced access to important databases to inform planning and decision-making; rapid dissemination of timely public health information; enhanced ability to communicate and develop solutions with one or many colleagues in any part of the country or most places in the world (enhanced referring to the speed and the cost of direct, informal, person-to-person communication); and rapid training in state-of-the-art public health strategies. Each function is illustrated through the presentation of several public health IDDSs.

CDC WONDER/PC is an on-line decision support service that provides users with access to two dozen important data bases (23, 24). These data sets include: (*a*) various types of surveillance data, (*b*) hospital discharges, (*c*) mortality information, (*d*) text of the Morbidity and Mortality Weekly Report, and (*e*) over 3000 references from the public health literature on cost-effectiveness and cost-benefit analyses. This information can be used to learn of breaking developments in a wide variety of public health areas, to access information on the efficacy of previous prevention and treatment efforts, and to plan the objectives of public health intervention efforts.

The CDC's Information Network for Public Health Officials (INPHO) is an IDDS currently under development that will be accessible through WONDER/PC. INPHO is an attempt to provide public health professionals with a single, integrated system to exchange essential information. As a unified health surveillance system, it will provide descriptions of the health status of communities to facilitate the delivery of preventive services, emergency reports on public health issues, guidelines on the delivery of preventive health services, training resources for agency personnel to develop the knowledge and skills needed to provide the recommended preventive services, and electronic mail to enhance communication among public health personnel. A multisectoral collaboration in the state of Georgia (between Georgia Division of Public Health, CDC, Woodruff Foundation, Georgia Center for Advanced Telecommunications Technologies, Medical College of Georgia, and Emory University) is the first attempt to implement and evaluate the system (29). The Public Health Training Network is a related CDC IDSS initiative that harnesses distance-learning technologies to meet the unique and diverse training needs of the public health workforce. Recent training topics for satellite video conferences have included smoking, HIV, nutrition, and health communication.

Nonprofit organizations are actively developing IDSSs as well. HandsNet, for example, is a national computer network that links over 3000 human service and public interest organizations via dial-in computer modem (31). HandsNet has forums on a number of public health topics including: funding and policy issues; health care reform; resources; and issues related to communities, youth, children, and families. AIDSNet, an outgrowth of HandsNet, specifically focuses on HIV- and AIDS-related issues. AIDSNet provides advocacy groups, service providers, researchers, and others with access to a network of information on policy, prevention, treatment, and funding issues. SCARCNet (Smoking Control Advocacy Resources Network), an IDSS developed by the Advocacy Institute, has been instrumental in organizing the forces of the antismoking movement (72). SCARCNet hosts daily strategy sessions on the latest tobacco news, distributes antitobacco legislation and other resources, and features biographies and positions taken by tobacco lobbyists. Similar systems are currently being developed by alcohol- and gun-control activists (72).

In summary, IDDSs are rapidly becoming an integral element of public health practice. Information acquisition, which formerly took days or weeks, and communication and training, which was time-consuming and/or expensive, can now be transacted rapidly with computers linked to modems or a network, and video monitors. This developing public health information infrastructure should enhance the practice and effectiveness of public health efforts in myriad ways.

CONCLUSION

We have introduced and reviewed the advances associated with five approaches to public health communication. We have also contended that these five (as well as other approaches that we have undoubtedly neglected) should be considered as a family of approaches to public health communication. This suggestion may be unacceptable to some public health professionals, including some authors whose work is cited in this chapter, because of perceived discrepancies in the inherent goals and objectives among the various approaches. A recent working group of experts on public health communication wrestled with the perceived discrepancies between individual versus social level change approaches (53). The group concluded that the most productive strategy was to consider public health communication on a continuum from strictly individual change strategies to strictly social change strategies. There is a marked overlap in the skills required to effectively conduct public health communication at both ends of the continuum (53).

Although much research is needed to further develop, refine, and integrate these approaches to public health communication, there is an even more pressing need to accelerate the diffusion of state-of-the-art public health communication practices into public health service agencies and organizations. Communication is a major programmatic activity in most health departments and other public and private-sector agencies concerned with the public's health (12, 21, 28). Yet even the casual observer is likely to notice the discrepancy between public health communication practices as recommended in this chapter and as typically implemented. If public health communication practices can be rapidly diffused into public health planning and delivery agencies over the remainder of this decade, it is our belief that public health will be stronger and better prepared to deal with the health challenges of the 21st century.

ACKNOWLEDGMENTS

We would like to sincerely thank Ann Bostrom and Eric Zook for helpful comments on a draft of this manuscript, and Caron Chess, Baruch Fischhoff, Ann Fisher, Charles T Salmon, and Paul Slovic for commenting on an earlier outline of the manuscript.

Literature Cited

1. Adams RJ, Jennings KM. 1993. Media advocacy: a case study of Phillip Sokolof's cholesterol awareness campaigns. *J. Consum. Aff.* 27:145–65
2. Altman L, Piotrow PT. 1989. Social marketing: does it work? *Popul. Rep.* 13:393–405
2a. Atkin C, Wallack L, eds. 1990. *Mass Communication and Public Health.* Newbury Park, CA: Sage

3. Bandura A. 1986. *Social Foundations of Thought and Action: A Social Cognitive Theory.* Englewood Cliffs, NJ: Prentice-Hall

4. Bandura A. 1991. Social cognitive theory of mass communication. In *Media Effects: Advances in Theory and Research,* ed. J Bryant, D Zillman. Hillsdale, NJ: Lawrence Erlbaum

5. Baranowski T. 1992–1993. Beliefs as motivation influences at stages in behavior change. *Int. Q. Community Health Educ.* 13:3–29

6. Breed WJ, DeFoe JR. 1982. Effecting media change: the role of cooperative consultation on media topics. *J. Commun.* 32:88–99

7. Campbell MK, DeVellis BM, Strecher VJ, Ammerman AS, Sandler RS. 1994. Improving dietary behavior: the effectiveness of tailored messages in primary care settings. *Am. J. Public Health* 84: 783–87

8. Catania JA, Kegeles SM, Coates TJ. 1990. Towards an understanding of risk behavior: an AIDS risk reduction model (ARRM). *Health Educ. Q.,* 17: 53–72

9. Centers for Disease Control and Prevention. 1994. *Using Entertainment-Education to Reach a Generation at Risk* Preliminary recommendations from a working group on Entertainment-Education. Feb. 12. Atlanta, GA: Off. Assoc. Dir., HIV/AIDS, CDC

10. Centers for Disease Control and Prevention. 1994. *It's your move: prevent AIDS.* Atlanta, GA: CDC

11. Chapman Walsh D, Rudd RE, Moeykens BA, Moloney TW. 1993. Social marketing for public health. *Health Aff.* Summer:104–19

12. Chess C, Salmone KL. 1992. Rhetoric and reality: risk communication in government agencies. *J. Environ. Educ.* 23: 28–33

13. Clift E. 1989. Social marketing and communication: changing health behavior in the Third World. *Am. J. Health Promotion* 3:17–24

14. Consumer Reports. 1994. New food labels: at last, you can trust them—most of the time. *Consum. Rep.* July: 437

15. Curry SJ, Kristal AR, Bowen DJ. 1992. An application of the stage model of behavior change to dietary fat reduction. *Health Educ. Res.* 7:97–105

16. Dawes RM. 1988. *Rational Choice in an Uncertain World.* San Diego: Harcourt Brace Jovanovich

17. DiClemente CC. 1993. Changing addictive behaviors: a process perspective. *Curr. Dir. Psychol. Sci.,* 2:101–5

18. Engelberg M. 1994. *Edutainment:* viewer goals and health persuasion effects of situation comedies.* PhD thesis. Stanford Univ., CA. 94 pp.

19. Fischhoff B. 1989. Making decisions about AIDS. In *Primary prevention of AIDS,* ed. VM Mays, GW Albee, SF Schneider, pp. 168–205. Newbury Park, CA: Sage

20. Fischhoff B, Bostrom A, Jacobs Quadrel M. 1993. Risk perception and communication. *Annu. Rev. Public Health* 14: 183–203

21. Flora JA, Wallack L. 1990. Health promotion and mass media use: translating research into practice. *Health Educ. Res.* 5:73–80

22. Flora JA, Maibach EW, Maccoby N. 1989. The role of mass media across four levels of analysis. *Annu. Rev. Public Health* 10:181–201

23. Friede A, Reid JA, Ory HW. 1993. CDC WONDER: a comprehensive on-line public health information system of the Centers for Disease Control and Prevention. *Am. J. Public Health* 83:1289–94

24. Friede A, Taylor WR, Nadelman L. 1993. On-line access to a cost-benefit/cost-effectiveness analysis bibliography via CDC WONDER. *Med. Care* 31:JS12–17 (Suppl.)

25. Galavotti C. 1992. Stages of behavior change: a conceptual framework for evaluating behavior. *CDC HIV/AIDS Prevent. Newsl.* 3:2–3

26. Galavotti C, Cabral R. 1993. Stages of change for condom and other contraceptive use: using theory to guide behavioral intervention and evaluation. *Conf. Behav. Res. Role Condoms Reprod. Health, NIH, Bethesda, MD.* May

27. Galavotti C, Cabral R, Grimley D, Riley GE, Prochaska JO. 1993. Measurement of condom and other contraceptive behavior change among women at high risk of HIV infection and transmission. *Abstr. #PO-D38-4416, 9th Int. Conf. AIDS, Berlin,* June

28. Gellert GA, Higgins KV, Lowery RM, Maxwell RM. 1994. A national survey of public health officers' interactions with the media. *J. Am. Med. Assoc.* 271:1285–89

29. Georgia Department of Human Resources. 1993. *Georgia Information Network for Public Health Officials.* Atlanta, GA: Georgia Dep. Hum. Resour. Dec.

30. Grimley DM, Riley GE, Bellis JM, Prochaska JO. 1993. Assessing the stages of change and decision-making for contraceptive use for the prevention of pregnancy, sexually transmitted diseases, and acquired immunodeficiency syndrome. *Health Educ. Q.* 20:455–70

31. HandsNet. 1994. Information packet. Cupertino, CA: HandsNet
32. Hawkins RP, Gustafson DH, Chewning B, Bosworth K, Day PM. 1987. Reaching hard to reach populations: interactive computer programs as public information campaigns for adolescents. *J. Commun.* 37:8–28
33. Hillman E, Hovell MF, Williams L, Hofstetter R, Burdyshaw C. 1991. Pregnancy, STDs, and AIDS prevention: evaluation of New Image teen theater. *AIDS Educ. Prev.* 3:328–40
34. Hogarth RM. 1987. *Judgment and Choice.* Chichester, England: Wiley. 2nd ed.
35. Hogarth RM, Reder MW. 1986. *Rational Choice: The Contrast Between Economics and Psychology.* Chicago: Univ. Chicago Press
36. Holtgrave DR, Tinsley BJ. 1992. *Risk Communication, Recycling and Young People.* Final Rep. US Environ. Prot. Agency, Coop. Agreem. No. 817465
37. Holtgrave DR, Weber EU. 1993. Dimensions of risk perception for financial and health risks. *Risk Anal.* 13:553–58
38. Holtgrave DR, Tinsley BJ, Kay LS. 1994. Encouraging risk reduction: a decision making approach to message design. See Ref. 52a. In press
39. Holtgrave DR, Tinsley BJ, Kay LS. 1994. Heuristics, biases and environmental health risk analysis. In *Applications of Heuristics and Biases in Social Issues. Vol. 3. Social Psychological Applications in Social Issues,* ed. L Heath, F Bryant, J Edwards, E Henderson, J Myers, E Posavac, Y Suarez-Balcazar, RS Tindale. New York: Plenum. In press
40. Hornik R, McDivitt J, Zimicki S, Yoder PS, Contreras-Budge E, McDowell J, Rasmuson M. Undated. *Communication for Child Survival: Pt. 1: Synthesis of Basic Results. Working Paper No. 1012.* Cent. Int. Health Dev. Commun., Annenberg Sch. Commun., Philadelphia, PA
41. Iyengar S. 1991. *Is Anyone Responsible? How Television Frames Political Issues* Chicago: Univ. Chicago Press
42. Kahneman D, Slovic P, Tversky A. 1982. *Judgment Under Uncertainty: Heuristics and Biases.* New York: Cambridge Univ. Press
43. Kaplan BJ, Shayne VT. 1993. Unsafe sex: decision-making biases and heuristics. *AIDS Educ. Prevent.,* 5:294-301
44. Kassler WJ, Dillon B, Haley C, Schenk T, Hutcheson D, et al. 1994. HIV prevention counseling using an on-site, rapid HIV assay. Paper accepted for presentation at 10th Int. Conf. AIDS, Yokohama, Japan
45. Kraus N, Slovic P. 1988. Taxonomic analysis of perceived risk: modeling individual and group perceptions within homogeneous hazard domains. *Risk Anal.* 8:435–55
46. Lefebvre RC, Flora JA. 1988. Social marketing and public health intervention. *Health Educ. Q.* 15:299–315
47. Lefebvre RC, Doner L, Johnston C, Loughrey K, Balch G, Sutton SM. 1994. Use of database marketing and consumer-based health communication in message design: an example from the Office of Cancer Communication's "5 A Day for Better Health" Program. See Ref. 52a. In press
48. Ling JC, Franklin AK, Linsteadt JF, Gearon SA. 1992. Social marketing: its place in public health. *Annu. Rev. Public Health* 13:341–62
49. Luce RD, Weber EU. 1986. An axiomatic theory of conjoint expected risk. *J. Math. Psychol.* 30:188–205
50. Maccoby N, Farquhar JW, Wood P, Alexander J. 1977. Reducing the risk of cardiopulmonary disease: effects of a community based campaign on knowledge and behavior. *J. Community Health* 3:100–14
51. Maibach E. 1993. Social marketing for the environment: using information campaigns to promote environmental awareness and behavior change. *Health Promot. Int.* 8:209–24
52a. Maibach E, Parrott RL, eds. 1995. *Designing Health Messages: Approaches from Communication Theory and Public Health Practice.* Newbury Park, CA: Sage. In press
53. Maibach E, Parrott RL, Long D, Salmon CT. 1994. Competencies of the public health communication specialist of the 21st Century. *Am. Behav. Sci.* 38:351–60
54. Malafarina K, Loken B. 1993. Progress and limitations of social marketing: a review of empirical literature on the consumption of social ideas. *Adv. Consum. Res.* 20:397–404
55. McCombs M, Shaw D. 1972. The agenda setting function of mass media. *Public Opin. Q.* 36:176–87
56. McKenna FP. 1993. It won't happen to me: unrealistic optimism or illusion of control? *Br. J. Psychol.,* 84:39–50
57. Montgomery KC. 1989. *Target: Prime Time* New York: Oxford Univ. Press. 272 pp
58. Montgomery KC. 1990. Promoting health through entertainment television. See Ref. 2a, pp. 114–28
59. Mostellor F, Youtz C. 1990. Quantifying probabilistic expressions. *Stat. Sci.* 5:2–34

60. Nariman HN. 1993. *Soap Operas for Social Change. Toward a Methodology for Entertainment-Education Television.* Westport, CN: Praeger. 143 pp.

61. Natl. Res. Counc. 1989. *Improving Risk Communication.* Washington, DC: Natl. Acad. Press

62. Nation's Health. 1994. *Public health struggles to merge onto Information Superhighway.* Am. Public Health Assoc. pp. 1, 20

63. Nowak GJ, Siska MJ. 1995. Using research to inform campaign development and message design: examples from the "American Responds to AIDS" campaign. See Ref. 52a. In press

64. O'Reilly KR, Higgins DL. 1991. AIDS community demonstration projects for HIV prevention among hard-to-reach groups. *Public Health Rep.* 106:714–20

65. Palmer CGS. 1993. Empirical testing of new theoretical framework of risk perception for the genetics reproductive decision problem. *Diss. Abstr. Int.* 54:1OB

66. Palmer CGS, Sainfort F. 1993. Toward a new conceptualization and operationalization of risk perception within the genetic counseling domain. *J. Genet. Couns.* 2:275–94

67. Parrott RL. 1994. Comic book heroes battle a tough enemy in AIDS. In *Mass-Mediated AIDS: Messages about Transmission and Risk* ed. LK Fuller. Amherst, MA: Human Resource Dev. Press. In press

68. Prochaska JO, DiClemente CC, Norcross JC. 1992. In search of how people change: applications to addictive behaviors. *Am. Psychol.* 47:1102–14

69. Prochaska JO, DiClemente CC, Veliver WF, Rossi JS. 1992. Criticisms and concerns of the transtheoretical model in light of recent research. *Br. J. Addict.* 87:825–28

70. Romer D, Hornik R, Maxfield, A. 1993. *Condom Social Marketing as an AIDS Prevention Strategy.* Work. Pap. No. 134, Cent. Int. Health Dev. Commun., Annenberg Sch. Commun., Philadelphia, PA

71. Shaffer R. 1994. Birth of a genre. *Forbes.* March 28, p. 114

72. Shapiro E. 1994. Tobacco firm seeks antismoking network's records. *Wall St. J.* March 30:B1, 8

73. Singhal A. 1994. *Social Change Through Entertainment.* Newbury Hills, CA: Sage. In press

74. Singhal A, Rogers E. 1988. Television soap operas for development in India. *Gazette* 41:109–26

75. Singhal A, Rogers E. 1989. Prosocial television for development in India. In *Public Information Campaigns,* ed. RE Rice, CK Atkin, pp. 331–50. Newbury Hills, CA: Sage

76. Skinner CS, Strecher VJ, Hospers H. 1994. Physicians' recommendations for mammography: do tailored message make a difference? *Am. J. Public Health.* 84:43–49

77. Slater MD. 1995. Choosing audience segmentation strategies and methods for health communication. See Ref. 52a. In press

78. Slater MD, Flora JA. 1991. Health lifestyles: audience segmentation analysis for public health intervention. *Health Educ. Q.* 18:221–33

79. Slovic P. 1987. Perception of risk. *Science,* 236:280–85

80. Spedden SE, Ryan PB. 1992. Probabilistic connotations of carcinogen hazard classifications: analysis of survey data for anchoring effects. *Risk Anal.* 12:535–41

81. Street Kids Int. 1990. *Karate Kids.* Street Kids Int.: Montreal

82. US Dep. Health Hum. Serv. 1989. *Media Strategies for Smoking Control: Guidelines.* Washington, DC: NIH Publ. #89–3013

83. Valdiserri RO, West GR, Moore M, Darrow WW, Hinman AR. 1992. Structuring HIV prevention service delivery systems on the basis of social science theory. *J. Community Health,* 17:259–269

84. Valenbuena V. 1987. *Using Traditional Media in Environmental Education.* Singapore: Asian Mass Commun. Res. Assoc. Inform. Cent.

85. Van der Velde FW, Hooykaas C, Van der Pligt J. 1992. Risk perception and behavior: pessimism, realism and optimism about AIDS-related health behavior. *Psychol. Health* 6:23–28

86. von Winterfeldt D, Edwards W. 1986. *Decision Analysis and Behavioral Research.* New York: Cambridge Univ. Press

87. Wallack L. 1990. Improving health promotion: media advocacy and social marketing approaches. See Ref. 2a, pp. 147–63

88. Wallack L. 1993. *Media Advocacy: a Strategy for Empowering People and Communities.* Presented at Shaping Futur. Public Health: Perspect. Berkeley Sch. Public Health, Berkeley

89. Wallack L, Sciandra R. 1991. Media advocacy and public education in the Community Intervention Trial to Reduce Heavy Smoking (COMMIT). *Int. Q. Community Health Educ.* 11:205–22

90. Wallack L, Dorfman L, Jernigan D, Themba M. 1993. *Media Advocacy and Public Health. Power for Prevention.* Newbury Hills, CA: Sage. 226 pp.

91. Watson SR, Buede DM. 1987. *Decision Synthesis: The Principles and Practice of Decision Analysis.* Cambridge, England: Cambridge Univ. Press

92. Weber EU. 1988. A descriptive measure of risk. *Acta Psychol.* 69:185–203

93. Weber EU, Bottom WP. 1989. Axiomatic measures of perceived risk: some tests and extensions. *J. Behav. Decis. Mak.* 2:113–31

94. Weber EU, Bottom WP. 1990. An empirical evaluation of the transitivity, monotonicity, accounting and conjoint axioms for perceived risk. *Organ. Behav. Hum. Decis. Process.*, 45:253–75

95. Weinstein ND, ed. 1987. *Taking Care: Understanding and Encouraging Self-Protective Behavior.* Cambridge, England: Cambridge Univ. Press

96. Weinstein ND. 1988. The precaution adoption process. *Health Psychol.* 7:355–86

97. Weinstein ND. 1989. Optimistic biases about personal risk. *Science* 246:1232–33

98. Weinstein ND, Klotz ML, Sandman PM. 1987. *Public Response to the Risk from Radon, 1986.* New Brunswick, NJ: Rutgers Univ., Environ. Commun. Res. Program

99. Weinstein N, Sandman PM. 1992. A model of the precaution adoption process: evidence from home radon testing. *Health Psychol.* 11:170–80

100. Yates JF. 1990. *Judgment and Decision Making.* Englewood Cliffs, NJ: Prentice-Hall

101. Yates JF. 1992. *Risk-Taking Behavior.* Chichester, England: Wiley

Annu. Rev. Public Health. 1995. 16:239–52

PUBLIC HEALTH INFORMATICS: How Information-Age Technology Can Strengthen Public Health*

Andrew Friede
Information Resources Management Office, Centers for Disease Control and Prevention, 1600 Clifton Road NE, Atlanta, Georgia 30333

Henrik L. Blum
University of California, 570 University Hall, Berkeley, California 94720

Mike McDonald
2600 Tenth Street, Suite 400, Berkeley, California 94710

KEY WORDS: computers, communications, education, informatics, public health, information systems, software

ABSTRACT

The combination of the burgeoning interest in health, health care reform and the advent of the Information Age, represents a challenge and an opportunity for public health. If public health's effectiveness and profile are to grow, practitioners and researchers will need reliable, timely information with which to make *information-driven decisions,* better ways to communicate, and improved tools to analyze and present new knowledge.

"Public Health Informatics" (PHI) is the science of applying Information-Age technology to serve the specialized needs of public health. In this paper we define Public Health Informatics, outline specific benefits that may accrue from its widespread application, and discuss why and how an academic discipline of public health informatics should be developed. Finally, we make specific recommendations for actions that government and academia can take to assure that public health professionals have the systems, tools, and training to use PHI to advance the mission of public health.

INTRODUCTION

The combination of the burgeoning interest in health, combined with health care reform and the advent of the Information Age, represent a challenge and an opportunity for public health. If public health's effectiveness and profile are to grow, practitioners and researchers will need reliable, timely information with which to make *information-driven decisions,* better ways to communicate, and improved tools to analyze and present new knowledge.

"Public Health Informatics" (PHI) is the science of applying Information-Age technology to serve the specialized needs of public health. Systems developed with PHI knowledge can help a county health office staff use surveillance data to estimate the number of doses of measles vaccine needed for an outbreak; make it easier for a regional planning commission to integrate census, surveillance, and hospitalization data to project the occupancy of AIDS hospice beds for a city, and prepare related funding requests for the state legislature; assist an epidemiologist in collecting and analyzing data to study malnutrition among homeless children and the impact of nutrition programs in different regions of the US; and facilitate a health educator's use of multimedia to communicate, in a compelling fashion, new knowledge to professional and lay audiences.

In 1990, Greenes & Shortliffe, in the *Journal of the American Medical Association,* presented an overview of Medical Informatics (10). In this paper we define Public Health Informatics, outline specific benefits that may accrue from its widespread application, and discuss why and how an academic discipline of public health informatics should be developed. Finally, we make specific recommendations for actions that government and academia can take to assure that public health professionals have the systems, tools, and training to use PHI to advance the mission of public health.

WHAT IS PUBLIC HEALTH INFORMATICS?

Public Health Informatics is the application of information science and technology to public health practice and research. Specifically, this means developing innovative ways to use inexpensive and powerful computers, on-line databases, the capacity for universal connection of people and computers, and multimedia communications to support the mission of disease prevention and health promotion. Practical PHI work, ideally guided by PHI professionals who are trained and experienced in both information technology and public health, involves bringing together specialists in both fields to conceptualize new ways of applying information technology to solve public health problems. The practice of public health informatics goes beyond applying known "computer science." Rather, it involves synthesizing knowledge from both disciplines, which is leading to new ways of thinking about and practicing public health.

Software and hardware developed for laboratory science or business often lack features required for public health. For example, standard statistical packages cannot easily be used to perform standardization, fit mathematical models to disease patterns, or calculate sample sizes for case-control studies; commonly available data-entry programs cannot handle the very long or complex questionnaires common in public health; general-purpose graphing programs make bar and pie charts but not histograms or county maps. Public health data files often contain many millions of records, and quickly accessing these very large files requires special database designs. Finally, there is an increasing need to search the full contents of massive text databases such as publications, reports and recommendations, tables of summary data, information about the Healthy People 2000 Objectives, etc. Typically, these documents are not key-worded, and their diversity, dynamic nature, and the unavailability of appropriate key words in the MeSH (Medical Subject Headings) system would preclude doing so; one of the challenges for public health informatics is to develop streamlined ways to access complex textual data.

CDC and other government agencies increasingly consider information dissemination to be central to their mission. These activities could be enhanced by building information systems specifically designed for public health data and various users: Synthesized knowledge can be easily communicated to the public through specialized voice and video systems (in addition to standard radio and television); summary data can be provided to the manager or public inquiries specialist via on-line information systems; researchers may wish to use more sophisticated systems to manipulate complex databases. Developing diverse systems that meet the full range of public health needs requires developing a cadre of professionals with training and experience in both public health and information technology.

Medical informatics has forged an analogous link between clinical medicine and information technology, focusing on hospital and clinical research information systems (automating medical charts, linking laboratory data to clinical data, etc), computerized diagnostic systems, biomedical engineering, patient and student education, and medical library automation (10). Clearly there is overlap between medical informatics and PHI. However, because public health has its foundations in epidemiology and prevention, public health informatics must focus on speeding and simplifying the conversion of hypotheses about the distribution and determinants of diseases in *populations* into usable information, and help to disseminate new knowledge in ways that will support public health practice. In addition, to the extent that clinicians of the twenty-first century incorporate epidemiology and public health principles into clinical medicine, and come to see the patient as part of a community, public health informatics will make important contributions to the work of practicing physicians (11).

Public health needs to make more effective use of information technology to support its mission. Modern businesses use information technology to update centralized databases from hundreds of retail stores located around the country several times a day, to predict and report elections as they are taking place, and to instantly make reservations on any airline in the world. Public health could make use of similar technology to enhance the timeliness and efficiency of survey and surveillance systems; rapidly and effectively communicate scientific findings to the public; and offer services (such as public health clinic appointments for childhood immunizations) to underserved populations. Public health leaders in academia and at all levels of government will thus be empowered to better evaluate prevention strategies, and allocate resources for services and research. This will require applying currently available knowledge, and making advances in: (*a*) data and information systems; (*b*) communications; and (*c*) specialized tools.

IMPROVED DATA AND INFORMATION SYSTEMS FOR INFORMATION-DRIVEN DECISIONS

Data Systems

Data systems are formal systems for data collection, collation, editing, and distribution. They benefit public health practice by standardizing data gathering and processing. Data systems produce data (i.e. raw observations or numbers). To generate reports (tables, graphs, or data subsets), the end-user must write computer programs. An example of a widely used data system is the National Vital Statistics System, which state vital registrars use to provide data to CDC for accumulation into a national data bank.

Data systems could be improved by making more effective use of technology to improve accuracy, timeliness, and confidentiality. Accuracy can be improved by more widespread use of computer-assisted personal interviewing, wherein the data are cross-checked as they are keyed (for example, if the interviewee is pregnant, then age = "73" cannot be entered). CDC has written and makes extensive use of programs that provide this feature, including Epi Info, SURVEY, and the data-entry modules of the AIDS Reporting System. Accuracy can also be enhanced by maintaining the data in databases during all phases of the data cycle, where records can be reviewed and edited upon receipt, and then can be used to update information systems. Timeliness can be enhanced by electronic data transmittal; for example, states now transmit notifiable diseases data every Monday to CDC for publication in that Friday's *Morbidity and Mortality Weekly Report.* They are later added to CDC WONDER, CDC's on-line public health information system, where they are available for more detailed analysis.

Preserving confidentiality can be facilitated by making wider use of computer programs that generate a pseudonym based on the phonetics of an individual's name combined with other information (e.g. birth date). The AIDS Reporting System uses this method to assure that information that could identify an individual is never transmitted to CDC, yet it allows a case to be tracked over time. Another way to guarantee confidentiality is to transfer the data to information systems where the data are stored in aggregate (summary) form only, which is how several surveillance data sets are stored in CDC WONDER.

INFORMATION SYSTEMS

Information systems are computer systems that provide routine mechanisms for converting data into information (e.g. summary statistics, tables, graphs). In contrast to data systems, information systems can be accessed without any computer programming by the user; rather, results are accessed via menus or simple commands. Information systems benefit public health practice by providing easy and rapid access to information. One example of a widely used information system is CDC's AIDS Reporting System used for AIDS surveillance data, which allows state and local health departments to input, verify, and prepare reports via menus. The reporting area, which may be a state or county, can use menus to quickly and easily prepare a profile of risk factors among AIDS cases reported this year as compared to last year. Because this system integrates data entry and reporting, it promotes both the uniformity of the national database, and facilitates state-level analysis, thereby putting timely information in the hands of local decision-makers.

A second example is CDC WONDER, which provides menu-driven access to more than 40 large on-line databases (7). CDC WONDER has been used to perform tasks such as updating reports in a few minutes (14), pulling together data on older Americans from a dozen different surveys and surveillance data sets in an afternoon (a task that would normally require weeks of computer programming); or searching the full text of the *Morbidity and Mortality Weekly Report* for all articles during the past 10 years that mention AIDS and Washington State, an assignment that would be virtually impossible unless the data were in a system that offered full-text searching.

To take on new public health challenges, such as tracking progress towards meeting the *Healthy People 2000 Objectives,* and understanding why goals are (or are not) being met, public health workers need to acquire and synthesize many more data about the public's health than are now available; information must be in formats that are directly usable for developing prevention strategies under frameworks such as those provided by the "Model Standards" (2). To be useful for the *Healthy People 2000* (6) and "Model Standards" processes (1), this information must contain concise, up-to-the-minute, age-, race-, and geography-specific syntheses of key data, recommendations, and supporting materials. Background tables and supporting documents must be available, but to facilitate rapid action, the bottom line needs to be crystal clear. PHI can be brought to bear on several aspects of data and information system development.

Information systems could be improved by increasing the number of data sets that are included, providing sophisticated facilities to help users identify pertinent data sources, and creating easier-to-use and more flexible statistical and graphing tools. Information systems vary in their objectives: CDC WONDER contains many data sets, but statistical analysis facilities are limited (7). In contrast, BWTRGR has data limited to Massachusetts births, but allows the user to perform regression (19); EPIGRAM provides access to detailed data about a single state (Texas) (9). Both kinds of systems have important roles to play.

Agencies that have had success in building public health information systems need to share their expertise. An unknown number of data-collection and information systems are currently in various stages of early consideration or planning, including a national system to track the immunization status of children, expanded cancer incidence surveillance, regional trauma registries (17), and registries of people exposed to substances suspected of being hazardous to health. Making any plans to develop similar systems widely known would promote collaborations, increase data accuracy, and reduce duplication.

Developing standards for communications protocols, data elements, interfaces (the appearance of the screen and keystrokes that a user needs to work a computer program), etc, will make both data and information systems easier to build and use. For example, if all public health systems used the same kind of modems, had compatible age groupings, and had screens that worked the same way, then encoding, transmitting, and accessing data would be greatly speeded, users would be less confused by programs that do not look and work alike, and user support costs would be reduced. With respect to interfaces, standardization would be promoted by moving towards the adoption of the emerging standard for commercial software (or using commercial products directly, when possible), which uses a graphical user interface with drop down menus, an enabled mouse, etc (as is found in Microsoft Windows, X-Windows, and the Apple Macintosh).

There are several systems created by various CDC departments to electronically collect, edit, analyze, and transmit laboratory, hospital-infection, human

Table 1 Recommendations for data and information systems

Time frame	Recommendations
Short term (1–2 Years)	*Data systems:* Implement more widespread electronic data collection and transmittal; link to information systems *Information systems:* Increase number of data sets; enhance analytical and reporting features to support *Healthy People 2000 Objectives* process
Long term (3–5 Years)	*Data systems:* Standardize data elements and equipment *Information systems:* Standardize interfaces; combine duplicative systems

immunodeficiency virus (HIV) and AIDS, and notifiable disease data from local and state health departments to CDC. These systems reduce the burden for reporting agencies and make data available sooner and in standardized form, which makes it easier to prepare timely reports and update information systems (3). However, they do not share common interfaces or communications protocols. France's computerized network for infectious disease surveillance has demonstrated that standardized equipment and data elements can greatly speed disease surveillance and feedback (18). Just as public health laboratorians have developed standard ways to manufacture vaccines, and the Advisory Committee on Immunizations Practices recommends doses and schedules, public health professionals are starting to hammer out proposed standards for technical features and implementation plans for data and information systems (12; Table 1).

IMPROVED COMMUNICATIONS FOR DYNAMIC ACCESS TO INFORMATION

Improved communications encompasses the technology and practices of enhancing, speeding, and simplifying the flow of information, whether that information is held by a human being or a machine, and whether the information is a number, a picture, a sound, or another representation of a fact or idea. PHI should enable the public health community to communicate more effectively in three domains: (*a*) human-to-human; (*b*) human-to-machine; and (*c*) machine-to-machine.

The application of new *human-to-human* communications technologies has already benefited public health by improving work efficiency. Electronic and voice mail eliminate telephone tag and make it easy to send the same message or computer file to many individuals simultaneously. For example, The Director of CDC uses electronic mail to transmit to all CDC staff the text of selected speeches and the minutes of executive staff meetings, thereby helping to unify

CDC. Another example is CDC's Voice Information System, which the public uses to access prerecorded information on hundreds of topics, including Chronic Fatigue Syndrome, Lyme disease, vaccination requirements for travelers, and AIDS. Since its inception in 1988, this system has been accessed millions of times; its benefits include giving more consistent information on a 24-hour basis, which frees CDC staff to answer more complex queries from health professionals.

Increased benefits will accrue by connecting more people to electronic mail; integrating electronic mail with bulletin boards and other information services; and by making wider use of video teleconferencing (which allows participants at both ends to see each other on a television screen) and satellite-based instruction (wherein the instructor appears on a television screen at remote sites). Video teleconferencing is used between CDC and other PHS offices in Atlanta, Washington, DC, and Cincinnati to reduce travel time and expense for meetings and classes; this technology also allows more people to participate, and thus speeds decision-making and reduces miscommunications. At the state level, Alabama's Department of Public Health is currently piloting satellite televised instruction to local health departments; early results are encouraging.

Improved *human-to-machine* communications have facilitated public health work by making user-friendly interfaces more widely available, a result of the availability of microcomputers, which are usually easier to use than mainframes. Increased benefits to public health will accrue during the next 2–4 years as more mainframe interfaces are supplanted by cooperative processing, wherein a microcomputer and mainframe work jointly on a single task. Under this system, the user has access to the power and massive storage of a mainframe computer (where the data are centrally stored and updated), but can manipulate data via the user-friendly microcomputer, which can offer a mouse, windows, color selection, and access to higher-resolution printers (8). Finally, because systems that look and work in a consistent fashion are easier to learn and use, human-to-machine communications will be promoted by standardizing interfaces.

The impact of messages directed at professional and lay audiences can be strengthened by more sophisticated use of sound, video, and modern graphics. During the next few years, putting large amounts of information in easy-to-use form into the hands of all public health workers will be facilitated by multimedia workstations (which integrate sound, video, and computerized databases). The challenge to public health leaders will be to channel this evolving technology for public health practice, by training staff to think in PHI terms, providing up-to-date workstations and software, and making it clear that new technology may require abandonment of old work patterns (and maybe some software and hardware that has not evolved).

Table 2 Recommendations for communications

Time frame	Recommendations
Short term (1–2 Years)	Make more widespread use of e-mail, bulletin boards, and voice information systems Develop cooperative processing for public health, video teleconferencing, and invest in better workstations and communications lines
Long term (3–5 Years)	Develop multimedia public health applications for public health Make cooperative processing widespread Develop and implement standards for interfaces and equipment

Improvements in *machine-to-machine* communications have benefited public health by providing increased reliability and reduced costs for data transmission and machine-to-machine connections. This is a result of the widespread availability of faster and less expensive modems, fiber-optic communications, and sophisticated electronic networks. In the future, machine-to-machine public health communications will benefit from faster data transmissions between data collection and synthesis/analysis points, and reducing the errors, labor, and losses associated with mailing disks and tapes. Clearly, the internet, although currently not suitable for transmitting sensitive information, will have an important role to play. PHI is being used to develop new surveillance systems, wherein computers receive data around the clock and automatically update the database, send an electronic mail message notifying both sender and recipient if the data contained errors (or failed to arrive), and return an edited report to the sender (8). These systems will speed the availability of accurate data for inclusion in truly timely information systems and reports (Table 2).

BETTER TOOLS FOR PUBLIC HEALTH PRACTICE

Public health informatics has been used to develop tools that serve public health's special needs for population-based information and communications. Examples that demonstrate the utility of such systems include:

- *Patient Flow Analysis,* a statistical analysis and graphing system based on software-driven simulations, is used in family planning clinics to optimize schedules and the order of service delivery, thereby reducing waiting time and increasing productivity;
- *Epi Info,* a microcomputer database and statistics program used by epidemiologists to collect, verify, and analyze epidemic data in the field (rather

than sending the data to a central office for analysis), thereby allowing quicker formulation of recommendations for control (4);

- *SUDAAN*, a statistical analysis system provides programs to analyze data from complex cluster surveys;
- *SETS*, a system to distribute CDC survey data and specialized analysis software on CD-ROM, which facilitates data analysis and saves mainframe resources for its users;
- *Arkansas' Early Intervention Services System*, which links several data-bases and integrates remote communications, facilitating the delivery of public health services (18);
- An *"electronic" extramural course in epidemiology* developed in Canada, which uses computer conferencing for distance-based education, allows students to continue their public health education without needing to move or change work schedules (16).

These examples demonstrate that PHI's function of applying information technology to public health practice can facilitate work at Federal, state, and local levels. Proposed new PHI applications include: better tools for authors of multimedia based training courses; public health clinic management software that emphasizes "walk-ins" and follow-up, and that is integrated with surveillance systems; mapping software that can be used to correlate information about health effects and the location of putative environmental risk factors (e.g. contaminated ground water or sources of radiation); improved systems to identify sources of survey data and associated laboratory samples that may be available for further analysis; and quick ways to get expert consultations.

It must be emphasized that the vast majority of public health software and hardware systems have been, and should continue to be, based on commercially available products. The best commercial products have large numbers of users. This large user base enables those manufacturers to provide customer support and upgrades, and to sponsor training and user groups. Large companies that stay in business tend to adhere to (or develop) emerging standards. Economies of scale tend to control prices, especially as compared to custom-built systems, in which most of the actual cost may go for specialized training or postpurchase modifications. PHI projects should build on what is available and tested whenever possible. New software should only be developed when a commercial alternative is not available or is too expensive (especially for very large scale applications when hundreds or thousands of copies may be required), or when modifying existing software to suit public health needs is not feasible.

Federal, state, and local agencies that have been successful in using information technology should now extend technical assistance to locales that are just getting started, with a special emphasis on promoting *local* systems development, which can be designed to suit specific local needs. For example,

Table 3 Recommendations for better tools

Time Frame	Recommendations
Short term (1–2 Years)	Develop new applications for public health practice: clinic management software, mapping tools for environmental exposures, etc Develop capacity for software development in state and local health departments
Long term (3–5 Years)	Develop and implement interface standards Assure that PHI is integrated into all public health activities

Washington State's Department of Health has developed a system to track its progress towards meeting the *Healthy People 2000 Objectives* that emphasizes the State's concerns (8). One problem with all this rich activity has been the resultant diversity in interfaces, tools, and underlying technology. If systems are too particularistic, they may fall into disuse (10). Standardizing interfaces and underlying technologies may promote the development of tools that have a lasting impact (17; Table 3).

THE DISCIPLINE OF PUBLIC HEALTH INFORMATICS

There are several reasons to develop a new academic discipline in informatics (10). First and foremost, it will help assure that new information technology and practices are developed to serve public health's specific needs, and that technology and an understanding of how best to use it will evolve along with public health itself. Second, having PHI in an academic setting will promote basic research. Third, a discipline provides a locus of expertise and support for students who need to be trained in subjects not currently well represented in public health faculties. Finally, it provides a career path, thus attracting talented students and professionals who can help build the field.

Supporting the triad of teaching, research, and service is a powerful way to encourage the growth of a new science. The components of service have been outlined in this paper. Teaching would include developing instructional and degree-granting programs in schools of public health, and offering seminars and courses in public health agencies and to academic collaborators. For those working in government or business, it means serving as adjunct faculty, precepting students in epidemiology, biostatistics, preventive medicine, nursing, information science, and engineering. CDC staff who work in this field teach an entire course at the Emory School of Public Health on using information systems, and one of Epi Info's developers teaches it to the epidemiology students. CDC has several engineering students from the Georgia Institute of

Technology working part-time on various projects; this experience has provided an exposure to public health that they would not otherwise have had and has stimulated career interests in human services.

Research activities should include investigating the applicability of new technology to public health via formal hypothesis generation and testing, and implementing new ideas and technologies. There is a need to insert basic research, rigor, and peer-review into a field that otherwise could become overly focused on meeting day-to-day needs. For example, CDC is collaborating with the University of Michigan to investigate new communications architectures for databases, and with the Georgia Institute of Technology on networking.

Traditional academic activities will be key to building credibility for public health informatics as a discipline, and will also greatly promote external collaborations. The preparation of results for publication and presentations at professional meetings is as important for PHI as it is for other disciplines. Much of the medical informatics literature is in paired articles: one for the medical result, another for the informatics significance; this model is directly applicable in public health.

Public health informatics programs in government and academia should develop the capacity to carry out consultations and collaborations on subjects ranging from the choice of appropriate software to the development of complex systems. Historically, an important engine of public health has been the injection of experts into new environments, such as Federal assignees to state and local health departments, schools of public health, and the World Health Organization; and university scholars coming to public health service agencies for sabbaticals. This results in cross-fertilization between government, academia, international agencies, and foreign governments.

A logical extension of consultation would be the creation of centers of academic and applied excellence in PHI to assure the development and sharing of expertise (Table 4). This model has been used by the National Library of Medicine, National Institutes of Health, which has funded academic medical centers to develop enterprise-wide information management systems under the Integrated Academic Information Program Management System (15). This project has contributed to nationwide interest in using medical informatics in medical centers and has helped move many projects out of the medical informatics laboratory into clinical use. Public health is poised to emulate this model, assuming sufficient funds are made available. One way to develop centers of excellence in PHI could be via promoting partnerships made up of Federal, state, and local governments; private foundations and nonprofit agencies; and private for-profit corporations. These Centers could evaluate and develop PHI strategies that would then be widely shared. One highly successful example has been the Georgia Information Network for Public Health Officials (INPHO) project, funded by a $5.2 million grant from the Robert W. Woodruff Foundation.

Table 4 Recommendations for the discipline of Public Health Informatics

Time Frame	Recommendations
Short term (1–2 Years)	The public health community should establish academic programs and centers in excellence in PHI
	PHI professionals should involve themselves in practice, teaching, and research; and publish and present their findings
	Academia, government, and business should develop collaborative and consultative activities
Long term (3–5 Years)	Consider establishing departments of PHI in schools of public health, and a journal
	Develop more formal programs for the exchange of scholars, sabbaticals, etc

Collaborators include the foundation; academia (Emory University, Medical College of Georgia, and Georgia Institute of Technology); and government (the Georgia Department of Public Health, CDC). This project has developed new strategies for networking, disease surveillance, and disseminating information, and represents a model that can be exported to other states.

CONCLUSION

Gaps in public health information and weaknesses in communications will be only partly ameliorated by the development of new technology. Rather, important gains will depend more on bold long-range planning, concerted and well-led efforts at standardization, documenting the contributions of PHI towards the improvement of public health, and garnering and properly aiming new resources. This, in turn, will require that governmental and academic public health leaders develop a commitment to public health informatics. A fully developed academic discipline must be the foundation stone of this initiative. To do less will make public health outmoded and will place it at risk.

Public health informatics is viewed today in the same light as were chronic disease epidemiology and advanced statistics 20 years ago: obscure, forbiddingly complex, something for the specialist, impractical, expensive, of doubtful general utility. Just as these other advances had salutary and indeed revolutionary impacts on epidemiology, so too could Public Health Informatics have profound benefits on public health practice.

ACKNOWLEDGMENTS

We would like to thank Lisa S Rosenblum, Daniel A Pollock, Andrew G Dean, Donna F Stroup, Howard W Ory, and Jeffrey R Harris, of the Centers for

Disease Control and Prevention, and Truls Østbye, of the University of Western Ontario, for their thoughtful comments on earlier drafts.

Literature Cited

1. American Public Health Association. 1991. *Healthy Communities 2000: Model Standards.* Washington, DC: Am. Public Health Assoc.
2. APEX*PH* Work Group. 1991. *Assessment protocol for excellence in public health.* Natl. Assoc. County Health Off.
3. Bean NH, Martin SM, Bradford H. 1992. PHLIS: an electronic system for reporting public health data from remote sites. *Am. J. Public Health* 82:1273–76
4. Dean AG, Dean JA, Burton AH, Dicker RC. 1991. Epi Info: a general purpose microcomputer program for public health information systems. *Am. J. Prev. Med.* 7:178–82
5. Eatmon JM. 1991. Hardware and software needs for coordination of early intervention services (Public Law 99–457). *Proc. Public Health Conf. Records Stat.,* pp. 514–19, July 15–17. Washington, DC
6. Friede A, Freedman MA, Paul JE, Rizzo NP, Pawate VI, Turczyn KM. 1994. DATA2000: a computer system to link HP2000 objectives, data sources, and contacts. *Am. J. Prev. Med.* In press
7. Friede A, Reid JA, Ory HW. 1993. CDC WONDER: a comprehensive online public health information system of the Centers for Disease Control and Prevention. *Am. J. Public Health* 83: 1289–94
8. Friede A, Rosen DR, Reid JA. 1994. CDC WONDER/PC cooperative processing for public health informatics. *J. Am. Med. Inform. Assoc.* 1:303–12
9. Goldman DA. 1994. The EPIGRAM computer for analyzing mortality and population data sets. *Public Health Rep.* 109:118–24
10. Greenes RA, Shortliffe EH. 1990. Medical informatics, an emerging academic discipline and institutional priority. *J. Am. Med. Assoc.* 263:1114–20
11. Greenlick MR. 1992. Educating physicians for population-based clinical practice. *J. Am. Med. Assoc.* 267:1645–48
12. Hughes JM, Teutch SM, Stroup NE, Friede AM, Garbe P, et al. 1991. *Surveillance Coordination Group Report: Recommendations for Electronic Systems for Public Health Surveillance.* Atlanta, GA: Cent. Disease Control
13. Kelso S. 1991. Developing a system to trace health objectives and indicators. See Ref. 5, pp. 534–38
14. Kleinman JC, Kiely JL. 1991. Infant mortality. *Stat. Notes* 1:1–11. Hyattsville, MD: Centers for Disease Control; US Dept of Health, Education, and Welfare Publ. 92–1237
15. Lindberg DA, West, RT, Corn M. 1991. IAIMS: an overview from the National Library of Medicine. *Bull. Med. Libr. Assoc.* 80:244–46
16. Østbye T. 1989. An "electronic" extramural course in epidemiology and medical statistics. *Int. J. Epidemiol.* 18: 275–79
17. Pollock DA, McClain PW. 1989. Trauma registries: current status and future prospects. *J. Am. Med. Assoc.* 262: 2280–83
18. Valleron A-J, Bouvet E, Garnerin P, Menares J, Heard I, et al. 1986. A computer network for the surveillance of communicable diseases: the French experiment. *Am. J. Public Health* 76: 1289–92
19. Wartenberg D, Agamennone VJ, Ozonoff D, Berry RJ. 1989. A microcomputer-based vital records data base with interactive graphic assessment for states and localities. *Am. J. Public Health* 79:1531–36

Annu. Rev. Public Health. 1995. 16:253–82

INTERNATIONAL ASPECTS OF THE AIDS/HIV EPIDEMIC*

Ann Marie Kimball[1], Seth Berkley[2], Elizabeth Ngugi[3], and Helene Gayle[4]

[1]Department of Health Services and Epidemiology, University of Washington, Seattle, Washington 98195; [2]Health Sciences Division, Rockefeller Foundation, 420 Fifth Avenue, New York, NY 10018-2702; [3]Department of Community Health, Strengthening STD/HIV Control Project, P.O. Box 19675, Nairobi, Kenya; [4]Centers for Disease Control and Prevention, 1600 Clifton Road, Atlanta, Georgia 30333

KEY WORDS: HIV transmission, global AIDS policy, HIV prevention

ABSTRACT

This review provides the reader with pertinent information on the epidemiology, prevention, and new technologies of the ongoing HIV pandemic. These aspects are key to international policy discussions surrounding the public health response to the international spread of HIV. Our understanding of the impact of AIDS on other diseases is evolving, as is our insight into the demographic and economic effects of the epidemic on the global community. Observations on the success of certain prevention strategies allow rational allocation of resources in newly affected epidemic areas. Information on the origin and nature of HIV transmission exemplifies the phenomenon of global emerging infections. As world populations are brought closer together through transportation, communication, trade, and commerce, insight into emerging infections of epidemic potential becomes increasingly important to the practitioner of public health. Although important, legal and social aspects of the epidemic will not be emphasized here. The epidemics of HIV/AIDS in the United States and Europe are not reviewed here. The global pandemic has recently been described in an overview in this publication to which the reader is also referred (15).

THE IMPORTANCE OF AIDS

The importance of AIDS is, in part, due to the societal effect of the prolonged course of the illness affecting young adults, and the eventual complete fatal outcome of the disease. Only now is the international development community becoming cognizant of the social, political, and economic impacts of AIDS worldwide. The World Health Organization has projected that over 13 million people are now infected and that 18 million people will succumb to clinical AIDS by the year 2000 (83). More than two million people have died thus far. Other authors characterize these estimates as too conservative (45). Moreover, the world population (estimated at 5.3 billion at the time of this writing) is not uniformly infected. Thus, as discussed below, some regions and certain population groups will be much more adversely affected by morbidity and mortality from AIDS. Nonetheless, the economic costs, estimated to reach $350 billion by the year 2000 (4), will be felt worldwide. This figure approximates the current gross national product of Australia.

The international policy dialogue has begun to reflect an understanding of the profundity of the challenge still before us, particularly as issues of equity are highlighted in vaccine development efforts (32). The coordination of multiple UN agency programs into a single effort is aimed at broadening and strengthening the international response (72) through a new joint cosponsored program. Nonetheless, intractable global economic and political questions remain: Are international strategies beyond promotion and advocacy needed to insure timely protective action by individual governments? What is the most appropriate form of international relief for those countries hardest hit by the pandemic? How will this relief be financed? How should counterproductive and ethically unacceptable strategies (e.g. quarantine of the HIV positive and restrictions on the travel and employment of infected persons) be met by the international public health community? We aim to provide a framework for this broad, ongoing dialogue.

THE TRANSMISSION OF HIV

It is now thought that the late 1970s were the apparent starting point of intense HIV spread (1). The initiation of HIV spread appears to have occurred simultaneously in at least two distinct geographic areas—Central Africa and the United States/Caribbean, but was not heralded until 1982 when the first cluster of clinical illness was reported in the medical literature (11a). In retrospect, endemic African disease patterns had clearly been shifting for some time during the 1980s, possibly in response to the incursion of HIV and resultant immunocompromise. For example, cryptococcal meningitis in tropical areas

Table 1 Patterns of HIV spread

Pattern I	Extensive spread of HIV began in the late 1970s/early 1980s. Homosexual males and intravenous drug users have been the predominantly affected populations, but heterosexual transmission is increasing.
Pattern II	Extensive spread of HIV began in the mid-to-late 1970s/early 1980s. Heterosexual transmission has and continues to predominate.
Pattern I/II	Extensive spread of HIV began in the late 1970s/early 1980s. Initially mostly homosexual men and IV drug users were affected, but heterosexual transmission became predominant in mid-to-late 1980s.
Pattern III	Introduction and/or extensive spread of HIV did not occur until mid-to-late 1980s. Extensive spread of HIV is now being documented in several countries in South-East Asia, but the prevalence of HIV in most countries classified within this pattern remains relatively low.

increased, with changing ecology of the agent (ref. 6a). The advent of more sophisticated diagnostic techniques revealed that sporadic cases of clinical AIDS occurred in North America and Africa prior to the reported cluster (27).

In the mid-1980s, WHO scientists classified regions into three patterns of epidemic spread of HIV in an attempt to clarify the distinct regional modes of HIV transmissions (Table 1). However, it has subsequently become apparent that such classification represents a "snapshot" of an epidemiologic global phenomenon that is characterized more by continual change than by its ability to be classified. For example, countries in Latin America designated as Pattern I began to display heterosexual transmission shortly after this scheme was published and thus became Pattern I/II countries. Because this epidemiological classification is based on the year when HIV was introduced or began to spread extensively, plus the predominant model of HIV transmission, a Pattern III country can never be reclassified as a Pattern I or a Pattern II. Pattern III countries where extensive spread of HIV had not yet been documented, but where high rates of sexually transmitted diseases (STDs) and/or where IV drug use existed, were projected to have a large HIV/AIDS epidemic during the 1990s.

The mechanisms of HIV transmission are limited: sexual intercourse; exposure to contaminated blood products or body fluids, including the use of unclean needles for injection; vertical transmission from an infected mother to her child prior to or at delivery; and transmission from an infected mother to her child through breast-feeding. Estimates of the efficiency for each route vary from about 0.1% per sexual contact to over 90% for blood-borne transmission via transfusion. However, wide regional variations occur—for reasons that remain unclear. For example, recent research in Thailand suggests there is a much higher risk of 3–6% per heterosexual contact compared with the estimate of 0.1% for North America (47). However, these findings have been recently questioned (20a). To calm fears of contagion, it has been as important to define the routes of nontransmission as to define the routes of transmission. Casual transmission is very rare even in settings of substandard hygiene and of direct nursing of the sick. Nor has transmission by mosquitoes been demonstrated (43). Malaria itself, rather than its vector, has contributed to HIV transmission through the anemia it causes. Transfusion of children with malaria promotes HIV transmission if blood screening for HIV is not available (34) and HIV is prevalent.

Insight gained through behavioral research and the application of microbiological tools indicates that the transmission dynamics of this global pandemic are more complex than initially suspected. Our understanding of the nature of different strains of HIV and their apparent segregation by certain transmission routes continues to evolve.

Heterosexual transmission accounts for an estimated 70–80% of global transmission of HIV. Nonetheless, other routes also figure prominently in the global picture because of their social repercussions. Infected mother-to-infant transmission of the virus is increasing worldwide. However, not all children born from infected mothers are infected. This rate of vertical transmission is estimated to be 25–50% in lesser developed countries (Table 2) compared with 20–30% in developed countries. Maternal-to-infant transmission can occur prepartum, and HIV has been found in fetuses aborted in the first trimester of pregnancy (59). Transmission definitely occurs during delivery; contrary to previous findings, a recent study of mode of delivery suggested caesarean section may decrease transmission by up to 50% (22a, 76), but these studies await confirmation.

The risk of transmission from mother to infant through breast-feeding is a difficult issue internationally. During the late 1970s, it was demonstrated that bottle-feeding clearly placed infants at increased risk of diarrheal disease mortality, especially during periods of epidemic diarrheal disease (28). In response, the World Health Organization, UNICEF, and other agencies

Table 2 Rates of maternal/infant transmission

Collected African studies		
Location	% Transmission	Reference
• Kinshasa, Zaire	39	63a
• Lusaka, Zambia	39	30a
• Brazzaville, Congo	52	41a
• Kigali, Rwanda	25.7	42a

recommended and actively promoted breast-feeding in the developing world as a means of improving child survival. The first definitive report of transmission of HIV through breast-feeding was published in 1985 (92). Subsequent studies have shown high rates of infant HIV infection through breast-milk transmission when the mother seroconverts during the breast-feeding period. A prospective study in Kigali of 212 mothers seronegative at delivery identified nine maternal seroconversions, of which five (56%) resulted in infant seroconversion via breast-milk transmission (75). In a recent review, Dunn et al estimated that additional risk of maternal-to-infant trans-mission from breast-feeding (above and beyond that incurred in delivery) to be 14% (21). Based on such data, the policy recommendation in favor of breast-feeding has been repeatedly re-examined (35). Latin American coun-tries are adopting guidance similar to that of the United States and the United Kingdom, which do not promote breast-feeding when the mother is infected with HIV. Universal recommendation of breast-feeding remains in countries where access to clean water and hygiene are problematic.

The role that infected blood plays in the spread of HIV worldwide varies by region. In Latin America, blood screening is virtually complete, whereas in Africa estimates of screened transfusions do not exceed 50%. In Africa the attributable risk of unscreened blood is thought to be small (less than 10% overall); nonetheless, this is a preventable route of transmission that contributes to transmission (10). Before the implementation of blood screening in 1985, large numbers of infections were transmitted by transfusions, particularly to infants where one donor could infect multiple patients. Other methods besides screening have been employed to reduce the risk of transmission through blood transfusion. These include decreasing the use of transfusions through early treatment of predisposing conditions, thereby eliminating unnecessary use of transfusion, and obtaining blood from low-risk donors.

Shared use of needles for recreational drug use is a major route of trans-mission. The use of injections for treatment worldwide is routine both in traditional and modern practice, and the reuse of needles is common in resource-poor settings because of limited supply and the absence of sterile technique. Concern that contaminated needles used in health care settings may play a major role in HIV transmission has not been borne out by research. A careful review of the limited data on parenteral transmission of HIV from epidemiologic studies and age-specific HIV infection rates suggests that, even if occasional transmission of HIV does occur, such injections are not a major route of transmission (5), with the possible exception of the Romanian epi-demic among insitutionalized children (90a). Certainly no link has been dem-onstrated between vaccination programs in Africa or Latin America and HIV transmission, probably due to the strong emphasis during training of medical personnel regarding the supply and use of sterile needles.

THE AIDS PANDEMIC: A SERIES OF REGIONAL EPIDEMICS

AIDS in Africa

At the same time that the first cases of AIDS were being identified in homosexual populations in the United States and Europe, cases of a wasting illness with a high mortality and an unknown etiology were occurring in villages in Central Africa (58, 66, 74). Physical examination, including routine examination of the oral cavity, plays a major role in diagnosing diseases in these communities. The occurrence of oro-pharyngeal candidiasis together with the occurrence of wasting disease in adults portended the appearance of a new disease for the region and was noted by clinicians in the early 1980s. The advent of HIV testing in 1985 enabled Eastern and Central African countries such as Rwanda, Tanzania, Uganda, and Zaire to confirm HIV and relate this illness to the newly described disease of AIDS in the United States and Europe.

Coincidentally, virology researchers in Senegal identified a similar virus, which was not initially associated with disease. This agent, now known as HIV2, was originally thought by some in the West African scientific community to be protective against HIV1, since HIV2 was present and HIV1 was not apparent in the mid-1980s in West Africa. Subsequent studies have demonstrated that HIV2 is pathogenic, and causes AIDS. Some studies suggest that the severity of HIV2 disease may be somewhat less than HIV1 disease (18).

These discoveries focused international attention on AIDS in Africa. Serologic testing using the early generation of tests led to excessive and inaccurate estimates of infection as a result of cross-reactivity with serum that had high concentrations of nonspecific antibodies from exposure to other infectious agents (65). As a result, Africa was unfairly identified as the origin of HIV infection worldwide. The results from these serologic surveys, later retracted, damaged international confidence in predictions of the epidemic. This mistrust may have facilitated denial once the true magnitude of infection became clear. Behaviors associated with transmission in the West, such as homosexuality, use of intravenous drugs, and anal intercourse, were absent in the vast majority of AIDS cases in Africa. Studies demonstrated a male-to-female ratio of close to 1:1—very different from the overwhelmingly male presentation seen at that time in North America and Europe. Subsequent studies in areas where the epidemic is long-standing, like Uganda and Tanzania, have shown infection rates to be higher in women than in men (2, 6). In addition, females are infected at a younger age than males—on average 5 years—in virtually all African populations studied, a finding also seen among populations in the Caribbean and South America.

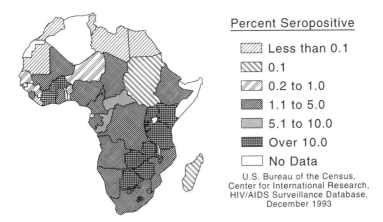

Percent Seropositive

Less than 0.1
0.1
0.2 to 1.0
1.1 to 5.0
5.1 to 10.0
Over 10.0
No Data

U.S. Bureau of the Census,
Center for International Research,
HIV/AIDS Surveillance Database,
December 1993

Figure 1   African HIV1 seroprevalence for low-risk urban populations. Reprinted with permission.

The epidemic has clearly spread much more widely in the heterosexual population in Africa than in North America or Europe. The relative rates of HIV infections for the continent is shown in Figure 1. Careful studies have suggested that the transmission cannot be explained solely by more sexual exposure but rather that the actual efficiency of transmission appears to be higher. This hypothesis has led to a search for risk factors that could explain a higher risk of transmission. Studies in Africa have shown other sexually transmitted infectious diseases (STDs) (both ulcerative and nonulcerative), male noncircumcision, and young age among females to increase the risk of transmission. Some studies have also shown sex during menses, use of in-travaginal preparations, and oral contraceptives to be risk factors. These effects are not consistent across studies. Female circumcision, although biologically plausible as a risk factor, is not common in the areas with the highest rate of transmission and probably contributes little to attributable risk.

The initial report of an almost exclusively urban location for HIV has been misleading. A study of Ebola fever conducted in a small rural, isolated community in Zaire in 1986 suggested that rural areas adhering to traditional village life would not be affected by the HIV epidemic (55). Using stored serum from the Ebola fever investigation, investigators showed a stable seroprevalence of 0.8% over a ten-year period (from 1976–1986) (55). However, by 1986, commercial sex workers in this rural area already had a seroprevalence of 11%, which suggested that seroprevalence would soon begin to rise. National and sentinel surveys have shown high rates of HIV infection throughout many sub-Saharan countries. In virtually all areas, infection rates in the largest cities still exceed those in smaller towns and rural areas. However, the infection is spreading to rural areas, and HIV infection can no longer be considered an "urban disease." In Uganda, a national serosurvey conducted as early as 1986 showed HIV rates in urban areas to be 2–3 times those in rural areas. Nonetheless, because 90% of the population lived in rural areas and infection rates were not trivial, over 80% of those with HIV infections were and are living in rural areas. Further studies in Uganda have shown a gradient in infection rates as one moves from larger population centers with easy access to transportation to rural villages. A study in a rural district, Rakai, indicated that the highest transmission rates were in main road trading centers (38%), with intermediate rates in rural trading villages on secondary roads (25%), and the lowest rates in rural agricultural villages (9%) (79). A study in Tanzania showed similar findings (36).

The spread of AIDS is devastating to individuals, families, communities, and countries. AIDS has a powerful effect beyond the actual numbers of infected and dying. It affects people during their economically most productive adult years when they are typically responsible for the support and care of others. The chronic nature of the illness and its high cost of treatment magnify its societal impact. In addition, because of its sexual spread there is clustering among certain households, with both the husband and wife—or wives, in a polygamous family—commonly infected. Simulations by the World Bank indicate an annual slowing of growth of income per capita by an average of 0.6 percentage point per country in the 10 worst affected countries in sub-Saharan Africa (87). One study in a rural community in Masaka, Uganda, has shown that 89% of the deaths in the 25–34 year age group can be attributed to HIV infection—an excess mortality of 13/1000 (50).

AIDS in the Western Hemisphere

In the Caribbean, the first reports of clinical AIDS in 1983 indicated that the initiation of infection in the United States and the Caribbean was temporally closely related. The earliest group at risk in the Caribbean, as in the United States, consisted of gay and bisexual men. In fact, reports of illness were confined to this group until 1985, when a transition to more heterosexual transmission began. As in the United States, the advent of HIV seroprevalence testing in the mid-1980s confirmed a high seroprevalence among gay and bisexual males, but also demonstrated a rapid rise among other high-risk groups such as commercial sex workers and intravenous drug users.

For reasons that are not completely understood, the transition to a heterosexual pattern of disease was extremely rapid in the Caribbean in the mid-1980s. This shift has been discussed in relation to a variety of factors: Bisexuality is more common than an exclusively homosexual orientation; populations are more proximate and urbanized in port city settings; there are high

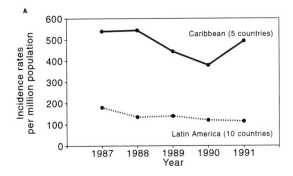

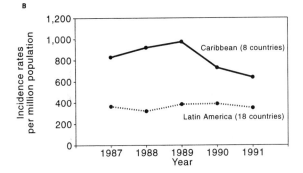

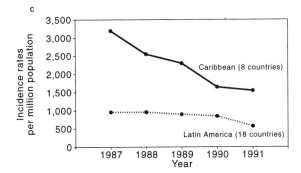

Figure 2   A: Median of annual incidence rates of syphilis (primary and secondary), by year, 1987–91, Latin America and the Caribbean; *B*: Median of annual incidence rates of syphilis (all forms), by year, 1987–91, Latin America and the Caribbean; *C*: Median of annual incidence rates of gonorrhea, by year, 1987–91, Latin America and the Caribbean. Reprinted with permission from Pan American Health Organization, PAHO Surveillance Data 1991.

levels of endemic sexually transmitted disease; the characteristics of the HIV strains that were introduced; and the background of other retroviruses that predated HIV in this population (3).

Synergistic linkage with sexually transmitted diseases (78) is one plausible mechanism behind the shift in risk to heterosexual populations, given the high rates of sexually transmitted diseases in the Caribbean (Figure 2). Biases for these data include the increased ascertainment that occurs in these island settings with relatively small, accessible populations. The rates of gonorrhea are threefold, for syphilis twofold, and for chancroid 15-fold higher in the Caribbean than in Latin America. In addition, an epidemic of crack cocaine in the Bahamas was shown to be closely related temporally to an epidemic of genital ulcer disease and a marked increase in HIV seroprevalence (26). These kinds of interactions among STDs are well-known contributors to infectivity and severity of HIV/AIDS (77).

The other countries in Central and South America have remained less affected by the pandemic than either the U.S. or the Caribbean. In general, rates of disease in Central America and in urban centers on the eastern coast of South America are two- to fourfold higher than those found elsewhere on the continent (Figure 3). In all areas, the annual incidence rates for clinical AIDS have been climbing year to year since reporting started in 1988. Within countries active commercial urban centers generally are foci of AIDS.

The transition to heterosexual transmission with increasing cases among women is seen in surveillance data from South America as well as the Caribbean. Two groups—bisexual males and intravenous drug users—are thought to serve as "bridge" groups in the generalization of transmission. The community of gay and bisexual men most affected in Latin America is difficult both to research and to reach with public health interventions because of social

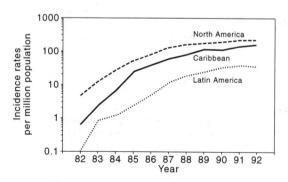

Figure 3   Annual incidence rates of AIDS in the Americas, (per million), three major regions 1982–92. Reprinted with permission from Pan American Health Organization, PAHO Surveillance Data 1992.

stigmatization. Recent studies in Mexico suggest that the risk of infection in partner pools is a stronger predictor of individual risk in that group than individual behavior (33), but research in gay populations is too limited to confirm this observation.

Seroprevalence rates among intravenous drug users in urban centers in Brazil and Argentina are similar to those of the eastern seaboard in the United States (38). As early as 1989, seroprevalences between 20% and 62% were reported in a series of surveys of intravenous drug injectors carried out in Buenos Aires, as well as 29% in Mexico City and 73% in Santos City, Brazil. Selection biases make international comparisons difficult. Because intravenous drug users in Latin America are socially stigmatized, with limited treatment available for their addiction, they are only identified late in their course. Thus studies of seroprevalence may reflect a heavier exposure to HIV through nonsterile needle use over a longer period of time than for North American users, who are often tested in the setting of drug-treatment centers. Nonetheless, the high infection rates seen in intravenous drug injectors in Latin America represent an important target group for prevention strategies. No recent studies have been published on this high-risk group.

The dramatic increase in HIV transmission to women in Central America is facilitated by their subservient social role. Perhaps the major risk factor for women is conduct by her sexual partner—conduct that she is not in a position to question, given the prevailing social norms. For example, a study in Costa Rica found the typical woman with AIDS was a housewife who reported no knowledge of any risk factors that may have caused her infection (30). This suggests that these women may have been unaware because the risky conduct was actually that of the husband.

The relationship between cervical pathology and HIV transmission merits study in this setting. Women in Latin America and the Caribbean have high rates of cervical disease including cervical cancer (Figure 4). The mortality rates from cervical cancer are between 1.6 and 6.1 times higher than in Canada, Cuba, and the United States. These data reflect a stagnation of services to women. A case control study carried out in the Honduran port city of San Pedro Sula (J Zelaya, M Rocha & AM Kimball, unpublished information) in 1991 associated HIV infection among women with sexual conduct of her partner, her own number of sexual partners, and, most significantly, the presence of dysplasia, inflammation, or HPV on her cervix. Regular gynecological examinations with appropriate early treatment of cervical lesions would be a strategy worth testing in these locations.

HIV transmission to women in Latin America was intensified by the earlier lack of blood screening. Mexico, as of 1991, attributed 63% of cumulative cases of AIDS in women to blood transfusion, whereas this route was cited for only 6% of men. The risk to women is higher because of the higher

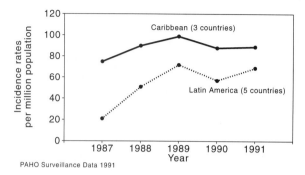

Figure 4   Median of annual incidence rates of cervical cancer, by year, 1987–1991, Latin America and the Caribbean. Reprinted with permission from Pan American Health Organization, PAHO Surveillance Data 1992.

incidence of transfusion at childbirth. Blood screening has been shown to be an effective strategy for reducing risk of HIV in women in Latin America (41). Systematic blood screening has been a cornerstone of most national programs in the region. Private blood banks, such as those operating in some Andean countries, have been more difficult to regulate than those in the public sector.

An alarming result of the shift of the epidemic to women is the consequent increase in perinatal transmission around the region. As shown in Figure 5, increasing numbers of such cases are being reported, although the absolute numbers remain small. Studies from Brazil suggest that a high proportion of transmission is related to intravenous drug use by the mother or her partner (30, 44).

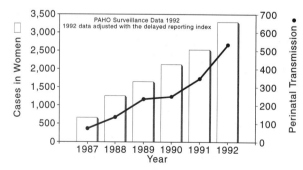

Figure 5   Number of reported cases in women, and cases due to perinatal transmission, Latin America and the Caribbean, 1987–92. Reprinted with permission from Pan American Health Organization, PAHO Surveillance Data 1992.

Prevention strategies for women in Latin America will be enhanced when barrier or virucidal methods under the control of women themselves are available (40). Social norms make disclosure of previous risk behavior by men to their female partners unlikely, and the ability of women to negotiate regular condom use even less likely. In this setting, the need for new research on HIV prevention that works for women is compelling.

NEWER EPIDEMICS

Asia and the Pacific

The history of the HIV/AIDS epidemic in the world cannot yet be written. The epidemic is continuing to advance, with the most dramatic recent growth occurring in Asia. Two major routes of transmission, intravenous drug use and sexual intercourse, have combined to create rapid increases in transmission in that region. Two countries, Burma and Thailand, are instructive as examples of this new epidemic; the US Census bureau has recently published a detailed discussion (80). Data from Burma suggest that the rate of infection in some groups of intravenous drug users increased from 17% in 1989 to 76% in 1991. Data for women at high risk (commercial sex workers) indicate recent seroprevalence has reached 11%.

Thailand put into place an extensive surveillance system for seroprevalence studies that has facilitated meticulous tracking of the epidemic. Incursion of the virus was seen first among intravenous drug users, gay males, and commercial sex workers in the Northern and Central regions of the country. Coincident surveillance documented a near doubling of infection in urban STD clinic attendees throughout the country between 1990 and 1993, with the highest level seen in the North, and 8% seroprevalence in 1992 among military recruits in the North. The prevalence among low-charge female commercial sex workers has increased steadily from 3% in 1989 to 29% in 1993 (5a).

There is continued paucity of surveillance information about high-risk groups from the rest of Asia. Serosurveillance among intravenous drug injectors reveals a high incidence of infection in China (15%) (91) and Malaysia (30%) (67), but not among injectors tested in Hong Kong (86). Other countries apparently are not reporting on seroprevalence in this high-risk group. Commercial sex workers in Bombay, India, are heavily infected, but information about other countries is lacking. Given the explosive rise in infection seen in these groups in Africa, the Caribbean, and Latin America, additional studies in the newer epidemic areas of Asia and Oceania are needed.

If seroprevalence is as low as the limited available information suggests, there is still opportunity for timely prevention campaigns. Singapore has mounted a particularly active educational campaign (67), conducted under the

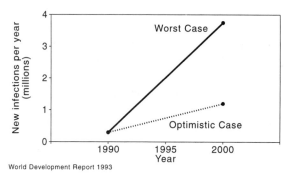

World Development Report 1993

Figure 6   New infections per year in Asia. Source: World Health Organization, Global Programme on AIDS.

close collaboration of government and nongovernmental sectors. Thailand has documented success with its "100% condom" campaign among prostitutes. Operations research in South China has demonstrated the potential efficacy of harm-reduction strategies using bleach for needles (89). Such efforts represent a hopeful start.

The World Health Organization estimates that the implementation of effective prevention in Asia could dampen the rate of transmission, with more than 2 million infections prevented by the year 2000 (Figure 6).

In Asia, the early development of a broad response to the epidemic, not limited to the health sector, is encouraging. Increasingly, the HIV/AIDS issue is being successfully incorporated into the policy agenda of development, trade, and commerce. The US/Japan Agreement for Cooperation for Economic Development includes AIDS cooperation in the Asia Pacific region as a point for the agenda (73). Both of these major economies have pledged several billion dollars in support of AIDS prevention. Business councils have been formed in the Asian capitals of Kuala Lumpur, Hong Kong, Taipei, Bangkok, and Djakarta to address the threat of AIDS. The 10th International Conference on AIDS in Yokohama, Japan, included satellite sessions on business and AIDS in the Asia Pacific region, including the founding of an intersectoral network of corporations and public health organizations (Asia Pacific Alliance Against AIDS). The costs of HIV/AIDS to business have been detailed (23). Business interests are central to the economic development of the Asia Pacific region, so the costs of an uncontrolled epidemic in this region may further spur prevention activity.

INFORMATION SYSTEMS/CASE REPORTING

Reporting completeness varies widely around the globe. Routine disease-reporting systems in most African countries are extremely limited. Estimates suggest that only 10–30% of actual AIDS cases are being reported. In Latin America and the Caribbean, it is estimated that between 30% and 50% of cases are reported. To monitor the spread of infection, WHO has piloted a number of sentinel reporting systems to follow infection rates over time in selected populations.

Differences in the presentation of the disease in Africa and the lack of sophisticated diagnostic facilities have made the use of the standard CDC/WHO case definition for AIDS problematic. In 1985 the World Health Organization convened a meeting in Bangui, Central African Republic, to develop a simple case definition for use in Africa (82). The Pan American Health Organization (PAHO) convened a similar meeting in Caracas, Venezuela, to tailor the definition of AIDS to regional diagnostic capabilities. The Bangui definition requires no laboratory or pathologic testing to establish the diagnosis, whereas that developed in Venezuela includes HIV testing. The Bangui definition is moderately specific (92%), but is not sensitive (52%) (85). The clinical diagnosis of pediatric cases of AIDS in international settings presents even more of a problem. A companion to the Bangui definition for children has a sensitivity of 35% and a specificity of 87%, modifications have not led to substantial improvements (16). It is hoped that a new generation of tests will improve the ability at least to diagnose infection in infants.

THEORIES OF EMERGENCE: A CONTINUING SEARCH

The emergence of HIV as a major human pathogen is an area of ongoing investigation. The close timing of the apparent initiation of transmission in Africa and the New World—two geographically remote sites—continues to provoke theories of origin, which are published both in the lay press and the scientific literature. Improving genetic techniques indicate that the HIV2 virus is close genetically to simian retroviruses. However, HIV1 is "centuries away" from SIV in genetic terms. The disparate sites of its first occurrence and additional genetic detailing through microepidemiologic techniques still leave questions about how this major pandemic started. Some level of man-made facilitation through the imperfect incubation of unrelated vaccines in monkey cells has been posited by some authors, but convincingly refuted by others (22). Recent modeling of genetic variation suggests that the rate of "escape mutant" production of HIV strains is higher than previously believed. This high degree of genetic variability may have figured in its emergence as a major pathogen.

HIV has been present in Africa for decades. The earliest documented infection with HIV in Africa was from a serum sample from Equateur Province in Northern Zaire from 1976. HIV was isolated from serum collected and frozen during a serosurvey investigation of the epidemic of Ebola fever in 1976. Another study of stored serum from Africa detected antibodies reactive to HIV by ELISA and Western blot from a frozen serum from Kinshasa from 1959 (51). However, virus isolation was never attempted.

The HIV pandemic can be seen as a sentinel event in the history of global disease. Given the increasing international linkages between communities through travel, trade, and migration, the emergence of new infectious diseases such as AIDS will become more frequent (42). Thus, gaining as much insight into the factors that brought the HIV pandemic to its current level of devastation will be central to our ability to cope with future pandemics.

THE INTERNATIONAL RESPONSE

Prevention Challenges

Prevention remains the only effective way to protect individuals, families, and communities from HIV transmission, and the eventual sequelae of AIDS. Despite a decade of research, cures and preventive vaccines remain elusive, and will remain so for resource-poor settings for the foreseeable future. Initial efforts at prevention in Africa were hampered by (a) unavoidably tardy initiation relative to the timing of transmission, (b) the "vertical" nature of the effort and its heavy reliance on external expertise, (c) the difficulty in defining culturally acceptable and appropriate interventions, and (d) the lack of cheap diagnostic testing or infrastructure for testing. As a result, current levels of infection are highest in Africa, and still rising, and the ongoing challenges to prevention continue to be very serious.

Despite its relative inefficiency, transmission of HIV through sexual intercourse is by far the most prevalent transmission worldwide. Most communities maintain a culture of silence about sexuality, and sexual practices that may increase the risk of HIV have been difficult to identify and are often culturally based (57). There is a general suspicion of the introduction of sexual education in schools, despite studies demonstrating the efficacy of this approach in delaying the initiation of sexual activity (90) and in promoting sexual responsibility, as evidenced by the use of contraceptives (64).

Accurate information is often particularly deficient for teenagers. For example, one schoolgirl in Kenya reported a classmate attempting to persuade her that her womb would burst in later pregnancy if she were not "cleansed" through sexual intercourse in girlhood (EN Ngugi, personal observation). Thus the provision of accurate and comprehensible information is, appropriately, a centerpiece of educational efforts to prevent AIDS around the world.

In the Americas, frank educational campaigns directed at young adults have been equally difficult to mount. School-based information campaigns have been successfully put in place in some countries, such as Bahamas.

Gender inequality is an obstacle to AIDS prevention internationally, as is

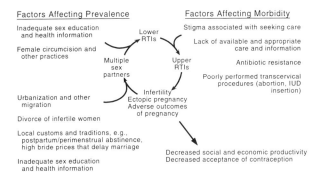

Factors Affecting Prevalence

Inadequate sex education
and health information

Female circumcision and
other practices

Urbanization and other
migration

Divorce of infertile women

Local customs and traditions, e.g.,
postpartum/perimenstrual abstinence,
high bride prices that delay marriage

Inadequate sex education
and health information

Factors Affecting Morbidity

Stigma associated with seeking care

Lack of available and appropriate
care and information

Antibiotic resistance

Poorly performed transcervical
procedures (abortion, IUD
insertion)

Lower
RTIs

Upper
RTIs

Multiple
sex
partners

Infertility
Ectopic pregnancy
Adverse outcomes
of pregnancy

Decreased social and economic productivity
Decreased acceptance of contraception

Figure 7 Interaction between sociocultural and physiological factors in reproductive tract infections in developing countries (77a).

generally true in political, economic, and social development. In Africa, the Caribbean, and Latin America (39), cases of AIDS occur earlier in life in women than in men. This difference, labeled the "demographic imperative" for enhancing prevention in women, has been ascribed to (*a*) male preference for younger partners less likely to already be infected, (*b*) the relative disfranchisement of young women in poor societies that makes them economically dependent on older men for survival, (*c*) traditional marriage practices which foster child marriage and emphasize fertility, and (*d*) physiologic increased risk of receptive sex especially with the presence of juvenile cervical ectopy. It has been documented that women have a relatively higher risk than men per sexual encounter with an infected partner. The interaction between sociocultural and physiological variables in perpetuating a high degree of risk for women is represented in Figure 7. In this model, factors affecting prevalence of reproductive tract infections (RTI) are shown to reinforce morbidity with the outcome of decreased productivity.

International prevention efforts are grappling with the need to address issues specific to women. Abstinence, reduction of sexual partners, and condom use are the three behavioral changes that have been associated with reduced HIV transmission. As seen in the discussion of the Latin American epidemic, participation in these strategies by women is not straightforward because of their position in their society. Some educational strategies can help some women, for example the increasing emphasis on client education in prevention programs for commercial sex workers. Female-based barrier or virucidal methods will be necessary additions if prevention is to be effective (68).

For the near future, the continuing social disparity of the sexes will continue to hamper effective prevention. Studies in Kenya show that economic and social barriers compel women to wait twice as long as men to address symptoms of sexually transmitted disease infection (48a). This delay prolongs the increased vulnerability to HIV transmission that such coinfection represents. Health service schemes to treat these diseases continue to be inaccessible financially and logistically, as well as culturally unacceptable in most international settings .

As we review the regional epidemics, the increasing infection of women has led in all settings to an increasing number of vertically transmitted infections in their infants. The successful use of AZT in chemical trials in the U.S. to interrupt such transmission could presage help in preventing such transmission. Given an early efficacy of over 60% (17), this intervention merits discussion and study in settings where vertical transmission is highest.

The concept of targeting "core group" members is gaining acceptance in international efforts. This concept, first put forward based on experience gained in New York City (63), has been refined in international modeling and research. A recent analysis by the World Bank contrasting "core" with "non-core" approach to prevention projected tenfold greater impact in averting cases of sexually transmitted diseases (56). Developing country researchers have confirmed the cost-effectiveness of focused interventions for core group transmitters (60). However, after a certain population prevalence is reached the effectiveness of such an approach is more difficult to demonstrate. In addition, in some settings the stigmatization of high-risk individuals as potential "core group" members has resulted in repeated and frequent testing without real programmatic benefit.

In Europe and the United States, counseling, testing, and partner notification are central and effective strategies in HIV-transmission control. These strategies have not been employed to any great extent in developing countries. Access to individual HIV testing is problematic because of cost and difficulties in defining appropriate counseling strategies. Thus prevention strategies in resource-poor settings are not focused as specifically on individuals at risk. Often caregivers are reluctant to reveal the results of HIV testing if such testing is positive, an overwhelming obstacle to public health workers who are attempting follow-up counseling (53). Even in some research studies in Africa, commercial sex workers have not been advised of their seropositivity, with the rationale that resources did not permit adequate counseling or support if the information was shared. Thus the targeting of core groups in many developing countries has relied on anonymous serosurveillance information and generalization of research results rather than on individual testing.

In Asia and Latin America, individual testing and counseling are available, although concerns over confidentiality render governmental involvement in such activities less acceptable. Most counseling and testing activity is being carried out by the nongovernmental sector. New testing technologies may make testing more accessible and less costly, for instance by using two different rapid tests and foregoing the more costly Western blot confirmation, as outlined by WHO (84).

Harm-reduction strategies are increasingly gaining acceptance and recognition for their effectiveness in developed countries (20). These strategies have also been successful when applied in resource-poor settings. Unfortunately, intravenous drug use prior to AIDS had been stereotyped internationally as a western, or US, problem. As HIV serosurveillance has unmasked the true extent of this public health problem worldwide, most countries face the AIDS pandemic without the diagnostic, prevention, or treatment capabilities to combat injection drug use. Politically, services for this group are not seen as a priority, with the result that the implementation of needle exchange or bleach programs has lagged far behind the imperative presented by the level of transmission. Many Latin American and Asian urban centers, particularly those located on illicit international drug-trafficking routes, are at tremendous risk of HIV transmission related to intravenous drug use in the next decade.

Condom promotion is one of the few effective strategies available to combat HIV transmission in developing countries. Because there is no knowledge of infection status, there is only general promotion of condoms, with more intense promotion for risk groups such as commercial sex workers and their clients. Work in population and family planning programs in the previous decade had resulted in a very low international acceptance of the condom as a method of birth control. More modern approaches of "social marketing" of condoms have had some additional success. Labor intensive condom promotion to certain groups has been successful among commercial sex workers in Zaire and Thailand. In the latter case, a "100% condom" program coupled with the authority and enforcement of law demonstrated a dramatic drop in sexually transmitted diseases as condom use increased (29).

In summary, the range of prevention strategies available to public health workers in the developing countries is limited. In fact, technical and financial resources available to prevent HIV transmission in most settings now witnessing the pandemic are inadequate to the challenge. An analysis of governmental expenditures on HIV/AIDS in the United States and the rest of the hemisphere revealed that at least $90 was spent in 1990 on HIV prevention and control in the U.S. for every one dollar spent in Latin America (69). This difference may well reflect the debt crisis that has severely limited public health expenditures in Latin American countries over the past decade. This international disparity of the ability to invest in the power of prevention will be further discussed below.

New Technologies

Although the origin of the HIV/AIDS pandemic continues to elude definition, new diagnostic tools have increased the understanding of transmission and pathophysiology of the disease. Increasingly scientists are able to map the genome of the HIV virus and define the variants that are affecting different geographical regions of the world. In addition, technology for detecting virus and identifying the number of virus particles ("viral load") affecting an individual has improved greatly (24, 70, 71). These technologic advances are allowing microepidemiologic studies of HIV as well as studies of the host response to infection. This technology is increasingly being applied to the areas where HIV transmission has proved most intractable to prevention, such as Africa through collaborative research efforts.

The developing countries of the world serve as source of genetic variants of HIV under study. Increasingly, researchers in these countries are participating in the application of these sophisticated techniques to the epidemiologic puzzles of transmission among their populations. Recent studies in Thailand, for example, have teamed Thai and US researchers in an effort to understand the significance of two separate strains of HIV isolated in Thailand. It appears that each strain has a preferred route of transmission, a finding which may, if confirmed, have implications for prevention.

Techniques being developed hold promise for improving the application of HIV diagnostic tests globally, as well as for defining the epidemiology of transmission. Current bariers to use such as cost, the need for centrifugation and refrigeration, and laboratory training may be mitigated as development moves forward. This could enhance the specificity of prevention targeting in resource-poor settings as discussed above.

HIV Vaccines

An affordable AIDS vaccine could significantly increase the capacity for prevention in resource-poor settings. Since the discovery of the responsible viral agent of AIDS in 1984, there has been a concerted effort to develop an AIDS vaccine. The limited success of behavioral and social prevention efforts makes it crucial to assure a continuing full-fledged effort to develop a vaccine for worldwide use. A vaccine is potentially most cost-effective in halting the spread of the epidemic. The initiative can be broadly divided into the development of a preventive vaccine (i.e. given before infection either to prevent infection or to prevent the development of disease in those infected), or a therapeutic vaccine (i.e. given to an infected person to slow or stop progression of disease).

There has been an unprecedented gain in knowledge about the virus, its biology, and its mechanisms of action over the past decade. Numerous vaccine strategies are being explored in the laboratory and in animal models. However, certain critical scientific obstacles have retarded the development of a vaccine:

1. There is not a good animal model of HIV disease. The Simian Immunodeficiency Virus model in macaques has some important differences from

HIV, and chimpanzees infected with HIV do not develop disease. We are therefore unable to rely on animal testing to determine the efficacy of different vaccine approaches.

2. The nature of the immune response needed to prevent HIV disease is not known; there have been no confirmed cases of clearance of HIV following natural exposure. There is intense interest in surrogate markers to determine the success of a vaccine (or drug), but no answers.

3. The diversity of virus sequences found in different countries is enormous. The immunologic relation between these different viruses is unknown, but studies suggest that to be effective, a vaccine must contain strains from multiple subtypes (46).

4. Infection may occur both through cell-associated and free virus particles either through mucosal or systemic routes of exposure. It is not known whether local mucosal immunity will be required for a successful preventive vaccine strategy.

Given these major problems, vaccine development should use traditional empirical approaches with early movement from the laboratory to testing in humans. Unfortunately, the long latency period from infection to illness, the fact that the virus integrates into host DNA, and the risk related to the oncogenic potential of retroviruses have made vaccine developers wary in their approach to vaccine development and testing in humans. As a result, such classical approaches of vaccine development as live attenuated or whole killed virus were given low priority for development. The long time required to develop, test, and register any vaccines has led many manufactures to accord low priority to HIV vaccine development in general. Most vaccines under development are protein or peptide subunit vaccines made from US or European strains, with the logic that companies need a proof of efficacy before increasing investment to deal with other strains. If these approaches are successful, the resultant vaccines will probably be expensive to produce, will have limited immunologic protection, and may not be useful for those with infections with non-US, non-European strains. Such vaccines will, therefore, have limited, if any, usefulness for those living in developing countries where 90% of the new HIV infections are occurring.

At this juncture, current product development activity should be supplemented with approaches and strains that are more likely to be useful for those living in developing countries, and with policy determinations to finance and distribute newly developed vaccines to those who need them most. A new international venture is underway that hopefully will provide some solutions to these difficult problems (62).

In summary, considerable progress has been achieved in understanding the biology of the Human Immunodeficiency Virus (HIV). Although the possibility of a vaccine remains elusive, there are encouraging signs. Various vaccine development strategies are under way in the laboratory, although their movement into testing is limited by scientific and economic forces. The current initiative on vaccine development is insufficient in scope given the magnitude of the problem. Furthermore, the gap between the spread of the disease and the amount of effort on vaccine development is widening. New strategies are imperative to speed this effort and to assure that any vaccines that are developed will be made available to those who need it most—those living in developing countries.

CARE: THE CHALLENGE BROADENS

Current Therapies

Outside of affluent countries, the response of caring for persons with HIV in developing countries has been limited. Use of antiretroviral therapies has been limited to the wealthy who are able to travel or import medicines for use in their treatment. Experience with these medications is minimal in most developing countries. One exception is the Brazilian program, which began purchasing zidovidine at public expense for HIV/AIDS patients in 1992, just as evidence for longterm benefit from AZT has become disappointing. Public expenditure on care in that country between 1992 and 1996 is estimated at $1.2 billion. Argentina has begun purchasing AZT through its national social security program.

Increasingly, the limitation of the international support to prevention has become unacceptable to health workers in developing countries. Strategies are needed to assist in coping with the care of persons with HIV/AIDS (19). This argument is reinforced with the finding that AZT may prove an effective tool to prevent vertical transmission. Pressure on valuable hospital resources, now monopolized by AIDS patients, could be eased by community nursing programs. This call for help has been met with concern that resources will be diverted from prevention to care, and the discussion continues (8).

Despite the reluctance to invest in care, there is eagerness to study the high-prevalence populations of the developing world. The resulting ethical crisis is being addressed through the leadership of WHO and other international organizations. Issues of research are being discussed at the international level. Minimum ethical standards have been defined, including the expectation that drugs or vaccines tested in poor populations will be made available on a continuous basis to such populations. These requirements may be playing some role in the slow pace of research for cure, and new incentives are being considered to promote research.

Tuberculosis

HIV is reversing the gains made in tuberculosis control throughout the world. The pervasive nature of tuberculosis as a coinfection with HIV is only now being documented. A recent study of wasting ("Slim's Disease") in Ivory Coast suggests that up to one half of such clinical cases are coinfection of TB and HIV (13). Based on notification and annual risk estimates, CDC and WHO estimate that 7.5 million incident cases of clinical tuberculosis occurred in 1990, and that this number will increase to 11.9 million by the year 2005. This global increase is due to changes in population age structure (77% of increase) and HIV infection (23% of increase) (12). As of 1992, WHO estimates that 4 million persons had been dually infected, 95% of whom live in developing countries. The urgency of strengthening tuberculosis control programs is obvious (52), although the utility of strategies such as BCG vaccination and preventive chemotherapy in developing countries is less clear. Recent studies have supported the cost-effectiveness of tuberculosis control programs in the face of the HIV epidemic even in heavily affected areas such as sub-Saharan Africa (11).

PREDICTING THE FUTURE OF THE HIV/AIDS PANDEMIC

Various sophisticated modeling techniques have been brought into play to help define the future of this ongoing international calamity. Opinion is not uniform, although most researchers predict the trends seen in Figure 8. As shown, Asia is predicted to show rapidly increasing incidence, with Africa continuing to see high incidence. Transmission is continuing in the earliest areas of the HIV/AIDS epidemic such as Uganda. The potential efficacy of prevention and control efforts will probably be greatest in new areas of epidemic activity. The World Bank has included scenarios based on differing investment assumptions

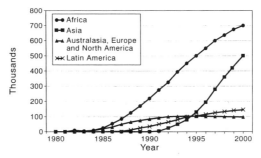

Figure 8   Estimated and projected annual AIDS incidences by "macro" region, 1980–2000. Reprinted from World Health Organization, Global Programme on AIDS, 1992, with permission.

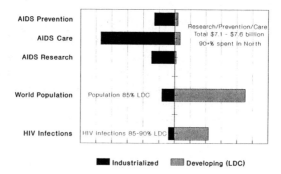

Figure 9   Relative worldwide resource allocations for AIDS, 1992. Reprinted by permission of the publishers from *AIDS in the World,* J Mann, DJM, Tarantola, TW Netter. Cambridge, MA: Harvard Univ. Press.

in the 1993 Development Report. As shown in Figure 6, increased resource availability could halve the annual infections projected for Asia in the year 2000. A great deal of work clearly remains if global efforts are to succeed. At present there is a mismatch with 90% of resources being spent where only 10% of global HIV infections occur (Figure 9, 10).

As the epidemic has widened in geographic reach and deepened in the number of persons and groups affected in each country, the economic and social toll has become more pronounced. Although global estimates vary, a recent estimate of $350 billion by the year 2000 has been put forward (4), based on a well-accepted proprietary trade-linked model of economic systems. The model allows the examination of shared impact among trading economies, reflecting the increasing interdependence of world economies. The weakness

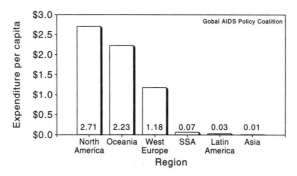

Figure 10   Annual expenditure on AIDS prevention per capita, 1991. Source: Global AIDS Policy Coalition.

of this work is its reliance on a proprietary tool which prevents independent validation of the methodology used. Nonetheless, there is general acceptance that the economic cost of AIDS is high. These costs include the following:

1. *Direct costs of treatment and care*   These costs include the opportunity cost in poor countries of using scarce hospital beds for an illness with no cure. In some areas in Central Africa 70–80% of beds are occupied by persons with AIDS (37). In Thailand, similar occupancy rates are seen in the Northern region according to recent unpublished reports.
2. *Indirect costs of the epidemic*   These costs are as much as ten times larger than the direct costs. They include the loss in productivity, loss in purchasing power through diversion of personal resources into care expense, and an increase in the dependency of societies through the loss of adults and increases in orphaned children and elderly with no identified support.

Indirect costs vary by economic setting. Experience in the United States has demonstrated the impact of AIDS on a developed, market economy, a harbinger for the effect on the market economies of Asia over the next two decades. Initial studies are underway (9).

Despite progressive recommendations by the United Nations organizations such as WHO, ILO, and others, the societal response to the deepening world crisis of HIV has created concerns about human rights and has not been cost-effective. Travel restrictions that mandate HIV testing for visitors or immigrants are widespread, as shown in Table 3. Although such screening of immigrants may limit care expenditure (93), this consideration can be effectively limited through other means. Travel restrictions serve no public health function in limiting the introduction or spread of HIV, and have a general "chilling" effect on international travel that is difficult to quantify. More restrictive measures have been put into place in Cuba: A system of sanatoria has been established and widespread mandatory testing has been carried out with over 10 million tests performed under governmental auspices since the initiation of the program. This system has proved to be unsustainable in its social and economic costs, and the recent efforts to reintroduce internees into society have met with difficulty. In addition, although rates of infection have remained relatively low in Cuba, similar rates are found in Nicaragua, which did not implement isolation programs. The similarity suggests that being off the route of trade and travel may be more responsible for the slow unfolding of the HIV epidemic in these settings. Thus, beyond the human rights concerns that sanitoria efforts provoke, there is increasing evidence that quarantine cannot serve as an efficient control of HIV transmission.

In summary, the international pandemic of HIV is continuing to progress in all regions of the globe. The epidemiological trends show that women and

Table 3 Countries screening migrants and travelers as of 1991

Returning nationals	Bhutan, Bulgaria, Burma, China, Cuba, Czechoslovakia, Hungary, Iraq, Jordan, Korea (DPR), Korea (Republic of), Mongolia, Pakistan, Philippines, Poland, Syria, Tunisia, USSR, Vietnam, Yugoslavia
Immigrants	Argentina, Australia, Burma, China, Costa Rica, Cuba, Hungary, Iraq, Rupublic of Korea, Mongolia, Philippines, South Africa, Syria, Thailand, United States, USSR
Applicants for long-term residence	Belize, Bulgaria, China, Costa Rica, Czechoslovakia, Germany (Bavaria), Jordan, Republic of Korea, Kuwait, Pakistan, Philippines, Poland, Syria, Thailand, Turks and Caicos Islands, United Arab Emirates, United States, USSR
Foreign residents	Bulgaria, Costa Rica, Dominican Republic, Germany (Bavaria), Iraq, Kuwait, Mongolia, Pakistan, Philippines, South Africa, Syria, Tunisia, USSR
Migrant workers	Bhutan, Czechoslovakia, Dominica, Dominican Republic, Jordan, Kuwait, Libya, Philippines, South Africa, Spain, Sri Lanka, St. Vincent and Grenadines, Suriname, Syria, Turks and Caicos Islands, United Arab Emirates, Vietnam
Foreign students	China, Czechoslovakia, Hungary, India, Kuwait, Poland, Syria, Tunisia, USSR
Applicants for asylum	Philippines, Spain, United States
Refugees	Belize, Hong Kong, Pakistan, Philippines, Sudan, Vietnam

children are increasingly affected. Asia has become the newest major area of epidemic activity. The epidemic has taught us that AIDS prevention strategies and the technologies they rely on need to be made accessible on a global basis for successful disease control. Early investment in effective strategies for prevention is cost-effective (7). Broadening the societal response to AIDS beyond the health sector may improve the world's ability to stem the inexorable transmission of HIV into new areas and new population groups.

Literature Cited

1. Anderson RM, May RM. 1992. Understanding the AIDS pandemic. *Sci. Am.* 266:58–66
2. Barongo LR, Borgdorff MW, Mosha FF, Nicholl A, Grosskurth H, et al. 1992. The epidemiology of HIV-1 infection in urban areas, roadside settlements and rural villages in Mwanza Region, Tanzania. *AIDS* 6:1521–28
3. Bartholemew C, Cleghorn G. 1989. Retroviruses in the Caribbean. In *AIDS: Profile of and Epidemic.* ed. F Zacarias. Washington, DC: PAHO
4. Behravesh N. 1993. *Measuring the global economic impact of the AIDS epidemic.* DRI/McGraw-Hill Insight Rep.
5. Berkley SF. 1991. Parenteral transmission of HIV in Africa. *AIDS* 5:S87–S92
6. Berkley S, Naamara W, Okware S, Downing R, Kondelule J, et al. 1990. AIDS and HIV infection in women in Uganda—are women more infected than males? *AIDS* 4:1237–42
7. Berkley S, Piot P, Schopper D. 1994. AIDS: Invest now or pay more later. *Fin. Dev.* 31:40
8. Biggar RJ. 1993. When ideals meet reality—the global challenge of HIV/AIDS. *Am. J. Public Health* 83: 1383–84
9. Bloom DE, Lyons JV. 1993. *Economic Implications of AIDS in Asia.* UN Dev. Program. Rep.
10. Butler D. 1994. Concern over the "invisible problem" of HIV blood in developing countries. *Nature* 369:429
11. Cantwell MF, Binkin N. 1994. *Tuberculosis in Subsaharan Africa: can a good tuberculosis control program make a difference?* Presented at 43rd Annu. EIS Conf., Cent. Dis. Control, Atlanta, April
11a. Cent. Dis. Control. 1982. Persistent, generalized lymphadenopathy among homosexual males. *Morbid. Mortal. Wkly. Rep.* 31:249–51
12. Cent. Dis. Control. 1993. Estimates of future global tuberculosis morbidity and mortality. 1993. *Morbid. Mortal. Wkly. Rep.* 42:961–64
13. Cent. Dis. Control. AIDS Clearinghouse. 1994. TB underestimated in HIV Wasting, Daily rep. June 11
14. Central Africa 1959. *Lancet* 1:1279–80
15. Chin J, Mann J. 1990. HIV infections and AIDS in the 1990s. *Annu. Rev. Public Health* 11:127–42
16. Colebunders RI, Greenberg A, Nguyen-Dinh P, Francis H, Kabote N, et al.

1987. Rapid communication: evaluation of a clinical case definition of AIDS in African children. *AIDS* 1:151–53
17. Connor EM, Sperling RS, Gelber R, Kiselev P, Scott G, et al. 1994. Reduction of maternal-infant transmission of human immunodeficiency virus type 1 with zidovudine treatment. *N. Engl. J. Med.* 331:1173–80
18. DeCock KM, Adjorlolo G, Ekpine E, Sibailly T, Kouadio J, et al. 1993. Epidemiology and transmission of HIV-2. Why there is no HIV-2 pandemic. *J. Am. Med. Assoc.* 270:2083–86
19. DeCock KM, Luca SB, Lucas S, Agness J, Kadio A, Gayle HD. 1993. Clinical research, prophylaxis, therapy and care for HIV disease in Africa. *Am. J. Public Health* 83:1385–89
20. Des Jarlais DC, Friedman SR, Ward TP. 1993. Harm reduction: a public health response to the AIDS epidemic among injecting drug users. *Annu. Rev. Public Health* 14:413–50
20a. Duerr A, Xia Z, Nagachinta T, Tovanabutra S, Tansuhaj A, et al. 1994. *Probability of male-to-female HIV transmission among married couples in Chiang Mai, Thailand.* Presented at Int. Conf. AIDS, 10th, Yokohama, Japan
21. Dunn DT, Newell ML, Ades AE, Peckham CS. 1992. Risk of human immunodeficiency virus type 1 transmission through breastfeeding. *Lancet* 340: 585–88
22. Editor. 1992. Poliovaccine and AIDS origin link very unlikely. *Lancet* 340: 1090–91
22a. European Collaborative Study. 1994. Caesarian section and risk of vertical transmission of HIV-1 infection. *Lancet* 343:1464–67
23. Farnham P. 1994. Defining and measuring the costs of the HIV epidemic to business firms. *Public Health Rep.* 109: 311
24. Ferre F, Marchese AL, Griffin SL, Daigle AE, Richieri SP, et al. 1993. Development and validation of a polymerase chain reaction method for the precise quantiation of HIV-1 DNA in blood cells from subjects undergoing a 1-year immunotherapeutic treatment. *AIDS* 7: S21–27 (Suppl. 2)
25. Getchell JP, Hicks DR, Svinivasan A, Heath JL, York, DA, et al. 1987. Human immunodeficiency virus isolated from a serum sample collected in 1976 in Central Africa. *J. Infect. Dis.* 156:833–37
26. Gomez P, Kimball A, Orlander H, Bain

RM, Fisher L, Hoemes K. 1995. Epidemic crack cocaine use, linked with genital ulcer disease and heterosexual HIV infection in the Bahamas. Submitted

27. Grmek M. 1990. *History of AIDS: The Emergence of a Modern Pandemic*, p. 124. Princeton, NJ: Princeton Univ. Press

28. Gunn RA, Kimball AM, Pollard RA, Feeley JC, Feldman RA, et al. 1979. Bottle feeding as a risk factor for cholera in infants. *Lancet* 2:730–32

29. Hanenberg RS, Rojanapithayakorn W, Kunasol P, Sokal DC. 1994. Impact of Thailand's HIV-control programme as indicated by the decline of sexually transmitted diseases. *Lancet* 344:243–45

30. Herrera G. 1990. *Characteristics of women with AIDS in Costa Rica.* Costa Rica Natl. AIDS Program. San Juan, Costa Rica

30a. Hira SK, Kamanga J, Bhat GJ, Mwale C, Tembo G, et al. 1989. Perinatal transmission of HIV1 in Zambia. *Br. Med. J.* 299:1250–52

31. Hughes A, Corrah T. 1990. Human immunodeficiency virus type 2 (HIV-2). *Blood Rev.* 4:158–64

32. Int. Forum AIDS Research. 1990. *Toward an AIDS Vaccine: The Policy Supporting the Research.* Washington, DC: Inst. Med. Proc., Sept.

33. Iszazola JA, Valdespino-Gomez SL, Gortmaker SL, Townsend J, Becker J, et al. 1991. HIV-1 seropositivity and behavioral and sociological risks among homosexual and bisexual men in six Mexican cities. *J. Acquired Immune Defic. Syndr.* 4:614–22

34. Jager H, Ngaly B, Perriens J, Nseka K, Davaci F, et al. 1990. Prevention of transfusion-associated HIV transmission in Kinshasa, Zaire: HIV screening is not enough. *AIDS* 4:571–74

35. Kennedy KI, Fortney JA, Bonhomme MG, Potts M, Lamptey P, Carswell W. 1990. Do the benefits of breastfeeding outweigh the risk of postnatal transmission of HIV via breastmilk? *Trop. Doctor* 20:25–29

36. Killewo J, Nyamuryekunge K, Sandstrom A, Bredbergraden U, Wall S, et al. 1990. Prevalence of HIV-1 infection in the Kagera Region of Tanzania: a population-based study. *AIDS* 4:1081–85

37. Kimball AM. 1991. *Impact of HIV/AIDS on social and economic development in Africa.* Testimony before the US House of Representatives, Comm. For. Aff., Subcommittee on Africa, Nov. 6. US. GPO

38. Kimball AM, González RS, Betts CM, eds. 1990. *Annu. HIV/AIDS Surveillance Rep., 1991.* Washington, DC: PAHO

39. Kimball AM, González RS, Zacarías F. 1991. AIDS among women in Latin America and the Caribbean. *Bull. PAHO* 25:367

40. Kimball AM, González RS, Zacarías F. 1993. Women and the AIDS epidemic: an impending crisis for the Americas. In *Gender, Women and Health in the Americas.* PAHO Sci. Publ. 541

41. Koifman R, Monteiro G, Rodriques R. 1990. *Epidemiologic characteristics of AIDS in women in Rio de Janeiro, Brazil.* Presented at 6th Int. Conf. AIDS, San Francisco

41a. Lallemant M, Cheynier D, Nzingoul S, Jourdain G, Sinet M, et al. 1992. Characteristics associated with HIV1 infection in pregnant women in Brazzaville, Congo. *J. Acquired Immune Defic. Syndr.* 5:270–85

42. Lederberg J, Shope RE, Oaks SC Jr, eds. 1992. *Emerging Infections: Microbial Threats to Health in the United States.* Washington, DC: Natl. Acad. Press

42a. Lepage P, Vandeper P, Msellati O, Hittimand DG, Simonon A, et al. 1993. Mother-to-child transmission of human immunodeficiency virus type 1 (HIV1) and its determinants: a cohort study in Kigali, Rwanda. *Am. J. Epidemiol.* 137: 589–99

43. Lifson AR. 1988. Do alternate modes for transmission of human immunodeficiency virus exist? *J. Am. Med. Assoc.* 259:1353–56

44. Lima ES, Bastos FI, Teller PR, Friedman SR. 1993. HIV infection and AIDS among drug injectors at Rio de Janeiro: perspectives and unanswered questions. *Bull. Narc.* 45:107–15

45. Mann J, Tarantola DJ, Netter TW, eds. 1992. *AIDS in the World: The Global AIDS Policy Coalition*, pp. 25–32. Cambridge, MA: Harvard Univ. Press

46. Mascola JR, Louwagie J, McCutchan FE, Fischer CL, Hegerich PA, et al. 1994. Two antigenically distinct subtypes of human immunodeficiency virus type 1: viral genotype predicts neutralization serotype. *J. Infect. Dis.* 169:48–54

47. Mastro TD, Satten GA, Nopkesorn T, Sangkharomya S, Logini IM. 1994. Probability of female-to-male transmission of HIV-1 in Thailand. *Lancet* 343: 204–7

48. Ministry of Health, Thailand 1992. *100% condom program.* Rep. to GPA/WHO

48a. Moses S, Ngugi EN, Bradley J, Njeru E, Eldridge G, et al. 1994. Health care-seeking behavior related to the transmission of sexually transmitted diseases. *Am. J. Public Health* 84:1947–51

49. Moss RB, Ferre F, Trauger R, Jensen FC, Daigle A, et al. 1994. Inactivated HIV-1 immunogen: impact on markers of disease progression. *J. AIDS* 7:S21–27 (Suppl. 1)

50. Mulder D, Kamali A, Nakyinge J, et al. 1993. HIV-1 associated mortality in a rural Ugandan Cohort: results at two year follow-up. *Proc. 9th Int. Conf. AIDS, Berlin* (Abstr. WS-CO3-6)

51. Nahmias AJ, Weiss J, Yao X, Lee F, Kodsi R, et al. 1986. Evidence for human infection with an HTLV III/LAV-like virus in Central Africa. *Lancet* 1:1279–80

52. Narain JP, Raviglione MC, Kochi A. 1992. HIV associated tuberculosis in developing countries: epidemiology and strategies for prevention. *Tubercle Lung Dis.* 73:311–21

53. Ngugi EN, Njenga E, Anderson S, et al. 1994. Preliminary results of a feasibility study to integrate community based care of people with HIV/AIDS into existing urban health services in Nairobi.

54. Nowak MA, McLean AR. 1991. A mathematical model of vaccination against HIV to prevent the development of AIDS. *Proc. R. Soc. London Ser. B* 246:141–46

55. Nzilambi N, DeCock KM, Forthal DN, Francis D, Ryder RW, et al. 1988. The prevalence of infection with human immunodeficiency virus over a 10 year period in rural Zaire. *New Engl. J. Med.* 318:276–79

56. Over M, Piot P. 1993. HIV infection and sexually transmitted diseases. In *Disease Control Priorities in Developing Countries.* New York: World Bank/Oxford Univ. Press

57. PANOS. 1994. *The Practice of Dry Sex.* World AIDS

58. Piot P, Taelman H, Minlangu KB, Mbendi N, Ndangi K, et al. 1984. Acquired immunodeficiency syndrome in a heterosexual population in Zaire. *Lancet* 2:65–69

59. Plebani A, Biolchini A, Bucceri A, Buscaglia M, Pardi G, Semprini AE. 1990. Prenatal immune status of fetuses of HIV-seropositive mothers. *Gynecol. Obstet. Invest.* 29:108–11

60. Plummer FA, Nagelkerke NJD, Moses A, Ndinya-Achola JO, Bwayo J, Ngugi E. 1991. The importance of core groups in the epidemiology and control of HIV-1 infection. *AIDS* 5:S169–76 (Suppl. 1)

61. Raggi R, Blanco GA. 1992. Epidemic model of HIV infection and AIDS in Argentina. Status in 1990 and predictive estimates. *Medicina* 52:225–35

62. Rockefeller Found. 1994. *HIV vaccines—accelerating the development of preventive HIV vaccines for the world,* Bellagio, Italy, March 7–11

63. Rothenberg RA. 1983. The geography of gonorrhae: empirical demonstration of core group transmission. *Am. J. Epidemiol.* 117:688–94

63a. Ryder RW, Nsa RW, Hassig SE, Behets F, Rayfield M, et al. 1989. Perinatal transmission of the human immunodeficiency virus type 1 to infants of seropositive women in Zaire. *New Engl. J. Med.* 320:1637–42

64. Sakondhavat C, Kanato M, Leung-tongkum P, Kuchaisit C. 1988. KAP study on sex, reproduction and contraception in Thai teenagers. *J. Med. Assoc. Thailand* 71:649–53

65. Saxinger WC, Levine PH, Dean AG, Dethe G, Langewantzin G, et al. 1985. Evidence for exposure to HTLV-III in Uganda before 1973. *Science* 227:1036–38

66. Serwaada D, Sewankambo NK, Caswell JW, Bayley AC, Tedders RS, et al. 1985. Slim disease: a new disease in Uganda and its association with HTLV-III infection. *Lancet* 2:849–52

67. Singh S, Crofts D, Gertig D. 1993. HIV infections among IDUs in North East Malaysia. *9th Int. Conf. AIDS, Berlin,* Poster Present.

68. Stein ZA. 1990. HIV prevention: the need for methods women can use. *Am. J. Public Health* 80:460–62

69. Suarez R, Kimball A. 1992. *What would be the cost of AZT for Latin America and the Caribbean.* Presented at 2nd Pan Am. Conf. AIDS, Santo Domingo

70. Trauger RJ, Ferre F, Daigle AE, Jensen FC, Moss RB, et al. 1994. Effect of immunization with inactivated gp120-depleted Human Immunodeficiency Virus Type 1 (HIV-1) immunogen on HIV-1 immunity, viral DNA, and percentage of CD4 cells. *J. Infect. Dis.* 169:1256–64

71. Trauger RJ, Giermakowska WK, Ferre F, Duffy PC, Wallace MR, et al. 1993. Cell-mediated immunity to HIV-1 in Walter Reed stages 1–6 individuals: correlation with virus burden. *Immunology* 78:611–15

72. UN Resolution. 1994. *(ECOSOC) E/1994/18/Rev 1,* July 20

73. US Japan Cooperative Framework for Economic Development 1993. Point 5

282   KIMBALL ET AL

74. Van de Perre P, Lepage P, Kestelyn P, Hekker AC, Pouvroy D, et al. 1984. Acquired immunodeficiency syndrome in Rwanda. *Lancet* 2:62–65
75. Van de Perre P, Simonson A, Msellati P, Hitimana DG, Vaira D, et al. 1991. Postnatal transmission of human immunodeficiency virus type one from mother to infant. *New Engl. J. Med.* 325:593–98
76. Villari P, Spino C, Chalmers TC, Lau J, Sacks HS. 1993. Cesarean section to reduce perinatal transmission of hu- man immunodeficiency virus. A metaanalysis. *J. Curr. Clin. Trials* July 8
77. Wald A, Corey L, Handsfield HH, Holmes HK. 1993. Influence of HIV infection on manifestations and natural history of other sexually transmitted diseases. *Annu. Rev. Public Health* 14:19–42
77a. Wasserheit JN. 1989. The significance and scope of reproductive tract infections among third world women. *Int. J. Gynecol. Obstet.* 3:145–68 (Suppl.)
78. Wasserheit JN. 1992. Epidemiologic synergy: interrelationships between human immunodeficiency virus infection and other sexually transmitted diseases. *Sex. Transm. Dis.* 19:61–77
79. Wawer MJ, Serwadda D, Musgrave SD, Kondelule JK, Musagara M, et al. 1991. Dynamics of spread of HIV-1 infection in a rural district of Uganda. *Br. Med. J.* 303:1303–6
80. Way P, Stanecki K. 1993. *Trends and Patterns of HIV/AIDS Infection in Selected Developing Countries.* Res. Note No. 12. US Census Bur.
81. Weninger BG, Quinhoes EP, Sereno AB, Deperez MA, Krebs JW. 1992. A simplified case definition of AIDS derived from empirical data. *J. Acquired Immune Defic. Syndr.* 12:1212–13
82. WHO. 1985. *Workshop on AIDS in Central Africa.* Bangui, Central African Republic, Oct. 22-24
83. WHO. 1994. Current global situation of the HIV/AIDS pandemic. *Wkly. Epidemiol. Rec.* 69:7–8
84. WHO Evaluation Unit. 1994. Strategies for laboratory HIV testing strategies that do not require use of the Western blot approach. *Bull. WHO* 72:129–34
85. Widy-Wirski R, Berkley S, Downing R, Okware S, Recine U, et al. 1988. Evaluation of the WHO clinical case definition for AIDS in Uganda. *J. Am. Med. Assoc.* 260:3286–89
86. Wong K, Lee SS, Lim WL. 1993. HIV surveillance among drug users in Hong Kong. *9th Int. Conf. AIDS, Berlin,* Poster Present.
87. World Bank. 1993. *Investing in Health, The 1993 World Development Rep.* New York: Oxford Univ. Press
88. *World Development Report.* 1993. New York: Oxford Univ. Press
89. Xia M, Kreiss J, Holmes K. 1993. *Risk factors for HIV infection among drug users in Yunan Province, China: association with intravenous drug use and protective effect of boiling reusable needles and syringes.* Presented at ISSTDR, Finland
90. Zabin LS, Hirsch MB, Smith EA, Street R, Hardy JB. 1986. Evaluation of a pregnancy prevention program for urban teenagers. *Fam. Plan. Perspect.* 18:119–26
90a. Zaknum D, Oswald HP, Zaknun J, Mayersbach P, Sperl W, et al. 1991. Effects of health and medical undertreatment on the clinical status and social behavior of infants and small children in a Romanian orphanage. *Padiatr. Padol.* 26:65–67
91. Zheng XW, Zhang JP, Tian CQ, Cheng HH, Yang XZ, et al. 1993. Cohort study of HIV infection among drug users in Ruili, Longchuan and Luxi of Yunnan Province, China. *Biomed. Environ. Sci.* 6:348–51
92. Ziegler JB, Johnson RO, Cooper DA, Gold J. 1985. Postnatal transmission of AIDS associated retrovirus from mother to infant. *Lancet* 1:896–98
93. Zowall H, Coupal L, Fraser RD, Gilmore N, Deutsch A, Grover SA. 1992. Economic impact of HIV infection and coronary heart disease in immigrants to Canada. *Can. Med. Assoc. J.* 147:1163–72

Annu. Rev. Public Health. 1995. 16:283–306

PSA SCREENING: A Public Health Dilemma

Margaret T. Mandelson, Edward H. Wagner, and Robert S. Thompson

Center for Health Studies and Department of Preventive Care, Group Health Cooperative, Seattle, Washington 98101

KEY WORDS: prostate cancer, screening, prostate-specific antigen, mass screening, PSA

ABSTRACT

Screening for prostate cancer with serum prostate specific antigen (PSA) is one of the most controversial practices in health care today and guidelines from professional and policy organizations are contradictory. Prostate cancer is unique because of a wide discrepancy between prevalent asymptomatic cancer and clinical disease and an uncertain natural history. Proponents and critics of mass screening agree that PSA can detect early cancer and that definitive data that PSA reduces prostate cancer mortality are not available. Differences in screening recommendations reflect distinct viewpoints regarding what constitutes screening benefit and what level of evidence is needed to endorse a screening practice. This review describes what is known about the areas most relevant to the conflicting perspectives: the epidemiology and natural history of prostate cancer, the ability of PSA to detect disease and operational characteristics of PSA as a screening test, and the efficacy of treatment of early disease.

INTRODUCTION

Screening for prostate cancer with serum prostate specific antigen (PSA) is one of the most controversial practices in health care today. PSA is accepted as a tumor marker for following patients with prostate cancer, but guidelines from professional and policy organizations for screening with serum PSA are contradictory (Table 1). All groups agree on two critical issues: (*a*) Serum PSA can detect early stage cancer with relatively high sensitivity; and (*b*) definitive data that PSA reduces prostate cancer mortality are not currently

283

0163-7525/95/0510-0283$05.00

Table 1 Screening PSA recommendations by professional organizations

Recommend	Decline to recommend
American Cancer Society (96)	National Cancer Institute (107)
American Urologic Society [a]	U.S. Preventive Services Task Force (140)
American College of Radiology [b]	Canadian Task Force on the Periodic Health Examination (29)
Canadian Urological Association (30)	British Columbia Office of Technology Assessment (64)

[a] Executive Committee Report. January 1992
[b] Resolution #36, approved October 1991

available. Differences in recommendations reflect distinct viewpoints regarding what constitutes screening benefit and what level of evidence is needed to endorse a screening practice. Groups that base recommendations on a formal process of evidence appraisal, the U.S. Preventive Services Task Force and the Canadian Task Force on the Periodic Health Examination, have concluded that the benefits of screening PSA are unknown at this time and there is sufficient evidence to exclude PSA screening from routine examination in asymptomatic men. This position is not expected to change in 1995 (S Woolf, personal communication) and is consistent with recommendations of the British Columbia Office of Technology Assessment (64). Professional organizations, including the American and Canadian Urological Associations and the American College of Radiology, advocate the use of PSA as a screening test.

Prostatic carcinoma is a significant public health problem, the leading cause of cancer-related morbidity in US men and the second leading cause of cancer mortality after lung cancer (21). Recommendations to screen for prostate cancer are based on two underlying hypotheses. First, substantial cure rates may occur when prostate cancer is treated at an early, organ-confined stage. Second, a significant proportion of prostate cancers follows a natural history of progressive disease that, if left untreated, will result in morbidity and death (7, 127). Survival rates of men with early stage prostate cancer are clearly superior to survival in men with late stage disease (101), so the ability of PSA to detect prostatic cancer at an early stage has raised hopes that screening will reduce mortality. However, the contribution of treatment to this survival pattern is unclear. Prostate cancer is unique because a high rate of undiagnosed, asymptomatic disease is found in elderly men at autopsy and the natural history of the disease is uncertain. Fifteen to thirty percent of men 50 and older and approximately 60% of men 70 and older have histologic evidence of disease, but only a small fraction of these cases are diagnosed each year or cause death (25, 139).

PSA is a protein found in epithelial cells of the prostate gland. It is a glycoprotein with one polypeptide chain, is 70% carbohydrate, and has a molecular weight of 33–34,000 dalton. PSA in the serum exists as a series of isoforms (at least 5), some of which function as serine proteases (147). As a relatively inexpensive blood test, PSA has advantages over digital rectal exam (DRE) alone, the oldest screening test for prostate cancer. DRE is limited to examination of the posterior and lateral surfaces of the prostate gland, whereas approximately half of all tumors arise in areas not palpable by DRE. Perhaps as a result, DRE sensitivity is low (33% to 69%), specificity ranges from 77% to 89%, and the interpretation of findings is subjective (67, 68). In contrast, serum PSA is an objective, noninvasive measure with higher sensitivity (83–96%) but with weak specificity and low positive predictive value (45). The health risks and medical costs of both false-positive and true positive screening PSA results are not insubstantial. Low PSA specificity results in a cascade of interventions in men without disease. "Over-diagnosis" of screen-detected prostate cancer may result in unnecessary treatment by radical prostatectomy that can result in permanent complications, such as impotence and incontinence. While the health benefits of PSA screening are debated, estimated first year national costs of a program of annual screening are $11.9 (83) and $12.7 billion (53).

The magnitude of prostate cancer incidence, prevalence, and mortality, the availability of a simple, relatively inexpensive blood test, the absence of other sensitive and specific tests, and the potential economic and human costs of prostate cancer make it one of the most important health care issues that face our delivery systems today. It is beyond the scope of this review to critique and summarize all of the available primary data related to prostate cancer screening with PSA. Here we briefly describe what is currently known about the areas most relevant to the conflicting perspectives described above: the epidemiology and natural history of prostate cancer, the ability of PSA to detect prostate cancer and operational characteristics of PSA as a screening test, and the efficacy of treatment of early stage disease. The current controversy between advocates and skeptics of PSA screening is not likely to be resolved soon but poses unique challenges in the delivery of primary care, given limited resources. We close this review with an example of one delivery system's response to the widespread adoption of PSA screening in the midst of continued scientific uncertainty.

EPIDEMIOLOGY AND NATURAL HISTORY OF PROSTATE CANCER

Prostate cancer is the most commonly diagnosed malignancy in men. An estimated 200,000 new cases will be diagnosed in the U.S. in 1994, accounting for 32% of all cancers in men, excluding nonmelanoma skin cancer and carcinoma in situ. Approximately 38,000 deaths will be attributed to this disease in 1994 (21). These figures were 106,000 and 30,000, respectively, in 1990 (133). Prostate cancer risk sharply rises with age, 92% of cases diagnosed in men 50 and older between 1986 and 1990 occurred after age 64 (101). Because of the high prevalence of asymptomatic disease, it is estimated that US males 50 and older have a lifetime risk of developing prostate cancer of 42%, but only a 13% lifetime risk of being diagnosed with clinical prostate cancer and a 3.2% risk of dying from the disease (101).

Incidence and Mortality

The U.S. is in the midst of an "epidemic" of prostate cancer. Population-based data from the National Cancer Institute's SEER (Surveillance, Epidemiology, and End Results) program show that age-adjusted prostate cancer incidence increased over 100% between 1973 and 1990, with a 65% increase in incidence since 1979 (Figure 1) (101). African American men have higher incidence rates of prostate cancer (163.6 per 100,000 in 1990) than Whites (128.5 per 100,000 in 1990), but their age-adjusted incidence has not increased as dramatically between 1979 and 1990: Blacks 33% increase; Whites 67% increase. Only two explanations can account for this tremendous growth in prostate cancer incidence: (a) a changing prevalence of disease risk factors or (b) improved ability to detect disease that would have previously been considered latent. These possibilities are reviewed below.

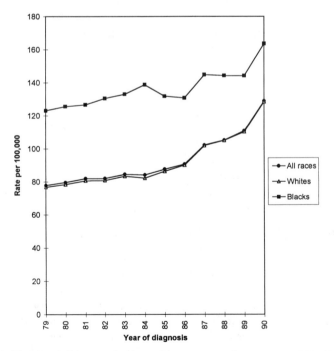

Figure 1 Time trends in cancer incidence. Rates are age-adjusted to the 1970 US standard population.

Deaths associated with prostate cancer account for 13% of all cancer deaths in US males (21). Prostate cancer mortality increased 17% between 1979 and 1990. The rate was lower among Whites (17%) than among Blacks (28%), although Blacks showed less increase in incidence (101), as noted above. A recent analysis of prostate cancer mortality 1950–89 by age and year of birth showed that prostate cancer mortality rates rose in men aged 85 and older, remained constant among Whites under the age of 80, and declined in Blacks and non-Whites under age 65 (74). Improved detection may partially account for this mortality trend in Whites, but is an unlikely explanation for the pattern observed in non-Whites since both the incidence rate and the proportion of localized disease remained steady during the study period, 1975–1989. Hsing & Devesa (74) hypothesized that the increase in mortality among older men may be at least partially attributable to a lack of age adjustment in the highest age interval of men 85 and older, a group that has shifted toward older ages as rates for competing causes of death have declined.

The ultimate measure of the population effectiveness of screening is a decline in disease-specific mortality, but reductions in mortality resulting from success-ful programs may not be detectable until years after a substantial proportion of at-risk people are screened. Day (48) and others (104, 119) argue that measures of advanced disease are an appropriate intermediate outcome for disease-specific mortality in the evaluation of cancer screening. Failure to consider two important sources of bias, lead-time bias and length bias, can result in erroneous conclu-sions of prostate cancer screening benefit (104). Lead-time bias is an apparent increase in survival because screening moves the date of detection earlier without changing the natural history of disease or age distribution of prostate cancer mortality. Length bias is a form of "over-diagnosis" that would occur if serum PSA identifies disease that is less aggressive, and thus less likely to cause mortality, than cancers detected without screening. Late stage disease incidence is considered an appropriate surrogate for mortality because it avoids lead-time bias associated with disease-specific survival and minimizes length bias associ-ated with the evaluation of screen-detected cases.

Table 2 shows that the rate of distant disease in US men did not decline between 1979 and 1987, the most recent year of available national information on stage, although well before the widespread use of PSA testing. More current data from the Seattle-based SEER registry fail to show evidence of a consistent decline in rates of distant stage prostate cancer incidence through 1992 (Table 2). Because of the effects of lead-time and length bias, if PSA were able to detect earlier cancers but not impact disease outcome (measured here by incidence of distant stage disease), widespread screening with PSA would result in a lower proportion of late-stage cancers even in the absence of a beneficial effect of early detection and treatment on the natural history of prostatic cancer. This pattern was observed in western Washington: The pro-

Table 2 Time trends in stage distribution and age-adjusted incidence of advanced prostate cancer among US men, 1979–1992

	Year of diagnosis						
	1979–80	81–82	83–84	85–86	87–88	89–90	91–92
Rate of distant stage cancer (per 100,000) [a,b,c]							
United States	13.8	14.5	14.6	15.5	14.9		
Western Washington	13.3	15.1	15.7	17.1	15.4	12.9	13.6
Western Washington stage distribution (%)							
Local	67.0	64.8	64.1	64.6	70.4	69.5	67.8
Regional	16.0	15.8	18.0	18.7	18.2	21.9	25.7
Distant	17.0	19.4	17.9	16.7	11.4	8.6	6.5

[a] Adjusted to the 1970 US standard population
[b] Stage-specific data available through 1987
[c] Restricted to whites

portion of prostate cancers diagnosed at a distant stage fell 62% between 1979 and 1992, with most of this decline occurring in the recent time periods studied, while the incidence of distant disease remained constant.

GEOGRAPHIC VARIABILITY IN INCIDENCE   Rates of prostate cancer vary widely among countries (20, 76, 106, 150), and several investigators have noted substantial geographic variation in incidence within the United States (91, 101, 118). Most recently, Lu-Yao & Greenberg (91) reported wide variation in prostate cancer incidence rates among white men aged 50–79 in nine SEER program areas between 1983 and 1989. While the overall average annual increase in age-adjusted incidence was 6.4% per year, the estimated annual percent increase in incidence ranged from 2.7 (Connecticut) to 12.0 (Seattle). Reasons related to geographic variation are discussed in greater detail below.

There is little evidence that the variability within the United States of increasing incidence rates of prostate cancer is related to geographic differences in the prevalence of disease risk factors over time. Instead, three medical care factors appear to account for much of the growth and variability in prostate cancer incidence. First, widespread use of TURP (trans-urethral resection of the prostate) to treat benign prostatic hypertrophy (BPH) and incidental detection of cancer in removed tissue (87, 118, 129) has increased the detection of early disease. Second, a surge in radical prostatectomy and associated lymph node dissections (91) has increased the detection of regional disease and a resulting shift in stage. Finally, increased use of PSA as a screening test (52) and for surveillance of patients on medical therapy for BPH has increased detection of both early and regional disease.

TURP and early stage disease   Both BPH and prostate cancer increase with age. Results from several studies show indirect evidence that incidental detection of prostate cancer in surgical specimens from TURPs increased the incidence rates of prostate cancer during the 1970s and 1980s. Surveys conducted by the American College of Surgeons found that TURP was the primary means of diagnosis in over half of all cases of prostate cancer reported between 1974 and 1983 (129). More recently, Potosky et al (118) reported a strong correlation between prostate cancer incidence in the United States between 1973 and 1986 and the use of TURP to relieve urinary obstruction due to BPH. Regression analyses of incidence data from four SEER sites and hospital discharge data on the number of TURPs performed in the same geographic areas showed that 88% of the variation in the total incidence and 82% of the variation in incidence of localized disease were explained by the variation in the TURP discharge rate. Similar findings have been reported from Canada, where a 55% increase in TURP rates occurred between 1970 and 1988 (87). During that same time period, both the rate of prostate cancer in men with symptoms of BPH and the rate of cancer found incidentally following TURP for suspected BPH rose by

11%. Observations of a relationship between population rates of TURP for BPH and prostatic cancer are consistent with previous findings from case series of a high rates of carcinoma in TURP specimens (122, 132).

Radical prostatectomy and regional disease   A second medical care factor associated with the dramatic surge in prostate cancer incidence is radical prostatectomy. A sharp increase in radical prostatectomy rates has been observed across age groups, with wide variation among geographic regions of the United States and among delivery systems, fee for service or managed care (HMO), within the same region (65, 92, 136). An analysis of Medicare data showed that radical prostatectomy rates rose nationwide more than 400% between 1984 and 1990, with the highest rates observed in the Pacific region and the lowest rates observed in the Mid-Atlantic region (92). This consistent pattern of geographic variation indicates not only differences in choices of treatment for prostate cancer, but also differences in the rates of detection (69). Similar increases and geographic variability were noted in younger men as well (136). The increase in US rates of regional disease (91) is likely associated with more aggressive surgery for small lesions and the subsequent upstaging of cancers that previously would have been classified as localized (17). Treatment patterns for prostate cancer in US men have changed dramatically over the past decade, with increased enthusiasm for early and aggressive treatment with radical prostatectomy (87, 91, 92, 136).

Increased use of PSA   Several lines of evidence point to a dramatic increase in the use of PSA testing for detection of prostatic cancer, although few direct data on the prevalence of PSA testing are available. A study of the impact of PSA use on prostate cancer incidence in Medicare men is currently under way; results have not been reported at this time (A Potosky, personal communication). The pattern of increase in prostate cancer incidence described above coincides with increased media coverage of prostate cancer and serum PSA (1, 94, 117). Diagnoses of prostate cancer in politicians (108, 109) and other public figures (26, 110, 141) have raised awareness of the disease. The recent sharp rise in incidence has been compared to patterns of breast cancer occurrence observed in 1974 following the diagnosis of two prominent women (120). PSA screening is supported by medical industry groups through sponsorship of Prostate Cancer Awareness Week, a program that offers free PSA testing to men 50 years of age and older. In addition, advertising and promotion of a newly-approved medical treatment for BPH, the 5-alpha reductase inhibitor finasteride, also promotes PSA screening since patients must undergo baseline PSA testing prior to treatment and periodic PSA testing while they receive the drug. Phase III clinical studies of finasteride showed that the rate of prostate cancer detection was more than twice the expected incidence in the general population among both placebo- and finasteride-treated patients (115). Increased surveillance of men on finasteride may substantially contribute to future detection of prostate cancer as this treatment for BPH becomes more widely adopted.

Two studies have reported direct evidence of increased use of PSA. Researchers from the Detroit SEER registry hypothesized that widespread use of PSA may account for a greater than doubling of local and regional prostate cancer rates observed in their region between 1990 and 1991. They found that this trend was mirrored by a more than 250% increase in PSA tests performed in five laboratories in the same geographic area (52). Population-based rates of serum PSA testing and rates of prostate cancer were also compared in a recent report from the British Columbia Office of Health Technology Assessment (64). PSA testing is approved by the British Columbia Commission of the Ministry of Health for diagnostic and monitoring purposes, but the volume of testing that occurred in fiscal years 1992–93 suggested that PSA was being used for indications not identified in the conditions of coverage. This observation was further supported by an analysis of physician specialty ordering patterns in 44,143 PSA tests for 38,161 patients during the same time period. General practitioners ordered 34 times more PSA tests than did urologists. Prostate biopsies also rose during the same period, and rates of prostate cancer increased through 1992, the most recent year of data available (64).

Etiology of Prostate Cancer

If strong risk factors were identified, they might explain the increase in incidence or offer opportunities for more selective screening. Unfortunately, the etiology of prostate cancer is unclear and, combined with uncertainties around the natural history, provides little direction for identifying high-risk groups that might benefit from targeted testing with serum PSA. Recent reviews (31, 95, 111, 116) have summarized what is known about the effects of race, diet, occupation, other medical conditions, environmental and hormonal factors, and family history on prostate cancer risk. Positive associations between dietary fat consumption and prostate cancer incidence and mortality have been reported by ecologic and case-control studies (9, 18, 63, 70, 73, 82, 100, 123–126, 138, 143), but evidence from cohort studies has been less consistent (72, 75, 102, 131, 135). Occupational studies of prostate cancer risk have reported excess risk in farmers or agricultural workers (27, 28, 38, 50, 55, 57, 146), although these findings are not uniformly observed in international studies. Increased risk has been reported in rubber and tire manufacture workers, particularly workers exposed to heavy metal oxides (49, 57, 65, 146), but links to other exposures have not been established. There is no evidence that the prevalence of established risk factors (older age, Black race, and family history of prostate cancer) has increased at a rate that would account for the dramatic rise in prostate cancer incidence.

Natural History of Prostate Cancer

Like other cancers, survival is better in patients with early stage disease than in patients with advanced prostatic cancer. Since screening by PSA can result in greater detection of localized disease than screening by DRE or diagnosis of cancer in men with symptoms, this pattern of improved survival is the foundation of support for PSA screening (46, 127). However, as discussed above, screening will identify aggressive cancers earlier in their progression, thus conveying an apparent benefit in survival even if treatment is ineffectual (lead-time bias) and early stage disease detected in screened men may have improved survival rates because this group of tumors includes low-risk, slow-growing cancers that are not life threatening (length bias sampling). For these reasons, public health justification of screening requires definitive evidence that treatment of screen-detected cases reduces mortality from the cancer.

Evaluation of screening by PSA poses additional challenges that are unique to prostate cancer. The discrepancies between estimates of tumor prevalence, incidence, and mortality are indicative of a large reservoir of undetected cases that may not be clinically significant or cause death. Skeptics of screening by PSA, or by any other method, point to results from autopsy studies in men who died from other causes and argue that screening will pick up cases that are not clinically significant and would not cause death. As noted above, studies conducted in the United States and elsewhere report prevalence rates of "indolent" or "latent" prostatic cancer of 15% to 30% percent in men 50 and older and 60% in men 70 and older, compared with a lifetime risk of dying of prostate cancer of about 3.2% (25, 54, 59, 66, 90, 101, 132, 148). In addition, many newly diagnosed cases of prostate cancer are incidental findings from trans-urethral resection (TURP) for benign prostatic hypertrophy (BPH) and the contribution of these cases to recent trends in incidence has been reviewed.

There is universal agreement that most prostate cancers have a long, presymptomatic, nonmetastatic phase and thus meet an important criterion for screening suitability. Unsuspected lesions found at autopsy, or in tissue from men treated by TURP for BPH, are more limited than clinically overt cancers, but are not morphologically or histologically distinct. Survival of men with untreated localized cancers may not differ from similar aged men in the population (2, 4, 42, 78), reflecting the slow growth of most prostate cancers; however, prostate cancer is considered incurable once penetration through the prostatic capsule has occurred. An ideal screening test would distinguish the large proportion of cancers that men would die "with" from the small fraction of cancers that men would die "from". Proponents of PSA screening point to factors that are associated with poor disease prognosis as justification for screening and treatment (79, 86, 89). However, currently available tests cannot readily distinguish between tumors that are life threatening and tumors that might remain clinically dormant.

TUMOR STAGE AND GRADE   There are multiple prostate cancer staging systems but two systems are most commonly used: Conventional Staging (also called the American Classification System or the A,B,C,D System) (144) and the TNM system (6). Conventional stages A, B, C, and D are further subdivided based on clinical presentation, pathologic focality, and Gleason score, a widely used system that quantifies pathologic grade and divides prostate cancer into five histologic patterns based on degree of tumor differentiation (61). Because of variability in prostate tumor staging, the SEER program collects data on extent of disease, coded as summary staging, instead of relying on a determination of stage specified in the medical record. Summary stage categories are (*a*) localized tumors confined within the prostate capsule; (*b*) regional tumors that have penetrated through the capsule or involve regional lymph nodes; and (*c*) distant tumors that have metastasized to distant organs, bones or lymph nodes. SEER data do not distinguish tumors that were clinically staged from those that were pathologically staged.

In prostate cancer, the two factors most closely correlated with outcome, tumor stage and histologic grade, cannot be reliably ascertained without surgical intervention. Clinical staging is often inadequate since 25% to 50% of cancers are pathologically "upstaged" at pelvic lymphadenectomy and radical prostatectomy (60). Similarly, histologic grade determined from biopsy specimens may differ from the grade determined after examination of an entire surgical specimen from the same patient (5). This unique and incompletely understood natural history is a source of immense debate and frustration to both the clinical and public health communities.

OPERATIONAL CHARACTERISTICS OF SCREENING PSA

The ideal serum tumor marker is one that is expressed only by cancer cells and can be reliably detected at the time the tumor achieves biological importance. PSA is a protein found in epithelial tissue of the healthy prostate, in benign hyperplastic tissue, and in prostate cancer. In this sense, PSA is not prostate-cancer specific, it is prostate-tissue specific. Benign conditions can influence serum concentrations. PSA levels of 0 to 4 ng/ml are considered normal; efforts are under way to establish more precise reference ranges by considering factors such as age (47, 59, 113), prostate volume (11, 22, 43), rates of increase in serial PSA determinations (32), and possible value of PSA isozyme fractionation (147). Professional groups that recommend PSA screening advocate its use in conjunction with digital rectal exam. If either test is abnormal, prostate ultrasound is recommended with biopsy of detected lesions.

To be suitable for screening, a test should have favorable operational characteristics such as high sensitivity, specificity, and positive predictive value in an asymptomatic sample that is representative of the underlying population at risk (13). There is a growing body of evidence that screening PSA, especially in conjunction with digital rectal examination (DRE), detects early stage cancers (23, 24, 34–37, 69, 84, 85, 97–99, 121). Nevertheless, determining measures of sensitivity and specificity for PSA has been difficult because studies to date have not subjected patients with negative tests to systematic biopsy. Thus the prevalence of false and true negatives are not known. Furthermore, the use of transrectal ultrasound (TRUS) and subsequent biopsy of detected lesions as a confirmatory examination is also problematic since cancerous lesions are not uniformly hypoechoic, or visible on ultrasound.

Studies of cancer detection using PSA have been conducted in asymptomatic populations of volunteers responding to direct mail advertising or press releases, and in patients in urologic practice settings who are generally symptomatic, so the PSA is performed as a diagnostic test and not a screening test. Among asymptomatic men, the sensitivity of PSA testing is 67–81% for assay values of 4.0 ng/dl and greater (10, 83, 85, 97) and increases as the criterion for a positive PSA increases (85). When the test is performed in conjunction with DRE and positivity is defined as abnormal on either examination, the sensitivity also increases, although the specificity will invariably decrease (83, 97). It is likely that these results overestimate the true screening sensitivity of PSA, since the prevalence of undetected disease in men who test negative and are not biopsied (false-negatives) may be quite high. Furthermore, the generalizability of these measures to a population-based screening program is probably limited. Participants in most of the studies cited above consisted of volunteers ranging in age from 45 to 80 who were presumably asymptomatic, but self-selection bias may result in a sample of men who are highly health conscious (51) or have a high rate of urinary complaints (97).

While high PSA sensitivity is cited by supporters of screening, low PSA specificity is a major concern to those who oppose mass screening with PSA. Rates of abnormal PSA levels in PSA cancer detection studies range from 8% (36) to 20% (96), while prostate cancer was detected in about 2–3% of men tested (24, 36, 69, 97). The diagnostic cascade that follows positive test results includes transrectal ultrasound and, in many cases, transrectal needle biopsies directed at palpably or ultrasonographically suspicious areas, or four to six biopsies that systematically sample the entire prostate. There is variability in follow-up of men with negative biopsies following a positive PSA test. Some urologists recommend repeating the entire set of biopsies at least once, particularly for a PSA of 10 ng/dl or higher, while others perform follow-up PSA tests at short intervals and rebiopsy for either persistent elevations in PSA or a rising PSA value. Complications occur in about 4% of patients biopsied, including urinary tract infections, bleeding, and needle biopsy–associated tumor tracking. (12, 19, 44). Thus, independent of considerations of treatment efficacy, poor PSA specificity contributes to the human and medical costs of a screening program.

Efforts to improve PSA test sensitivity are at the expense of specificity, the proportion of persons without disease who test negative. From a public health standpoint, high test specificity is particularly important to avoid invasive evaluative procedures in asymptomatic individuals who falsely test positive. PSA is clearly elevated in prostate cancer; however, there is substantial overlap with PSA values in men with benign prostatic hypertrophy (BPH). Depending on the PSA assay used, 28% to 86% of men with BPH and without evidence of prostate cancer were found to have abnormal PSA levels (11, 56, 112, 128). In addition, both DRE and TRUS have been shown to elevate PSA levels (81, 128, 149).

Efforts to improve PSA specificity are under way. One possibility is to use serial PSA measurements to more accurately distinguish benign from malignant prostatic disease (32). While this method may show promise for surveillance of men with minimal PSA elevation and no clinical or ultrasonographic evidence of disease, its usefulness in a screening setting is questionable. A second method that accounts for both PSA value and the volume of prostate tissue is the PSA density (PSAD) or PSA index. PSAD has been studied in urologic populations of men with persistently elevated PSA values in an intermediate range (11, 14, 15), with inconsistent results. Its application in mass screening is also limited since it requires transrectal ultrasound to estimate prostatic volume.

EFFICACY OF EARLY TREATMENT

Treatment of Localized Disease

The central question in the current debate about screening for prostate cancer with PSA is whether early detection and subsequent treatment results in reduced prostate cancer mortality (39). The current controversy appears to have less to do with interpretation of treatment data than with philosophical differences between patients, clinicians, and policy makers. From a policy perspective, many believe that mass screening is not justified until evidence of benefit from clinical trials is available (16, 71, 130, 140). From a clinical perspective, many advocate the responsibility to undertake whatever measures possible to reduce the risk of cancer until results from those studies are available (8, 60, 112).

In the absence of data from clinical trials, nonexperimental studies have assessed outcomes of treatment of localized disease. Men with localized disease confined to the prostate have five-year survival rates of 92%, compared with 82% in men with regional extension beyond the prostatic capsule and approximately 28% in men with distant metastases (101). Reported ten-year survival follows a similar gradient and is approximately 75%, 55%, and 15% for local, regional, and distant disease, respectively. (83). Although these observations suggest a high curative potential for early disease, the contribution of treatment to this pattern is unknown.

Geographic variation in treatment within the U.S. and internationally underscores the controversy around optimal therapy for clinically localized prostate cancer. Only one randomized trial has reported results from a comparison of surgery and observation, watchful waiting (93). While this study reported no difference in mortality between the treatment groups, it was too small and lacked adequate statistical power, thus limiting interpretation of these results. In the absence of data from randomized trials, case series, pooled analyses, and, more recently, decision analysis studies (58, 103) have evaluated the impact of initial therapy on treatment outcome.

Outcome measures from six large case series (3, 62, 77, 78, 80, 105, 145) of patients treated conservatively were recently reported (42) to generate reliable measures of survival and mortality in subgroups of men with clinically localized prostate cancer. Five- (97–98%) and ten-year (87%) survival rates in men with grade 1 and grade 2 tumors were comparable to similar aged men in the population, suggesting that these early stage tumors do not influence survival even in the absence of treatment. Based on currently available data, these results argue against aggressive therapy for older men and highlight the need for randomized clinical trial evidence to resolve issues of the relative benefit of treatment.

Wasson et al (142) reviewed 144 reports of patients treated by surgery, radiation therapy, and watchful waiting to estimate mortality and rates of metastatic disease. Currently available literature did not provide evidence of benefit of one treatment over another, but the lack of standardized reporting of measures such as age, stage of disease, tumor grade, and follow-up limits pooling of data on study endpoints and contributes to the uncertainty of optimal treatment of localized disease. The literature was generally adequate for evaluating rates of complications following treatment, which were substantial following surgery or radiation therapy. This review highlights some of the flaws in the prostate cancer clinical literature. Differences in treatment settings, definitions of disease progression and treatment failure, staging criteria, and noncomparability of historical controls are factors that impair critical evaluation of the benefits of treating early stage disease.

Watchful Waiting

Treating some men with prostate cancer is debated, since treatment may be associated with complications that compromise quality of life and override small improvements in survival. Watchful waiting, or expectant management, is a strategy that reserves treatment for symptoms or complications related to prostate cancer without necessarily attempting a cure (33, 40). Until recently, most men with prostate cancer diagnosed incidentally at surgery for BPH were treated in this manner and it is still widely used in western Europe. Although watchful waiting may allow patients to avoid immediate complications of surgery or radiation therapy such as impotence and incontinence, there are adverse consequences associated with this treatment strategy. These include the psychological stress to the patient that an opportunity for cure may be lost and the risk of suffering from metastatic disease in patients whose tumors may progress (41). Additional complications of watchful waiting are associated with hormonal therapy used to treat progressive disease and include hot flashes and decreased libido and sexual potency (33).

Two decision analytic models of the risks and benefits of alternative treatment strategies have been reported (58, 103). Each concluded that watchful waiting is a reasonable alternative to surgery or radiation for many men, particularly older men with well-differentiated tumors. In each analysis, adjustment for quality of life that accounted for the effects of treatment-related complications such as impotence, incontinence, and bowel injury resulted in substantially lower estimates of potential gain in life expectancy associated with treatment relative to watchful waiting. In the analysis by Mold et al (103), the gain in absolute life expectancy averaged 1.1 months, but declined to a loss of 3.5 months if definitive therapy were performed and associated complications were considered. Results reported by Fleming et al (58) showed that invasive treatment was associated with less than a one-year improvement or a decrease in quality-adjusted life expectancy. The Fleming model has been criticized for using overly conservative estimates of treatment outcomes that may be inferior to results obtained under current practice (33); nevertheless, mortality rates have not declined nationally or in states with high rates of radical prostatectomy. In fact, in western Washington State, an area with the highest national rates of radical prostatectomy (91), prostate cancer mortality slightly increased during the past ten years (1984: 21.7 per 100,000; 1993: 23.7 per 100,000; J Stanford, unpublished data).

A MANAGED CARE SYSTEM'S APPROACH TO PSA SCREENING

The current controversy between advocates and skeptics of PSA screening is unlikely to be resolved until results are available from randomized trials that are under way. In the meantime, primary care physicians are faced with conflicting recommendations, patient demand, and medical industrial support for PSA screening within and outside of the clinical setting. A delivery system's response to a potential crisis created by widespread adoption of PSA screening is illustrated through the experience of a health maintenance organization, Group Health Cooperative of Puget Sound (GHC). GHC serves over 388,000 enrollees in western Washington State, an area covered by a local SEER registry. Following the publication of Catalona's landmark study in the *New England Journal of Medicine* in March 1991 (36) and the associated publicity in the lay press, physician and patient demand for PSA screening increased dramatically. The number of PSA tests ordered by GHC primary care physicians and the rate of testing in men 40–79 years of age more than doubled between March and

September of 1991 (Figure 2). Sharpest increases were observed in men 60–69 and 70–79, an older age group less likely to benefit from treatment of localized lesions. Using estimates from the Catalona study—13% positive PSA tests, 27% positive predictive value, 79% sensitivity, and 59% specificity—internal analysis based on 1991 enrollment of 35,516 men 50–74 years of age showed that approximately 4200 men would test positive and would require additional evaluation by TRUS and biopsy to detect about 863 cases of localized prostate cancer of varying clinical significance (RS Thompson, personal communication). Stuart et al (137) expanded these analyses and applied rates of complications from evaluation of false positive examinations and treatment for detected cases of prostate cancer, used in a decision analysis by Optenberg & Thompson (114), to show expected outcomes in a cohort of age-eligible GHC men. The projected first-year impact of PSA screening GHC men 50–74 years of age based on radical prostatectomy treatment for stage A2 and B disease included 30 surgical deaths, 362 cases of postoperative impotence, 268 cases of urinary stricture, 89 cases of incontinence, and 49 cases of rectal injury. Estimated costs to GHC would exceed $56 million (137).

A literature synthesis of prostate cancer screening and treatment of early disease conducted by the GHC Committee on Prevention concluded that PSA did not meet the six evidence-based criteria GHC considers before endorsing primary or secondary prevention measures. In light of increasing use of a practice of uncertain health benefit and potentially enormous health costs, the GHC Department of Medical Education mounted an academic detailing program directed at primary care physicians to discourage PSA testing in asymptomatic men (137). This project was initiated in October 1991 and was associated with an immediate and dramatic decline of PSA tests ordered by primary care physicians (Figure 2). It included educational materials directed at the physician that reviewed the scientific evidence and addressed potential concerns regarding litigation and pressure from colleagues. Patient education was an additional important component of this program's success. This program is ongoing, and new physician and patient education materials are prepared as research in PSA efficacy continues (M Stuart, personal communication). A predicted increase in rates of localized disease has occurred in the GHC population (Figure 3). Trends in testing and cancer occurrence continue to be monitored. A similar effort has been reported in a fee-for-service setting (134). However, the experience at GHC contrasts with that of other health maintenance organizations that report rising rates of PSA screening in the absence of an internal evaluation program (A Glass, J Thompson, S Van Den Eeden personal communications).

FUTURE RESEARCH

It is clear that aggressive screening with PSA will find more prostate cancers and that evidence of benefit of early detection on prostate cancer mortality has not

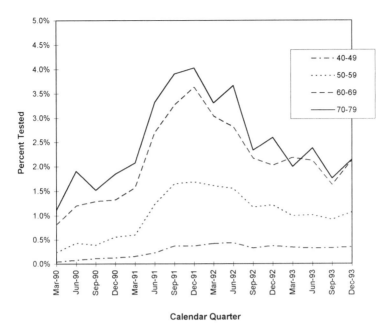

Figure 2 Frequency of PSA testing in males 40–79 by primary care physicians at Group Health Cooperative of Puget Sound, 1993–1994.

been demonstrated. This dilemma highlights the most important areas of ongoing research: (*a*) laboratory studies to identify biomarkers that will predict prognosis; (*b*) prospective randomized controlled trials (RCTs) to compare alternative treatment strategies: expectant management, radiation therapy, and surgery for localized disease; and (*c*) RCTs to evaluate the efficacy of screening using serum PSA. Screening efficacy of PSA is being studied through a major screening trial launched by the National Cancer Institute, the Prostate, Lung, Colorectal, and Ovarian (PLCO) trial, a ten-center study designed to measure early detection techniques for cancers at these sites. The prostate portion of this study entails randomization of 74,000 men to an intervention arm that consists of four annual screens by DRE and PSA, or to a control arm of "usual care." This study began subject accrual in 1993 and will need to proceed for at least 10 years to have sufficient power to detect a 20% decrease in prostate-cancer mortality (83). Furthermore, particularly because of possible increased use of PSA in the community but also because of potential non- compliance in the intervention group, the sample size may need to be increased to account for "dilution" in the intervention group and "crossover" among controls.

   The problem of early detection of prostate cancer is complex, and data from

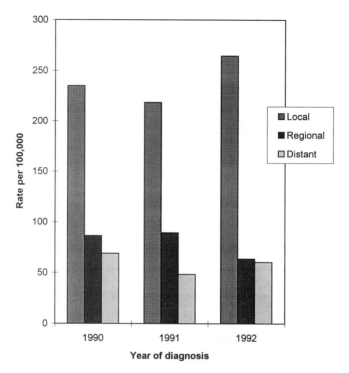

Figure 3 Stage-specific incidence of prostate cancer among Group Health Cooperative of Puget Sound men 40 and older, 1990–1992. Age-adjusted to the 1970 US standard population.

randomized trials will not be available in the immediate future. In the meantime, observational studies and decision analyses will have to provide direction for balancing the understandable desire of patients and clinicians to leave no stone unturned with the human and economic costs of a screening modality that has such a weak scientific basis. Given the absence of a national standard package of health care benefits and limited resources of the health care system, individual health systems and states face a difficult choice about prostate cancer screening.

Literature Cited

1. Adler J. 1993. The killer we don't discuss. *Newsweek,* Dec. 27. 122:40–42
2. Adolfsson J, Carstensen J, Lowhagen T.
   1992. Deferred treatment in clinically localised prostatic carcinoma. *Br. J. Urol.* 69:183–87

3. Adolfsson J, Carstensen J. 1991. Natural course of clinically localized prostate adenocarcinoma in men less than 70 years old. *J. Urol.* 146:96–98

4. Adolfsson J, Steineck G, Whitmore WF Jr. 1993. Recent results of management of palpable clinically localized prostate cancer. *Cancer* 72:310–32

5. Aihara M, Wheeler TM, Ohori M, Scardino PT. 1994. Heterogeneity of prostate cancer in radical prostatectomy specimens. *Urology* 43:60–67

6. American Joint Committee on Cancer. 1988. *Manual for Staging of Cancer.* Philadelphia, PA: Lippincott. 3rd ed.

7. Andriole GL. 1993. The case for prostate cancer screening. *Semin. Urol.* 11:50–53

8. Andriole GL, Catalona WJ. 1993. Using PSA to screen for prostate cancer: the Washington University experience. *Urol. Clin. North Am.* 20:647–51

9. Armstrong B, Doll R. 1975. Environmental factors and cancer incidence and mortality in different countries, with special reference to dietary practices. *Int. J. Cancer* 15:617–31

10. Babaian RJ, VonEschenbach AC, Miyashita H, Ramirez EI, Evans RB. 1991. Early detection program for prostate cancer: results and indentification of high-risk patient population. *Urology* 37:193–97

11. Bare R, Hart L, McCullough DL. 1994. Correlation of prostate-specific antigen and prostate-specific antigen density with outcome of prostate biopsy. *Urology* 43:191–96

12. Bastacky SS, Walsh PC, Epstein JI. 1991. Needle biopsy associated tumor tracking of adenocarcinomas of the prostate. *J. Urol.* 145:1003–7

13. Battista RN, Grover SA. 1988. Early detection of cancer: an overview. *Annu. Rev. Public Health* 9:21–45

14. Benson MC, Whang IS, Olsson CA, McMahon DJ, Cooner WH. 1992. The use of prostate specific antigen density to enhance the predictive value of intermediate levels of serum prostate specific antigen. *J. Urol.* 147:817–21

15. Benson MC, Whang IS, Pantuck A, Ring K, Kaplan SA, et al. 1992. Prostate specific antigen density: a means of distinguishing benign prostatic hypertrophy and prostate cancer. *J. Urol.* 147:815–16

16. Bentvelsen FM, Schroder FH. 1993. Modalities available for screening for prostate cancer. *Eur. J. Cancer* 29A:804–11

17. Black WC, Welch HG. 1993. Advances in diagnostic imaging and overestimations of disease prevalence and the benefits of therapy. *New Engl. J. Med.* 328:1237–43

18. Blair A, Fraumeni JF Jr. 1978. Geographic patterns of prostate cancer in the United States. *J. Natl. Cancer Inst.* 61:1379–84

19. Blight EM Jr. 1992. Seeding of prostate adenocarcinoma following transrectal needle biopsy. *Urology* 39:297–98

20. Boffetta P, Parkin DM. 1994. Cancer in developing countries. *CA Cancer J. Clin.* 44:81–90

21. Boring CC, Squires TS, Tong T, Montgomery S. 1994. Cancer statistics, 1994. *CA Cancer J. Clin.* 44:7–26

22. Brawer MK, Aramburu EAG, Chen GL, Preston SD, Ellis WJ. 1993. The inability of prostate specific antigen index to enhance the predictive value of prostate specific antigen in the diagnosis of prostatic carcinoma. *J. Urol.* 150:369–73

23. Brawer MK, Beatie J, Wener MH, Vessella RL, Preston SD, Lange PH. 1993. Screening for prostatic carcinoma with prostate specific antigen: results of the second year. *J. Urol.* 150:106–9

24. Brawer MK, Chetner MP, Beatie J, Buchner DM, Vessella RL, Lange PH. 1992. Screening for prostatic carcinoma with prostate specific antigen. *J. Urol.* 147:841–45

25. Breslow N, Chan CW, Dhom G, Drury AB, Franks LM, et al. 1977. Latent carcinoma of prostate at autopsy in seven areas. *Int. J. Cancer* 20:680–88

26. Brooks NR. 1993. Milken says he has cancer of prostate. *Los Angeles Times*, Feb. 24, 112:D1

27. Brownson RC, Chang JC, Davis JR, Bagby JR Jr. 1988. Occupational risk of prostate cancer: a cancer registry-based study. *J. Occup. Med.* 30:523–26

28. Burmeister LF, Everett GD, Van Lier SF, Isacson P. 1983. Selected cancer mortality and farm practices in Iowa. *Am. J. Epidemiol.* 118:72–77

29. Canadian Task Force on the Periodic Health Examination. 1991. Periodic health examination, 1991 update: 3. secondary prevention of prostate cancer. *Can. Med. Assoc. J.* 145:413–28

30. Canadian Urological Association. 1992. *Guidelines for Early Detection of Prostate Cancer.* Winnipeg: Can. Urol. Assoc.

31. Carter BS, Bova GS, Beaty TH, Steinberg GD, Childs B, et al. 1993. Hereditary prostate cancer: epidemiologic and clinical features. *J. Urol.* 150: 797–802

32. Carter HB, Pearson JD. 1993. PSA velocity for the diagnosis of early prostate cancer. *Urol. Clin. North Am.* 20:665–70

33. Catalona WJ. 1994. Drug therapy: man-

agement of cancer of the prostate. *New Engl. J. Med* 331:1000–3

34. Catalona WJ, Richie JP, Ahmann FR, Hudson MA, Scardino PT, et al. 1994. Comparison of digital rectal examination and serum prostate specific antigen in the early detection of prostate cancer: results of a multicenter clinical trial of 6,630 men. *J. Urol.* 151:1283–90

35. Catalona WJ, Smith DS, Ratliff TL, Basler JW. 1993. Detection of organ-confined prostate cancer is increased through prostate-specific antigen-based screening. *J. Am. Med. Assoc.* 270:948–54

36. Catalona WJ, Smith DS, Ratliff TL, Dodds KM, Coplen DE, et al. 1991. Measurement of prostate-specific antigen in serum as a screening test for prostate cancer. *New Engl. J. Med.* 324:1156–61

37. Chadwick DJ, Kemple T, Astley JP, MacIver AG, Gillatt DA, et al. 1991. Pilot study of screening for prostate cancer in general practice. *Lancet* 338:613–16

38. Checkoway H, DiFerdinando G, Hulka BS, Mickey DD. 1987. Medical, lifestyle, and occupational risk factors for prostate cancer. *Prostate* 10:79–88

39. Chodak GW. 1993. Questioning the value of screening for prostate cancer in asymptomatic men. *Urology* 42:116–18

40. Chodak GW. 1994. The role of conservative management in localized prostate cancer. *Cancer* 74:2178–81

41. Chodak GW. 1994. Treatment of early stage prostate cancer: conservative management—delayed therapy. In *Important Advances in Oncology,* ed. VT DeVita, S Heilman, SA Rosenberg, pp. 241–44. Philadelphia: Lippencott

42. Chodak GW, Thisted RA, Gerber GS, Johansson JE, Adolfsson J, et al. 1994. Results of conservative management of clinically localized prostate cancer. *New Engl. J. Med.* 330:242–48

43. Collins GN, Lee RJ, McKelvie GB, Rogers ACN, Hehir M. 1993. Relationship between prostate specific antigen, prostate volume and age in the benign prostate. *Br. J. Urol.* 71:445–50

44. Collins GN, Lloyd SN, Hehir M, McKelvie GB. 1993b. Multiple transrectal ultrasound-guided prostatic biopsies—true morbidity and patient acceptance. *Br. J. Urol.* 71:460–63

45. Crawford ED, DeAntoni EP. 1993. PSA as a screening test for prostate cancer. *Urol. Clin. North Am.* 20:637–46

46. Cupp MR, Oesterling JE. 1993. Prostate-specific antigen, digital rectal examination, and transrectal ultrasonography: their roles in diagnosing early prostate cancer. *Mayo Clin. Proc.* 68:297–306

47. Dalkin BL, Ahmann FR, Kopp JB. 1993. Prostate specific antigen levels in men older than 50 years without clinical evidence of prostatic carcinoma. *J. Urol.* 150:1837–39

48. Day NE, William DRR, Khaw KT. 1989. Breast cancer screening programmes: the development of a monitoring and evaluation system. *Br. J. Cancer* 59:954–58

49. Decoufle P, Stanislawczyk K, Houten L. 1977. A retrospective survey of cancer in relation to occupation. *NIOSH Res. Rep. DHEW publ. no. (NIOSH)* 77–178

50. Delzell E, Grufferman S. 1985. Mortality among white and nonwhite farmers in North Carolina, 1976–1978. *Am. J. Epidemiol.* 121:391–402

51. Demark-Wahnefried W, Catoe KE, Paskett E, Robertson CN, Rimer BK. 1993. Characteristics of men reporting for prostate cancer screening. *Urology* 42:269–75

52. Demers RY, Swanson GM, Weiss LK, Kau TY. 1994. Increasing incidence of cancer of the prostate: the experience of black and white men in the Detroit metropolitan area. *Arch. Intern. Med.* 154:1211–16

53. Dorr VJ, Williamson SK, Stephens RL. 1993. An evaluation of prostate-specific antigen as a screening test for prostate cancer. *Arch. Intern. Med.* 153:2529–37

54. Edwards CN, Steinthorsson E, Nicholson D. 1953. An autopsy study of latent prostatic cancer. *Cancer* 6:531–54

55. Elghany NA, Schumacher MC, Slattery ML, West DW, Lee JS. 1990. Occupation, cadmium exposure, and prostate cancer. *Epidemiology* 1:107–15

56. Ercole CJ, Lange PH, Mathisen M, Chiou RK, Reddy P, Vessella RL. 1987. Prostatic specific antigen and prostatic acid phosphatase in the monitoring and staging of patients with prostatic cancer. *J. Urol.* 138:1184–84

57. Ernster VL, Selvin S, Brown SM, Sacks ST, Winkelstein W Jr, Austin DF. 1979. Occupation and prostatic cancer: a review and retrospective analysis based on death certificates in two California counties. *J. Occup. Med.* 21:175–83

58. Fleming C, Wasson JH, Albertsen PC, Barry MJ, Wennberg JE. 1993. A decision analysis of alternative treatment strategies for clinically localized prostate cancer. *J. Am. Med. Assoc.* 269:2650–58

59. Franks LM. 1954. Latent carcinoma of the prostate. *J. Pathol. Bacteriol.* 68:603–16

60. Garnick MB. 1993. Prostate cancer: screening, diagnosis and management. *Ann. Intern. Med.* 118:804–18

61. Gleason DF. 1966. Classification of prostatic carcinomas. *Cancer Chemother. Rep.* 50:125–28

62. Goodman CM, Busuttil A, Chisholm GD. 1988. Age, and size and grade of tumour predict prognosis in incidentally diagnosed carcinoma of the prostate. *Br. J. Urol.* 62:576–80

63. Graham S, Haughey B, Marshall J, Priore R, Byers T, et al. 1983. Diet in the epidemiology of carcinoma of the prostate gland. *J. Natl. Cancer Inst.* 70:687–92

64. Green CJ, Hadorn D, Bassett K, Kazanjian A. 1993. *Prostate-Specific Antigen in the Early Detection of Prostate Cancer.* Vancouver, BC: BC Off. Health Technol. Assess.

65. Greenwald HP, Henke CJ. 1992. HMO membership, treatment, and mortality risk among prostatic cancer patients. *Am. J. Public Health* 82:1099–104

66. Guileyardo J, Johnson W, Welsh R, Akazaki K, Correa P. 1980. Prevalence of latent prostatic carcinoma in two U.S. populations. *J. Natl. Cancer Inst.* 65:311–16

67. Guinan P, Bush I, Ray V, Vieth R, Rao R, Bhatti R. 1980. The accuracy of the rectal examination in the diagnosis of prostate carcinoma. *New Engl. J. Med.* 303:499–503

68. Guinan P, Ray P, Bhatti R, Rubenstein M. 1987. An evaluation of five tests to diagnose prostate cancer. *Prog. Clin. Biol. Res.* 243A:551–58

69. Gustaffson O, Norming U, Almgard LE, Fredriksson A, Gustavsson G, et al. 1992. Diagnostic methods in the detection of prostate cancer: a study of a randomly selected population of 2,400 men. *J. Urol.* 148:1827–31

70. Heshmat MY, Kaul L, Kovi J, Jackson MA, Jackson AG, et al. 1985. Nutrition and prostate cancer: a case-control study. *Prostate* 6:7–17

71. Hinman, F Jr. 1991. Screening for prostatic carcinoma. *J. Urol.* 145:126–30

72. Hirayama T. 1979. Epidemiology of prostate cancer with special reference to the role of diet. *Natl. Cancer Inst. Monogr.* 53:149–55

73. Howell MA. 1974. Factor analysis of international cancer mortality data and per capita food consumption. *Br. J. Cancer* 29:328–36

74. Hsing AW, Devesa SS. 1994. Prostate cancer mortality in the United States by cohort year of birth, 1865–1940. *Cancer Epidemiol. Biomarkers Prevent.* 3:527–30

75. Hsing AW, McLaughlin JK, Schuman LM, Bjelke E, Gridley G, et al. 1990. Diet, tobacco use, and fatal prostate cancer: results from the Lutheran Brotherhood Cohort Study. *Cancer Res.* 50:6836–40

76. International Agency for Research on Cancer. 1987. *Cancer Incidence in Five Continents,* 5:170–766. Lyon: IARC

77. Johansson JE. 1994. Watchful waiting for early stage prostate cancer. *Urology* 43:138–42

78. Johansson JE, Adami HO, Andersson SO, Bergstrom R, Holmberg L, Krusemo UB. 1992. High 10-year survival rate in patients with early, untreated prostatic cancer. *J. Am. Med. Assoc.* 267:2191–96

79. Johansson JE, Adami HO, Andersson SO, Bergstrom R, Krusemo UB, Kraaz W. 1989. Natural history of localised prostatic cancer. *Lancet* 2:799–803

80. Jones GW. 1992. Prospective, conservative management of localized prostate cancer. *Cancer* 70:307–10 (Suppl.)

81. Klomp ML, Hendrikx AJ, Keyzer JJ. 1994. The effect of transrectal ultrasonography (TRUS) including digital rectal examination (DRE) of the prostate on the level of prostate specific antigen (PSA). *Br. J. Urol.* 73:71–74

82. Kolonel LN, Hankin JH, Lee J, Chu SY, Nomura AMY, Hinds MW. 1981. Nutrient intakes in relation to cancer incidence in Hawaii. *Br. J. Cancer* 44:332–39

83. Kramer BS, Brown ML, Prorok PC, Potosky AL, Gohagan JK. 1993. Prostate cancer screening: what we know and what we need to know. *Ann. Intern. Med.* 119:914–23

84. Labrie F, Dupont A, Suburu R, Cusan L, Tremblay M, et al. 1992. Serum prostate specific antigen as pre-screening test for prostate cancer. *J. Urol.* 147:846–52

85. Labrie F, Dupont A, Suburu R, Cusan L, Gomez JL, et al. 1993. Optimized strategy for detection of early stage, curable prostate cancer: role of pre-screening with prostate-specific antigen. *Clin. Invest. Med.* 16:425–39

86. Lerner SP, Seale-Hawkins C, Carlton CE Jr, Scardino PT. 1991. The risk of dying of prostate cancer in patients with clinically localized disease. *J. Urol.* 146:1040–45

87. Levy IG, Gibbons L, Collins JP, Perkins DG, Mao Y. 1993. Prostate cancer trends

in Canada: rising incidence or increased detection? *Can. Med. Assoc. J.* 149:617–24

88. Lloyd JW, Lundin FE, Redmond CK, Geiser PB. 1970. Long-term mortality study of steelworkers: IV. Mortality by work area. *J. Occup. Med.* 12:151–57

89. Lowe BA, Listrom MB. 1988. Incidental carcinoma of the prostate: an analysis of the predictors of progression. *J. Urol.* 140:1340–44

90. Lundberg S, Berge T. 1979. Prostate carcinoma: an autopsy study. *Scand. J. Urol. Nephrol.* 4:93–97

91. Lu-Yao GL, Greenberg ER. 1994. Changes in prostate cancer incidence and treatment in USA. *Lancet* 343:251–54

92. Lu-Yao GL, McLerran D, Wasson J, Wennberg WE for the Prostate Patient Outcomes Research Team. 1993. An assessment of radical prostatectomy: time trends, geographic variation, and outcomes. *J. Am. Med. Assoc.* 269: 2633–36

93. Madsen PO, Graversen PH, Gasser TC, Carle DK. 1988. Treatment of localized prostatic cancer: radical prostatectomy versus placebo: a 15-year follow-up. *Scand. J. Nephrol.* 110:95–100 (Suppl.)

94. Marbach WD. 1991. Prostate cancer: sounding an early alarm. *Business Week* May 6, 3212:130

95. Meikle AW, Smith JA. 1990. Epidemiology of prostate cancer. *Urol. Clin. North Am.* 17:709–17

96. Mettlin C, Jones G, Averette J, Gusberg H, Murphy GP. 1993. Defining and updating the American Cancer Society's guidelines for the cancer-related checkup: prostate and endometrial cancers. *CA Cancer J. Clin.* 43:42–46

97. Mettlin C, Lee F, Drago J, Murphy GP, Investigators of the American Cancer Society National Prostate Cancer Detection Project. 1991. The American Cancer Society National Prostate Cancer Detection Project: findings on the detection of early prostate cancer in 2425 men. *Cancer* 67:2949–58

98. Mettlin C, Murphy GP, Lee F, Littrup PJ, Chesley A, et al. 1993. Characteristics of prostate cancers detected in a multimodality early detection program. *Cancer* 72:1701–8

99. Mettlin C, Murphy GP, Ray P, Shanberg A, Toi A, et al. 1993. American Cancer Society—National Prostate Cancer Detection Project: results from mutiple examinations using transrectal ultrasound, digital rectal examination, and prostate specific antigen. *Cancer* 71:891–98 (Suppl.)

100. Mettlin C, Selenskas S, Natarajan N, Huben R. 1989. Beta-carotene and animal fats and their relationship to prostate cancer risk: a case-control study. *Cancer* 64:605–12

101. Miller BA, Ries LA, Hankey BF, Kosary CL, Harras A, et al. 1993. SEER cancer statistics review 1973–90. *Natl. Cancer Inst. NIH Publ. No. 93–2789*

102. Mills PK, Beeson WL, Phillips RL, Fraser GE. 1989. Cohort study of diet, lifestyle, and prostate cancer in Adventist men. *Cancer* 64:598–604

103. Mold JW, Holtgrave DR, Bisonni RS, Marley DS, Wright RA, Spann SJ. 1992. The evaluation and treatment of men with asymptomatic prostate nodules in primary care: a decision analysis. *J. Fam. Prac.* 34:561–68

104. Morrison AS. 1982. The effects of early treatment, lead time, and length bias on the mortality experienced by cases detected by screening. *Int. J. Epidemiol.* 11:261–67

105. Moskovitz B, Nitechi A, Richter-Levin D. 1987. Cancer of the prostate: is there a need for aggressive treatment? *Urol. Int.* 42:49–52

106. Muir CS, Nectoux J, Staszewski J. 1991. The epidemiology of prostatic cancer. *Acta Oncol.* 30:133–40

107. National Cancer Institute. 1993. *PDQ Cancer Screening Guidelines. Screening for Prostate Cancer. Information for Physicians.* Bethesda, MD: Natl. Cancer Inst. Publ. No. cn-304727

108. New York Times. 1991. Senator Helms says doctors are treating him for cancer. *NY Times,* Sept. 24, 141:A14

109. New York Times.1991. Full recovery seen for Dole in Surgery for prostate cancer. *NY Times,* Dec. 19, 141:pA15

110. Neely K. 1992. Frank Zappa stricken with cancer. *Rolling Stone,* Jan. 9, 621:22

111. Nomura AMY, Kolonel LN. 1991. Prostate cancer: a current perspective. *Am. J. Epidemiol.* 13:200–27

112. Oesterling JE. 1991. Prostate specific antigen: a critical assessment of the most useful tumor marker for adenocarcinoma of the prostate. *J. Urol.* 145:907–23

113. Oesterling JE, Jacobsen SJ, Chute CG, Guess HA, Girman CJ, et al. 1993. Serum prostate-specific antigen in a community-based population of healthy men: establishment of age-specific reference ranges. *J. Am. Med. Assoc.* 270: 860–64

114. Optenberg SA, Thompson IM. 1990. Economics of screening for carcinoma of the prostate. *Urol. Clin. North Am.* 17:719–37

115. Peters DH, Sorkin EM. 1993. Finasteride: a review of its potential in the treatment of benign prostatic hyperplasia. *Drugs* 46:177–208
116. Pienta KJ, Esper PS. 1993. Risk factors for prostate cancer. *Ann. Intern. Med.* 118:793–803
117. Podolsky D. 1992. Should you get tested? *US News World Rep.,* May 4, 112:74–76
118. Potosky AL, Kessler L, Gridley G, Brown CC, Horn JW. 1990. Rise in prostatic cancer incidence associated with increased use of transurethral resection. *J. Natl. Cancer Inst.* 82:1624–28
119. Prorok PC, Hankey BF, Bundy BN. 1981. Concepts and problems in the evaluation of screening programs. *J. Chron. Dis.* 34:159–71
120. Reynolds T. 1993. Prostate cancer rates climbed sharply in 1990. *J. Natl. Cancer Inst.* 85:947–48
121. Richie JP, Catalona WJ, Ahmann FR, Hudson MA, Scardino PT, et al. 1993. Effect of patient age on early detection of prostate cancer with serum prostate-specific antigen and digital rectal examination. *Urology* 42:365–74
122. Rohr LR. 1987. Incidental adenocarcinoma in transurethral resections of the prostate: partial versus complete microscopic examination. *Am. J. Surg. Pathol.* 11:53–58
123. Rose DP. 1993. Diet, hormones, and cancer. *Annu. Rev. Public Health* 14:1–17
124. Rose DP, Boyar AP, Wynder EL. 1986. International comparisons of mortality rates for cancer of the breast, ovary, prostate, and colon, and per capita food consumption. *Cancer* 58:2363–71
125. Ross RK, Shimizu H, Paganini-Hill A, Honda G, Henderson BE. 1987. Case-control studies of prostate cancer in blacks and whites in southern California. *J. Natl. Cancer Inst.* 78:869–74
126. Rotkin ID. 1977. Studies in the epidemiology of prostatic cancer: expanded sampling. *Cancer Treat. Rep.* 61:173–80
127. Scardino PT, Weaver R, Hudson MA. 1992. Early detection of prostate cancer. *Hum. Pathol.* 23:211–22
128. Schellhammer PF, Wright GL. 1993. Biomolecular and clinical characteristics of PSA and other candidate prostate tumor markers. *Urol. Clin. North Am.* 20:597–606
129. Schmidt JD, Mettlin CJ, Natarajan N, Peace BB, Beart RW Jr, et al. 1986. Trends in patterns of care for prostatic cancer, 1974–1983: results of surveys by the American College of Surgeons. *J. Urol.* 136:416–21
130. Schroder FH, Boyle P. 1993. Screening for prostate cancer—necessity or nonsense? *Eur. J. Cancer* 29A:656–61
131. Severson RK, Nomura AMY, Grove JS, Stemmermann GN. 1989. A prospective study of demographics, diet, and prostate cancer among men of Japanese ancestry in Hawaii. *Cancer Res.* 49:1857–60
132. Sheldon CA, Williams RD, Fraley EE. 1980. Incidental carcinoma of the prostate: a review of the literature and critical reappraisal of classification. *J. Urol.* 124:626–31
133. Silverberg E, Boring CC, Squires TS. 1990. Cancer statistics, 1990. *CA Cancer J. Clin.* 40:9–26
134. Skelton NK, Skelton WP III. 1994. Changing physician PSA ordering patterns through education. *Arch. Intern. Med.* 154:819–20
135. Snowdon DA, Phillips RL, Choi W. 1984. Diet, obesity, and risk of fatal prostate cancer. *Am. J. Epidemiol.* 120:244–50
136. Steele GD, Osteen RT, Winchester DP, Murphy GP, Menck HR. 1994. Clinical highlights from the national cancer data base: 1994. *CA Cancer J. Clin.* 44:71–80
137. Stuart ME, Handley MA, Thompson RS, Conger M, Timlin D. 1992. Clinical practice and new technology: prostate-specific antigen (PSA). *HMO Pract.* 6:5–11
138. Talamini R, LaVecchia C, Decarli A, Negri E, Franceschi S. 1986. Nutrition, social factors and prostatic cancer in a Northern Italian population. *Br. J. Cancer* 53:817–21
139. Tulinius H. 1982. Latent malignancies. 1982. In *Cancer Campaign, Cancer Epidemiology,* ed. E Grundman, 6:129–37. Stuttgart: Fischer
140. US Preventive Services Task Force. 1994. Screening for prostate cancer: commentary on the recommendations of the Canadian Task Force on the Periodic Health Examination. *Am. J. Prev. Med.* 10:187–93
141. Wall Street Journal. 1991. Time Warner's Ross beginning treatment for prostate cancer. *Wall St. J.* Nov. 27, pB2 (W), pB6 (E)
142. Wasson JH, Cushman CC, Bruskewitz RC, Littenberg B, Mulley AG, et al. 1993. A structured literature review of treatment for localized prostate cancer. *Arch. Fam. Med.* 2:487–93
143. West DW, Slattery ML, Robison LM, French TK, Mahoney AW. 1991. Adult dietary intake and prostate cancer risk in Utah: a case-control study with special emphasis on aggressive tumors. *Cancer Causes Control* 2:85–94

144. Whitmore WF Jr. 1956. Hormone therapy in prostatic cancer. *Am. J. Med.* 21:697–713
145. Whitmore WF Jr, Warner JA, Thompson IM Jr. 1991. Expectant management of localized prostatic cancer. *Cancer* 67:1091–96
146. Williams RR, Stegens NL, Goldsmith JR. 1977. Associations of cancer site and type with occupation and industry from the Third National Cancer Survey Interview. *J. Natl. Cancer Inst.* 59:1147–51
147. Wu JT. 1994. Assay for prostate specific antigen (PSA): problems and possible solutions. *J. Clin. Lab. Anal.* 8:51–62
148. Yatani R, Chigusa I, Akazaki K, Stemmermann GN, Welsh RA, Correa P. 1982. Geographic pathology of latent prostatic carcinoma. *Int. J. Cancer* 29:611–16
149. Yuan JJ, Coplen DE, Petros JA, Figenshau RS, Ratliff TL, et al. 1992. Effects of rectal examination, prostatic massage, ultrasonography and needle biopsy on serum prostate specific antigen levels. *J. Urol.* 147:810–14
150. Zaridze DG, Boyle P, Smans M. 1984. International trends in prostatic cancer. *Int. J. Cancer* 33:223–30
151. Gann PH, Hennekens CH, Meir JF. 1995. A prospective evaluation of plasma prostate-specific antigen for detection of prostatic cancer. *J. Am. Med. Assoc.* 273:289–94
152. Lange, PH. 1995. New information about prostate-specific antigen and the paradoxes of prostate cancer. *J. Am. Med. Assoc.* 273:336–37

NOTE ADDED IN PROOF

Since this review went to press, Gann et al (151) reported findings from a case-control study that compared baseline PSA values from stored blood in 366 men with prostate cancer and 1098 controls. "Aggressive" and "nonaggressive" tumors were distinguished by stage, grade, and Gleason score. PSA sensitivity was higher for "aggressive" tumors diagnosed within 4 years (87%) than for "nonaggressive" tumors (53%). Specificity was approximately 91%. This report of high sensitivity for "aggressive" disease attracted considerable attention as Gann (151) and others (152) recommend the identification of cost-effective PSA screening strategies while we await results from ongoing prospective trials of screening and treatment of early disease. This recommendation seems premature because early and late cancers were grouped together as "aggressive," and the aim of screening is to identify localized cancer with high malignant potential. The clinical implications of these findings are therefore unclear. Other factors that may have resulted in overestimates of sensitivity and specificity in this study include inclusion of control men with occult cancer and the discrepancy between elevated PSA in clinical practice, where some men may have tumors not detectable at ultrasound or biopsy, and elevated PSA in a retrospective study.

Annu. Rev. Public Health. 1995. 16:307–26

TUBERCULOSIS, PUBLIC HEALTH, AND CIVIL LIBERTIES

Ronald Bayer

School of Public Health Columbia University and The HIV Center for Clinical and Behavioral Studies, New York State Psychiatric Institute, 600 West 168th Street, New York, NY 10032

Laurence Dupuis

Division of Bioethics, Montefiore Medical Center, 111 East 210th Street, Bronx, NY 10467-2490

KEY WORDS: tuberculosis, ethics, civil liberties, coercion, public health law

ABSTRACT

The resurgence of tuberculosis confronts policy-makers with difficult legal and ethical questions about the proper use of state power and resources to protect public health. This chapter examines the implications of expanded use of invasive or coercive measures—including directly observed therapy, involuntary detention of noncompliant patients, and forced administration of medications—designed to reduce the risk of tuberculosis transmission and to ensure that those with TB are fully treated. These measures focus attention on the limitations of government power and obligation and on the delicate balance between the demands of civil liberty and the demands of public health.

INTRODUCTION

Tuberculosis, a scourge referred to in the seventeenth century as the "captain of all these men of death" (11), has returned to plague contemporary America, just when medical and public health measures seemed poised to consign the disease to the pages of history. In 1989, the Center for Disease Control's

307

Advisory Council for the Elimination of Tuberculosis established a goal of eliminating tuberculosis in the United States by 2010 (15). But as early as 1985, the long trend of declining tuberculosis cases had already reversed itself, and by 1992, there were 52,000 more cases than would have been expected had the downward trend continued (2).

The dramatic return of this disease poses serious questions about the failures of public health policy during the 1970s and 1980s (37, 45). The new epidemic has also forced a reappraisal of the legal and ethical implications of disease-control measures that might be marshaled to combat the spread of contagious disease (8). This chapter first briefly reviews the medical and epidemiological background of the current tuberculosis epidemic and the influence of AIDS on traditional approaches to disease control. The remainder of the chapter focuses on the specific ethical and legal questions surrounding tuberculosis control, with a particular emphasis on the civil-liberties implications of four approaches to disease control: the provision of supportive services to encourage patients to complete therapy; the use of directly observed therapy to monitor adherence to therapy; the involuntary detention of noncompliant patients; and the forced administration of tuberculosis medications.

THE RETURN OF TUBERCULOSIS

Tuberculosis is a communicable disease caused by *Mycobacterium tuberculosis,* an organism that is most commonly transmitted by inhaling airborne droplets expelled by the cough of a person with infectious tuberculosis (15). In most cases, people infected with *M. tuberculosis* do not develop clinical disease, but remain noninfectious, asymptomatic carriers (15, 49). Among infected persons with noncompromised immune systems, there is an estimated 5–10% *lifetime* risk of developing clinical disease. People with both *M. tuberculosis* and HIV infection, by contrast, have a 5–10% *annual* risk of developing clinical disease (49). Clinical disease most commonly affects the lungs, but may affect other sites as well (15). Treatment of active disease ordinarily involves taking several drugs, at least two to three times per week, for a period of 6–9 months (18). Such treatment is generally highly effective, and results in long-term cure in about 95% of cases (55). Treatment of HIV-infected tuberculosis patients, however, is complicated by the unusually rapid progression from initial infection to active disease, which results in a high incidence of treatment failure and mortality (33, 49).

Tuberculosis was among the leading causes of death in western society throughout the nineteenth century (51), and remains one of the most common infectious diseases worldwide. Approximately one third of the global population carries *M. tuberculosis*, 8 million new cases are reported annually, and each year nearly 3 million die from the disease (11). In the United States, however, the prevalence of the disease declined steadily, beginning in the early part of the century and continuing until the mid-1980s (51). The historical decline in TB morbidity and mortality has been attributed to a number of factors. Prior to the introduction of antibiotic therapy in 1946 (38), the decline in tuberculosis probably was the result of improvements in nutrition and housing that accompanied rising wages and improved living standards in the first half of the century, as well as specific public health interventions—such as education, isolation, and quarantine—that contained the spread of the disease (51). From 1953, the year after the introduction of the antituberculosis drug, isoniazid, through 1984, the number of tuberculosis cases reported decreased from 84,304 to 22,255, an average decline of 5% per year (15, 16).

Despite the overall decline in tuberculosis in the United States, the disease continued to be a significant problem among people of color and in low-income communities. For example, in 1984, when the tuberculosis case rate had dropped to 9.4 new cases per 100,000 population in the United States, the case rate in central Harlem—a predominantly African-American community with high rates of poverty—was 90.7 per 100,000 (14).

Beginning in 1985, the downward trend in reported cases of tuberculosis in the United States was reversed. From 1985 through 1991, the number of reported TB cases increased 18% (18). The HIV epidemic is certainly a major factor in the resurgence of tuberculosis. In New York City, nearly 50% of tuberculosis patients in 1988–89 were also infected with HIV; this suggests that many reported cases are the result of reactivation of latent infection in immune-suppressed individuals (49). While reactivation of latent disease has contributed to the increase in reported tuberculosis cases, recent studies indicate that more than one third of active cases in New York City and San Francisco are the result of recent transmission (2, 30, 52). Dramatic cutbacks in public funding and in facilities for TB control and treatment, as well as increasing poverty, homelessness, overcrowded housing and drug abuse have all played critical roles in the emerging epidemic (14).

The resurgence of tuberculosis is primarily afflicting those disadvantaged communities where the disease had persisted despite the overall national decline. From 1985 through 1990, the number of tuberculosis cases increased dramatically among Hispanics, African-Americans, and Asian/Pacific Islanders, while reported cases among non-Hispanic whites continued to decline (16). By 1990, the TB case rate in central Harlem approached 200 per 100,000, approximately 4 times the New York City rate and 20 times the national rate (49). These are also the communities that have borne much of the weight of the continuing HIV/AIDS epidemic (49).

Exacerbating the ominous increase in tuberculosis is the emergence and proliferation of strains of the disease that resist one or more of the medications typically used to treat TB patients. In a national survey of culture-positive TB cases reported in the first quarter of 1991, investigators found that 9.5% of cases were resistant to rifampin and/or isoniazid, two of the safest and most effective first-line antituberculosis drugs, and that 3.5% of cases were resistant to both drugs (10). A study in New York City found that 19% of culture-positive cases during April 1991 were resistant to both rifampin and isoniazid (23). Multidrug-resistant tuberculosis (MDR-TB) is considerably more difficult and expensive to treat than nonresistant disease, and is associated with much greater mortality, particularly among patients infected with HIV (33). In a report on 171 carefully treated and monitored non-HIV patients with multidrug-resistant disease, only 56% of the patients had successful drug-therapy outcomes (negative sputum cultures without relapse) and 37% died, about half from tuberculosis (25). In investigations of nine outbreaks of multidrug-resistant tuber- culosis in hospitals and prisons, the CDC found mortality rates ranging from 72% to 89%. Between 20% and 80% of the cases in those outbreaks were HIV infected (18).

The rise of multidrug-resistant tuberculosis is ultimately attributable to inadequate drug therapy, which results either from inappropriate treatment by the physician or poor adherence to recommended therapy by the patient (23, 33). Although the current system for tracking rates of treatment completion is inadequate (9, 11), available data indicate that in some of the cities hardest hit by drug-resistant strains of tuberculosis, completion rates have been dismally low. For example, in New York City between 1986 and 1990, only 53.6% of patients completed six continuous months of therapy, whereas San Francisco, Dallas, and El Paso all had completion rates above 90% during the same period (11). At one location in New York, 89% of tuberculosis patients were lost to follow-up before they had completed therapy (14). Although drug-resistant strains initially develop as a result of inadequate therapy, it must be underscored that such strains can be transmitted directly to previously healthy individuals. One study in New York concluded that most patients with drug-resistant tuberculosis did not acquire drug-resistant disease through inadequate treatment of a susceptible strain, but were initially infected with a drug-resistant strain transmitted to them by another person (23).

DISEASE CONTROL AFTER AIDS

Responses to the resurgence of tuberculosis must be understood in the context of the AIDS epidemic, which has shaped popular as well as professional conceptions of the appropriate public health approaches to epidemic disease.

As the public policy responses to AIDS took shape in the United States and in other democratic nations, a consensus emerged against using coercive state interventions long associated with the practice of public health (7). Rather, a voluntaristic strategy took hold that focused on eliciting the cooperation of those at risk for HIV infection. Mass education, voluntary testing and counseling, the protection of the rights of privacy of those with HIV, and the prohibition against unwarranted acts of discrimination were essential elements of this approach. The roots of this strategy, broadly endorsed by public health officials at the federal, state, and local levels, were many. HIV transmission typically takes place in intimate or secretive settings between consenting adults during sexual intercourse or drug use, not through casual contact. Public health and clinical medicine have no magic bullet to cure the disease; only voluntary personal risk-reduction behavior is effective in preventing further transmission. AIDS primarily affects marginalized populations—gay and bisexual men, intravenous drug users, social and ethnic minorities—with a long history of suspicion about the intentions and practices of government. The shaping of AIDS policy was singularly affected by the capacity of one of these groups—urban, middle-class gay men—to articulate their concerns about the dangers of using the AIDS epidemic as a pretext for undermining their hard-won, but still fragile, rights of privacy and liberty.

But tuberculosis is not AIDS. It is an airborne disease that can be transmitted to contacts who may be largely unaware that they are being placed at risk, or who may be unable to take precautions to protect themselves. Unlike AIDS, tuberculosis is generally curable. Even drug-resistant tuberculosis may be treated effectively, particularly in cases where the disease is susceptible to at least one of the first-line medications. The availability of effective therapy makes it possible to interrupt the spread of infection to the general population through medical intervention with the individual patient. Finally, while legislation and practice surrounding AIDS reflected the transformation that had occurred in American constitutional law over the previous three decades, which had expanded the rights of the individual to challenge the exercise of state authority, TB surveillance and control were still governed "by antiquated laws that predate modern concepts of constitutional law and the need for a flexible range of public health powers" (27).

It is an unfortunate irony that AIDS and tuberculosis—the former a new threat that has evoked a radical rethinking of public health practices stressing principles of voluntarism, the latter an ancient threat, the control of which epitomized the coercive tradition in public health—have been superimposed upon each other for epidemiological and biological reasons. The resurgence of tuberculosis in the midst of the AIDS epidemic challenges us to revisit the legal and ethical principles that guide public health practices and to navigate a course between a return to broad and relatively unfettered coercive state action and a reliance on solely voluntary measures that may not prove sufficient to protect vulnerable communities (8).

THE ETHICAL AND LEGAL FOUNDATIONS OF TUBERCULOSIS CONTROL

The threat of tuberculosis to the public health provides the ethical and legal basis for government intervention in decision-making regarding an individual's health care. In contemporary ethical theory, and in biomedical ethics, strong emphasis is placed on the rights of the individual and on principles of autonomy and self-determination. But as central as those values are, the legitimacy of limiting them has long been recognized. Although conflict does exist about the nature and justification of those limits, there is no controversy in liberal democratic cultures over the principle that when the exercise of one person's freedom may result in harm to another, the state may intervene. Known as the "harm principle," this universally recognized limitation on autonomy was given its most potent expression by the nineteenth-century philosopher John Stuart Mill:

> [T]he only purpose for which power can be rightfully exercised over any member of a civilized community, against his will, is to prevent harm to others. His own good, either physical or moral, is not a sufficient warrant (40).

This principle clearly provides an ethical foundation for establishing public health programs designed to require those with communicable diseases to behave in ways that are likely to reduce the risk of transmission. It is sufficiently robust to justify requiring those with infectious tuberculosis to avoid public places where exposure to others would occur, and to authorize state action to enforce such requirements.

The public health authority to limit individual freedom when disease threatens has long been recognized in constitutional jurisprudence. Nearly ninety years ago, in *Jacobson v. Massachusetts*, a case that centered on the question of compulsory vaccination, the Supreme Court held that the U.S. Constitution permitted states to enact "such reasonable regulations ... as will protect the public health and the public safety" as long as such efforts did not "contravene the Constitution of the United States, nor infringe any right granted or secured by that instrument" (36). *Jacobson* also reiterated the rule that courts should give deference to a state's exercise of the police powers designed to protect the public health. Such measures could be invalidated only if they had "no real or substantial relation" to their ostensible goals. This extraordinary deference to government action prevailed throughout much of the 20th century, persisting as late as the 1960s (46). The past three decades of constitutional development, however, particularly in the area of involuntary confinement of psychiatric patients, have seen increased scrutiny of the exercise of the police powers, raising questions about the constitutionality of statutes relating to communicable disease and tuberculosis control, many of which were enacted before the profound shift in the balance between individual liberties and state authority (6, 27, 46).

Although the law gave considerable latitude to public health officials, virtually all TB control measures were focused on the necessity of identifying, treating, and limiting the activity of those whose tuberculosis was infectious. In 1992, the Centers for Disease Control undertook a broad review of state laws governing tuberculosis control, and found that 43 states provided for the quarantine of TB patients within their own homes, 35 specifying that the quarantine should last until the person was no longer infectious. Forty-two states permitted the commitment of TB patients to treatment facilities, 24 permitting such confinement until the individual no longer posed a health threat to others (19).

The resurgence of tuberculosis and the emergence of drug-resistant strains among inadequately treated patients have compelled public health officials to recognize the necessity of efforts to assure that patients with tuberculosis be treated beyond the period of infectiousness until they are cured. In 1992, a panel meeting under the auspices of the United Hospital Fund of New York made the attainment of "treatment until cure" the centerpiece of its recommendations (22). The Advisory Council for the Elimination of Tuberculosis underscored the necessity of treatment until cure in its 1993 report on the status of TB control laws throughout the United States (19).

The ethical, legal, and constitutional principles that justify public health efforts to control tuberculosis seem broad enough to justify efforts to assure that all patients with tuberculosis are treated until cured. Legal commentators have endorsed the goal of treatment until cure (24, 27, 46), as have advocates acting on behalf of individuals with HIV infection and AIDS (31, 35). There has been sharp controversy, however, over the nature of the public health interventions that might be employed to achieve the goal of treatment completion, and the extent to which the legal and ethical principles that guide medical and public health practice should constrain the exercise of those interventions.

ETHICAL AND LEGAL ISSUES IN ENHANCING PATIENT ADHERENCE TO TREATMENT

Although there may be exceptions, patients diagnosed with acute infectious tuberculosis tend to be compliant with treatment because of the desire to be rid of the unpleasant symptoms of the disease—weakness, fever, cough, and nightsweats. Much more complex is the attainment of compliance during the postacute phase of tuberculosis, when symptoms no longer motivate the patient to take his or her medication. Poor patient compliance with treatment is not unique to tuberculosis, although failure to complete therapy for many other diseases does not have the same dire individual and public health consequences.

Any effective approach to improving adherence to therapy must be sensitive to the obstacles to treatment that face the economically disadvantaged and socially marginalized people among whom tuberculosis is most common. The prevalence of homelessness, drug abuse, alcoholism, and psychiatric comorbidity are factors that must be considered in shaping policies to enhance treatment completion. Brudney, who has been particularly concerned with tuberculosis among the homeless, has written:

> Homelessness, by definition, means lack of permanent shelter. Whether a person lives on the streets, wanders from one SRO to another, or moves in and out of a congregate facility, medical care is rarely his or her first priority. The daily search for food and shelter belie the possibility of an organized schedule, appointment keeping or routine medical ingestion as is necessary with TB treatment. Alcoholism, drug dependence and psychiatric disturbances affect anywhere from 50 to 90 percent of the homeless, and the notion that persons so affected can remember and comply with clinic appointments and medication regimens is laughable (13).

In ethics there is a dictum that states "ought implies can." A person cannot be held morally accountable for failing to adhere to ethical or legal standards if he or she cannot do so, or if he or she faces insuperable obstacles to adherence. This ethical principle compels us to recognize that the elimination of impediments that impinge on the capacity of an individual to cooperate in his or her own care for tuberculosis is essential. This is especially so given the prospect of the imposition of compulsory measures and the potential loss of liberty for those who are not compliant. What are the practical implications of "ought implies can"?

The goal of treatment completion and the ethical norms that should shape the measures used to attain that goal require that homeless individuals not be discharged from hospitals to the streets or to chaotic and often dangerous mass shelters after treatment for their acute infectious tuberculosis. They cannot reasonably be expected to comply with their care unless they are provided with a secure residence and, in many instances, with other social supports. That is also true of prisoners with tuberculosis whose sentences come to an end before their treatment has been completed. Individuals with drug or alcohol addiction must be provided with referrals and access to treatment programs. So too must individuals with psychiatric illnesses that could impair their capacity to comply with long-term, often complex, treatment regimens. Unfortunately, hospital discharge plans rarely, if ever, assure access to such supportive services that facilitate treatment. The provision of such services will be costly, but will ultimately be less costly than the consequences of treatment failure—the spread of tuberculosis and the potential development of drug-resistance. Furthermore, effective outpatient services are less costly than the confinement of patients in secure facilities.

The ethical requirement that the government provide supportive services to enhance the prospect of compliance may find legal expression in the constitutional principle that requires the state to use the least restrictive means possible to achieve its goals when individual liberties are at stake. More than three decades ago the U.S. Supreme Court held in *Shelton v. Tucker*:

> Even though the governmental purpose be legitimate and substantial, that purpose cannot be pursued by means that broadly stifle fundamental personal liberties when the end can be more narrowly achieved. The breadth of legislative abridgment must be viewed in the light of less drastic means for achieving the same basic purpose (50).

In *Lessard v. Schmidt*, a Federal District Court decision handed down in 1972, the implications of this standard were further defined. The state "must bear the burden of proving (1) what alternatives are available; (2) what alternatives were investigated; and (3) why the investigated alternatives were not deemed suitable" (39).

Public health authorities now generally recognize that it is preferable, from both an ethical and a practical perspective, to make affirmative efforts to encourage voluntary compliance with health precautions before resorting to coercive action. In the context of tuberculosis, federal, state, and local health authorities acknowledge the importance of providing social supports and other "enablers"—such as car fare, meals, and even small cash payments—for undergoing care (19, 29). However, it remains unclear whether what is accepted in principle will be put into practice by health officials. Also unclear is whether a court would *legally* require the state to expend public resources to enhance the prospect of compliance with TB therapy before taking more coercive action.

For some advocates for patients with tuberculosis, the case for requiring the provision of services before depriving a patient of liberty is clear. The New York City Tuberculosis Working Group, for example, has argued:

> In deciding whether the prescription against forced detention had been overcome by clear and convincing evidence, the court would consider any evidence of mitigating circumstances including failures by the City to provide services or benefits to which the patient was entitled .... It is unethical, illegal, and bad public policy to detain "non-compliant" persons before making concerted efforts to address the numerous systematic deficiencies that make adherence to treatment virtually impossible for many New Yorkers (42).

From the perspective of the Working Group, the government that fails to provide adequate social supports for the most vulnerable loses the legal as well as the moral authority to threaten with a deprivation of liberty those whose behavior poses a health risk.

However, poor public policy—even unethical public policy—is not neces-sarily unconstitutional. A court would have to consider whether a failure on the part of the government to provide a particular service—for example, a stable apartment, as opposed to a bed in a dangerous shelter—renders an effort to impose restrictions on individual liberty constitutionally suspect. At a time when government resources are limited, a court would also have to consider whether the claims of those with tuberculosis, who are threatened with a deprivation of liberty, are always to be given precedence over those who are equally needy but who do not have tuberculosis. Must the state always give priority to those with tuberculosis who find themselves on long waiting lists for drug treatment? Or for minimally decent living conditions? Must they be given priority over those who may have waited for extended periods and who may be quite desperate, perhaps even more desperate? The legal question posed here is whether the doctrine of the least restrictive alternative, which initially served as a negative limit on government action (i.e. the state cannot hospitalize if outpatient care would have been as effective) can also be interpreted to impose positive obligations on government, such as an obligation to provide social supports that may facilitate compliance?

Although recent decisions make clear the reluctance of the U.S. Supreme Court to find in the Constitution an affirmative governmental obligation to provide social services to the general public (21), it is not as clear that the Constitution would be held to allow the state to restrict the liberty of a person who has not been convicted of a crime without providing such services first (24, 43). It is also conceivable that state courts would construe state constitu-tions more generously than the Supreme Court has interpreted the U.S. Con-stitution.

Some commentators have further suggested that the Americans with Dis-abilities Act (ADA), which protects people with disabling health conditions (including infectious diseases) from discrimination, might obligate health au-thorities to take reasonable affirmative steps to "accommodate" a person with a communicable disease before restricting certain liberties (26, 42). Providing social services or referrals to existing entitlement programs might be viewed as reasonable steps for the state to take before initiating coercive action. Ball & Barnes, however, contend that the exercise of coercive public health powers to detain noncompliant individuals does not come within the purview of the ADA, because the restrictive action is based on the patient's noncompliant behavior, not on the patient's disabling health condition. They also suggest that the legislative history of the ADA indicates that the Act was not intended to affect public health measures designed to reduce the transmission of infec-tious diseases (6).

The extent of the government's legal obligation to provide social support to patients with tuberculosis is for now unresolved, but is likely to be addressed in the coming years as courts attempt to articulate the limits of both government action against and obligation toward people with tuberculosis.

DIRECTLY OBSERVED THERAPY

Among the strategies designed to enhance patient compliance is directly observed therapy (DOT), a practice that involves having the patient take his or her medications in the presence of a health care provider or other responsible third party. First proposed for individuals with poor records of treatment adherence and for those whose demographic or psychological profile suggested a high risk of treatment failure, directly observed therapy has emerged as a standard of care (18). Recently, the Centers for Disease Control and Prevention, a number of prominent physicians, and others have recommended that all tuberculosis patients be placed on a regime of directly observed therapy, at least in localities where rates of completion fall below an acceptable level (18, 22, 34). Indeed, the Advisory Council for the Elimination of Tuberculosis calls for DOT in areas where treatment completion falls below 90% (18).

The primary rationale for the administration of medications under direct supervision is the recognition that nonadherence is common among patients who must take medication over an extended time period (22, 55). In the case of tuberculosis, such noncompliance has the grave consequence of leading to drug resistance and reactivation of clinical disease. The CDC recommends that DOT "be considered for all patients because of the difficulty in predicting which patients will adhere to a prescribed treatment regimen" (18). In addition, the recommendation for universal, rather than selective, DOT is motivated by a desire to avoid discrimination based on race, social class, and other factors that providers may perceive to have an effect on compliance (22).

The practice of directly observed therapy has been efficacious from a public health perspective. It has contributed to increasing rates of treatment completion (17, 18). In addition, a recent study in Texas found substantial declines in the rates of drug resistance and relapse after the institution of a county-wide program of universal directly observed therapy (55). The rate of primary drug resistance (i.e. the patient contracted a drug-resistant strain from another person) decreased from 13.0 percent to 6.7 percent, while the rate of acquired resistance (i.e. a patient's initially drug-sensitive strain became resistant, probably due to a treatment failure) declined from 14.0% to 2.1%. The relapse rate declined from 20.9% to 5.5% (55).

From an ethical, legal, and constitutional perspective, the important question is not who should be *offered* the support of DOT, but rather, when may DOT be *imposed* by the state.

Faced with the dramatic rise of multidrug-resistant tuberculosis and data that suggested very high rates of treatment failure, Iseman, Cohn & Sbarbaro put forth a public health argument for universal directly observed therapy.

> We believe it is time for entirely intermittent directly observed treatment programs ... to be used for all patients. Some will argue that it will be impossible to treat every patient with directly observed therapy and that many people with tuberculosis do comply with treatment and would be offended by having to submit to direct observation while they swallow medications. Unfortunately, the literature is replete with studies demonstrating ... that professionals are not able to distinguish the compliant from the noncompliant in advance (34).

Given the price of failure, in morbidity, mortality, and the cost of treating resistant strains of TB, they conclude, "we cannot afford not to try it." The case for universal directly observed therapy, at least at the outset of treatment, has also been made by the United Hospital Fund Working Group on Tuberculosis and HIV. It too was concerned by the failure of other approaches to achieve high rates of treatment completion and by the inability of professionals to predict treatment adherence. Though fully aware of the burdens that DOT would entail for some individuals, the working group concluded that, on ethical and legal grounds, universal DOT was desirable:

> The fact that all start their post-hospitalization treatment under a common program of supervision should help to reduce the stigma of treatment and create an effective public health plan for the control of TB. Such an approach will also limit the extent to which initial treatment decisions violate the principle of justice which seeks to preclude acts of invidious discrimination (22).

The call for universal directly observed therapy has provoked sharp opposition. First, it has been argued that such an effort would entail an enormous waste of scarce resources. Funds that could best be used to provide services to those most in need would be diverted to the supervision of those who would be compliant on their own (22, 31). But most critically, universal directly observed therapy has been challenged as an unethical intrusion upon autonomy, as "gratuitously annoying" (3); as a violation of the constitutional requirement that the least restrictive alternative be used; and as contrary to the requirements of the Americans With Disabilities Act that decisions involving restrictions on those with disabilities be based on an individualized assessment. The Policy Director for the Gay Men's Health Crisis, D Hansel, has written:

> I cannot see how mandatory directly observed therapy can be reconciled with the principle of the least restrictive alternative in the exercise of governmental power, since it would require the imposition of a coercive treatment regime in a class of people without any showing that they, as individuals will fail voluntarily to follow a course of medical treatment. Nor does it comport with basic Constitutional due process principles, which require an individualized determination before state sanctions are imposed (22).

Legal commentators too have generally rejected mandatory DOT as overly broad and thus violative of constitutional principles (6, 27, 46). However, this opposition to *universal* DOT should not be construed as a rejection of *mandatory* DOT in all cases. Even advocates for patients' civil liberties accept mandatory, court-ordered DOT in cases of clear noncompliance, especially when the alternative appears to be involuntary confinement (12).

In its 1993 revision of the New York City Health Code, the City's Board of Health rejected universal mandatory DOT and instead authorized the Commissioner of Health to impose DOT on patients who were noncompliant with treatment during the noninfectious stage of their illness (41).

DETENTION OF NONCOMPLIANT PATIENTS

As noted earlier in this chapter, ethical, legal, and constitutional principles have long recognized the authority of the state to confine individuals with infectious tuberculosis when they pose a threat to the health of others. This power to deprive an individual of his or her liberty in the name of public health has vested public health officials with an authority that, from the perspective of the individual, may be indistinguishable from that wielded by the criminal justice system. Yet until relatively recently, the protections accorded to defendants in criminal prosecutions have not been extended to those viewed as a threat to the public health. As late as 1966, a California appellate court upheld the confinement of a TB patient pursuant to a law that provided virtually no procedural protections for the patient. In its ruling, the court, quoting an earlier case, stated:

> Health regulations enacted by the state under its police power and providing even drastic measures for the elimination of disease ... in a general way are not affected by constitutional provisions, either of the state or national government (5).

This broad deference to the legislature and to the exercise of public health powers would come to look archaic just a few years later, as the jurisprudence of confinement underwent a radical revision in the wake of a series of far-reaching constitutional challenges to the power of the state to confine patients with psychiatric disorders to mental hospitals (6, 27, 46). By 1979, Chief Justice Burger would state in *Addington v. Texas*:

> This Court has repeatedly recognized that civil commitment for any purpose constitutes a significant deprivation of liberty that requires due process protection. Moreover, it is indisputable that involuntary commitment to a mental hospital ... can engender adverse social consequences to the individual. Whether we label this phenomena "stigma" or choose to call it something else is less important than that we recognize that it can occur and that it can have a very significant impact on the individual (1). (Citations omitted)

It was on the basis of such developments in mental health law, rather than as a result of challenges to the actions of public health officials in responding to tuberculosis cases, that it became possible to assert successfully that TB patients be accorded the procedural protections guaranteed by the Constitution. In 1980, in the only reported appellate court decision to date upholding the procedural rights of a tuberculosis patient, the Supreme Court of Appeals in West Virginia articulated a standard that expressly followed the developments in mental health law. The state's Tuberculosis Control Act was ruled unconstitutional because it did not guarantee the right to counsel, did not provide for the right to cross examine, confront and present witnesses, and failed to hold the state to the stringent "clear and convincing" standard of proof required by *Addington* (28, 46).

Although the West Virginia decision is not controlling in other states, the social transformation in the legal and political context within which issues of confinement were considered in the 1970s and 1980s did shape policy and practice in the United States. In 1993, when the Advisory Council for the Elimination of Tuberculosis recommended changes in state tuberculosis control laws, it declared:

> As in commitment proceedings under state mental health laws, any law under which a person may be examined, isolated, detained, committed and/or treated for TB must meet due process and equal protection requirements under state and federal statutes and constitutions. Also, all patients who are subject to these legal proceedings should be represented by legal counsel (19).

Reflecting the doctrine of the least restrictive alternative, discussed above, the Council recommended:

> Before committing TB patients for inpatient treatment, states should adopt step-by-step interventions beginning with DOT and supplemented by incentives and enablers (19).

The Council's incorporation of both procedural due process protections and the doctrine of the least restrictive alternative into its recommendations were especially crucial, because it was calling for the expansion of existing tuberculosis laws to "permit the involuntary isolation and detention of non-infectious patients" who "refuse to adhere to a treatment regimen or to complete treatment" (19).

This expansion on the conceptions of who posed a threat to the public health, driven by concerns about MDR-TB, represented a move of great significance. No longer did the person to be confined have to represent an immediate threat of transmission. Rather it was the *prospect* of reactivation and the *prospect* of the development of drug-resistance that provided the grounds for state intervention. Here the concept of "threat" was informed by the population-based concerns of public health. It was concern about the collective consequence of permitting many individuals to conduct themselves in a way that posed some threat that motivated the extension of public health powers to reach noninfectious TB patients. But this was a calculus far different from one that would center on the potential risk posed by a given individual. Nevertheless, legal commentators (3, 27, 46) have, by and large, agreed that "confinement until cure would probably be found constitutional for noninfectious patients who did not adhere to treatment" (3).

A striking reflection of the expansion of the concept of what constitutes a public health threat was the adoption in 1993 of treatment until cure regulations by the New York City Board of Health. Under the newly enacted Section 11.47 of the City's Health Code, the Commissioner may confine an individual for whom there is a "substantial likelihood, based on such person's past and present behavior, that he or she cannot be relied upon" to complete treatment. Under the amended code, a court review must be accorded to a confined patient within five business days, and even if the individual does not request release, the Department of Health must seek judicial review within the first 60 days of detention, and subsequently at 90-day intervals. Upon requesting release, the confined individual is entitled to a lawyer, and, if too poor to afford counsel, must be provided with one at public expense (41).

Most controversial in the City's Code is the way in which the requirement of the least restrictive alternative standard has been applied. During the hearing process that preceded the adoption of the amended code, civil liberties advocates claimed that the proposed new regulations were unconstitutional because they did not require the city to "exhaust" all less restrictive alternatives prior to seeking the involuntary confinement of a persistently noncompliant TB patient. The Department of Health responded to this challenge by stating:

> For all patients for whom compulsory measures are considered, we will perform an individual assessment and give priority to less restrictive treatment alternatives *where appropriate* (that is where there is a substantial probability of success) *and available* ... At the same time the Department cannot and should not be required to exhaust a pre-set, rigid, hierarchy of alternative measures that would ostensibly encourage voluntary compliance, but then be compelled to wait for the patient to fail each of them, regardless of the patient's individual circumstances and regardless of the potentially adverse consequences to the public health (47). (Emphasis added)

For those challenging the city's perspective, the "where appropriate and available" standard represented a profound threat to individual rights and an evisceration of the least restrictive alternative standard, which required that "no person may be detained until authorities have made a good faith attempt to employ every available less restrictive means to reduce the person's risk of harm to an insignificant level" (42).

This broad interpretation of the least restrictive alternative doctrine formed the basis for a constitutional challenge brought against New York City's Health Department in early 1994 (32). In that challenge, the patient, who was confined pursuant to the new health code provisions, and a number of *amici,* including the American Civil Liberties Union, argued that a distinction should be made between the latitude that should be available to the Commissioner of Health when confronting a patient with infectious tuberculosis and a noncompliant patient who was not contagious:

> The due process guarantees of the United States and New York Constitutions require that less restrictive alternatives be exhausted prior to involuntary commitment. For people with *contagious* TB disease, where there is an imminent risk of contagion, the Commissioner may be able to prove by clear and convincing evidence that confinement is the only effective means of protecting the public health. For people with *non-contagious* TB disease, however, there is an array of less restrictive alternatives to commitment that may facilitate completion of treatment. These less restrictive alternatives include education about the disease and its treatment, stable housing, substance abuse treatment, mental health treatment, food coupons and mandatory directly observed therapy. Because New York City Health Code Section 11.47 does not require that the Commissioner *exhaust* less restrictive alternatives prior to involuntary commitment, it should be declared unconstitutional (12). (Emphasis added)

The distinction between contagious and noncontagious patients, given such prominence here, was precisely the distinction that the public health authorities, concerned about the rise in drug resistance, had sought to erase because of the importance of "treatment to cure," regardless of current infectiousness.

Here the inevitable tension between public health and civil liberties perspectives on disease control is placed in bold relief. For the former, given a history of noncompliance and reasonable grounds for believing that a given patient would continue to be noncompliant, even with additional support, the option of confinement had to be available to prevent repeated treatment failures, recurrence of infectiousness, and the development of drug resistance. From the perspective of civil liberties, the burdens of uncertainty had to be distributed differently. In the face of a deprivation of liberty, the burden of proving that a particular less restrictive intervention will not work must fall upon the health department. That burden cannot be met by "reasonable" clinical impressions, but only by "clear and convincing" evidence.[1]

---

[1] On June 30, 1994, the New York Supreme Court, Appellate Division, First Department, entered a decision affirming the contested detention, on the grounds that the city had proved by clear and convincing evidence that less restrictive measures would have failed (32). However, the Court did not expressly rule on the argument that the statute itself was unconstitutional.

FORCED MEDICATION

Remarkably, the very New York Health Code that extended the scope of the Commissioner's authority to isolate noncompliant patients despite their non-infectious status states that the regulations are "not to be construed to permit or require the forcible administration of any medication without a prior court order" (41). In part, this restraint is simply a reflection of prevailing constitutional doctrines that recognize the rights of psychiatric patients, even criminally or civilly committed patients, to refuse treatment (20, 48, 54). It also reflects the importance of general principles of autonomy and informed consent (4). At the heart of judicial rulings that have established the right to refuse medication is the assumption that individuals may retain the right to some self-determination even when confined because they pose a risk to themselves or others. In *Rivers v. Katz,* the New York Court of Appeals held that a civilly committed patient can be compelled to accept medication only after a judicial determination that the individual lacked the capacity to make a reasoned decision about the particular treatment. The determination of capacity was to be made at a hearing at which the patient was afforded representation by a lawyer (48).

What holds for a patient whose mental capacities are impaired is certainly true for those who are confined for tuberculosis, where no assumption about such impairment can be made. A decisionally capable patient may choose to forgo treatment even at the risk of death. That is the bedrock of the principle of informed consent. But such a patient does not have the right to endanger others. That is the bedrock of the statutory authority to confine noncompliant TB patients. It is, of course, possible that in a given case the refusal to accept medication may reflect psychiatric impairment. Under such circumstances, and after appropriate judicial review, compulsory treatment of the psychiatric disorder might be undertaken to enhance the prospect that the patient would be able to make an informed judgment about whether to cooperate in the treatment of his or her tuberculosis (22). But the ultimate paradox may remain: The state may confine a noncompliant individual because of the failure to undergo treatment, but may not impose treatment on the confined patient. This paradox underscores the fundamental limits of state power in a liberal society: The government may act to protect the public, but not to protect the competent individual from his own willful, perhaps foolish, choices.

CONCLUSION

From both an ethical and legal perspective, the state has an obligation to assure that the population is protected against the ravages of infectious disease. That responsibility in the context of tuberculosis is best exercised by the development of programs and strategies designed to facilitate the identification and treatment of those with disease. In large measure, the central public health goals can be achieved by encouraging the cooperation of patients with tuberculosis. The expanded provision of directly observed therapy, indeed the establishment of directly observed therapy as a standard of care, may also be crucial. There will, however, be occasions when recourse to coercion will be necessary to protect the public health. Such occasions come at a price both because of the public costs of confinement and the individual's loss of liberty. But acknowledging that it may be necessary to rely on coercion should not be confused with making compulsion the centerpiece of a tuberculosis program. For pragmatic and principled reasons, coercion must be viewed as a last resort.

Much has been learned since the resurgence of tuberculosis took a place on the national agenda in the early 1990s. It has become clear that the rise in the number of cases, and, more centrally, the increase in the number of multidrug-resistant cases stemmed, at least in part, from the erosion of the public health infrastructure and the intensification of poverty and overcrowding in urban areas (14, 51). With public alarm providing the motivation, governmental expenditures on TB control rose sharply. Those funds made possible a rapid expansion of local health department initiatives, including the broadening of voluntary directly observed therapy. In New York City, for example, the number of TB patients receiving directly observed treatment increased from fewer than 100 in 1991 to more than 1200 in 1993 (30). The fruits of those efforts may be reflected in 1993 statistics, which for the first time in eight years on a national level and the first time in 14 years in New York City indicate that new cases of tuberculosis declined (30, 53). It is too soon to know whether these numbers represent a trend or a statistical adjustment. But what is certain is that if stabilizing or declining tuberculosis cases provoke another cycle of budgetary retrenchment, the foundations for yet another upsurge in cases will have been laid (44). This time history will repeat itself not as tragedy but as farce.

ACKNOWLEDGMENTS

R Bayer's work on this chapter was supported in part by the Robert Wood Johnson Foundation, and in part by NIMH Center Grant 2-P50-MH43520 NIMH/NIDA, Anke A Ehrhardt, Principle Investigator.

Literature Cited

1. *Addington v. Texas*, 441 U.S. 418, 425–26 (1979)
2. Alland D, Kalkut GE, Moss AR, McAdam RA, Hahn JA, et al. 1994. Transmission of tuberculosis in New York City: an analysis by DNA fingerprinting and conventional epidemiologic methods. *New Engl. J. Med.* 330:1710–16
3. Annas GJ. 1993. Control of tuberculosis—the law and the public's health. *New Engl. J. Med.* 328:585–88
4. Annas GJ, Densberger JE. 1984. Competence to refuse medical treatment: autonomy vs. paternalism. *Toledo Law Rev.* 15:561–96
5. *Application of Halko*, 54 Cal. Report. 661 (1966). See Ref. 46
6. Ball CA, Barnes M. 1994. Public health and individual rights: tuberculosis control and detention procedures in New York City. *Yale Law Policy Rev.* 12:38–67
7. Bayer R. 1989. *Private Acts, Social Consequences: AIDS and the Politics of Public Health.* New York: Free Press
8. Bayer R, Dubler NN, Landesman S. 1993. The dual epidemics of tuberculosis and AIDS: ethical and policy issues in screening and treatment. *Am. J. Public Health* 83:649–54
9. Bellin E. 1994. Failure of tuberculosis control: a prescription for change. *J. Am. Med. Assoc.* 271:708–9
10. Bloch AB, Cauthen GM, Onorato IM, Dansbury KG, Kelly GD, et al. 1994. Nationwide survey of drug-resistant tuberculosis in the United States. *J. Am. Med. Assoc.* 271:665–71
11. Bloom BR, Murray CJ. 1992. Tuberculosis: commentary on a reemergent killer. *Science* 257:1055–64
12. Brief *Amici Curiae* of the American Civil Liberties Union, Brooklyn Legal Services Corp. B, Gay Men's Health Crisis, et al. *In re Application of the City of New York v. Mary Doe* (No. 400770/94) (1994)
13. Brudney K. 1993. Homelessness and TB: a study in failure. *J. Law Med. Ethics* 21:360–67
14. Brudney K, Dobkin J. 1991. Resurgent tuberculosis in New York City: human immunodeficiency virus, homelessness and the decline of tuberculosis control programs. *Am. Rev. Resp. Dis.* 144:745–49
15. Cent. Dis. Control. 1989. A strategic plan for the elimination of tuberculosis in the United States. *Morbid. Mortal. Wkly. Rep.* 38(Suppl. S-3):1–23
16. Cent. Dis. Control. 1992. Prevention and control of tuberculosis in U.S. communities with at-risk minority populations: recommendations of the Advisory Council for the Elimination of Tuberculosis. *Morbid. Mortal. Wkly. Rep.* 41(Suppl. RR-5):1–11
17. Cent. Dis. Control. 1993. Approaches to improving adherence to antituberculosis therapy—South Carolina and New York, 1986–1991. *Morbid. Mortal. Wkly. Rep.* 42:74–75, 81
18. Cent. Dis. Control. 1993. Initial therapy for tuberculosis in the era of multidrug resistance: recommendations of the Advisory Council for the Elimination of Tuberculosis. *Morbid. Mortal. Wkly. Rep.* 42(Suppl. RR-7):1–8
19. Cent. Dis. Control. 1993. Tuberculosis control laws—United States, 1993: recommendations of the Advisory Council for the Elimination of Tuberculosis. *Morbid. Mortal. Wkly. Rep.* 42(Suppl. RR-15):1–28
20. Cichon DE. 1992. The right to "just say no": a history and analysis of the right to refuse antipsychotic drugs. *Louisiana Law Rev.* 53:283–426
21. *DeShaney v. Winnebago Co. Dep. Soc. Serv.*, 489 U.S. 189 (1989)
22. Dubler NN, Bayer R, Landesman S, White A. 1992. Tuberculosis in the 1990s: ethical, legal and public policy issues in screening, treatment and the protection of those in congregate facilities: a report from the Working Group on TB and HIV. In *The Tuberculosis Revival: Individual Rights and Societal Obligations in a Time of AIDS*, pp. 1–42. New York: United Hospital Fund New York
23. Frieden TR, Sterling T, Pablos-Mendez A, Kilburn JO, Cauthen GM, Dooley SW. 1993. The emergence of drug-resistant tuberculosis in New York City. *New Engl. J. Med.* 328:521–26
24. Gittler J. 1994. Controlling resurgent tuberculosis: public health agencies, public policy, and law. *J. Health Polit. Policy Law* 19:107–47
25. Goble M, Iseman MD, Madsen LA, Waite D, Ackerson L, Horsburgh CR. 1993. Treatment of 171 patients with pulmonary tuberculosis resistant to iso-

niazid and rifampin. *New Engl. J. Med.* 328:527–32

26. Gostin LO. 1991. Public health powers: the imminence of radical change. *Milbank Q.* 69(Suppl. 1/2):268–90

27. Gostin LO. 1993. Controlling the resurgent tuberculosis epidemic: a 50-state survey of TB statutes and proposals for reform. *J. Am. Med. Assoc.* 269:255–61

28. *Greene v. Edwards,* 263 S.E.2d 661 (W. Va. 1980). See Ref. 46

29. Hamburg MA. 1993. Rebuilding the public health infrastructure: the challenge of tuberculosis control in New York City. *J. Law Med. Ethics* 21:352–59

30. Hamburg MA, Frieden TR. 1994. Tuberculosis transmission in the 1990s. *New Engl. J. Med.* 330:1750–51

31. Hansel DA. 1993. The TB and HIV epidemics: history learned and unlearned. *J. Law Med. Ethics* 21:376–81

32. *In re Application of the City of New York v. Doe* (No. 40770/94) (1994)

33. Iseman MD. 1993. Treatment of multidrug-resistant tuberculosis. *New Engl. J. Med.* 329:784–91

34. Iseman MD, Cohn DL, Sbarbaro JA. 1993. Directly observed treatment of tuberculosis: we can't afford not to try it. *New Engl. J. Med.* 328:576–78

35. Jacobs SL. 1993. Legal advocacy in a time of plague. *J. Law Med. Ethics* 21:382–89

36. *Jacobson v. Massachussets,* 197 U.S. 11, 25 (1907) See Ref. 46

37. Joseph S. 1993. Editorial: tuberculosis, again. *Am. J. Public Health* 83:647–48

38. Lerner BH. 1993. New York City's tuberculosis control efforts: the historical limitations of the "war on consumption." *Am. J. Public Health* 83:758–66

39. *Lessard v. Schmidt,* 349 F. Suppl. 1078, 1096 (E.D. Wis. 1972)

40. Mill JS. *On Liberty.* In *Prefaces to Liberty: Selected Writings of John Stuart Mill,* ed. B Wishy. 1959. Lanham, MD: Univ. Press Am.

41. New York, NY, Health Code, Article 11, Section 11.47

42. New York City Tuberculosis Work. Group. 1992. Developing a system for tuberculosis prevention and care in New York City. In *The Tuberculosis Revival: Individual Rights and Societal Obligations in a Time of AIDS,* pp. 51–58. New York: United Hospital Fund New York

43. Parmet WE. 1993. Health care and the Constitution: public health and the role of the state in the framing era. *Hastings Const. Law Q.* 20:267–335

44. Reichman LB. 1991. The u-shaped curve of concern. *Am. Rev. Resp. Dis* 144:741–42

45. Reichman LB. 1993. Fear, embarrassment, and relief: the tuberculosis epidemic and public health. *Am. J. Public Health* 83:639–40

46. Reilly RG. 1993. Combating the tuberculosis epidemic: the legality of coercive treatment measures. *Columbia J. Law Soc. Probl.* 27:101–49

47. Respondent's Brief. *In re Application of the City of New York v Mary Doe* (No. 400770/94) (1994)

48. *Rivers v. Katz,* 495 N.E.2d 337 (N.Y. 1986)

49. Selwyn PA. 1993. Tuberculosis and AIDS: epidemiologic, clinical and social dimensions. *J. Law Med. Ethics* 21:279–88

50. *Shelton v. Tucker,* 364 U.S. 479, 488 (1960)

51. Sidel VW, Drucker E, Martin SC. 1993. The resurgence of tuberculosis in the United States: societal origins and societal responses. *J. Law Med. Ethics* 21:303–16

52. Small PM, Hopewell PC, Singh SP, Paz A, Parsonnet J, et al. 1994. The epidemiology of tuberculosis in San Francisco: a population-based study using conventional and molecular methods. *New Engl. J. Med.* 330:1703–9

53. Tuberculosis figures decline, but U.S. unsure it's a trend. *New York Times,* May 26, 1994, p. A19

54. *Washington v. Harper,* 494 U.S. 210 (1990)

55. Weis SE, Slocum PC, Blais FX, King B, Nunn M, et al. 1994. The effect of directly observed therapy on the rates of drug resistance and relapse in tuberculosis. *New Engl. J. Med.* 330: 1179–84

Annu. Rev. Public Health 1995. 16:327–54

THE STATUS OF HEALTH ASSESSMENT 1994

John E. Ware Jr.

The Health Institute, New England Medical Center Hospitals, 750 Washington Street #345, Boston, Massachusetts 02111

KEY WORDS: health status assessment, health-related quality of life, condition-specific measures, generic health measures

ABSTRACT

General health status and a broader concept of quality of life are discussed and methods of widely used surveys are reviewed. A consensus regarding the inclusion of measures of physical, mental, social, and role functioning and general health perceptions is noted for comprehensive assessments of health. A schematic of relationships among condition-specific and generic measures is presented along with results expected for objective and subjective measures of physical and mental dimensions of health. Suggestions are offered for the labeling of disease-specific and generic measures and ways to avoid confounding of content. Applications of health surveys in general population monitoring, health policy evaluation, clinical trials of alternative treatments, monitoring and improving of health care outcomes, and in everyday clinical practice are exemplified and discussed. A unified measurement strategy is proposed and arguments in favor of standardizing the content of health surveys across applications are offered.

INTRODUCTION

Now is a good time to take stock of state-of-the-art methods for assessing health from the patient's point of view because these methods are being used more widely in 1994 than ever before. Much has taken place since the last *Annual Review* of assessment methods in 1987 (7). In 1989, the U.S. Congress passed the Patient Outcome Research Act, which called for the establishment of a broad-based, patient-centered outcomes research program. In addition to

327

0163-7525/95/0510-0327$05.00

WARE

traditional measures of survival, clinical endpoints, and disease- and treatment-specific symptoms and problems, the law mandated measures of "functional status and well-being and patient satisfaction." Previously, the debate about using and interpreting such assessments was conducted chiefly by method-ological researchers. More recently, the debate has been joined by health-care managers and policymakers whose concern about the content, use, and inter-pretation of health indices has become as intense as that of academics. This has been stimulated by the widespread use of short-form measurement tools such as the COOP Charts (59) and the MOS short-forms (87, 107) in health-care settings. These measures make it practical to look beyond traditional measures of biologic functioning to larger issues of functioning and well-being.

A health-care outcome has come to mean the extent to which the results of treatment meet a patient's needs or expectations. These ideas are not new (18, 48). Lembcke expressed the sentiment well earlier in the century:

> The best measure of quality is not how well or how frequently a medical service is given, but how closely the result approaches the fundamental objectives of prolonging life, relieving distress, restoring function and preventing disability.

These objectives are now echoed by those who argue that the goal of medical care is to achieve a more effective life (52) and preserve function and well-being (28, 80, 90). Although patients are the best source of information re-garding the achievement of these goals, their experiences of disease and treat-ment are not a part of the medical record and are not part of the health-care database.

DEFINING GENERAL HEALTH STATUS

Life has two dimensions: quantity and quality (70, 96). Quantity of life is expressed in terms of average life expectancy, mortality rates, death due to specific causes, and numerous other indicators (70). These indicators have little value in understanding how *well* people live in developed countries (27). The primary sources of this information are standardized patient surveys of functioning and well-being and general health perceptions that have proven to be useful during the past decade.

Against the urgings of some (8), it has become fashionable to lump all measures that define health beyond traditional indicators of biologic function-ing into a single category of quality-of-life measures. This practice offers a shorthand method of referring to a collection of concepts both more broad and more qualitative than traditional measures of clinical endpoints. However, quality of life as traditionally defined is a much broader concept than health (15, 96). Quality of life encompasses standard of living, quality of housing and neighborhood, job satisfaction, health, and other factors (15). If we look at U.S. health-care and domestic policy more broadly, using quality-of-life nomenclature without qualification is likely to cause some confusion.

General health status—the terminology adopted here—has also been referred to as health-related quality of life (96). The World Health Organization definition of health as a "state of complete physical, mental, and social well-being and not merely the absence of disease or infirmity" (120) continues to be useful as a gross conceptual framework for health (88). Dictionary definitions emphasize both physical and mental dimensions of health and refer to the body and bodily needs and its emotional and intellectual status. Health also connotes completeness—nothing is missing from the person—and proper function—all is working efficiently. Well-being—including soundness and vitality—is also part of the dictionary definition (96). Among the attributes of these definitions most important in constructing measures are dimensionality, particularly the distinction between physical and mental components, and the full range of health levels implied.

WIDELY USED SURVEYS

The content and other characteristics of general health surveys reveal much about the evolution of definitions in the nascent field of health assessment. Table 1 presents a summary of information about ten widely used general health surveys. These surveys are considered *generic* to the extent that they assess health concepts that represent basic human values relevant to functional status and well-being (96, 98). Most concepts that they represent are universally valued and have been linked to personal evaluations of health across age, disease, and treatment groups (23, 53, 109). Generic *health* measures also emphasize outcomes thought to be most directly affected by disease and treatment, as opposed to quality of life in general (98, 109). Generic measures provide a common yardstick to compare chronically ill patients with the general population for purposes of estimating the burden of disease and providing a basis for comparing the benefits of alternative treatments (70, 109).

The top panel (first 12 rows) of Table 1 lists the health concepts represented in two or more of the ten surveys. Questions were classified according to published definitions (96). Concepts represented by each survey were considered regardless of whether the survey yields a separate score. The bottom panel summarizes information about other important characteristics including administration, scale construction, questionnaire length, and scoring options. The ten questionnaires (columns of the table) are ordered according to initial publication date. Instruments from the 1970s include the Quality of Well-Being (QWB) Index (68), the Sickness Impact Profile (SIP) (6), scales analyzed in the Health Insurance Experiment (HIE) (12, 101). Instruments from the 1980s include the Nottingham Health Profile (NHP) (38), the Quality of Life Index

Table 1 Summary of information about widely used general health surveys

	QWB	SIP	HIE	NHP	QLI	COOP	EURO-QOL	DUKE	MOS FWBP	MOS SF-36
CONCEPTS [a]										
Physical functioning	•	•	•	•	•	•	•	•	•	•
Social functioning	•	•	•	•	•	•	•	•	•	•
Role functioning	•	•	•	•	•	•	•	•	•	•
Psychological distress		•	•	•	•	•	•	•	•	•
Health perceptions (general)			•	•		•	•	•	•	•
Pain (bodily)	•	•	•	•		•	•	•	•	•
Energy/fatigue			•	•					•	•
Psychological well-being		•	•					•	•	•
Sleep				•					•	
Cognitive functioning		•	•						•	
Quality of life						•		•	•	
Reported health transition						•				•
CHARACTERISTICS										
Administration method (S = self, I = interviewer, P = proxy)	I, P	S, I, P	S, P	S, I	S, P	S, I	S	S, I	S, I	S, I, P
Scaling method (L = Likert, R = Rasch, T = Thurstone, U = utility)	U	T	L	T	L	L	U	L	L	L, R
Number of questions	107	136	86	38	5	9	9	17	149	36
Scoring options (P = profile, SS = summary scores, SI = single index)	SI	P, SS, SI	P	P	SI	P	SI	P, SI	P	P, SS

QWB = Quality of Well-Being Scale (1973) (40, 67)
SIP = Sickness Impact Profile (1976) (5, 6)
HIE = Health Insurance Experiment surveys (1979) (12, 100)
NHP = Nottingham Health Profile (1980) (38, 39)
QLI = Quality of Life Index (1981) (85, 119)

COOP = Dartmouth Function Charts (1987) (47, 59)
EUROQOL = European Quality of Life Index (1990) (29)
DUKE = Duke Health Profile (1990) (65)
MOS FWBP = MOS Functioning and Well-Being Profile (1992) (88)
MOS SF-36 = MOS 36-Item Short-Form Health Survey (1992) (107, 109)

[a] Note: Rows are ordered in terms of how frequently concepts are represented; only concepts represented in two or more surveys are listed. Analyses of content were based on published definitions (96). Columns are roughly ordered in terms of date of first publication.

(QLI) (85), and the COOP Charts (59), the only survey that uses illustrations. Four of the surveys were published in the 1990s: the EuroQol Index (29), the new Duke Health Profile (65), the MOS Functioning and Well-Being Profile (MOS-FWBP) (88), and the MOS 36-Item Short-Form Health Survey (MOS-SF-36) (107). A 20-item short form (MOS-SF-20) derived from HIE measures (108) was initially used in the MOS (86, 87) and is compared with these and other measures elsewhere (88, 109).

The rows of Table 1 are ordered according to the number of surveys representing each concept. Consensus regarding inclusion is greatest for the three physical-, social-, role-functioning concepts, which are represented in all measures. Psychological distress is represented in all but the QWB. It should be noted that the Symptom Problem Complex, which is part of the QWB, sometimes includes depression or other mental health symptoms (41); however, this does not satisfy the standard of content applied to the forms in Table 1. As a consequence, the empirical validity of the QWB as a measure of mental health is weak (73). Eight of the ten forms (all but QWB and QLI) measure bodily pain, although the SIP includes its pain items in the Emotional Behavior (EB) scales. This may explain why the SIP global psychosocial index score has been found to be more responsive than other mental health measures to changes following total hip arthroplasty (44). Eight of the ten forms (all but the QWB and SIP) measure general health perceptions and six of the ten forms measure energy/fatigue, also referred to as vitality. Less frequently represented, but represented in two or more forms, are psychological well-being, sleep problems, cognitive functioning, quality of life, and self-reported health transitions.

Unlike the other questionnaires, the HIE survey was one of the first compilations of modules developed independently, as documented in detail elsewhere (12, 13, 22, 23, 25, 75, 100, 101). Most of the HIE analyses focused on five of these modules (physical, mental, social, role, and general health) constructed from 86 items in a 249-item questionnaire (101). Psychometric studies of these modules had noteworthy impact on the way they were analyzed in the HIE (88, 115). Innovations included the combination of a wide range of physical functioning items in the same scale (89), from self-care to strenuous physical activities, and the construction of global mental (94) and general health scales (23). HIE studies of the Psychological General Well-Being (PGWB) Index (26), fielded initially to measure mental health, had considerable impact on subsequent measurement models (88, 101). Factor analytic studies confirmed the hypothesized physical and mental components of health and revealed that two of the PGWB psychological well-being scales, General Health and Vitality, did not discriminate mental from physical health components (101). These studies are mentioned here to illustrate the usefulness of factor analytic studies. Some have argued that factor analysis is inappropriate for use in constructing health measures (40, 41). HIE factor analytic studies led to a reformulation of the PGWB and to a two-dimensional conceptualization of physical and mental health that has served as the basis for much hypothesis testing (88, 101, 103, 104, 109). Four PGWB scales became the foundation for various forms of the Mental Health Inventory (MHI) (22, 88, 103, 110). Although the PGWB General Health and Vitality measures were removed from the MHI, they have proven to be among the most useful general health measures (109, 110) and became the basis for subsequent short-form measures (22, 59, 88, 107, 108, 109).

Table 1 also includes one of the first widely used short-form generic health measures, the Quality of Life Index (QLI) (85). Although this survey was developed primarily for use in comparing patients with cancer, it is a forerunner of the current generation of comprehensive short-forms used across conditions. Although the QLI has only five items, it represents five of the six most frequently measured concepts listed in Table 1. The QLI is noteworthy also because it was developed by an international team of investigators, an approach being tried by others (102).

Not shown in Table 1 are symptom inventories included in three of the questionnaires. The QWB, HIE, and MOS forms all include lists of specific symptoms although they are analyzed quite differently. The QWB scores symptoms and other specific problems in the overall index score using population weights (40, 68). In contrast to the QWB, which ignores differences in symptom severity across individuals, the HIE and MOS scored the severity of symptoms in terms of their frequency on an individual basis and analyzed them in various symptom scores in parallel with the generic measures (13, 22, 81, 99, 100, 101, 104). Measuring specific symptoms in parallel with generic health concepts is becoming widely accepted (19, 33, 42, 69, 81, 92, 95, 101, 113).

Four different methods of scale construction and item/scale scoring are represented in Table 1; the most popular is the Likert method of summated ratings (50), which has been used for six of the ten questionnaires. Also represented are two Thurstone (93) methods of constructing interval scales used in the SIP and NHP. The utility and visual analogue methods of scoring an aggregate index are also represented, in the QWB and EuroQoL, respectively. Several factors probably account for the popularity of the Likert method, including the simplicity of scale construction and scoring, the elimination of the second step in data collection in estimating scale values or weights (as required by the Thurstone and utility methods), and the proven track record of the Likert method in empirical studies. The need for population-specific weights has been an issue in translations of Thurstone scales (82). The Rasch scaling method, widely used in constructing interval scales in other fields, has recently been applied successfully in measuring health (35).

Whereas the QWB offers the advantage of a single utility index appropriate for use in economic evaluations, it is one of the least comprehensive measures in Table 1. The SIP, which includes six additional scales not listed in Table 1 (6), is one of the most comprehensive. The SIP is entirely a measure of sickness-related behavioral dysfunctions. It uses dichotomous items weighted to achieve 12 interval scales, as well as three summary measures (6). In contrast, the HIE and MOS add more subjective measures (e.g. general health perceptions), in addition to behavioral dysfunctions, and use multilevel rating items (88).

Differences in the *range* of health levels represented in the questionnaires listed in Table 1 should also be noted. In contrast to the WHO definition of health (120), three of the first four questionnaires (SIP, QWB, NHP) define perfect health and well-being as the absence of functional limitations and/or specific symptoms and problems (6, 38, 68). The result is a potential for substantial information loss (10, 109). The situation is analogous to a weight-measuring scale that stops at 100 pounds. All objects weighing more are assigned the highest score. This would be satisfactory in a world where nothing weighs more than 100 pounds. This shortcoming of these scales has not gone unnoticed (24). In health, relying solely on a negative perspective has been equated with "defining the economy only in terms of debt, never balance or surplus, and business only in terms of loss, never profits or redistribution" (24). Although observers have predicted that measures defining health more completely eventually will "transform the context of medicine" (24), the immediate and practical reality is that scales restricting the range of measurement are inferior to scales that do not. Clues for evaluating this important feature are the concepts represented (e.g. Table 1), content of the questions, and the resulting score distributions. Measures tapping the full range of health will yield a greater variability of score distributions; fewer people will score at the ceiling or floor (10).

Table 1 reflects considerable consensus regarding a *minimum* standard of comprehensiveness (content validity) in a health questionnaire. To be comprehensive in terms of the first six concepts, a generic health survey must include, at a minimum, physical functioning; mental health (psychological distress); limitations in social and role functioning due to health problems; and general health perceptions. Objective reports of behavioral functioning and more subjective ratings of health and well-being are both required for comprehensiveness (96). It is important to note that energy/fatigue, psychological well-being, and cognitive functioning are among the important concepts left out of this minimum set.

Finally, in addition to the articles cited in this review, there are other highly useful sources of information about the questionnaires in Table 1, as well as other general health measures. For example, two books published since 1990 present accurate, comprehensive, and up-to-date summaries of information about widely used measures (70, 115). Other books focus specifically on assessments in clinical trials (14, 83); another focuses on cancer research (63); and one focuses on MOS short- and long-form measures (88).

IMPROVING HEALTH SCHEMATICS AND METRICS

Models help to understand the relationships of health concepts to health determinants and consequences, e.g. life stress and utilization of health-care services, respectively. Modeling efforts to date have placed health concepts in the broad context of the structure and process of care, as well as factors outside the health-care system (71), including social, cultural, and geographic determinants (4). Recent modeling efforts have depicted relationships among risk factors, the disabling process and quality of life (72), clinical parameters (diagnosis and specific symptoms) and general functioning and well-being (117), and proximal variables (indicators of diagnosis, severity of disease, and specific symptoms) as opposed to more distal health concepts (role functioning and general health perceptions) (11). Health schematics and more elaborate models are important and useful because they facilitate scoring and interpretation of measures and help clarify hypothesized relationships that should be formally tested.

Figure 1 focuses on three generic health concepts: physical health (physical limitations and physical well-being); mental health (psychological distress and psychological well-being); and personal evaluations of health in general (past, present, and future outlook). As documented in detail elsewhere (96), these concepts have been measured using a wide range of operational definitions including: self-reports of behavioral functioning in the areas of physical, role, and social activity; subjective ratings of well-being; and an array of physical, mental, and general health problems. Classification of measures in terms of Figure 1 is a matter of content (96) and empirical validity (37, 53, 101, 104). The schematic of relationships among health concepts shown in Figure 1 differs from previous formulations in several respects. First, it distinguishes between physical and mental health at both specific and generic levels. This distinction follows from two discoveries: (a) physical and mental dimensions of health account for 80–85% of the reliable variance in generic health surveys such as those used in the MOS (37, 53, 104) and they have been confirmed in studies of the SIP (5), and (b) generic measures of physical and mental health tend to have distinctly different relationships to clinical measures of physical and mental disease (54, 104, 109). Second, the schematic of relationships among health concepts portrays a specific-generic *continuum* rather than a simple categorization of specific and generic concepts and measures. Measures at level 1 are viewed as specific to a condition (i.e. a diagnostic test specific to one cause), specific to a generic component of health (level III),

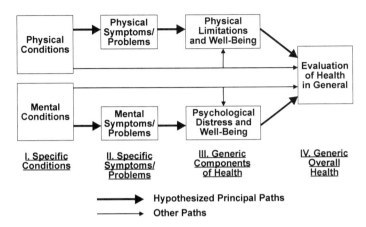

Figure 1   Relationships among specific and generic health concepts.

but not specific to a particular disease, and the most generic of all (level IV, e.g. an evaluation of health in general). Finally, Figure 1 implies much about the results expected from studies of the relationships among specific and generic concepts, regardless of which measures are used.

From Figure 1, more serious *physical* conditions, such as congestive heart failure, are hypothesized to go hand-in-hand with physical symptoms that impact most on generic measures of the *physical component* of health. In contrast, more serious mental conditions, such as depressive disorders, are hypothesized to go hand-in-hand with mental (emotional) symptoms that impact most on generic measures of the *mental component* of health. Rankings of patient groups based on clinical measures of physical morbidity are hypothesized to correspond (sometimes substantially) with rankings of patient groups based on generic measures of physical health (e.g. levels I and III of the schematic). A similar correspondence would be expected between rankings of patient groups based on clinical and generic measures of mental health (levels I and III). At least preliminary support for these hypotheses exists (34, 86, 104).

The same logic applies to hypotheses about relationships among measures at levels II and III of the schematic. Examples of specific symptoms more strongly associated with generic measures of the physical component of health include shortness of breath when climbing stairs, stiffness and pain in muscles, and chest pains brought on by activity (109). Specific symptoms more strongly associated with generic measures of the mental component of health include symptoms of depression and anxiety (103). Specific symptoms and problems that do *not* appear to be useful in predicting whether physical or mental components of health are most likely to be affected are heart pounding or palpitations, feeling drowsy or sedated, waking up early or being unable to sleep, and fainting (109). Specific conditions and symptom/problem inventories appear to explain about 1/4 to 1/3 of the variance in generic health concepts (86, 104, 112). Information about specific conditions, including presence and severity, is necessary to understand the two generic components of health as well as evaluations of health in general.

The bolded arrows in Figure 1 show the hypothesized relationships between specific conditions and symptoms and generic components of physical and mental health. There is support for these hypothesized relationships (86, 97, 104, 111, 112). Alternative paths have also been proposed (49), and cause and effect relationships in both directions are likely. Further, mental conditions have been shown to be associated with substantial decrements in measures of physical functioning (53, 104, 112). As hypothesized from Figure 1, measures of limitation in role functioning that distinguish between the physical and mental causes have proven to be more useful than those measures that do not in capturing and distinguishing differences in physical and mental health outcomes (88). MOS measures of role functioning, for example, have been shown to measure the physical spectrum (top half of the figure) or the mental spectrum (bottom half of the figure), depending on whether respondents attribute limitations to physical health or to personal and emotional problems (88, 104).

Associations between indicators of specific conditions and measures that are more conceptually proximal have been hypothesized to be stronger, compared to those that are more conceptually distal (11). For example, a measure of dyspnea would be more strongly associated with a measure of physical functioning than with a measure of general health perceptions. On average, for more distal measures, both the magnitude of associations and the size of *mean differences* could be smaller between groups with and without dyspnea. If associations are weaker for more distal measures, as hypothesized by others (11), is the explanation weaker effects or greater within-group variability resulting from multiple causality? With the hypothesis of multiple causality for more distal measures, weaker associations are expected owing to greater within-group variations, but mean differences in more distal measures (general health) are also expected to be substantial for groups differing in dyspnea. For example, role functioning presumably is less *related* than physical functioning to the severity of physical disease, because role functioning is determined by more factors than is physical functioning (96). This hypothesis follows from the principle underlying the distinction among measures along the specific-generic continuum, illustrated in Figure 1. A specific measure is, by definition, much closer to a specific cause. The most specific identifies a single cause; these are the best tools for diagnostic purposes. In contrast, generic measures are measures of outcomes, largely without regard to specific health-related causes. In testing hypotheses about more proximal and more distal measures, it is critical that proximal-distal not be confounded with the distinction between physical and mental components of health. The problem of confounding is illustrated below.

The historical confounding of physical health concepts with more objective (e.g. observable) phenomena and the confounding of mental health concepts with more subjective measures of well-being are noteworthy sources of confusion in the literature. For example, the report of one study of patients with end-stage renal disease (ESRD) criticized subjective measures because they did not correspond with objective measures (30). This study used the Karnofsky Index (43) as an objective indicator of functional impairment and ability to work. Measures of psychological affect, well-being, and life satisfaction (15) were the subjective indicators. The report's conclusion stated that patients with end-stage renal disease have a relatively poor quality of life as defined objectively, but not as defined subjectively. These findings led the authors to conclude that the assessment of the subjective aspects of quality of life is "highly problematic" (30). It is doubtful that the study actually compared objective and subjective measures of the same component of health.

In light of Figure 1, the ESRD study results might have been interpreted with the wrong schematic. An alternative explanation is that associations tend to be weak between physical and mental health concepts. Consistent with Figure 1, ESRD has much greater impact on the physical component of health as measured by the Karnofsky Index than on the mental component of health as defined by subjective measures of psychological well-being. Had that study included both objective and subjective indicators of the physical component of health, it might have observed substantial decrements in both. Likewise, more objective measures of the mental component of health status most likely would have agreed with the subjective measures in finding less impact of end-stage renal disease on mental health. Examples of subjective and objective measures of physical and mental health are discussed elsewhere (96, 97).

Another important feature of the schematic in Figure 1 is the absence of the third WHO health dimension (120), namely the social component of health. This feature of the schematic follows from the author's earlier proposition that the concept of health status at an *individual level* should "end at the skin" (99, p. 621), and concepts of physical and mental health are defined accordingly. In contrast, the concept of social functioning or activity extends beyond the individual to include the quantity of social contacts and the quality of social resources (25). A change in social circumstances, such as the loss of a job, would define a change in an individual's social circumstance, but not health status, according to this proposition.

Following the failure of HIE attempts to use subjective evaluations of social circumstances (e.g. feeling cared for, loved, and wanted by others) (101, 103) to distinguish the social dimension from the mental dimension of health, a strategy of defining social activity more objectively was tried (25). Measures of social integration (57), including more objective measures of the frequency of visits with friends and relatives, and participation in group activities, were hypothesized to define the third health dimension (factor) distinct from physical and mental health (25). The three factors were confirmed empirically. But contrary to hypotheses for the concept of *health*, the social dimension was very weakly related to personal evaluations of health in general. Thus, social contacts (as defined in the HIE) were not given nearly as much weight as physical and mental health in the personal equation used to evaluate health in general by HIE participants. The resulting HIE conceptualization of health recognized the importance of social activities, social resources, and stressful life events as external factors determining health status (116) without equating such differences in social circumstances with health. Similarly, health risk behaviors and health promotion activities are important health determinants (4). To improve the validity of social indicators as measures of health status, the MOS focused on limitations in social contacts *attributed to health* (88). This strategy markedly improved their usefulness in detecting differences in health status, particularly *mental* health (54). The third factor in the WHO physical, mental, and social conceptualization of health (120) remains to be operationalized.

Disease-Specific and Generic Measures

As discussed above, there is great value in measuring symptoms and problems unique to specific diseases and treatments in parallel with generic measures (42, 69). An ideal measurement and interpretation strategy is one capturing the burden of disease and treatment benefits in specific terms as well as in terms of general health outcomes (20, 42, 60, 69, 92, 95). Questionnaires that confound them in their scoring have potential for abuse. For example, a comparison of outcomes between two drugs is biased if the health index utilized included side effects of one drug but not those of another. An index including symptoms relieved by one treatment but not another is also biased.

How would scales constructed from the ten questionnaires in Table 1 be classified in terms of the schematic in Figure 1? The classification for most is straightforward, involving only levels III or IV and primarily the physical or mental components of health, depending on the scale (96, 97). For two of the measures, the QWB and the SIP, the classification is complicated by confounding generic and specific measures. Many disease-specific symptoms and problems are included in the QWB (e.g. upset stomach, loose bowel movements, joint problems, and pain at specific bodily sites) (41, 68). Relative to the large number of items contained in the SIP, only a few appear to be condition specific (e.g. problems with bladder control, drinking less fluids, and going only to places with rest rooms nearby) (6), which are symptoms of diabetes and prostate disease (33, 36). Scale scores are more affected by diseases associated with symptoms represented. The burden of one disease relative to another and the benefit of one treatment relative to another are most validly estimated from truly generic scales. To estimate the public health implications for a particular condition or disease, a *general* health measure should either equally represent all specific symptoms of all diseases, a seemingly impractical undertaking, or it should represent none of them. These issues warrant further study.

In conclusion, two dilemmas must be resolved: (*a*) minimum standards of content for generic measures, and (*b*) how to handle measures reflecting specific medical conditions or treatments. Standards for definitions are needed both with respect to comprehensiveness (Table 1) and genericity (Figure 1). Standards should be established and adhered to in *labeling* health status surveys. Warnings to potential users should be noted where necessary. The label generic measure should be limited to measures of core health concepts proven to be sensitive to the impact of a wide range of diseases, which also implies a lack of specificity. Given the availability of measures useful in measuring generic health concepts, it is practical to include them in studies seeking to draw conclusions about general health outcomes.

APPLICATIONS OF HEALTH SURVEYS

Applications of general health surveys include: (*a*) monitoring the health of the general population; (*b*) evaluating health-care policy; (*c*) conducting clinical trials of alternative treatments; (*d*) designing systems for monitoring and improving health-care outcomes; and (*e*) making clinical decisions in medical practice. Each is discussed briefly below.

General Population Monitoring

Standardized health surveys are necessary to monitor the general population because the available information has many shortcomings. Mortality statistics tell little about the health of the general population in developed countries (27) and therefore do not apply to the great majority of patients who survive. Utilization rates are difficult to interpret as indicators of health status because they reflect differences in access to services and other factors distinct from the health status of those affected. For example, in *Health United States 1990*, the only mental health data were reports of changes in utilization rates of inpatient admissions to mental health organizations from 1983 to 1988—an increase of 17% (58, pp. 3, 158). Does this reflect an improvement in health? A worsening? Neither? Mental health measures (as opposed to suicide rates) were not included in the 1990 report and have not been routinely reported over the past ten years.

Federal leadership has been conspicuously lacking in defining health comprehensively, in advancing assessment methods, and in promoting the adoption of common standards across federal agencies. For example, annual health reports prepared by the U.S. Department of Health and Human Services do not offer a definition of health. Nor do they offer updates on advances in understanding of health concepts or state-of-the-art improvements in measurement. Methods used in National Health Interview Surveys have numerous shortcomings including: (a) emphasis on negative definitions of health status; (b) reliance on utilization of health-care services and access as an indicator of health status; (c) omission of general mental health measures; and (d) reliance on relatively crude single item and categorical definitions rather than *measurement* scales. As a result, these national surveys do not yield comprehensive national norms and are of little or no value in the norm-based interpretation of widely used health status measures. The usefulness of such norms has been demonstrated in numerous publications (5, 64, 70, 86, 87, 109). Australia appears to be ahead of the U.S. in this regard (2).

All health survey applications would benefit from national norms for at least the consensus generic health concepts. Normative data are necessary to document normal health status, to estimate the burden of different medical and psychiatric conditions, and to chart the course of changes in population health status over time. A committee of the Institute of Medicine (IOM) has offered specific recommendations to achieve these objectives (72) including: (a) revising the National Health Interview Survey to better represent general health concepts, particularly mental health; and (b) conducting a comprehensive longitudinal survey of functional limitations and disability.

Health-Care Policy Evaluation

Assessing health outcomes in health-care policy evaluations is a high priority because the U.S. health-care system is being restructured to contain rising health-care expenditures. Those persons implementing cost-containment strategies have given little attention to the health effects of these strategies. Yet accountability demands this kind of information (74). This is the logic of the effectiveness initiative and outcomes management (28, 76). Both require a transition from relying on utilization of health-care services and a narrow set of clinical endpoints—traditionally measured to evaluate treatment effectiveness—to a broader set of health-outcome measures incorporating human, not just biologic, criteria (96, 97).

The Health Insurance Experiment (HIE)—the largest comprehensive health-care policy evaluation to date—examined the effects of different approaches to organizing and financing health-care services on general health outcomes for children and adults. The HIE demonstrated the feasibility of standardized surveys in monitoring outcomes on a large scale over a five-year follow-up period. As summarized from reports published over a ten-year period (67), the HIE demonstrated that two cost-containment strategies—cost-sharing in a fee-for-service (FFS) system and a prepaid HMO-type group practice—reduced health-care expenditures substantially relative to FFS free care. For middle- and upper-income groups participating in the HIE, reductions were gained without harm to health, as defined by a wide range of health status measures (13, 101). These results seem to have played a role in increasing the adoption rate of patient cost-sharing in the insurance industry during the period immediately following the HIE's publication (61). Both clinical and general health status measures also suggested some harmful effects of both FFS cost-sharing and HMO care, relative to free FFS care, among poorer and sicker study participants, contributing to concerns about implementing managed care under Medicaid (13, 45, 101). An implication is that outcomes studies must be designed so that high-risk groups can be analyzed separately and with precision.

Among the most common and influential applications of health-outcome assessment in the 1990s will be those that attempt to demonstrate reductions in health-care costs without harm to health. Such attempts require valid assessment methods, appropriate study designs, and a high level of statistical precision in estimating health effects. A high level of precision for the methods used is necessary because they seek to accept the null hypothesis that cost-containment does not harm health. To be confident that clinically and socially relevant decrements in health are not missed, very small confidence intervals around estimates of health effects must be achieved. In analyzing health outcomes, the HIE was precise enough to detect a one-point difference (on a 100-point scale) in health outcomes between health plans (12). Studies that cannot rule out clinically and socially relevant differences in the range of 2–5 points or smaller are not satisfactory to determine whether changes in health-care policies result in harm to health.

During the past decade, the potential of nonexperimental approaches in evaluating health outcomes has been demonstrated. These quasi-experimental studies compare groups that are not formed randomly. Examples include studies of outcomes under Medicaid (51), the ongoing MOS studies (46, 91), and studies of specific treatments discussed below. One study demonstrated the potential of clinical and general health-outcome measures in estimating the health effects of policy changes for California's Medicaid system. Outcomes measures revealed that those who lost their benefits experienced poorer health outcomes compared to those who retained their benefits. These differences in outcomes were linked to medical care process. The MOS, which is attempting to link variations in practice styles in different health-care delivery systems to outcomes for chronically ill patients, offers a prototype of how outcomes-monitoring systems might be implemented across practice settings (91). Research priority should be given to advances in methods of improving and analyzing nonexperimental databases to evaluate outcomes under different health-care policies. Such mastery is crucial for practical and ethical reasons. Data collection for the HIE ended ten years ago. There have been no subsequent large-scale randomized trials addressing policy issues, although it has been estimated that the immediate cost savings resulting from decisions the HIE stimulated more than equaled total study costs (61). Policymakers seem to lack the will and foresight to support large-scale prospective studies of health-care outcomes.

Clinical Trials

Another pressing application of health surveys is clinical trials that evaluate pharmaceuticals and other new treatments and technologies (14). Comprehensive health-outcome assessments have rarely been included in clinical trials, with some noteworthy exceptions (9, 19, 31, 33). Alternative treatment regimens and health-care technologies can and should be compared in terms of their impact on patient functioning and well-being, in addition to traditionally defined biologic endpoints (16). One reason is that a treatment might represent a trade-off between an improvement in one or more clinical parameters or even length of life versus a deterioration in quality of life. For example, chemotherapy for small cell lung cancer may lower the quality of life of all of those treated while curing less than 10% (3). Another reason is that two drugs, equally efficacious in achieving normal biologic functioning (e.g. blood pressure control), might differ in their impact on quality of life (19). Though no systematic tracking of clinical trials exists in terms of the nature and number of assessments of functioning, well-being, and other health-status outcomes, it appears from informal surveys that such outcomes are assessed in a relatively small minority (less than 10%) of NIH-sponsored trials. In the 1990s, alternative treatments will be evaluated increasingly in terms of cost and health utility, in addition to clinical efficacy, before they are adopted by health-care organizations and those who pay for health-care services.

Documenting the value of a specific health-care intervention would be greatly facilitated by greater use of common standards for measuring general health outcomes in clinical research. Being market driven, the pharmaceutical industry in the U.S. seems to have an eye on the health-care needs and expectations of the public. Since it seeks to support claims about the value of its products in terms mattering most to the public and those who employ them, the industry is beginning to broaden general health-outcome assessment in the clinical trials it supports (14, 19, 31, 64, 83). The same logic applies to the NIH research program. Congressional review of the products of the NIH research program is likely to focus more specifically on evidence regarding what human life is like with different diseases and treatments. Congress has requested more information about the impact of NIH programs in terms of human functioning and not just organ functioning. Health-care purchasers also want this information. However, noteworthy gaps exist in the procedures for conducting and evaluating clinical trials that address outcomes in terms of general health status. High priority should be given to improving the comprehensiveness of health-outcome assessments, the scientific validity of clinical trials addressing health-status outcomes, and the decision-making processes relying on such information. Perhaps an advisory panel could review assessment methods and comment on the state-of-the-art of assessment methods related directly to the conduct of clinical trials. The panel could exemplify standards for evaluating and disseminating information about the strengths and weaknesses of assessment methods and critical study-design features. Such efforts could improve communication among manufacturers, investigators conducting clinical trials, the FDA and other federal agencies evaluating study findings, scientific and clinical audiences, and the general public.

Monitoring and Improving Health-Care Outcomes

This decade's most exciting and promising agendas require a new health-care database and improved models for monitoring and improving health-care outcomes (21). The challenge is to achieve an assessment system yielding interpretable and programmatically useful information. A major shortcoming of the existing health-care database is its lack of information about performance, particularly in terms of outcomes from the patient point of view. In the estimated 10–15 billion pieces of paper produced nationally during health-care visits annually (55), little is recorded about benefits.

The advantage of using general health assessments to monitor outcomes is their sensitivity to positive and negative effects associated with treatment benefits and burdens of chronic disease, respectively. A disadvantage is the difficulty of interpretation. Health status at any point in time is an outcome of numerous factors, including health-care services delivered prior to that point. The research community's challenge is to develop models that measure and statistically control for the effects of factors that might bias conclusions of specific health-care outcomes.

Controlling rising health-care costs will continue to be the dominant issue of the 1990s. The goal will be to accept the null hypothesis that health status before policy implementation equals health status after policy implementation (after adjusting for decline due to aging), or that any harm to health is worth the dollars saved. The focus of health-status assessment during the remainder of this decade will not be on producing optimal health status. We do not have a crisis in health-status outcomes throughout the American population. The universal problem is the cost of health care and organizational access (78). Experience in monitoring health-status outcomes, in conjunction with implementing cost-containment strategies, will serve as the foundation for the next health assessment stage—the era of improving health benefits.

It appears the American public is aggressively shopping for health plans that serve their needs best at the lowest price. Health plans offer a trade-off between price and access and quality (78). Individuals bet on their health needs. One would thus expect the healthiest individuals to more readily accept plans offering fewer services at lower prices and those needing more services to accept the higher prices associated with greater accessibility (62). Attempts to achieve financial objectives will further exacerbate differences in patient mix across health-care plans. All parties will thus become more interested in systems to measure and interpret differences in patient mix—a factor that should be given high priority in the research agenda of the 1990s.

One of the most useful methods of measuring patient mix is a standardized health survey representing multiple health dimensions. This was well demonstrated in the analysis of the three- and five-year general health outcomes in the HIE (13, 101, 105). The precision of predicting health-status outcomes was substantially increased with a baseline measure of each outcome, as well as baseline measures of other general health concepts. These baseline assessments are also essential to interpreting health outcomes across health-care delivery organizations based on self-selected populations.

Research priority must be given to the use of clinical data, including clinical severity in estimating general health outcomes. Though evidence is accumulating that average differences in functional status and well-being are substantial across different clinical severity levels at a point in time (46, 113, 114), it is not clear if clinical measurements are useful in understanding general health outcomes over time. This is both good news and bad news. From the perspective of employee benefit–plan managers and other health-care managers seeking to monitor general health outcomes, it may be good news because it suggests that changes in general health status may be interpretable without expensive clinical measures. This could revolutionize systems for population monitoring of general health outcomes. Yet the results also can be seen as bad news. They suggest that treatments narrowly targeting biological functioning, as opposed to functional status and well-being, are less likely to produce large differences in general health outcomes. This should not be a surprise. Treatments equally efficacious in controlling blood pressure, for example, may differ significantly in their impact on functioning and well-being; some may lead to a decreased quality of life, albeit a longer life (19). An important research agenda should be achieving a greater understanding of the interaction between biologic and human phenomena in terms of functioning and well-being as they are affected by medical intervention.

Research should also focus on the key predictive variables for three different uses of health assessments: monitoring and interpreting health-status outcomes;

health-care service expenditures; and survival. Different explanatory models will likely be required for different predictions. Although further research is needed, it appears likely that standardized measures of functional status and well-being, even short-form measures, will prove useful in all three predictive models (97).

Clinical Practice

Standardized health surveys have the potential to become the new laboratory tests of medical practice. Without these tests, patient functioning and well-being affected by disease and treatment are unlikely to be discussed during a typical medical visit. Two thirds to three fourths of adults in the U.S. reported that physicians rarely or never ask about the extent of their limitations in performing everyday activities, even in the presence of chronic conditions (79). As a result, doctors are not well informed about their patient's functional status, well-being, or changes over time. Practicing physicians are unaware of relatively concrete impairment manifested by observable physical limitations in physical, social, and role functioning (77). Differences in severity of psychological distress also are not apparent to treating physicians (111). Even the most severely psychologically distressed patients suffering from psychiatric disorders are unlikely to be recognized and treated (105, 111).

One solution might be the standardization of functional status and well-being assessments in everyday medical practice (1). Such routine assessments would be useful to: (a) ensure that all important dimensions of functional status and well-being are considered consistently; (b) detect, explain, and track changes in functional capacity over time; (c) make it possible to better consider the patient's total functioning when choosing among therapies; (d) guide the efficient use of community resources and social services; and (e) predict more accurately the course of chronic disease. Such data would also make it possible for physicians to better inform patients about the clinical and functional trade-offs involved in alternative treatments (33).

Standardized assessments also provide a view of the patient's complete status, complete impairment associated with all diseases, and complete benefits of all treatments in terms of functional status and well-being. Specific measures of disease and treatment do not have this breadth or sensitivity; they analyze the function of one organ in the body. Generic health surveys monitor the individual's total functioning. Standardization is essential to monitor the disease course and treatment benefits over time for a given patient. Recently reported results for individual hemodialysis patients illustrate both the feasibility and usefulness of periodic health profiles in managing patients during the progression from advanced renal failure to end-stage renal disease (56).

Finally, standardized assessments and normative data will ultimately make it possible for providers to assess today's functional status and well-being in relation to what is expected for a person of the same age, gender, and medical or psychiatric condition (17). Clearly, a great potential exists for standardized measures of functional status and well-being administered routinely as part of the clinical database.

A UNIFIED MEASUREMENT STRATEGY

The above applications have in common the surveying of at least a core set of generic health concepts. Standardizing these concepts conceptually and methodologically would benefit all applications. In contrast, little or no relationship currently exists between the concepts and methods used in national health interview surveys, clinical trials, effectiveness research, health-care management and policy evaluations, and everyday medical practice. A review of methods across applications reveals that some are very similar, often differing only enough to preclude meaningful comparisons. Much could be gained from inclusion of consensus general health measures in surveys fielded across these applications. The past decade has shown glimpses of the synergy achievable with measurement standardization (5, 7, 64, 88, 112).

The standardization of assessment methods for a core set of concepts might place a priority on the first six consensus generic health concepts listed in the top panel of Table 1. To make this approach practical, forms should vary in length according to the application requirements. To guarantee comparability of comparisons, short measures should be imbedded in longer form measures. For example, a 32-item mental health scale used in studies requiring the greatest precision would include an 5-item alternate form used for larger group-level analyses, which in turn would include the best available single-item version used in large-scale population monitoring. It is clear that both short-form multi-item scales and single-item measures can be calibrated to optimally reproduce the best full-length measures of those concepts (106, 109). The advantage of including shorter measures in the longer forms is that the normative data from a census or other large general population survey based on that measure will be of great value to all studies that include the measure in longer versions. Further, validation studies focusing on full-length versions will advance understanding of how to interpret scores for all shorter forms because they will be imbedded in longer forms. Analyses of single-item, 5-item, 18-item, and 32-item versions of the MOS Mental Health scale illustrate the potential of this strategy (54).

SUMMARY AND FUTURE DIRECTIONS

Debate about the uses of health assessment is spreading beyond the arcane realm of methodologists. Policy analysts and health-care managers—intent on getting the best value for their dollar—have joined the intellectual fray. Clinical investigators evaluating new treatments and technologies and practicing clinicians seeking better patient outcomes are also demanding useful assessment methods. The results are making the American public sit up and take notice (32, 118).

Despite advances in survey methods, the current state of outcomes research and health-care monitoring in general is woefully deficient. Comprehensive health assessments are not included in national health surveys, management information systems used by health-care delivery organizations, databases analyzed in most clinical trials, and inpatient or outpatient medical records. When it comes to health concepts, definitions, and measures, federal health agencies function without coordination and without comprehensiveness of health assessment methods. This country critically needs a coherent health-status–assessment strategy that integrates monitoring methods for Medicare and Medicaid benefits, health-care delivery results, and outcomes of clinical trials and biomedical research.

To meet future needs, information about general health outcomes must be added to the nation's health-care database. Minimum standards of comprehensiveness should be adopted to monitor the health of the general population and evaluate the impact of health-care policies. Federally sponsored biomedical research and clinical trials, as well as national health interview surveys, neither of which reflect the state-of-the-art of assessment methods (72), also should adhere to minimum standards.

We can finish out the 1990s with great potential for agreement regarding the conceptual framework and the measurement standards for physical and mental health concepts. The foundation for conceptual agreement includes but is not limited to several elements: (a) consensus regarding concepts represented in the most widely used health status measures; (b) widely accepted operational definitions of health status; and (c) recommendations for defining health by the field's most respected practitioners (7, 66, 84, 96). What we suffer from most is the lack of a database.

A core set of generic health-outcomes measures should be standardized and adopted for inclusion in the databases across all applications discussed here. This core set must: (a) well represent truly generic, universally relevant outcomes for defining health; and (b) exclude from the generic measure any outcome unique to a specific disease. Only if these two requirements are met will estimates of the burden of different diseases and comparisons among alternative treatments be comprehensive and unbiased. Specific measures should be analyzed in parallel with generic measures.

To be comprehensive, a generic health-outcome assessment must include: physical functioning; general mental health (psychological distress and well-being); limitations in social and role functioning due to health problems; and general health perceptions. Objective reports of behavioral functioning and subjective assessments of health and well-being are both required for comprehensiveness.

Priority should be given to deriving comprehensive health norms for the general population. Longitudinal surveys are required for the monitoring of health outcomes over time. The beneficiaries of these norms would be policymakers, health-care delivery organizations, purchasers, clinical researchers, and medical practitioners.

It is possible to include a standardized *core* set of health measures across applications (e.g. general population surveys, clinical trials), while supplementing this core with other general or specific measures according to the special needs of a given application. The resulting comparisons will greatly advance understanding of the interpretation of health measures for all applications. Adoption of a standardized core set of health measures should be given high priority.

In the future, a major use of health-status assessments will be to identify the health-care cost-containment strategies that have harmful health effects. Unless the assessments relied upon achieve a high degree of precision, relevant effects are likely to be missed. To assure this does not occur, evaluations must be precise enough to rule out adverse health outcomes.

The health consequences of managed care and other cost-containment strategies may be unequal across population subgroups. Socioeconomically disadvantaged individuals and those most burdened with treatable medical and psychiatric conditions may be most likely to experience adverse health outcomes. Health-policy evaluations should be designed to permit precise tests of whether adverse health outcomes occur in such subgroups.

Research should focus on the dynamics of biological functioning and physical and mental health status. To advance understanding of these dynamics, generic health outcomes should be assessed in conjunction with disease-specific measures; neither can be accepted as a substitute for the other. New models are required to evaluate trade-offs involved in treatment. It is hoped that the physical and mental health schematic offered here will prove useful in evaluating alternative treatment strategies with the goal of improving general health outcomes.

Although psychometric methods appear to produce the most valid health assessments, additional factors must be considered to make economic evaluations. To advance economic assessments of health benefits, research should integrate psychometric methods for assessing health status with methods of aggregating scales appropriate for economic evaluations. This would enhance crucial health-care decision-making.

Priority should also go to research that makes measurement methods easier to use. Since research findings may apply to the use of a method in one application and not another, research should focus on specific uses of assessment methods. The field is limited by the lack of translated forms of proven validity for use with minority groups (e.g. Chinese-, Japanese-, and Spanish-speaking Americans). User-friendly manuals and other supporting documents, as well as training necessary to assure their proper use and interpretation, should be readily available. Given that health assessment methods are being widely used by people not trained in assessment methods, better documentation is particularly important.

In summary, health-outcome–assessment methods have come a long way. The problem in 1994 is twofold: that health-outcome assessments are not being used to their full potential and coherent programs of basic and applied methodological research are not under way. To gain the most value, two paths must be pursued simultaneously: (*a*) Methodologists must continue to advance the state-of-the-art; and (*b*) Health-care decision-makers must use the best available assessment methods. In this highly imperfect world, decision-makers cannot wait for methodologists to perfect their craft. If they do, progress will be held hostage to perfection.

ACKNOWLEDGMENTS

Preparation of this chapter was supported by unrestricted research grants for the International Quality of Life Assessment (IQOLA) Project received from Glaxo Research Institute and Schering-Plough Corporation and by The Health Institute at New England Medical Center from its own research fund. The author's reviews of this field have also been sponsored by grants from the Henry J. Kaiser Family Foundation, Robert Wood Johnson Foundation, Pew Charitable Trusts, Agency for Health Care Policy and Research, and the National Institute on Aging. Many of the observations summarized in this chapter were made following a review of the field supported by the Association of Health Services Research and the Health Care Financing Administration as reported previously (JE Ware, *The Use of Health Status and Quality of Life Measures in Outcomes and Effectiveness Research,* 1991). The author also gratefully acknowledges Susan D. Keller, Martha Bayliss, Barbara Gandek, Mark Kosinski, Rebecca Voris, and Kathy Clark for their assistance in the preparation of this chapter.

Literature Cited

1. American College of Physicians. 1988. Comprehensive functional assessment for elderly patients. *Ann. Intern. Med.* 109:70–72
2. Australian Institute of Health. 1994. *Health Outcomes Bulletin.* Canberra: Australian Inst. Health Welfare. Vol. 2
3. Bergman B. 1991. *Quality of Life and Related Issues in Small Cell Lung Cancer.* Gotberg, Sweden: Univ. Gotborg
4. Bergner M. 1985. Measurement of health status. *Med. Care* 23:696–704
5. Bergner M, Bobbitt RA, Carter WB, Gilson BS. 1981. The Sickness Impact Profile: development and final revision of a health status measure. *Med. Care* 19:787–805
6. Bergner M, Bobbitt RA, Kressel S, Pollard WE, Gilson BS, et al. 1976. The Sickness Impact Profile: conceptual formulation and methodology for the development of a health status index. *Int. J. Health Serv.* 6:393–415
7. Bergner M, Rothman ML. 1987. Health status measures: an overview and guide for selection. *Annu. Rev. Public Health* 8:191–210
8. Bice TW. 1976. Comments on health indicators: methodological perspectives. *Int. J. Health Serv.* 6:509–20
9. Bombardier C, Ware J, Russell IJ, Larson M, Chalmers A, et al. 1986. Auranofin therapy and quality of life in patients with rheumatoid arthritis: results of a multicenter trial. *Am. J. Med.* 81:565–78
10. Brazier JE, Harper R, Jones NMB, O'Cathain A, Thomas KJ, et al. 1992. Validating the SF-36 health survey questionnaire: new outcome measure for primary care. *Br. Med. J.* 305:160–64
11. Brenner MH, Curbow B, Legro M. 1994. The proximal distal continuum in multiple health outcome measures. *Med. Care.* In press
12. Brook RH, Ware JE, Davies-Avery A, et al. 1979. Overview of adult health status measures fielded in RAND's Health Insurance Study. *Med. Care* 17:1–131 (Suppl. 7)
13. Brook RH, Ware JE, Rogers WH, Keeler EB, Davies AR, et al. 1983. Does free care improve adults' health? Results from a randomized controlled trial. *New Engl. J. Med.* 309:1426–34
14. Bungay KM, Ware JE. 1993. *Current Concepts: Measuring and Monitoring Health-Related Quality of Life.* Kalamazoo, MI: Upjohn
15. Campbell A, Converse PE, Rodgers WL. 1976. *The Quality of American Life: Perceptions, Evaluations, and Satisfactions.* New York: Russell Sage Found.
16. Chobanian AV. 1986. Antihypertensive therapy in evolution. *New Engl. J. Med.* 314:1701–2
17. Cluff LE. 1981. Chronic disease, function and the quality of care. *J. Chronic Dis.* 34:299–304
18. Codman EA. 1914. The product of a hospital. *Surg. Gynecol. Obstetr.* 18:491–96
19. Croog SH, Levine S, Testa MA, Brown B, Bulpitt CJ, et al. 1986. The effects of antihypertensive therapy on the quality of life. *New Engl. J. Med.* 314:1657–64
20. Damiano AM, Steinberg EP, Cassard SD, Bass EB, Diener-West M, et al. 1994. Comparison of generic versus disease-specific measures of functional impairment in patients with cataract. *Med. Care.* In press
21. Davies AR, Halpern R. 1993. *Health Care Outcomes: An Introduction. A VHA White Paper.* Irving, TX: VHA
22. Davies AR, Sherbourne CD, Peterson JR, Ware JE. 1988. *Scoring Manual: Adult Health Status and Patient Satisfaction Measures Used in RAND's Health Insurance Experiment.* Rand Corp., Santa Monica, CA
23. Davies AR, Ware JE. 1981. *Measuring Health Perceptions in the Health Insurance Experiment.* Rand Corp., Santa Monica, CA
24. Davis SM. 1987. *Future Perfect.* New York: Addison-Wesley
25. Donald CA, Ware JE. 1982. *The Quantification of Social Contacts and Resources.* The RAND Corp., Santa Monica, CA
26. Dupuy HJ. 1984. The Psychological General Well-Being (PGWB) index. See Ref. 112a, pp. 170–83
27. Elinson J, Mattson ME. 1984. Assessing the quality of life in clinical trials of cardiovascular therapies: introduction to the panel presenters. See Ref. 112a, pp. 143–45
28. Ellwood PM. 1988. Outcomes management: a technology of patient experience. *New Engl. J. Med.* 318:1549–56
29. EuroQOL Group. 1990. EuroQOL—a new facility for the measurement of health-related quality of life. *Health Policy* 16:199–208
30. Evans RW, Manninen DL, Garrison LP, Hart LG, Blagg CR, et al. 1985. The quality of life of patients with end-stage

renal disease. *New Engl. J. Med.* 312: 553–79

31. Evans RW, Rader B, Manninen DL, Cooperative Multicenter EPO Clinical Trial Group. 1990. The quality of life of hemodialysis recipients treated with recombinant human erythropoietin. *J. Am. Med. Assoc.* 263:825–30

32. Faltermayer E. 1992. Yes, the market can curb health costs. *Fortune* (Dec. 28) 84–88

33. Fowler FJ, Wennberg JE, Timothy RP, Barry MJ, Mulley AG, et al. 1989. Symptom status and quality of life following prostatectomy. *J. Am. Med. Assoc.* 259:3018–22

34. Garratt AM, Ruta DA, Abdalla MI, Buckingh JK, Russell IT. 1993. The SF-36 health survey questionnaire: an outcome measure suitable for routine use within the NHS? *Br. Med. J.* 306–1440–44

35. Haley SM, McHorney CA, Ware JE. 1994. Evaluation of the MOS SF-36 Physical Functioning scale (PF-10): II. Comparison of relative precision using Likert and Rasch scoring methods. *J. Clin. Epidemiol.* 47:671–84

36. Hammond GS, Aoki TT. 1992. Measurement of health status in diabetic patients. *Diabet. Care* 15:465–76

37. Hays RD, Stewart AL. 1990. The structure of self-reported health in chronic disease patients. *Psychol. Assess. J. Consult. Clin. Psychol.* 2:22–30

38. Hunt SM, McEwen J. 1980. The development of a subjective health indicator. *Sociol. Health Illn.* 2:231–46

39. Hunt SM, McKenna SP, McEwen J, Williams J, Papp E. 1981. The Nottingham Health Profile: subjective health status and medical consultations. *Soc. Sci. Med.* 15a:221–29

40. Kaplan RM, Anderson JP. 1988. The Quality of Well-Being Scale: rational for a single quality of life index. In *Quality of Life: Assessment and Application*, ed. SR Walker, RM Rosser, pp. 51–78. Lancaster: MTP Press

41. Kaplan RM, Bush JW, Berry CC. 1976. Health status: types of validity and the Index of Well-Being. *Health Serv. Res.* 11:478–507

42. Kantz ME, Harris WJ, Levitsky K, Ware JE, Davies AR. 1992. Methods for assessing condition-specific and generic functional status outcomes after total knee replacement. *Med. Care* 30 (5): S240–52

43. Karnofsky DA, Burchenal JH. 1949. The clinical evaluation of chemotherapeutic agents in cancer. In *Evaluation of Chemotherapeutic Agents*, ed. CM

MacLeod, pp. 191–205. New York: Columbia Univ. Press

44. Katz JN, Larson MG, Phillips CB, Fossel AH, Liang MH. 1992. Comparative measurement sensitivity of short and longer health status instruments. *Med. Care* 30:917–25

45. Keeler EB, Brook RH, Goldberg GA, Kamberg CJ, Newhouse JP. 1985. How free care reduced hypertension in the health insurance experiment. *J. Am. Med. Assoc.* 254:1926–31

46. Kravitz RL, Greenfield S, Rogers W, Manning WG, Zubkoff M, et al. 1992. Differences in the mix of patients among medical specialties and systems of care: results from the Medical Outcomes Study. *J. Am. Med. Assoc.* 267:1617–23

47. Landgraf JM, Nelson EC, Hays RD, Wasson JH, Kirk JW. 1990. Assessing function: does it really make a difference? A preliminary evaluation of the acceptability and utility of the COOP function charts. In *Functional Status Measurement in Primary Care*, ed. M Lipkin, pp. 150–65. New York: Springer

48. Lembcke PA. 1952. Measuring the quality of medical care through vital statistics based on hospital service areas: 1. Comparative study of appendectomy rates. *Am. J. Public Health* 42:276–86

49. Liang J. 1986. Self-reported physical health among aged adults. *J. Gerontol.* 41:248–60

50. Likert R. 1932. A technique for the measurement of attitudes. *Arch. Psychol.* 140:5–55

51. Lurie N, Ward NB, Shapiro MF, Brook RH. 1984. Termination from Medi-Cal: does it affect health? *New Engl. J. Med.* 311:480–84

52. McDermott W. 1981. Absence of indicators of the influence of its physicians on a society's health: impact of physician care on society. *Am. J. Med.* 70: 833–43

53. McHorney CA, Ware JE, Raczek AE. 1993. The MOS 36-Item Short-Form Health Status Survey (SF-36): II. Psychometric and clinical tests of validity in measuring physical and mental health constructs. *Med. Care* 31:247–63

54. McHorney CA, Ware JE, Rogers W, Raczek A, Lu JFR. 1992. The validity and relative precision of MOS short- and long-form health status scales and Dartmouth COOP Charts: results from the Medical Outcomes Study. *Med. Care* 30:MS253–65 (Suppl.)

55. Meier B. 1991. Rx for a system in crisis. *Good Health Magazine: The NY Times Magazine* Part 2:18–21

56. Meyer KB, Espindle DM, DeGiacomo

JM, Jenuleson CS, Kurtin PS, et al. 1993. Monitoring dialysis patients' health status. *Am. J. Kidney Dis.* 9:42

57. Myers JK, Lindenthal JJ, Pepper MP. 1975. Life events, social integration and psychiatric symptomatology. *J. Health Soc. Behav.* 421–29

58. Natl. Cent. Health Statistics. 1989. *Health, United States.* GPO: DHHS

59. Nelson EC, Wasson J, Kirk J, Keller A, Clark D, et al. 1987. Assessment of function in routine clinical practice: description of the COOP chart method and preliminary findings. *J. Chronic Dis.* 40:55S–63S (Suppl. 1)

60. Nerenz DR, Repasky DP, Whitehouse FW, Kahkonen DM. 1992. Ongoing assessment of health status in patients with diabetes mellitus. *Med. Care* 30 (5): MS112–24

61. Newhouse JP. 1991. Controlled experimentation as research policy. In *Health Services Research: Key to Health Policy*, ed. E Ginzberg, pp 161–94. Cambridge: Harvard Univ. Press

62. Newhouse JP. 1994. Patients at risk: health reform and risk adjustment. *Health Aff.* 13:132–46

63. Osoba D. 1991. *The Effect of Cancer on Quality of Life.* Boca Raton, FL: CRC Press

64. Osterhaus JT, Townsend RJ, Gandek B, Ware JE. 1994. Measuring the functional status and well-being of patients with migraine headaches. *Headache* 34:337–43

65. Parkerson GR, Broadhead WE, Tse CJ. 1990. The Duke health profile: a 17-item measure of health and disfunction. *Med. Care* 28:1056–72

66. Patrick DL. 1990. Assessing health-related quality of life outcomes. In *Effectiveness and Outcomes in Health Care: Proc. Invit. Conf. Inst. Med., Div. Health Care Serv.*, ed. KA Heithoff, KN Lohr, pp. 137–51. Washington, DC: Natl. Acad. Press

67. Patrick DL, Bush JW, Chen MM. 1973. Methods for measuring levels of well-being for a health status index. *Health Serv. Res.* 8:229–34

68. Patrick DL, Bush JW, Chen MM. 1973. Toward an operational definition of health. *J. Health Soc. Behav.* 14:6–21

69. Patrick DL, Deyo RA. 1989. Generic and disease-specific measures in assessing health status and quality of life. *Med. Care* 27 (3):S217–32

70. Patrick DL, Erickson P. 1993. *Health Status and Health Policy: Allocating Resources to Health Care.* New York: Oxford Univ. Press

71. Patrick DL, Stein J, Porta M, Porter CQ,

Ricketts TC. 1988. Poverty, health services, and health status in rural america. *Milbank Mem. Fund Q.* 66:105–36

72. Pope AM, Tarlov AR. 1991. *Disability in America.* Washington, DC: Natl. Acad. Press

73. Read JL, Quinn RJ, Hoefer MA. 1987. Measuring overall health: an evaluation of three important approaches. *J. Chronic Dis.* 40(1):7S–22S

74. Relman AS. 1988. Assessment and accountability: the third revolution in medical care. *New Engl. J. Med.* 319: 1220–22

75. Rogers WH, Williams KN, Brook RH. 1979. *Conceptualization and Measurement of Health for Adults in the Health Insurance Study: Vol. 7. Power Analysis of Health Status Measures.* RAND Corp., Santa Monica, CA. 25 pp.

76. Roper WL, Winkenwender W, Hackbarth GM, Krakauer H. 1988. Effectiveness in health care: an initiative to evaluate and improve medical practice. *New Engl. J. Med. 319* (18):1197–202

77. Rubenstein LV, McCoy JM, Cope DW, Barrett PA, Hirsch SH, et al. 1991. *Improving patient functional status: a randomized trial of computer-generated resource and management suggestions.* Abstr. presented at Am. Fed. Clin. Res.

78. Safran D, Tarlov AR, Rogers W. 1994. Primary care performances in fee-for-service and prepaid health care systems: results from the Medical Outcomes Study. *J. Am. Med. Assoc.* 271:1579–86

79. Schor EL, Lerner DJ, Malspeis S. 1994. Physician's assessment of functional health status and well-being: the patient's perspective. *Arch. Intern. Med.* In press

80. Schroeder SA. 1987. Outcome assessment 70 years later: are we ready? *New Engl. J. Med.* 316:160–62

81. Shapiro MF, Ware JE, Sherbourne CD. 1986. Effects of cost sharing on seeking care for serious and minor symptoms: results of a randomized controlled trial. *Ann. Intern. Med.* 104:246–51

82. Shumaker SA, Anderson R, Hays R, Berzon R, eds. 1993. International use, application and performance of health-related quality of life instruments. *Qual. Life Res.* 2:367–495

83. Spilker B. 1990. *Quality of Life Assessments in Clinical Trials.* New York: Raven

84. Spitzer WO. 1987. State of science 1986: quality of life and functional status as target variables for research. *J. Chronic Dis.* 40:465–71

85. Spitzer WO, Dobson AJ, Hall J, Chesterman E, Levi J, et al. 1981. Measuring

the quality of life of cancer patients: a concise QL-index for use by physicians. *J. Chronic Dis.* 34:585–97

86. Stewart AL, Greenfield S, Hays RD, Wells K, Rogers WH, et al. 1989. Functional status and well-being of patients with chronic conditions: results from the Medical Outcomes Study. *J. Am. Med. Assoc.* 262:907–13

87. Stewart AL, Hays RD, Ware JE. 1988. The MOS Short-Form General Health Survey: reliability and validity in a patient population. *Med. Care* 26:724–35

88. Stewart AL, Ware JE, eds. 1992. *Measuring Functioning and Well-Being: The Medical Outcomes Study Approach.* Durham, NC: Duke Univ. Press

89. Stewart AL, Ware JE, Brook RH. 1981. Advances in the measurement of functional status: construction of aggregate indexes. *Med. Care* 19:473–88

90. Tarlov AR. 1983. The increasing supply of physicians, the changing structure of the health-services system, and the future practice of medicine. *New Engl. J. Med.* 398:1235–44

91. Tarlov AR, Ware JE, Greenfield S, Nelson EC, Perrin E, et al. 1989. The Medical Outcomes Study: an application of methods for monitoring the results of medical care. *J. Am. Med. Assoc.* 262:925–30

92. Temkin NR, Dikmen S, Machamer J, McLean A. 1989. General versus disease-specific measures: further work on the Sickness Impact Profile for Head Injury. *Med. Care* 27:S44–53 (Suppl.)

93. Thurstone LL. 1928. Attitudes can be measured. *Am. J. Sociol.* 33:529–54

94. Veit CT, Ware JE. 1983. The structure of psychological distress and well-being in general populations. *J. Consult. Clin. Psychol.* 51:730–42

95. Wagner AK, Keller SD, Kosinski M, Baker GA, Jacoby A, et al. 1994. Advances in methods for assessing the impact of epilepsy and antiepileptic drug therapy on patients' health-related quality of life. *Qual. Life Res.* In press

96. Ware JE. 1987. Standards for validating health measures: definition and content. *J. Chronic Dis.* 40:473–80

97. Ware JE. 1991. Measuring functioning, well-being and other generic health concepts. In *The Effect of Cancer on Quality of Life*, ed. D Osoba, pp. 17–23. Boca Raton, FL: CRC Press

98. Ware JE. 1992. Measures for a new era of health assessment. In *Measuring Functioning and Well-Being: The Medical Outcomes Study Approach*, ed. AL Stewart, JE Ware, pp. 3–11. Durham, NC: Duke Univ. Press

99. Ware JE, Brook RH, Davies AR, Lohr KN. 1981. Choosing measures of health status for individuals in general populations. *Am. J. Public Health* 71:620–25

100. Ware JE, Brook RH, Davies-Avery A, Williams KN, Stewart AL, et al. 1980. *Conceptualization and Measurement of Health for Adults in the Health Insurance Study:* Vol. 1. *Model of Health and Methodology.* Rand Corp., Santa Monica, CA. 49 pp.

101. Ware JE, Brook RH, Rogers WH, Keeler EB, Davies AR, et al. 1986. Comparison of health outcomes at a health maintenance organization with those of fee-for-service care. *Lancet* 2:1017–22

102. Ware JE, Gandek B, the IQOLA Project Group. 1994. The SF-36 Health Survey: development and use in mental health research and the IQOLA Project. *Int. J. Mental Health* 23:49–73

103. Ware JE, Johnston SA, Davies-Avery A, Brook RH. 1979. *Conceptualization and Measurement of Health for Adults in the Health Insurance Study:* Vol. 3. *Mental Health.* Rand Corp., Santa Monica, CA. 162 pp.

104. Ware JE, Kosinski M, Bayliss MS, McHorney CA, Rogers WH, et al. 1995. Comparison of methods for the scoring and statistical analysis of SF-36 health profiles and summary measures: results from the Medical Outcomes Study. *Med. Care.* In press

105. Ware JE, Manning WG, Duan N, Wells KB, Newhouse JP. 1984. Health status and the use of outpatient mental health services. *Am. Psychol.* 39:1090–1100

106. Ware JE, Nelson EC, Sherbourne CD, Stewart AL. 1992. Preliminary tests of a 6-item general health survey: a patient application. See Ref. 88, pp. 291–308

107. Ware JE, Sherbourne CD. 1992. The MOS 36-item short-form health survey (SF-36): I. Conceptual framework and item selection. *Med. Care* 30:473–83

108. Ware JE, Sherbourne CD, Davies AR. 1992. Developing and testing the MOS 20-item short-form health survey: a general population application. See Ref. 88, pp. 277–90

109. Ware JE, Snow KK, Kosinski M, Gandek B. 1993. *SF-36 Health Survey Manual and Interpretation Guide.* Boston, MA: New Engl. Med. Center, Health Inst.

110. Weinstein MC, Berwick DM, Goldman PA, Murphy JM, Barsky A. 1989. A comparison of three psychiatric screening tests using Receiver Operating Characteristic (ROC) analysis. *Med. Care* 27:593–607

111. Wells KB, Hays RD, Burnam MA, Rog-

ers W, Greenfield S, et al. 1989. Detection of depressive disorder for patients receiving prepaid or fee-for-service care: results from the Medical Outcomes Study. *J. Am. Med. Assoc.* 262:3298–3302

112. Wells KB, Stewart A, Hays RD, Burnam MA, Rogers W, et al. 1989. The functioning and well-being of depressed patients: results from the Medical Outcomes Study. *J. Am. Med. Assoc.* 262: 914–19

112a. Wenger NK, Mattson ME, Furberg CD, Elinson J, eds. 1984. *Assessment of Quality of Life in Clinical Trials of Cardiovascular Therapies.* New York: Le Jacq Publ.

113. Wenneker MB, Greenfield S, McHorney CA, et al. 1990. The validity of a severity scale for hypertension in predicting functional status and well-being: results from the Medical Outcomes Study. *Clin. Res.* 38:228A

114. Wenneker MB, McHorney CA, Kieszak SM, et al. 1991. The impact of diabetes

severity on quality of life: results from the Medical Outcomes Study. *Clin. Res.* 39:612A

115. Wilkin D, Hallam L, Doggett MA. 1992. *Measures of Need and Outcomes for Primary Health Care.* Oxford: Oxford Med. Press

116. Williams AW, Ware JE, Donald CA. 1981. A model of mental health, life events, and social supports applicable to general populations. *J. Health Soc. Behav.* 22:324–36

117. Wilson I, Kaplan S. 1994. Clinical practice and patient's health status: how are the two related? *Med. Care.* In press

118. Winslow R. 1989. Patient data may reshape health care. *Wall Street J.,* pp. B-1, April 17

119. Wood-Dauphinee S, Williams JI. 1987. Reintegration to normal living as a proxy to quality of life. *J. Chronic Dis.* 40: 491–99

120. World Health Organization. 1948. World Health Organization constitution. In *Basic Documents.* Geneva: WHO

Annu. Rev. Public Health 1995.16:355–79

INCIDENCE, RISK FACTORS AND PREVENTION STRATEGIES FOR WORK-RELATED ASSAULT INJURIES:
A Review of What Is Known, What Needs To Be Known, and Countermeasures for Intervention

Jess F. Kraus, Bonnie Blander, and David L. McArthur

School of Public Health, University of California Los Angeles, Los Angeles, California 90095-1772

KEY WORDS: violence at work, injury, homicide, assault, epidemiology

ABSTRACT

This review organizes available data to address current epidemiological understanding of injuries from workplace assaults. We describe the incidence and general populations at risk for fatal and nonfatal work-related injury, and assess available information on risk factors and countermeasures considered important in reducing injury occurrence. Overall rates of occurrence of work-related homicides and nonfatal injuries are estimated, and those factors that appear to be consistent across studies are explored.

   Much of what is known about occupations at high risk for assaults and injuries comes from a small number of documents and special studies within subsets of workplaces. Unfortunately, the potency of specific countermeasures for prevention of violence-related injury in work settings continues to be largely unknown. Numerous fundamental questions remain to be answered: Critical is a full assessment of risk, identification of situations and circumstances amenable to intervention, and evaluations to demonstrate effectiveness.

355

INTRODUCTION

The Occupational Safety and Health Act, passed by the US Congress in 1970, sought to "assure so far as possible every working man and woman in the nation safe and healthful working conditions" (43). The prime focus of this Act was on the hazards pertaining to machinery and toxic chemicals in industry. Protection from workplace violence, however, was never mentioned.

During the 1980s interest began to grow concerning the frequency and circumstances of work-related violent injury. In 1982, Baker and associates (2) showed that workers were being murdered on the job. A 1982 report from the Centers for Disease Control described homicide among work-related deaths (10). In 1984, researchers from British Columbia (19) and Oklahoma (18) described the relative importance of work-related homicide among all occupational fatalities. The first epidemiologic reports on incidence and features of homicides in work settings appeared in the public health literature in 1987 (15, 26). Prompted by these findings and their own assessment, in the late 1980s the National Institute of Occupational Safety and Health (NIOSH) began to systematically collect data about occupational fatalities (44).

Objectives of the Review

This review organizes and synthesizes the available data on violence-related injury in the workplace in order to address three questions: What do we currently know about the problem, epidemiologically; what additional information is needed before effective interventions can be proposed; and what is the nature and effectiveness of countermeasures? This review describes the incidence and general populations at risk for fatal and nonfatal work-related injury, and assesses available information on risk factors and countermeasures considered important in reducing injury occurrence.

Background

Public interest in workplace violence has been piqued by media reports of numerous instances of workplace homicide. The popular media have been consistent in presenting stories about disgruntled workers who have attacked co-workers and/or supervisors. With few exceptions, the focus of media reports has been on events notable precisely because they are relatively rare. Not unexpectedly, journalists speculate that violent injury reflects the stresses of an increasingly harsh business environment, poverty, layoffs, and disgruntlement among workers. Additionally, the proliferation of guns and abuse of drugs and alcohol are frequently cited as exacerbating factors (5, 25, 37, 42).

Journalists have suggested that workplace violence is predictable and preventable since workers never just snap, but instead break down gradually under stress, leaving behind a series of subtle and not-so-subtle signals (5, 42). A general profile of a potentially dangerous employee has been proposed as a white male at least 35 years of age, with few interests outside of work, few social supports, holding grudges and extremist opinions, and preoccupied with guns. These employees are loners, have nonexemplary job performances, question authority, and often make overt threats (37). Unfortunately, the predictive quality of these attributes has not been tested analytically. Moreover, for every worker-on-worker homicide that appears in print or on screen, scores of injuries, beatings, stabbings, shootings, rapes, suicides, near-suicides, and psychological traumas go unreported.

METHODS

This review is limited to literature in English available since 1980 in US peer-reviewed journals, state and federal government documents, and publications from private companies and the popular press. All industries and occupations are considered with the exception of medical treatment facilities (see 9, 21, 28, 29 for analyses of injury in these environments). It is noteworthy that while the topic is of considerable interest in both academic and nonacademic settings, the descriptive language of key parameters varies considerably.

Definitions

Type of violence   Workplace violence with or without injury has been classified into several basic types. However, classification of type (exposure) of work-related violence has been difficult because of extensive overlap of a number of important characteristics of the event. For example, motivation of the perpetrator, action of the victims, and relationship between perpetrator and victim are not mutually exclusive factors.

The US Bureau of Labor Statistics (BLS) (50) has classified workplace homicide according to the type of circumstance: (*a*) business disputes (including actions of a co-worker or former co-worker); (*b*) customer or client disputes; (*c*) personal disputes involving a relative of the victim (primarily spouse or ex-spouse, boyfriend or ex-boyfriend, or significant other); (*d*) incidents involving police or security guards in the line of duty; and (*e*) incidents in which death occurred during a robbery or miscellaneous crime. The California Division of Occupational Health and Safety (Cal/OSHA) (6) has specified three types of workplace violence: Type I involves assailants with no legitimate relationship to the workplace (generally in the course of a robbery or other criminal act); Type II involves customers of a service provided by an establishment or clients, patients, passengers, criminal suspects, or prisoners; and Type III involves current or former employees, supervisors, managers, and other persons with employment-related involvement with an establishment, such as an employee's spouse, boyfriend, friend, relative, or a person who has a dispute with an employee. Although the perpetrator-victim relationship is an extremely important discriminator of violence and related homicide and non-fatal injury, sufficient detailed information rarely exists on reported cases to correctly classify all events.

Work-relatedness   One major difficulty in assessing the scope, dimensions, and characteristics of work-related assault injury is the definition of a work-related activity. The fact that a violent event occurs at a work-site does not necessarily mean that the event is a direct result of work-related activity (6). (Because workplace precursors of suicide cannot be separated from factors not associated with work, suicide is not addressed in this review.) Work-relatedness of an event is defined here as an injury or fatality caused by activity on the employer's premises or at other locations where employees are engaged in work activities or are required to be present as a condition of employment (6).

Employee   A person who is required or directed by an employer to engage in any work or to be at work, or at work site, at any time of employment (6).

Occupational injury   Injury resulting from a work-related exposure involving a single incident in the work environment (26).

Assault   An unlawful attack, or attempted attack, by one person upon another for purpose of inflicting severe or aggravated bodily injury. Assault often involves use of a weapon or other means likely to produce death or great bodily harm. Here, assault incidents are limited to those involving physical injury and thus exclude rape, verbal assault, harassment, and related outcomes.

MAJOR FINDINGS ON OCCURRENCE

Findings on Incidence: Homicide, U.S.

Several reports provide data for various external causes including motor vehicle, highway, machinery, homicide, falls, electrocution, struck by or caught in objects, and others (Table 1). All but one of the reports in Table 1 show that, aside from the aggregate of all miscellaneous causes of death, motor vehicle-related crashes (including pedestrians being struck by motor vehicles) have the highest percentage of occurrence. In California in 1993, homicide was the leading cause of work-related injury death, followed by motor vehicle–related causes (7). Figure 1 shows the distribution of homicide as a percent of all work-related fatalities in these same studies, indicating an average of

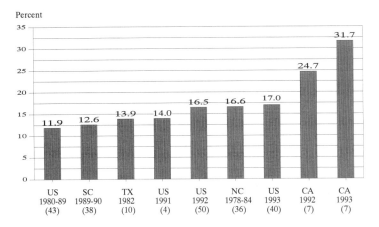

Percent

Figure 1   Work-related homicide as a percent of all work-related fatalities: selected US studies.

12% in the U.S. for 1980–89 to almost 32% in California in 1993. Note that the proportions by external cause across these studies have not been adjusted for age, gender, or race. Because of variations in definition and external cause classification, findings from different reports may not be readily comparable.

NIOSH, a unit of the US Department of Health and Human Services, Centers for Disease Control and Prevention, developed the National Traumatic Occupational Fatalities (NTOF) surveillance system in the mid-1980s to provide epidemiologic information on occupational fatal injuries (4, 8, 24, 45). Using death certificates from all 50 states plus New York City and the District of Columbia, information on industry, occupation, cause of death, demographics, and injury description has been collected and tabulated. A key finding from this national survey of occupational fatalities was that the homicide rate of 0.71 per 100,000 workers (Table 2) was the third leading cause of injury death, accounting for about 12% of all occupational injury deaths.

Following National Research Council recommendations (34), BLS undertook a careful review of all procedures used in data acquisition and analysis to improve its estimates of the numbers of US occupational fatalities. Procedures were developed in Texas in 1988, tested in Texas and Colorado in 1990–91, and put into place for a national survey in 1992 (41). The result of this work is the BLS Census of Fatal Occupational Injuries (CFOI), which utilizes validation of work-relatedness from at least two sources and assesses data from death certificates, state workers compensation reports, coroner/medical examination records, OSHA reports, news media, follow-up questionnaires, state motor vehicle reports, and other sources. Motor vehicle (highway)

Table 1 Percent of work-related fatal injuries by external causes, selected US studies

External cause	Sniezek & Horiagon, N.C. 1978–84 (36)	NIOSH, U.S. 1980–89 (43)	CDC, TX. 1982 (10)	Stone, S.C. 1989–90 (38)	Bell et at, U.S. 1991 (4)	Cal/OSHA CA (7) 1992	Cal/OSHA CA (7) 1993	Windau & Toscano U.S. 1992 (50)	Toscano,[a] 1993 (40)
Machinery[b]	9	14	15	9	7	5	3	5	5
Motor vehicle[c]	18	23	22	32	24	28	26	24	26
Homicide	17[e]	12	14	13	14	25	32	17	17
Falls	10	10	12	11	11	9	8	10	10
Electrocution	8	7	11	7	6	5	4	5	5
Struck by, against	11[f]	7	—	9	6	5	5	9	9
All others[d]	27	27	26	19	32	24	22	39	28

[a] Includes only 31 states
[b] BLS and California do not classify fatalities involving machinery but "caught in or compressed by equipment" is chosen as an approximate equivalent.
[c] Includes highway collisions and pedestrians struck by vehicle
[d] Includes drowning, fires, water and aircraft, etc
[e] Defined as "gun"
[f] Defined as falling object
— Not reported

Table 2 Number of and work-related homicide rate per 100,000 workers, selected US and state-specific studies

Author/Source (reference)	Location	Years	Total number of cases	Rate/ 100,000	Comment
Castillo & Jenkins (8)	U.S.	1980–89	7581	0.71	Average annual rate
Windau & Toscano (50)	U.S.	1992	1004	0.84[a]	Uses CFOI for case finding (see reference)
Toscano (40)	U.S.	1993	1063	0.88[a]	Uses CFOI for case finding (see reference)
Kraus (26)	CA	1979–81	466	1.5	Average annual rate using death certificate plus verification
Cone et al (12)	CA	1983	131	1.05	Death certificate and investigative files of Cal/OSHA
Sniezek & Horiagon (36)	NC	1978–84	181	0.99	Average annual rate based on medical examiner records
Davis (15)	TX	1975–84	964	1.53	Average annual rate derived from original papers
Richardson (35)	TX	1990–91	199	1.25[a]	Average annual rate derived from original report and separate BLS employment data
Stone (38)	SC	1989–90	35	1.12	Average annual rate using death certificates
Hales et al (20)	Ohio	1983–85	50	1.3	Average annual rate using workers compensation data

[a] Rates calculated using published case numbers and 1992 and 1993 BLS US employment data (40, 50)

and other vehicles were combined as transportation and ranked first in occurrence. Homicide was the second most commonly found cause (17%), followed by falls (10%), and contact with or struck by objects and equipment (9%).

Findings on Incidence: Homicide, States

Maryland   Baker and associates published an evaluation in 1982 of all work-related fatal injuries in 1978 in the state of Maryland (2). Records of the office of the Chief Medical Examiner of Maryland were searched. Case finding excluded suicides and children under 15 years of age. Shootings accounted for 11% of the total of 148 cases identified. No rates were calculated.

California and Texas   In 1987, two reports appeared in the public health literature identifying for the first time work-related homicide and their unique characteristics. In the California study an algorithm was developed utilizing the death certificate, and where appropriate, query of pertinent county coroners (26). Texas death certificates were studied similarly (15, 16). In California, Kraus reported an average annual work-related homicide rate of 1.5/100,000 workers for 1979–81 (26), whereas in Texas, Davis reported an average annual rate of 1.53 per 100,000 workers per year (15, 16) (see Table 2).

North and South Carolina   Sniezek & Horiagon reported that homicide accounted for about 17% of the 1091 work-related injury deaths in North Carolina in 1978–84 (36). Stone evaluated deaths in South Carolina for 1989 and 1990 (38). Homicide was the second leading cause with an overall rate of 1.12 per 100,000 workers, or about 13% of the total.

Texas   Results of the CFOI pilot study undertaken in Texas for 1990 and 1991 (35) showed an overall average annual incidence of homicide while at work of 1.25 per 100,000 employed persons per year.

Findings from these four states (California, Texas, North and South Carolina) are not strictly comparable because of differences in times of study, methods used for case identification, and qualifications for eligibility. However, despite these difficulties, the overall rate of occurrence of work-related homicide can be estimated at from 0.7 to 1.5 per 100,000 employed persons per year.

Findings on Nonfatal Work-Related Assault Injuries

Table 3 summarizes the years of data collection, the number of cases reported, and the average annual rate per 1000 employed persons for five reports on nonfatal work-related assaultive injuries. An elevated estimate of nonfatal

Table 3 Number and rate per 100,000 of nonfatal work-related assaultive injuries, selected US studies

Author/Source (reference)	Location	Year(s)	Number of cases reported	Rate or average annual rate per 1000	Comment
Bachman (1)	U.S.	1987–92	159,094	2.4[a]	Self-reported survey, rate based on 1990 work-force
Hales et al (20)	Ohio	1983–85	192	0.43	Excludes rape and homicide
Northwestern National Life Insurance (33)	U.S.	July 92–July 93	18	2.2	Survey of 600 persons with response to "physical attack"
Cal/OSHA (7)	California	1992	6549	0.47[b]	Based on OSHA 200 log cases
BLS (47)	U.S.	1992	22,400	0.18[c]	Includes rape, threats—all cases resulting in at least one day away from work

[a] Based on 109,419,000 employees in nonfarm US workforce of 1990 (46).
[b] Based on 13,805,000 employed persons in California, 1992 (48).
[c] Based on 119,583,000 employed persons in US workforce in 1992 (50).

injuries from the Northwestern National Life Insurance Company survey (33) was based on a sample of only 18 individuals.

According to data from the National Crime Victimization Survey of 1987–1992 (1), approximately 1 million victimizations occurred annually while persons were at work. Slightly less than 160,000 (16%) of these resulted in injuries, 10% of which required medical care. Simple asaults, which constituted more than two thirds of the total, resulted in injuries to one out of every seven victims; aggravated assaults resulted in injuries to one out of every five victims; robberies resulted in injuries to one out of every four victims. These data from approximately 100,000 persons in the United States were self-reported and not verified. Multiple episodes to the same person were not identified and half of all episodes were *not* reported to police.

Risk Markers

GENDER-SPECIFIC HOMICIDE OCCURRENCE   Work-related homicide rates are disproportionate to the percentage of the workforce by gender. Work-related homicide rates are 3.0 to 5.6 times higher for males compared with females

Table 4 Rate, rate ratios, and percent of all work-related injury deaths due to homicide, by gender, selected US studies

Source/Author (reference)	Year(s)	Homicide rate per 100,000 Male	Female	Rate ratio Male to female	Homicide as a percent of all work-related injury deaths Male	Female
Castillo & Jenkins (8)	1980–89	1.02	0.33	3.1	10	41
Windau & Toscano[a] (50)	1992	1.17	0.32	3.7	15	40
Kraus (26)	1979–81	2.2	0.5	4.2	11	44
Davis (15)	1975–84	2.1	0.7	3.0	13	53
Richardson (35)	1990–91	1.9	0.4	4.8	—	—
Sniezek (36)	1978–84	1.7	0.3	5.6	15	57
Cal/OSHA (7)	1992–93	1.95	0.40	4.9	30	48
Stone (38)	1989–90	—	—	—	10	56
Toscano[a] (40)	1993	1.32	0.35	3.8	15	40

[a] Rates calculated using published case numbers and employment data for 1992 and 1993 (references).
—Not reported

(see Table 4). However, proportionate mortality due to homicide is significantly higher for females compared with males. For example, approximately 10 to 30% of all male work-related fatal injury deaths are due to homicide compared with between 40 to 57% of female work-related deaths.

AGE- AND GENDER-SPECIFIC HOMICIDE WORK-RELATED RATES   To date only three published studies have given age-specific at-work homicide rates. US data (44, 50) show age-specific rates of 0.4 to 0.9 per 100,000 employed until age 65 when the rates increase appreciably to 1.7 to 1.9 per 100,000. California

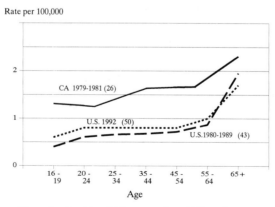

Figure 2 Age-specific work-related homicide rates; selected US studies.

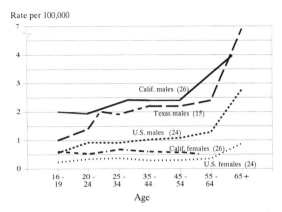

Rate per 100,000

Figure 3   Age- and sex-specific work-related homicide rates; selected US studies.

data (26) are consistently higher and show little variation across age groups (1.25 to 1.67 per 100,000) until over age 64 when the rate exceeds 2.25 per 100,000 employed (see Figure 2).

Figure 3 shows age- and gender-specific rates from three studies. The highest rates are for Texas and California males over age 65. Rates are about at the same level by age from about 25 to age 64 in all studies. The rates for females are appreciably lower than males for all ages.

HOMICIDE AND RACE/ETHNICITY   Little information is available on the incidence (or rate ratio) of homicide in the workplace according to racial or ethnic group. Using NIOSH data from 1980–1985, Bell reported that the rate for employed non-whites was 1.8 times higher than the rate for employed whites (4). Later data from NIOSH for 1980–89 show the rate for employed Blacks is 2.4 times higher than for employed whites and slightly less than the rate for all other races (45).

Data for Texas males show that the rate was highest among employed of "other" racial or ethnic groups (15). The rate for Black employed persons was 1.6 times higher than for whites, and the rate for Hispanics was 1.3 times higher than the rate for "other" whites. In North Carolina, the rate for non-white employed were only slightly higher than for white employed (1.1 vs 0.9 per 100,000 workers) (36). Recent data for 1992 and 1993 from the BLS for the U.S. show the frequencies (and rates) are higher for employed Black persons compared with employed white persons and the rate for employed Hispanics is higher than other employed whites or Blacks (40, 50).

MAJOR FINDINGS ON RISK FACTORS

Industries, Occupations, and Work-places at High Risk

GENERAL INDUSTRY DIVISIONS   Data from the U.S., California, and Texas are generally comparable in reporting homicide rates for general US Industry Divisions (see Table 5). The findings also show general agreement in rank; for example, rates are highest across all reports for persons employed in retail trade. All reports but the California and Texas studies show elevated homicide rates for those employed in transportation, communication, and public utilities. Rates exceed the overall average in most reports for those employed in public administration (a category that includes police and protective services). Homicide rates are consistently below the overall rate for those employed in manufacturing, finance/real estate, agriculture/forestry/fisheries/mining, and construction. Homicide rates by industry division, unfortunately, do not give precise information about tasks/activities or exposures.

GENERAL OCCUPATIONAL DIVISIONS   Only three reports are completely consistent in classifying occupational divisions, so comparisons of homicide rates across occupation are necessarily limited (see Table 5). US findings for 1980–89 show those employed as laborers or material handlers or involved in sales, transportation, service of all kinds, and executive/administrative/managerial positions are at highest risk of homicide while at work. Data from the BLS for 1992 and 1993 generally show similar rates by occupations listed above. One exception is that of executive/administrative/or managerial occupations, where the rate is about the same or lower than the overall average rates. Data from California are consistent with highest rates in service and laborer/material handling occupations.

Although findings on general industrial or occupational divisions give some clues as to the general types of workplace settings that may be at elevated risk of homicide, information on specific industries and occupations is far more useful for identifying high-risk exposures and possible interventions. Six reports identify police/detectives with very high rates, and five of the six reports show that taxicab drivers and chauffeurs are at extreme risk (see Table 6). Five reports show homicide risks are excessive to those employed in eating and drinking places. Several reports show sheriffs, bailiffs and other law enforcement officials, security guards, service station employees, stock handlers and baggers, bartenders, and sales personnel to be at high risk of homicide. While these findings give additional information on occupations and occupational settings that are hazardous, specific details of exposure remain largely unknown.

Table 5 Rate of work-related homicide deaths by industry and occupational divisions, selected US studies

Industry	Castillo NIOSH 1980–89 (8)	Kraus CA 1979–81 (26)	Davis[a] TX 1975–84 (15)	Sniezek & Horiagon[a] NC 1978–84 (36)	Windau & Toscano BLS 1992 (50)	Toscano & Windau BLS 1993 (40)
Agriculture/Forestry/ Fishing/Mining	0.54	1.09	1.0	**1.2**	0.38	0.29
Construction	0.38	1.13	1.4	0.3	0.39	0.31
Manufacturing	0.28	0.67	0.4	0.5	0.18	0.22
Transport	**0.93**	1.43	**2.0**	**1.1**	**2.00**	**1.86**
Wholesale Trade	0.25	1.33	0.5	—	0.37	0.46
Retail Trade	**1.57**	**3.30**	**6.2**	**3.6**[d]	**2.50**	**2.57**
Finance/Real Estate	0.35	0.73	1.3	0.3	0.53	0.41
Service	0.39	0.80	**1.8**[b]	**3.1**	0.57	0.50
Public Administration	**1.42**	**2.93**	**4.6**	—	0.57	0.64
Managerial/professional	0.24	1.31	—	—	0.26	0.31
Executive/administrative	**0.85**	—	—	—	**0.91**	0.76
Technical	0.13	—	—	—	—	—
Sales	**1.33**	1.13	—	—	2.13	**2.46**
Administrative support	0.18	—	—	—	0.18	0.23
Service	**0.98**	2.99	—	—	**1.40**	1.29
Farm/fish/forest	0.51	1.17	—	—	0.40	—
Prod/craft/repair	0.38	1.14	—	—	0.31	0.48
Machine operators	0.19	—	—	—	0.09	—
Transportation	**1.23**	—	—	—	2.76	2.56
Handlers . . . laborers	**1.37**	**1.64**	—	—	1.32	1.15
Overall[c]	0.71	1.50	1.67	1.02	0.84	0.88

[a] Male work-related homicides
[b] Combines business/repair/personal and/professional services using original published data
[c] Includes all other occupations not specifically listed
[d] Includes wholesale trade
— Not reported
Bold = in excess of overall average rate

WAGE/SALARY VS SELF EMPLOYED   One approach to identifying and describing high-risk workers is to stratify the workforce as wage and salary earners or self-employed. Data from the 1992 and 1993 CFOI and California suggest that the self-employed have over three times the risk of homicide while at work compared with wage and salary earners (26, 40, 50).

EMPLOYED POPULATIONS AT EXTREME RISK   The public health literature of the past decade has suggested that two employed populations are at extreme risk of homicide while at work: women and men at least age 65. These two groups are especially vulnerable because they may be viewed as easy targets

Table 6 Occupations and workplaces with highest homicide rates per 100,000 employed persons, selected US studies

Occupations	Castillo US 1980–89 (8)	Toscano US 1993 (40)	Windau & Toscano US 1992 (50)	Kraus CA 1979–81 (26)	Davis TX[a] 1975–84 (15)	Hales et al OH 1983–85 (20)
Taxicab drivers[b]	15.1	42.7	40.2	19.0	36.9	—
Police/detectives	9.0	6.1	5.3	20.8	25.7	25.2
Sheriffs & related	10.9	—	—	—	44.4	—
Hotel clerks	5.1	—	—	—	—	—
Service station	4.5	—	—	—	11.4	—
Security guards	3.6	—	—	16.5	11.0	17.2
Stockhandlers/baggers	3.1	—	—	—	11.0	—
Supervisors/proprietors	2.8	—	—	9.7	15.9	—
Managers/administrators	—	—	—	—	3.7	—
Bartenders	2.1	—	—	3.7	—	—
Sales personnel	2.1	—	—	4.6	—	—
Bus drivers	—	—	—	3.2	—	—
Janitors	—	—	—	2.7	—	—
Truck drivers	—	—	—	2.4	—	—
Construction/laborers	—	—	—	—	51	—
Barbers	2.2	—	—	—	—	—
Correctional officers	1.5	—	—	—	—	—
Workplaces						
Liquor stores	8.0	—	—	—	—	—
Food stores[c]	3.2	3.0	5.0	—	11.9	6.1
Eating/drinking places	1.5	2.5	2.1	—	7.0	2.0
Gasoline/service stations	5.6	2.6	1.9	—	14.2	17.7
Jewelry stores	3.2	—	—	—	—	—
Hotel/motels	1.54	—	—	—	7.5	24.1
Overall[d]	0.7	0.8	0.9	1.5	2.1	1.3

[a] Includes chauffeurs
[b] Male employed
[c] Includes grocery stores
[d] Includes all occupations and industries
— Not reported

offering no resistance, or perceived as having less of an inclination to interfere in the course of a robbery.

Women   In assessing homicide rates for employed women, it must be kept in mind that, on average, women may work fewer hours than men; hence the lower rates found for females may not properly reflect person/time exposure. Social acceptance notwithstanding, the highest-risk occupation (based on informal conversation with police agencies) is prostitution. Although in parts of the US prostitution is a legal enterprise, consistent practice in city and county agencies investigating homicides of prostitutes has been to avoid classifying them as "work-related" or "injury at work."

Homicide is the leading work-related external cause of death for all females in reports from Texas (16) and in the entire U.S. (3, 45). Davis reports that except for construction, transportation, and manufacturing, homicide was the leading external cause of injury deaths for females in all industries in Texas (16). Davis reports further that the rates among females were exceptionally high among women involved in sales, clerking, or management of food stores, bars, and cafes. NIOSH has reported that 30% of all fatal injuries at work for employed females involve homicide and are concentrated in three major industries: grocery stores, eating and drinking establishments, and public safety (8).

The older employed   All reports that provide age information on work-related homicide rates show that those 65 years of age and older have the highest rates recorded (27, 36). Especially vulnerable to assault and murder are those working as cooks, bartenders, and security guards. These persons are generally retired from their usual occupation and work part-time to enhance retirement income or to keep active. For persons in this age group, effective interventions may require assessment of workplace circumstances and exposures and reassignment of such persons to less hazardous times, workplaces, and activities.

Other Risk Factors

Only a single study has reported blood or cerebral spinal fluid alcohol levels among homicide victims killed while at work (15). Eighty-one percent of those who were tested within 4 hours of the time of death showed zero blood alcohol or cerebral spinal fluid levels. Ten percent showed a level of 0.10 gms/dl or higher, prima facie evidence of intoxication in most states. Alcohol levels were particularly high among males working in eating and drinking places, where more than 31% of employed in such businesses had an alcohol level of 0.10 gms/dl or higher. Much more information is needed on this factor, particularly among those exposed to opportunity for consumption of alcohol during their normal work-shift.

Findings from Cross-Sectional Surveys of Injury at Work from Violence-Related Causes

Virginia   A survey undertaken in 1991 of police department and sheriff's offices throughout the state of Virginia sought to determine the extent and severity of violent crime in convenience stores (49). Ninety-six percent of the

1020 violent crimes reported involved robbery or attempted robbery. Since a reference population was not indicated, the rates of events could not be calculated and interpretation of the findings is necessarily constrained.

United States   Between 1989 and 1990 the National Association of Convenience Stores (NACS) analyzed 1204 questionnaires from its members (31). Ratios of 1.1 (1989) and 1.4 (1990) homicides per 1000 convenience stores were reported. Two thirds of the homicides involved a robbery, 65% occurred at night from 11 p.m. to 6 a.m., and firearms were used in more than 70% of the cases.

The Northwestern National Life Insurance Company undertook a telephone survey of a sample of 600 full-time employees in the United States, excluding military or those who were self-employed (33). Details of the sample base and the response rate were not provided, and the numbers reported suggest wide confidence intervals. Information was requested from each respondent for both the previous 12 months and for life-time occurrence. Fifteen percent of workers said that they had been physically attacked sometime during their working life and of this group 18% were attacked with a lethal weapon. Among the respondents, 44% indicated that the perpetrator was a customer or client and 27% that the perpetrator was a co-worker or supervisor.

Time, Place, and Circumstances of Work-Related Injuries

Time   Seven studies report either month, day-of-week, or hours of peak occurrence of fatal and nonfatal work-related assault or injuries (3, 15, 20, 24, 26, 35, 36). While the distribution of homicides over the months of the year is relatively even, three reports providing data on day-of-the-week have inconsistent findings. North Carolina data show that homicides were evenly distributed over the week (36), whereas data from Texas for 1975–84 show that over 70% of all homicides occurred between Monday and Friday (15). A later report from this same state suggests highest frequency days were Mondays, Wednesdays, and Saturdays (35). Across all seven studies occurrence of homicide or nonfatal assault was far more frequent in the afternoon and evening hours than late morning or early afternoon hours. It must be noted, however, that a substantial proportion of all cases in the various studies had no hour of occurrence reported.

Place (state or city)   Data from NIOSH for 1980–89 show that the highest reported work-related homicide rate is found in the state of Florida (45). Furthermore, homicide accounts for more than 30% of all work-related fatal injuries in Florida, New York, Nevada, and California, as well as New York City and Washington, D.C. Caution must be exercised in interpreting these

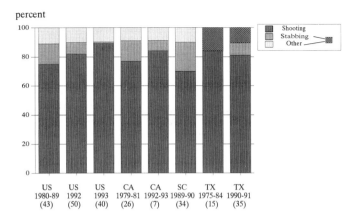

percent

Figure 4   Percent homicide while at work by manner of death; selected US studies.

findings since rates and proportions have not been adjusted for age, gender, and race.

The BLS has reported homicides for 10 of the largest Metropolitan Statistical Areas (MSA) in the United States for 1992 (50). Rates are much higher than the overall average for the United States (0.84/100,000) for New York City–Northern New Jersey–Long Island (1.7), Los Angeles–Anaheim–Riverside (1.2), Dallas–Fort Worth (1.6), and Miami–Fort Lauderdale (1.4). Work-related homicide in these four Metropolitan Statistical Areas are 45, 31, 29, and 33% of all work-related fatalities in these MSAs, respectively.

Manner of death   The exact cause of homicide has been reported in eight reports and includes shooting, stabbing, or other external causes. All reports are consistent in one finding: In excess of 70% of all work-related homicides involve a firearm (see Figure 4). Stabbing or cutting with sharp and piercing objects is the second most frequently reported cause in most studies. Other but much less frequent causes include blunt objects such as clubs.

Circumstances   According to BLS data for 1992 and 1993, homicide while at work was a direct result of a robber or other felon in from 75 to 82% of the cases (40, 50) (see Table 7). Findings for California and Texas are substantially less, from 37 to 48% (15, 16, 26). Worker-on-worker homicides committed by current or former employees is only from 4 to 10%. Note, however, that a high percent of cases in the California and Texas reports have no known motivation for homicide. These findings have particular significance for guiding exploration of potential interventions. For example, efforts at curtailing

Table 7   Homicide victim-perpetrator relationship, percent of cases in selected US studies

	Study (references)				
Victim-perpetrator relationship	Toscano & Windau U.S. 1992 (50)	Windau & Toscano U.S. 1993 (40)	Cal/OSHA CA 1992–1993 (7)	Davis TX 1975–84[a] (15)	Richardson TX 1990–91 (35)
Robber/other felon	82	75	45	48	37
Client/customer	4	4	14	21	3
Current/former co-worker	4	6	5	10	6
Relative/acquaintence	4	4	3	3	—
Others/unknown	6[a]	11[a]	34	18	54[b]

[a] Male employed
[b] Includes safety personnel killed in line of duty
— Not reported

robberies at the worksite would be far more effective in reducing the overall magnitude of the injury problem than trying to identify employees with a significant grudge who might choose to express their hostility at work.

Summary of High-Risk Markers, Factors, and Circumstances for Assault While at Work

Table 8 summarizes factors from available evidence to date that may be indisputably important in formulation of specific countermeasures. Unfortunately, most of these factors are vague in description and provide little from which to fashion specific interventions. Much more detailed study about risk factors is needed. Other important evidence is available, although not in the form of measures of effect, within a group of studies of convenience store robberies over the past 20 years.

Evidence of Risk Factors for Convenience Stores

Although not gleaned through standard epidemiologic methods, much of what is known about risk factors for homicide in the workplace is derived from two decades of studies of convenience stores in the United States. Some findings are provocative and informative, and may shed light on directions for future research.

The first study to identify potential risk factors for robbery and assault was undertaken by Crow & Bull in the early 1970s (13). Their approach was to analyze reports of over 17,600 robberies to convenience stores in the five counties of southern California. In addition, on-site surveys of 120 stores were

Table 8   Summary of high-risk markers, factors, and circumstances for homicide at work

Risk markers	
Age	Highest rates among older employed
Gender	Male rate 3–6 times rate of females but females are more likely to be murdered at work than males
Race/Ethnicity/ Place	Black and Hispanic employed have higher rates than white employed
Risk factors	
Manner of Death	Those killed while at work are more frequently shot
Industry	Employed in retail trades (sales), public administration (security, safety, protection) or transportation
Occupation/worksite	Employed as sales/clerk personnel in food stores, liquor stores, eating or drinking places; taxi drivers; police; sheriff or security guards; laborers, workers, or supervisors in gas stations or hotels and motels
Time	Hours of highest risk are late afternoon, evening, or late at night, especially from 10 P.M. to 2 A.M.
Location	Rates are high in one state and several metropolitan statistical areas
Circumstances	
Type of exposure	Killed in course of robbery

undertaken with an ex-robber as a member of the survey team. Some of the salient features of robbery/homicide from this evaluation were:

- The ratio of homicide in the workplace to robberies was 1: 256
- Ninety-five percent of reported robberies resulted in no physical injury
- The average number of robberies per day was highest in the months of November and September
- Robberies were most frequent on Sundays but occur every day
- Sixty-five percent of robberies were from 9 p.m. to 3 a.m., the period with fewest customers
- Robbery is perpetrated by strangers, not acquaintances
- Socioeconomic status of the neighborhood was not related to robbery frequency.

On the basis of those studies, the following were proposed as important risk factors for a robbery and, hence, murder and assault in convenience stores: amount of cash available; poor lighting levels at remote points and on-site; obstructions and reduced visibility in and around the store; lack of security devices such as mirrors; and easy accessibility and escape routes, among others (see Table 9). Strategies to correct these factors were ultimately adopted by 60 experimental stores and tested against a control group of 60 similar stores chosen randomly. The group of countermeasures, termed "crime-prevention

Table 9 Risk factors associated with convenience store robberies, selected US Studies

Risk factors	Crow & Bull (13)	Crow, Erickson, & Scott (14)	Swanson (39)	Jeffery, Hunter, & Griswold (23)	Clifton & Callahan (11)	NACS (31)	Virginia Crime Prevention Center (49)
Lots of money	yes	yes	yes	yes	—	—	—
Easy access and getaway	yes	yes	yes	yes	—	—	—
Female clerk	—	no	yes	—	—	yes	yes
Obstructed windows/no visibility	yes	yes	yes	yes	—	—	yes
No back room	—	—	yes	—	—	—	—
Type of safe/easily accessible	yes	yes	yes	—	—	—	—
Single clerk on duty	—	no	yes	yes	yes	no	yes
No customers in store	—	no	yes	—	yes	—	—
No alarm system	—	no	yes	—	—	—	—
Poor exterior lighting	yes	yes	yes	yes	—	—	—
Cash register/service area not visible from street/not in center of store	yes	yes	—	yes	—	—	—
Remote location of business/no other businesses or traffic	yes	yes	yes	yes	—	—	—
Only one car in front	—	—	yes	—	—	—	—
No gas pumps in front	—	—	yes	yes	—	—	—
Late store hours	—	—	—	no	yes	yes	yes
No mirrors in store	yes	—	—	no	—	—	—
No video in store	—	no	yes	—	—	—	—
No camera system	—	no	—	yes	—	—	—
No armed clerk	—	no	—	—	—	—	—
Likelihood of interference/lack of anonymity	—	yes	yes	—	—	—	—

—Not reported

measures," resulted in reduction in robberies of 13 to 18% (depending on the form of analysis), during an eight-month period following their introduction.

In a continuation of this work, Crow, Erickson & Scott interviewed 181 inmates in Texas, California, Illinois, Louisiana, and New Jersey state prisons (14). Although all the interviewees had been convicted for robbery offenses, only 22% of the sample had committed a convenience store robbery, hence the findings were not directly applicable to convenience stores per se. On the basis of these interviews a set of factors were ordered in attractiveness from the robber's point of view. The most important factors were amount of money available, escape route, anonymity, and likelihood of interference. Factors judged least attractive (i.e. deterrents) were an armed clerk, number of clerks in the store, number of customers in the store, a camera system, and alarm system or video recording system. Based upon this information an intervention program was implemented for which follow-up data showed a 65% decrease in robberies. The impact of the program on assault-related injuries was not recorded, however.

Following this early work, a study was undertaken by Swanson using the same interview methodology, focusing exclusively on 65 inmates in four Florida prisons incarcerated for robberies of convenience stores (39). From a very long list of characteristics, the ten most common factors that were "least appealing" to a robbery were: many customers, heavy traffic in front of store, two or more clerks, a back room, male clerk, one-way mirrors, limited escape routes, alarms, clear visibility into the store, and stores that sell gasoline. The most appealing factors for robberies were: store in remote area, only one clerk, no customers, easy access/get-away, lots of cash, female clerks, no back room, obstructed windows, type of safe, and no alarm. (see Table 9). Unfortunately, none of these factors has been shown unequivocally to be an independent factor in robbery or assault. Swanson concluded that the probability of robbery was lower for work-shifts with more than one clerk, for stores with limited times of operation, for stores with visible cameras, if there were other twenty-four hour stores nearby, and if the store had a time-release safe and the robber knew that fact.

In 1985, the Gainesville, Florida, police department analyzed all information available on convenience store robberies (which represented 50% of all business robberies) (11). Of 47 stores, all but two had been robbed at least once and all but nine had had multiple instances of robbery. At the urging of the police department, a city ordinance was enacted that included the following components: an unobstructed view of the cash register and sales area through windows, conspicuous signs in the windows indicating less than fifty dollars on hand and that a drop-time release safe was present that could not be removed, parking lots lit with an intensity of approximately two-foot candles per square foot, security cameras of a type and number approved by the city manager, and mandatory robber prevention training for all employees who work between 8 p.m. to 4 a.m. While it is not possible to ascertain which factor or combination of factors was effective in the reductions claimed, in one year Gainesville experienced a 64% reduction in convenience store robberies and a 75% reduction in the number of robberies from 8 p.m. to 4 a.m. It should be noted further that the prevented fraction of robberies associated with each factor or combination of factors has not been experimentally tested. Much of the approach in countermeasure development and implementation stems from either common sense or law enforcement experience in robbery deterrence.

Other studies focused on convenience stores have shown similar results. For example, based upon an assessment of environmental factors in a sample of stores, Jeffrey, Hunter & Griswold surmised that high visibility, multiple clerks, internal unobstructed views from outside the store, other commercial property in the vicinity, and stores with good cash-handling were less likely to be robbed (23). Another factor identified by Hunter was the availability of an easy escape route as one of the most important factors in convenience store robbery (22). In addition, Hunter identified the presence of gas pumps, amount of vehicular traffic, increased number of clerks, decreased hours of operation, and locating the cashier in the center of the store as deterrents to robbery and assault.

In 1991, a report by the National Association of Convenience Stores (NACS) presented results of three separate studies on convenience store security (31). The first study was a national survey of robbery experiences of 1256 NACS members during 1989–90. Some of the survey's findings were that robberies were not equally frequent across all stores; fourteen percent of the stores had one robbery, and seven percent had two or more robberies. From the second study it was determined that convenience store homicide rate was 1.05 per 1000 stores in 1989, and 1.37 per 1000 stores in 1990. Almost two thirds of the homicides occurred between 11 p.m. and 6 a.m., and almost thirty percent occurred between 3 a.m. and 4:30 a.m. Almost three quarters of the stores where homicides occurred had been robbed in the past. Eighty-nine percent of the victims were employees while the remainder were customers, and handguns were used in over seventy percent of the cases. The third study found that two clerks on duty, particularly during the night shift, had an effect on reducing the robbery rate, and that one robbery was the best single predictor for a second robbery. Data were insufficient to assess the deterrent effect of bullet-resistant barriers, but color-monitor systems in some stores produced a reduction in robberies of over fifty percent.

Florida's Convenience Store Security Act of 1990 (11) required convenience stores to include silent alarms, security cameras, drop-safes, and cash management devices, and specified security lighting standards for parking lots, signs on limited cash availability, unobstructed views of cash registers, as well as prohibition against window-tinting, height markers for windows and store entrances, robbery training for employees, and limited cash from 9 p.m. to 6 a.m. Further legislation was adopted in 1992 addressing businesses open between 11 p.m. and 5 a.m., especially businesses experiencing murder or robbery. The 1992 Act required additional security measures such as two or more employees on the premises at all times from 11 p.m. to 5 a.m., bullet-resistant safety enclosures, security guard on the premises, and the conduct of business only through an indirect pass-through window or closure the business at all times between the hours of 11 p.m. and 5 a.m. Results of this legislation, which became effective December 30, 1992, are not yet published.

The information on an array of risk factors and countermeasures is confusing and sometimes contradictory. This is not to detract from the importance of these findings but suggests that the sheer variety of information sources may explain disparities between results and differences of opinion. Robbery prevention programs rely on an aggregate of many simultaneous countermeasures aimed at different factors (32). Hence it is not possible to isolate which group of factors is more or less important in deterring robbery and assault.

In terms of countermeasures from a public health perspective, several identified in the contexts of convenience stores may, by extension, have applicability to other businesses such as fast-food restaurants, grocery stores, gas stations, or other businesses.

SUMMARY

Much of what is known about occupations at high risk for assaults and injuries comes from a few peer-reviewed articles and a number of relatively obscure documents or special studies within subsets of exposures (e.g. convenience stores). The literature on violence in health care settings and to police and security personnel is growing. There is reference to violent injury in Canada (30) and recent recognition of the problem in parts of Europe.

The prospects for control and reduction of violence while people work are probably better than most because of the potential to incorporate environmental, behavioral, training, and regulatory approaches to reduce risk. Unfortunately, in large measure the potency of specific countermeasures for prevention of violence-related injury remains unknown. Seldom have experimental "trials" been designed as randomized trials of specific risk-factor modifications. Numerous fundamental questions remain: Critical is a full assessment of risk, identification of situations and circumstances amenable to intervention, and evaluations to demonstrate effectiveness.

ACKNOWLEDGMENT

The authors wish to thank Carmen Mendoza for suggestions on earlier drafts and Dena Herman for assistance in graphic design.

Literature Cited

1. Bachman R. 1994. *Violence and Theft in the Workplace.* US Dep. Justice, Bur. Justice Stat., No. NCJ-148199
2. Baker SP, Samkoff JS, Fisher RS, Van Buren CB. 1982. Fatal occupational injuries. *J. Am. Med. Assoc.* 248:692–97
3. Bell CA. 1991. Female homicides in United States workplaces, 1980–1985. *Am. J. Public Health* 81:729–32
4. Bell CA, Stout NA, Bender TR, Conroy CS, Crouse WE, Myers JR. 1990. Fatal occupational injuries in the United States, 1980 through 1985. *J. Am. Med. Assoc.* 263:3047–50
5. Braverman M, Braverman SR. 1994. Seeking solutions to violence on the job. *USA Today,* May, 122(2588):29
6. Calif. Dep. Ind. Relat., Div. Occup. Saf. Health. 1994. *Cal/OSHA Guidelines for Workplace Security*
7. Calif. Dep. Ind. Relat., Div. Labor Stat. Res., 1992–93. Manuscript in preparation
8. Castillo DN, Jenkins EL. 1994. Industries and occupations at high risk for work-related homicide. *J. Occup. Med.* 36:125–32
9. Cembrowicz SP, Shepherd JP. 1992. Violence in the accident and emergency department. *Med. Sci. Law* 32:118–22
10. Cent. Dis. Control Prev. 1985. Fatal occupational injuries—Texas, 1982. *Morbid. Mortal. Wkly. Rep.* 34:130–39
11. Clifton W Jr, Callahan PT. 1991. *Convenience Store Robberies: An Intervention Strategy by the City of Gainesville, Florida.* Gainesville FL Police Dep.
12. Cone JE, Daponte A, Makoofsky D, Reiter R, Becker C, et al. 1991. Fatal injuries at work in California. *J. Occup. Med.* 33:813–16
13. Crow WJ, Bull JL. 1975. *Robbery Deterrence: An Applied Behavioral Science Demonstration.* La Jolla, CA: West. Behav. Sci. Inst.
14. Crow WJ, Erickson RJ, Scott L. 1987. Set your sights on preventing retail violence. *Secur. Manag.* 31:60–64
15. Davis H. 1987. Workplace homicides of Texas males. *Am. J. Public Health* 77:1290–93
16. Davis H, Honchar PA, Suarez L. 1987. Fatal occupational injuries of women, Texas 1975–84. *Am. J. Public Health* 77:1524–27
17. Dietz PE, Baker SP. 1987. Murder at work. *Am. J. Public Health* 77:1273–74
18. Duh RW, Asal NR. 1984. Mortality among laundry and dry cleaning workers in Oklahoma. *Am. J. Public Health* 74:1278–80
19. Gallagher RP, Threlfall WJ, Spinelli JJ, Band PR. 1984. Occupational mortality patterns among British Columbia farm workers. *J. Occup. Med.* 26:906–8
20. Hales T, Seligman PJ, Newman SC, Timbrook CL. 1988. Occupational injuries due to violence. *J. Occup. Med.* 30:483–87
21. Howell E, Brown K, Atkins J. 1990. Trauma in the workplace. An overview. *AAOHN J.* 38:467–74
22. Hunter R. 1988. *The relationships of selected environmental characteristics to the incidence of convenience store robbery within the state of Florida.* PhD thesis. Florida State Univ.
23. Jeffrey CR, Hunter RD. 1992. Preventing convenience store robbery through environmental design. In *Situational Crime Prevention: Successful Case Studies,* ed. RV Clarke, chap. 6. Albany, NY: Harrow & Heston
24. Jenkins EL, Layne LA, Kisner SM. 1992. Homicide in the workplace. The U.S. experience, 1980–1988. *AAOHN J.* 40:215–18

25. Johnson DL. 1993. The best defense against workplace violence. *Wall Street J.*, July 19, A14(10), A10(E)
26. Kraus JF. 1987. Homicide while at work: Persons, industries, and occupations at high risk. *Am. J. Public Health* 77:1285–89
27. Kraus JF, Macurda J, Sahl J, Anderson C. 1990. Work-related fatal injuries in older California workers, 1979–1985. *J. Occup. Accid.* 12:223–35
28. Lavoie FW, Cater GL, Danzl DF, Berg RL. 1988. Emergency department violence in United States teaching hospitals. *Ann. Emerg. Med.* 17:1227–33
29. Lipscomb JA, Love CC. 1992. Violence toward health care workers. An emerging occupational hazard. *AAOHN J.* 40: 219–28
30. Liss GM, Craig CA. 1990. Homicide in the workplace in Ontario: occupations at risk and limitations of existing data sources. *Can. J. Public Health* 81:10–15
31. Natl. Assoc. Convenience Stores. 1991. *Convenience Store Security: Complete Text Reports with Summary.* Alexandria, VA: Natl. Assoc. Conv. Stores
32. Natl. Safe Workplace Inst. 1987. *Understanding Crime Prevention.* Stoneham, MA: Butterworth
33. Northwest. Natl. Life Insur. Co., Employee Benefits Div. 1993. *Fear and Violence in the Workplace.* Minneapolis, MN
34. Pollack ES, Gellerman Keimig D, eds. 1987. *Counting Injuries and Illnesses in the Workplace: Proposals for a Better System.* Washington, DC: Natl. Acad. Press
35. Richardson S. 1993. Workplace homicides in Texas, 1990–91. *US Dep. Labor, Bur. Labor Stat. Rep. 845*
36. Sniezek JE, Horiagon TM. 1989. Medical-examiner-reported fatal occupational injuries, North Carolina, 1978–1984. *Am. J. Ind. Med.* 15:669–78
37. Solomon J, King P, Friday C, Annin P, De Silva DR, et al. 1993. Waging war in the workplace. *Newsweek,* July 19, 22(3):30
38. Stone PW. 1993. Traumatic occupational fatalities in South Carolina, 1989–90. *Public Health Rep.* 108:483–88
39. Swanson R. 1986. *Convenience store robbery analysis: A research study of robbers, victims, and environment.* Gainesville FL Police Dep.
40. Toscano G. 1994. National census of fatal occupational injuries, 1993. *US Dep. Labor, Bur. Labor Stat., USDL-94-384*
41. Toscano G, Windau J. 1993. Fatal work injuries: Results from the 1992 national census. *Mon. Labor Rev.* Oct:39–48
42. Toufexis A. 1994. Workers who fight firing with fire. *Time,* April 25, 143(17): 34
43. United States Code, Section 651(b) (The Occupational Health and Safety Act, 1970)
44. US Dep. Health Hum. Serv., Public Health Serv., Cent. Dis. Control Prev., Natl. Inst. Occup. Saf. Health. 1993. *Fatal Injuries to Workers in the United States, 1980–1989: A Decade of Surveillance.* Cincinnati: DHHS (NIOSH) Publ. No. 93–108
45. US Dep. Health Hum. Serv., Public Health Serv., Cent. Dis. Control and Prevention, Natl. Inst. Occup. Saf. Health. 1993. *NIOSH Alert: Request for Assistance in Preventing Homicide in the Workplace.* DHHS (NIOSH) Publ. No. 93–109
46. US Dep. Labor, Bur. Labor Stat. 1994. *Employment and Earnings,* Vol. 41, no. 8
47. US Dep. Labor, Bur. Labor Stat. 1994. *Violence in the Workplace Comes under Closer Scrutiny.* Summary 94–10
48. US Dep. Labor, Bur. Labor Stat. 1993. *Geographic Profile of Employment and Unemployment.* Bull. 2428
49. VA Crime Prevention Cent., Dep. Crim. Justice Serv. 1993. *Violent Crimes in Convenience Stores: Analysis of Crimes, Criminals and Costs.* Richmond, VA. House Doc. No. 30
50. Windau J, Toscano G. 1994. *Workplace Homicides in 1992.* US Dep. Labor, Bur. Labor Stat.

Annu. Rev. Public Health 1995.16:381–400

METHODOLOGICAL CHALLENGES IN INJURY EPIDEMIOLOGY AND INJURY PREVENTION RESEARCH

Peter Cummings, Thomas D. Koepsell, and Beth A. Mueller

Department of Epidemiology, School of Public Health and Community Medicine, University of Washington and the Harborview Injury Prevention and Research Center, Seattle, Washington 98104-2499

KEY WORDS: accidents, classification, epidemiologic methods, research design, social class

ABSTRACT

In the past decade there has been increasing attention to the public health importance of injuries. Public health agencies seeking to reduce injuries need methods for counting injuries, calculating injury rates, identifying the causes of injuries, and measuring outcomes of interventions. All of these areas present problems for injury epidemiologists and injury prevention programs. This paper provides a framework for classifying these problems into five categories: (*a*) numerator problems; (*b*) denominator problems; (*c*) causation; (*d*) exposure measurement problems; and (*e*) multiplicity. For most problems, we identify proven or potential solutions, using examples from the literature of injury epidemiology.

INTRODUCTION

The Centers for Disease Control and Prevention and many state and local health departments have made prevention of intentional and unintentional injuries a high priority (9, 86, 112, 115). Epidemiologists in public health agencies and their academic colleagues increasingly are involved in injury research, in the belief that a public health approach can decrease injury morbidity and mortality. This paper reviews challenges in research design and analysis that have special importance to the study of the causes of injuries.

381

0163-7525/95/0510-0381$05.00

Numerator problems include definition, classification, and ascertainment, complicated by the wide spectrum of injury severity, the multiple dimensions for categorization, and the need to consider intent. *Denominator problems* include matching numerators to denominators and choosing the most appropriate among several candidate denominators. *Causation* issues involve implications of the multicausal nature of injuries for study design, especially choice of the unit of study. *Exposure measurement problems* entail the use of proxy information for the study of injuries that may be rapidly fatal or disabling, the socially sensitive nature of some exposures, and the need to consider and measure social class as a key confounder. Finally, *multiplicity* refers to the fact that one person may sustain multiple injuries simultaneously, injuries may recur for the same individual, and multiple cases can arise from the same catastrophic event.

Although none of these issues is unique to injury research, all have particular relevance to the study of injuries. Our purpose is to familiarize investigators with these special problems and to describe some approaches for dealing with them. We also call attention to areas in which further methodological research would be fruitful.

NUMERATOR PROBLEMS

Numerator issues are related to our ability to count injuries.

Definition of Injury

Just defining some injuries can be a problem. The dictionary defines drowning as death due to suffocation in liquid. The International Classification of Diseases, 9th Revision (ICD-9), has one diagnostic code, 994.1, which covers both drowning and nonfatal submersion (84). Some authors in the medical literature use the term "drowning" to refer to death within 24 hours of submersion, whereas they use "near-drowning" to refer to patients who suffer submersion injury, receive medical care, and survive at least 24 hours (28, 63). This terminology is confusing, because it implies that some people die because of near-drowning. No clear way has been found to define milder episodes of submersion that do not result in either death or medical care. Many people have been underwater at some time in their lives and have experienced a craving for air before surfacing. The dividing line between underwater fun and a mild submersion injury is not clear!

The definition of injury is generally less clear for milder injuries. Death due to motor-vehicle crashes is relatively straightforward. Hospitalization for a crash-related injury depends on the standards used for admission; admission criteria used in the 1970s may not apply in the more cost-conscious era of the 1990s. The introduction of computerized tomography has changed admission practices in some hospitals; patients with head trauma who are neurologically normal and have normal CT scans are now sometimes released, rather than admitted for observation. If emergency department visits are used as a measure of crash-induced injury, then the definition of injury becomes entangled with availability of care and factors that influence care-seeking behavior, including personality, pain tolerance, and anxiety. It is not rare for uninjured patients to come to the emergency department after a car crash because of a desire for reassurance or because of the advice of an insurance agent or attorney.

While most would agree that a gunshot wound and a burn are injuries, it is not so clear that deaths due to poisoning should be classified as injury deaths, although this is commonly done (4). This division, which is used in the ICD-9 manual (84), sometimes draws a fine line; if a child dies from eating foxglove, this is coded as an injury death, but if a child dies from eating botulinum toxin, this is coded as an infectious disease death. Classifying iatrogenic complications as injuries, as is done by the ICD-9, may also not be ideal for some purposes. If a heavy smoker undergoes angiography in preparation for coronary bypass surgery and dies from a reaction to contrast media, the death will be classified as an injury. In one study of risk factors for death due to injury in infants, the researchers chose to exclude iatrogenic deaths, which they felt would not share the same risk factors as deaths that are not caused by complications of medical care (20).

Large cohort studies sometimes report mortality for various causes of death, and customarily classify as injuries all deaths with ICD-9 diagnosis codes between 800 and 999 or any death with an ICD-9 code for external cause of injury. This spectrum of diseases is very broad—lumping deaths due to dental extraction and medications with deaths due to homicide, vehicular crashes, and falls (33, 49). Some cohort studies are so large that they have been able to subdivide their analysis of injury deaths by intent (homicide, suicide, and unintentional) (87), but even these categories are broad. Because etiologic mechanisms may differ among the various injury types within these broad categories, causal associations between particular risk factors and injuries can easily go undetected.

Classification

Depending on the aim of the research, injuries may be classified in several ways. Each scheme has certain strengths and weaknesses and the profusion of schemes can lead to confusion and make it difficult to compare findings between different studies. The most common schemes are based on:

1. Anatomy: e.g. head injury, spinal injury
2. Pathologic mechanism: e.g. fracture, laceration, burn
3. Etiologic mechanism: e.g. gunshot wound, bite wound, iron poisoning

4. Intent: e.g. unintentional, self-induced, assault-related, related to medical treatment
5. Severity: e.g. fatal/nonfatal, Injury Severity Score, revised Trauma Score
6. Event: e.g. car crash, plane crash
7. Location: e.g. work, school
8. Activity: e.g. sports.

The issue of intent uniquely distinguishes injuries from other diseases; no effort is made to classify cancers or infections by intent. Because injuries can be inflicted deliberately on one person by another or on oneself, the study of injuries has strong ties to the criminal justice system and the social and behavioral sciences. The ICD-9 manual includes a list of codes for "external causes of injury and poisoning," commonly referred to as "E-codes." The E-code classification system reflects the desire to assign blame, in keeping with a legal approach to injury. The ICD-9 manual has only one disease code for poisoning due to iron medication (964.0), whereas there are five E-codes for the same poisoning depending on whether it is classified as due to accident (E858.2), suicide attempt (E950.4), assault (E962.0), therapeutic use (E934.0), or undetermined intent (E980.4) (84). [The ICD-9 manual and MEDLINE use the word "accident" for unintentional injuries. Most injury epidemiologists and public health leaders prefer to avoid this word, because they feel it implies that injuries are due to chance and cannot be prevented (86, 115).]

Some health care professionals and others view the prevention of intentional injuries as a social issue that lies outside the field of public health. When injuries are classified solely by intent, as suicides or homicides, many feel the problem must be addressed by experts in psychology or criminology. Classifying injuries by etiologic mechanism may make it easier to see how a more traditional public health approach may apply, including consideration of modifiable environmental and agent-related causes. For example, mortality due to suicide in Birmingham, England, fell by 45% from 1963 to 1969 (47). During this time the average carbon monoxide content of domestic coal gas in the city was reduced from 20% to 2.5%. When suicides were analyzed by method used, investigators found that suicides by coal gas declined from 144 in 1963 to 64 in 1970. Suicides by other methods did not show any compensatory increase. These findings were replicated in other areas of Britain (2, 58). Clearly, some suicides can be prevented without recourse to any mental health or social intervention.

Classifying disease by intent is not a comfortable role for many physicians. Nor is it always an easy task, even for those who are specially trained in forensic pathology. With the introduction of the eighth revision of the *International Classification of Diseases* in 1967 (83), a new category for intent was introduced; "Injury undetermined whether accidentally or purposely inflicted."

With this coding change, the homicide rate for infants (but not other age groups) showed a 25% drop between 1967 and 1968, as many deaths in infants were assigned to the new undetermined category (50). Misclassification of injuries by category of intent is common in some situations. For example, 161 children who died in Connecticut from 1980 to 1985 had a death certificate ICD-9 code for homicide, yet a detailed review of the records for each case failed to find evidence of homicidal intent in 29% of the cases (60). Conversely, investigators in Missouri reviewed deaths among children younger than age 5 and concluded that many deaths caused by homicide or abuse were erroneously coded as unintentional, of undetermined intent, or due to natural causes on the death certificate (27, 75). For children less than one year of age there is the special problem of Sudden Infant Death Syndrome (SIDS); SIDS can be mistaken for either homicide or unintentional injury, and death due to injury can be misclassified as SIDS (111a). One study of 26 cases of apparent SIDS found evidence for injury death due to overlying, asphyxia, or hyperthermia in the majority of cases after investigation of the scene of death (5a). Just how much misclassification occurs and in what direction is not known.

Suicidal intent can be difficult to determine (101); there can be pressure to code acts due to suicidal intent as being unintentional because some family members fear reproach or because some insurance policies will not pay for self-inflicted injuries. Without a suicide note or other evidence of intent, it may be impossible to distinguish unintentional from suicidal death in many automobile crashes. Jobes and colleagues asked medical examiners to classify by intent a real account of a death due to a car crash, and found that among 195 responses, 33% classified the crash as unintentional, 39% felt the crash was an act of suicide, and 28% assigned it to the undetermined category (51).

Grouping injuries by severity is important for studies of outcome. Over a dozen severity scales have been devised, and considerable research has been devoted to this area (13, 14, 36, 71). Despite progress, scoring systems still have problems with inter-observer reliability (36, 123) and missing data in patient records (14, 36). Zoltie and colleagues (123) tested the ability of 15 observers to assign trauma scores to 16 patients and found that survival probability, calculated from the assigned scores, varied by over 0.2 for six of the cases and over 0.5 in three cases. Sometimes patients cannot be properly coded; e.g. Glasgow Coma Score and respiratory rate cannot be measured for intubated or paralyzed patients (36). The Glasgow Coma Score was developed in an era when patients were not brought to the hospital intubated (111); this is now common, so newer scales need to take into account this change in treatment (72). Because patients frequently have more than one injury, it may be difficult to separate the effect of one injury from comorbidity due to other injuries (79).

Because of classification difficulties, authors who use national mortality data find it difficult to determine the number of deaths related to any one illicit drug (103, 121). Heroin-related deaths may be coded as poisoning by opiates or "intravenous narcotism," and they may be coded as unintentional, of undetermined intent, or as being due to "natural causes," depending on information on the death certificate (4, 121). If death is attributed to a substance that contributed to the causal pathway, then many AIDS deaths are classified as poisonings because of the role of intravenous narcotics in transmitting HIV (108, 121).

It is sometimes of interest to study the causes of an injury event rather than the causes of injury, given that an event has occurred. For example, a study might concentrate on the causes of car crashes, plane crashes, or major catastrophes on oil rigs (16), regardless of how many injuries might be caused by each event, or even whether any injuries occur. In such a study the numerator would be the number of events, rather than the number of persons with injuries. To measure the effectiveness of antilock braking systems, it would probably be ideal to compare the incidence of crashes for cars with and without this feature. To determine the effectiveness of seat belts, however, most studies compare the injury experience of belted occupants to that of unbelted occupants, given that a crash has occurred. The investigators' decision to use individuals or events as the unit of study will depend entirely on which class of risk factors is regarded as being of primary interest.

Ascertainment

Some diseases, such as breast cancer or leukemia, almost always result in either a medical encounter and/or death, so complete case ascertainment is a realistic goal. But many injuries do not result in a visit to a health care provider; it is not rare for patients with lacerations or even some kinds of fractures to fail to seek care, and it is common for patients to see no one for contusions or sprains. Thus injury research is usually limited to the tip of the iceberg—those injured persons who die or receive medical care. This situation is illustrated by research on drowning; nearly all studies of submersion have been based on case series of hospitalized patients (18, 21, 80, 91). Population-based studies either have reviewed mortality due to submersion (41, 90, 120) or have collected information on submersion-related deaths and hospitalizations (55, 96). In King County, Washington, investigators found that among 135 children who received prehospital care for submersion, cardiopulmonary resuscitation time greater than 25 minutes or estimated submersion time greater than 25 minutes were always associated with either death or severe neurologic damage (96b), a finding that they confirmed in a series of 77 patients (96a). Thus the study of drowning epidemiology has been the study of patients who either die or are hospitalized due to submersion. Patients who received lesser degrees of care or no care at all after submersion have not been studied, even though their experience might be useful in finding ways to prevent serious injury due to submersion.

Conversely, some studies have focused on minor injuries. Early studies of injuries to children in day care utilized injury event logs kept by the facilities (15, 24, 61, 105). Most of these injuries are trivial; in the words of one study (105), "Washing, ice, or Tender Loving Care were sufficient treatment for 96% of the injuries." Several authors have limited their studies of day-care injuries to patients who seek medical attention (8, 42, 59, 98, 102), while recognizing that seeking care is often determined by factors other than injury severity. Some of these studies have provided evidence that the risk of injury is less in day care than in the home (42, 98, 102).

Study of minor injuries may sometimes be justified and desirable if they share the same causes as serious injuries, because they are often more frequent and thus present opportunities to increase statistical power without greater population size or study duration. For example, most hip fractures in the elderly occur after a fall. One way to prevent hip fracture may be to identify and intervene on modifiable risk factors for falls, which are much more common than hip fractures. However, most falls do not lead to medical care, and recall of falls decays with time. To detect falls in a cohort of elderly subjects, some investigators have used a system of weekly mail-back postcards with telephone follow-up (44).

Even if we are willing to accept ascertainment of only those injuries that result in medical care, the problem confronting those in the field of injury research is substantial. It is rare that injuries are collected in a population-based registry that allows for identification of cases, and rarer still for such a registry to provide all the information needed for epidemiologic research. However, some studies have made clever use of existing data to answer important questions. For example, Ray and colleagues used computerized Medicaid hospitalization and pharmacy files, which are collected for financial purposes, to assess the association between certain medications and the risk of hip fracture (97). Hip fracture is well suited for this type of study: The injury is serious; it nearly always results in hospitalization; and, even if it leads to death, a period of hospitalization will usually precede the death, so a hospitalization database will capture virtually all the cases. The investigators found evidence that long-half-life anxiolytics, such as flurazepam and diazepam, tricyclic antidepressants, and antipsychotics were all associated with a twofold increase in risk of hip fracture.

One population-based data source for injury cases is hospital discharge tapes. Washington State, for example, maintains the Comprehensive Hospital Abstract Reporting System, a computerized record of all civilian hospital discharges that contains up to five ICD-9 diagnosis codes, up to three ICD-9 procedure codes, and up to two ICD-9 E-codes. Using this information along with death certificate records, one can identify all deaths and civilian hospitalizations recorded as due to injury in the state. Most states now have hospital discharge data systems, although only a few states require the use of E-codes (10, 104). It has been estimated that E-code information can be added to discharge data at an annual cost of about $600 per hospital (99).

Occasionally, special population-based registries have been established to capture information about injuries. In 1977, a large amount of valuable information was collected about trauma-related emergency department visits in a region of Ohio; 41 hospitals participated in this effort (5). A registry of all pediatric drowning deaths and hospitalizations has been maintained in King County, Washington, since 1974 (96). A study currently under way is collecting data on all patients who present to any emergency department for an injury due to a firearm or die from such an injury, in the cities of Memphis, TN, Galveston, TX, and Seattle, WA (11). Massachusetts has recently established a statewide weapon-injury reporting system that collects data on nearly all shootings and stabbings (74).

Trauma registries play an important role in auditing the quality of care given to victims of trauma. But they only capture part of a population's trauma experience, and it is hard to associate most registries with a defined population at risk (95). Typically, they are maintained by a trauma hospital and the catchment area covered by the emergency medical services system that brings patients to the hospital is not well defined. Epidemiologic studies based solely on trauma registries are subject to selection biases because patients who die before admission are not included, referral patterns influence the type of trauma patient seen at the hospital with the registry, and most trauma hospitals see only a poorly characterized fraction of the patients hospitalized for trauma in a geographic region (93, 116).

A potentially useful source of information that can be tapped with some special effort is emergency department data. Most emergency departments still use handwritten registration logs with a single discharge diagnosis, so recovering these data is time consuming. For some injuries, such as gunshot wounds, it is usually possible to identify cases from the log. But a motor-vehicle crash victim with fractures and lacerations may be impossible to identify by etiologic mechanism if the chief diagnosis is fracture.

Sometimes it is preferable to use several sources of data. Stout & Bell summarized the usefulness of four different data sources for fatal work injuries: Workers' compensation records identified 57% of the cases found by all the sources; medical examiner records identified 68%; fatality reports of the Occupational Safety and Health Administration identified 32%; and death certificates identified 81% (109). Poisoning is another injury that requires more than one source of data for full ascertainment. The American Association of Poison Control Centers has published extensive annual reports since 1984 (69). These data are skewed by the characteristics of the population that uses poison control centers; over one half of all poison center calls involve children under age 5, a group that accounts for less than 1% of poisoning mortality (4, 113). Only one fourth of hospital emergency department visits for poisoning (6, 46), half of hospitalizations for poisoning (6), and less than 5% of poisoning deaths are reported to poison control centers (4, 37, 68, 107). In Washington in 1990, 111 deaths due to nonmedicinal poisoning were identified by state vital records (117), while only 17 poisoning deaths were reported in that year to all poison control centers in the state (3). Hospital records are a poor single source of poisoning mortality data, since three fourths of poisoning deaths occur outside the hospital (107).

Researchers frequently use law enforcement data (39). Studies of motor-vehicle crashes rely on police records to identify crashes (35, 62), and sometimes to assess the degree of injury sustained by the occupants (110). Because police reports of injury severity are usually based on brief observations at the scene or in the emergency department, their accuracy and detail are limited (1). The Fatal Accident Reporting System (FARS) of the US Department of Transportation provides valuable data for many studies of vehicular crashes (25, 26). It is possible to link 85% of FARS deaths to multiple cause of death data from the National Center for Health Statistics, thus linking crash information to anatomic injuries on the death certificate (29).

Some injuries are underreported because of social sanctions related to the perpetrator and fears of reprisal and social stigma related to the victim. Domestic violence may be underdiagnosed in emergency departments, even when the victim is asked about the cause of the injuries and recall is not a factor (77, 78). Undocumented aliens may not seek treatment for some injuries if they fear that they will be reported to immigration authorities. In contrast, whiplash and back injuries may be prone to overreporting because of secondary economic gain.

DENOMINATOR PROBLEMS

Denominator issues are related to our ability to calculate injury rates.

Matching Numerators and Denominators

For studies of geographic variation in injury incidence it is not always clear how to identify or obtain the appropriate denominator. Motor-vehicle collision injuries, for example, are typically examined using the number of events in a region in the numerator and the population of the region in the denominator. This approach exaggerates the injury rate of a region that has many visitors who drive and underestimates the rate for a region that has few visitors, but many residents who drive outside the region. Another approach, which has been used to describe the epidemiology of drowning (96), uses the population of a county as the denominator and within-county drownings *only of residents* in the numerator. This approach allows calculations of accurate age-specific rates of *within-county* drowning incidence, but does not describe the full population-based incidence of injury, since drownings outside the county are excluded.

If the question of interest is whether residents of a particular area have characteristics that place them at increased risk of injury, it may be best to use all injuries that they experience regardless of place of occurrence (89). To study area-specific environmental risk factors for injury (23), the best strategy may be to count all events that occur there, whether to residents or nonresidents, and use some other measure of at-risk experience besides size of the resident population. For motor-vehicle crashes, for example, we should perhaps try to get vehicle-miles traveled in each study area. For many situations, the ideal denominator may not be available.

Choosing the Best Denominator

Sometimes there are several choices for an appropriate denominator, so the choice depends on the question of interest. Motor-vehicle collision injuries have different relationships with age, depending on whether all people, licensed drivers, or miles driven are used as the denominators (48). Drivers age 75 and older have the highest rate of fatal crashes per mile driven, but they drive much less than younger drivers, so that their incidence of fatal crashes per capita is only slightly greater than that of middle-aged drivers and much less than that of teenagers. If one wishes to know if engineering advances and other measures have made driving safer, then miles driven is the best choice of denominator (38).

CAUSATION

We review here some issues involved in teasing out the multicausal nature of injuries.

Some injuries are defined in such a way that a certain component cause is assumed to be necessary. This occurs when we define injuries by etiologic mechanism, such as gunshot wounds, motor-vehicle crashes, or drownings. Defining injuries in this way requires exposure to a necessary cause, such as a moving bullet, a moving car, or liquid. Investigators may need to focus on risk factors for exposure to the necessary cause (118) in addition to identifying other cofactors that might interact with the cause. For example, to make valid comparisons across age groups with regard to the risk of being fatally injured as a car driver, we need to allow for the fact that older people are less likely to have a driver's license and on the average drive less.

Injuries generally result from an interplay of agent, host, and environment, and the element of this triad that we choose to focus on typically determines the unit of analysis. In studying pedestrian injuries caused by motor vehicles, factors about the driver (7), vehicle (7), pedestrian (43), and street (81) all influence risk. If the researcher is interested in characteristics of crosswalks as risk factors for pedestrian injury, then crosswalks where injuries occurred may be chosen as cases and other crosswalks as controls. In investigating the causes of airplane crashes, some studies might choose the pilot as the unit of study, others might choose the airport, and still others might choose the plane.

In some ways injuries resemble infectious diseases. A person's risk of infection may be affected not only by characteristics or behaviors of the person, but by the vaccination status of their neighbors or the activities of their sexual partners. Similarly, the risk of being hit by a car may be related to the amount of alcohol consumed in a neighborhood, and the risk of being shot may be related to the number of guns owned by other people who live in the same area. Thus, injury epidemiologists may wish to seek information not only about the individuals in a study, but also about other family members, or other people in their community. Obtaining this information is difficult, but it can sometimes be done; in some studies, adjustment is made in the analysis using census tract information, whereas in other studies, cases and controls are matched on neighborhood of residence, a topic we discuss below.

In some studies of injuries, the exposure of it terest is a disease. There is obvious public interest in knowing, for example, if persons with epilepsy are at increased risk for traffic accidents. A cohort study that examined the experience of licensed drivers in Marshfield, Wisconsin, estimated that drivers with epilepsy had only a small elevation in risk for traffic accidents compared to other drivers: relative risk 1.33 (95% confidence interval 1.00 to 1.73) (45). A population-based study of epilepsy as a risk factor for fatal drowning among children estimated a large relative risk of 13.8 (95% confidence interval 7.0 to 27.0) (22).

EXPOSURE MEASUREMENT PROBLEMS

Proxy Respondents

In performing epidemiologic studies, it is frequently necessary to interview cases or controls about their experience with potential risk factors. In cancer epidemiology, this may be done by performing structured in-person interviews (119). But in studies of injuries where the outcome of interest is often rapid death or severe injury, an interview may be impossible; by the time the cases are identified they are dead or have severe brain injury and therefore cannot be interviewed. This problem was faced by investigators who wished to study risk factors for suicide (54) and homicide (53). By definition, the cases were all dead and the investigators obtained information about the cases from close relatives; these are known as "proxy respondents."

Several techniques have been devised to assist studies that make use of proxy respondents (88). In studies where exposure information on many or all cases must be obtained from proxies, it may be ideal to gather information about all controls both from the actual controls and proxy controls. This approach allows measurement of the degree of agreement between proxy respondents and the index subjects and may shed light on the direction and size of any misclassification bias due to the use of proxy-provided information. Studies that rely on proxy respondents generally need larger sample sizes because the estimated odds ratio is likely to be biased towards unity owing to less accurate reporting, and the rate of nonresponse is likely to be higher. These factors should be taken into account when sample size calculations are made. By keeping the data collection methods simple and structured, nonresponse may be reduced. In the analysis, it is wise to stratify the results by respondent category and to assess this as a potential confounder and effect modifier (114).

Sensitive Exposure Information

Measuring certain exposures may be difficult because the information that is sought has certain social or legal connotations. Examples include inquiries about gun ownership, alcohol use, domestic violence, arrest record, immigration status, and sexual behavior. Placing sensitive questions at the end of the interview may increase the response rate. Two studies that dealt with sensitive issues used the technique of introducing the question with a permissive statement: for example, "Half of all homes in America contain one or more firearms. Are guns of any kind kept in your home?" (54), and "Many people have quarrels or fights. Has anyone in this household ever been hit or hurt in a fight in the home?" (53).

One method that can help in eliciting an item of sensitive information is the randomized-response technique (40). In North Carolina in 1968, researchers wanted to know what fraction of women had had an abortion. They feared that most women who had experienced an abortion would not admit it. They handled this problem by using a simple mechanical device that randomly presented one of the following written statements to each woman in the study: (a) "I was pregnant at some time during the past 12 months and had an abortion;" (b) "I was born in the month of April." The woman was asked if the presented statement was true, but, although both the woman and the interviewer knew that there were two possible questions, only the woman knew which of the two statements had been presented. By using this method, each individual subject was assured of privacy. The investigators knew, on average, how often the mechanical device presented each statement and they knew, from another source of information, the expected frequency of "Yes" responses to the benign second statement. With this knowledge, they could estimate the overall proportion of "Yes" responses to the question about abortions and even calculate a confidence interval for that proportion, yet they could not know the answer to the question about abortion for any individual woman in the study.

Confounding by Socioeconomic Status

The incidence of many diseases varies by strata of social class (73). Disease risk factors related to social class may include occupation, residential neighborhood, access to health care, diet, crowding, psychological stress, alcoholism, and drug abuse. Controlling for social class has special importance to the study of injuries because the association between injuries and poverty is strong, especially for unintentional injuries and homicides (4). In Maine, a population that was 98.7% white in 1980, children from poor families had a relative risk of unintentional injury death of 2.6 and a relative risk of intentional injury death of 5.0, compared to other children (89). An analysis of data from the National Health Interview Surveys of 1985, 1986, and 1987 reported that fractures, lacerations, contusions, and burns were more common among those with family incomes less than $10,000, compared to persons in higher income categories (17). Two studies concluded that for children under age 16 poverty is a risk factor for burns (65) and gunshot deaths (57). Failure to control for socioeconomic status may confound many studies of the causes of injuries.

The measurement of social class usually involves collecting information about occupation, education, or income, or some combination of these items (66). Obtaining this information often requires direct questioning of study subjects. In many of the datasets used for injury studies, such as death certificates, hospital discharge data, or police reports, information about socioeconomic status is absent or limited. In this situation, other measures are sometimes used to represent social class; for example, median family income of census tract of residence, a measure that may be too crude to adequately control for socioeconomic status.

In the United States, race frequently has been used as a surrogate measure for social class. It is common to see rates for injury death broken down by sex and race, two variables that are readily available from death certificates (4, 30–32, 85, 100, 106). Although some real differences in disease incidence are related to race, for many diseases the association with race is reduced when some adjustment is made for social class (56, 94). A study of domestic homicides in Atlanta, GA, concluded that rates were the same when blacks and whites from census tracts with similar household crowding were compared (12). In Ohio, differences in homicide rates between black and white children under the age of 4 years were greatly reduced after adjustment for socioeconomic status (82).

Some authors have pointed out that reporting disease incidence rates by race has several drawbacks (52, 76, 92). Classification by race may obscure an underlying relationship between disease and poverty, a relationship that suggests that improving the economic situation of poor people might improve their health. By characterizing the issue as racial, the results may be interpreted as if race were the variable of interest. Because of these problems, studies that address the issue of race and injuries should consider why they are measuring race; if they are using it as a surrogate measure for socioeconomic status, perhaps they should say so (34). If social class is really the variable of interest, they might try to measure that instead.

In some studies, neighborhood has been used to control for socioeconomic status. When data from the 1988 National Household Survey on Drug Abuse were analyzed by stratifying on neighborhood, the authors found that the use of crack cocaine did not differ significantly for African Americans or Hispanic Americans compared to whites (67). In two recent studies of the risk of suicide (54) and homicide (53) in relation to gun ownership, the authors matched cases and controls on neighborhood and race, as well as age and sex. They did this by conducting a census of neighborhood households using a method developed by cancer epidemiologists (70, 122). While this methodology was time consuming, expensive, and required numerous trips to neighborhoods with high crime rates, it resulted in two groups that were very similar in regard to socioeconomic status. The study of suicides in the home estimated a relative risk of 4.8 for persons with a gun in the home compared to other persons (54). The relative risk for homicide in a home was 2.7 for persons with any firearm in the home (53). The results of these studies are more plausible because of the effort invested in selecting controls from the same neighborhood as the cases.

MULTIPLICITY

The problem of multiplicity can complicate the analysis of injury data: The same person can sustain multiple injuries at one time; some injuries can occur repeatedly in the same person over time; and one event can result in multiple injured persons. For example, 8% of a group of elderly residents of St. Louis, Missouri, reported having two or more falls in the previous year (19). This problem is also encountered in the study of infections. If we study assaults on workers in convenience stores or injuries to children in day care, it is very likely that more than one event will occur at the same location. When this happens, the assumption that events are statistically independent may not be correct. It is natural to assume that a person who falls once or a convenience store that has one assault may be more likely to have a second episode compared to a person or store that has not experienced the event of interest. When the correlation or clustering of recurrent events is ignored in analysis of the data, the calculated confidence intervals may be incorrect and study power may be reduced. Regression models, known as generalized estimating equations, have been devised to calculate a variance that takes recurrent events into account (64). We hope that these models will become available in commonly used statistical software packages.

SUMMARY

This review has concentrated on problem areas in the study of injuries. Taken together, these problems may seem daunting, but each has potential solutions that we have tried to identify. Injury epidemiology has made enormous progress in recent years, adopting increasingly sophisticated research methods from more established branches of epidemiology. Important challenges exist for epidemiologists to enhance public health practice in this field. Injury classification schemes are still evolving. Efforts to improve existing data sources, such as death certificates and hospital discharge registries, should be supported. We hope that more population-based injury registries will exist in the future to provide information for prevention programs devised by state and local health departments. Clever study designs will undoubtedly expand knowledge of injury causes. Better techniques for exposure measurement are needed in some injury research, including better measures of socioeconomic class. Future studies of injuries that solve the difficulties we have reviewed will make important contributions to the prevention of injuries and the control of medical care costs.

ACKNOWLEDGMENTS

Support for this work was provided by grant R49/CCR002570 from the Centers for Disease Control and Prevention.

Literature Cited

1. Agran PF, Castillo DN, Winn DG. 1990. Limitations of data compiled from police reports on pediatric pedestrian and bicycle motor vehicle events. *Accid. Anal. Prev.* 22:361–70
2. Ashford JR, Lawrence PA. 1976. Aspects of the epidemiology of suicide in England and Wales. *Int. J. Epidemiol.* 5:133–44
3. Assoc. Washington State Poison Control Centers. 1991. Annual Report
4. Baker SP, O'Neill B, Ginsburg MJ, Li G. 1992. *The Injury Fact Book.* New York: Oxford Univ. Press. 2nd ed.

5. Barancik JI, Chatterjee BF, Greene-Cradden YC, Michenzi EM, Kramer CF, et al. 1986. Motor vehicle trauma in northeastern Ohio. I: Incidence and outcome by age, sex, and road-use category. *Am. J. Epidemiol.* 123:846–61

5a. Bass M, Kravath RE, Glass L. 1986. Death-scene investigation in sudden infant death syndrome. *New Engl. J. Med.* 315:100–5

6. Blanc PD, Jones MR, Olson KR. 1993. Surveillance of poisoning and drug overdose through hospital discharge coding, poison control center reporting, and the Drug Abuse Warning Network. *Am. J. Emerg. Med.* 11:14–19

7. Brison RJ, Wicklund K, Mueller BA. 1988. Fatal pedestrian injuries to young children: a different pattern of injury. *Am. J. Public Health* 78:793–95

8. Briss PA, Sacks JJ, Addiss DG, Kresnow M, O'Neil J. 1994. A nationwide study of the risk of injury associated with day care center attendance. *Pediatrics* 93: 364–68

9. Brown ST, Foege WH, Bender TR, Axnick N. 1990. Injury prevention and control: prospects for the 1990s. *Annu. Rev. Public Health* 11:251–66

10. Centers for Disease Control and Prevention. 1992. External cause-of-injury coding in hospital discharge data United States, 1992. *Morbid. Mortal. Wkly. Rep.* 41:249–51

11. Centers for Disease Control and Prevention. 1994. *Report of current progress, extramural research findings, fiscal year 1993.* US Dep. Health Hum. Serv.

12. Centerwall BS. 1984. Race, socioeconomic status, and domestic homicide, Atlanta, 1971–72. *Am. J. Public Health* 74:813–14

13. Champion HR, Copes WS, Sacco WJ, Lawnick MM, Bain LW, et al. 1990. A new characterization of injury severity. *J. Trauma* 30:539–46

14. Champion HR, Sacco WJ, Copes WS, Gann DS, Gennarelli TA, Flanagan ME. 1989. A revision of the trauma score. *J. Trauma* 29:623–29

15. Chang A, Lugg MM, Nebedum A. 1989. Injuries among preschool children enrolled in day-care centers. *Pediatrics* 83:272–77

16. Clemmer DI, Diem JE. 1985. Major mishaps among mobile offshore drilling units, 1955–1981: time trends and fatalities. *Int. J. Epidemiol.* 14:106–12

17. Collins JG. 1990. Types of injuries by selected characteristics: United States, 1985–1987. *Natl. Cent. Health Stat. Vital Health Stat.* 10(175):25

18. Conn AW, Montes JE, Barker GA, Edmonds JF. 1980. Cerebral salvage in near-drowning following neurological classification by triage. *Can. Anaesth. Soc. J.* 27:201–10

19. Cumming RG, Miller JP, Kelsey JL, Davis P, Arfken CL, et al. 1991. Medications and multiple falls in elderly people: the St. Louis OASIS study. *Age Aging* 20:455–61

20. Cummings P, Theis MK, Mueller BA, Rivara FP. 1994. Infant injury death in Washington State, 1981 through 1990. *Arch. Pediatr. Adolesc. Med.* 148:1021–26

21. Dean JM, Kaufman ND. 1981. Prognostic indicators in pediatric near-drowning: the Glasgow Coma Scale. *Crit. Care Med.* 9:536–39

22. Diekema DS, Quan L, Holt VL. 1993. Epilepsy as a risk factor for submersion injury in children. *Pediatrics* 91:612–16

23. Durkin MS, Davidson LL, Kuhn L, O'Conner P, Barlow B. 1994. Low-income neighborhoods and the risk of severe pediatric injury: a small-area analysis in northern Manhattan. *Am. J. Public Health* 84:587–92

24. Elardo R, Solomons HC, Snider BC. 1987. An analysis of accidents at a day care center. *Am. J. Orthopsychiatry* 57: 60–65

25. Evans L. 1986. The effectiveness of safety belts in preventing fatalities. *Accid. Anal. Prev.* 18:229–41

26. Evans L, Frick MC. 1992. Car size or car mass: which has greater influence on fatality risk? *Am. J. Public Health* 82:1105–12

27. Ewigman B, Kivlahan C, Land G. 1993. The Missouri child fatality study: underreporting of maltreatment fatalities among children younger than five years of age, 1983 through 1986. *Pediatrics* 91:330–37

28. Fields AI. 1992. Near-drowning in the pediatric population. *Crit. Care Clin.* 8:113–29

29. Fife D. 1989. Matching Fatal Accident Reporting System cases with National Center for Health Statistics motor vehicle deaths. *Accid. Anal. Prev.* 21:79–83

30. Fingerhut LA. 1993. *Firearm mortality among children, youth, and young adults 1–34 years of age, trends and current status: United States, 1985–90. Advance data from vital and health statistics. No. 281.* Hyattsville, MD: Natl. Cent. Health Stat.

31. Fingerhut LA, Kleinman JC. 1989. *Firearm mortality among children and youth. Advance data from vital and health statistics. No. 178.* Hyattsville, MD: Natl. Cent. Health Stat.

32. Fingerhut LA, Makuc DM. 1992. Mortality among minority populations in the United States. *Am. J. Public Health* 82:1168–70

33. Frantz ID, Dawson EA, Ashman PL, Gatewood LC, Bartsch GE, et al. 1989. Test of effect of lipid lowering by diet on cardiovascular risk. The Minnesota coronary survey. *Arteriosclerosis* 9:129–35

34. Fullilove MT. 1993. Perceptions and misperceptions of race and drug use. *J. Am. Med. Assoc.* 269:1034

35. Gallaher MM, Sewell M, Flint S, Herndon JL, Graff H, et al. 1989. Effects of the 65-mph speed limit on rural interstate fatalities in New Mexico. *J. Am. Med. Assoc.* 262:2243–45

36. Gibson G. 1981. Indices of severity for emergency medical evaluation studies: reliability, validity, and data requirements. *Int. J. Health Serv.* 11:597–622

37. Goldfrank LR. 1993. Data, epidemiology, and the future strength of emergency medicine. *Ann. Emerg. Med.* 10:1859–60

38. Graham JD. 1993. Injuries from traffic crashes: meeting the challenge. *Annu. Rev. Public Health* 14:515–43

39. Graitcer PL. 1992. Injury surveillance. In *Public Health Surveillance,* ed. W Halperin, EL Baker Jr, RR Monson, pp. 142–56. New York: Van Nostrand Reinhold

40. Greenberg BG, Abernathy JR, Horvitz DG. 1970. A new survey technique and its application in the field of public health. *Milbank Mem. Fund Q.* 48 (Suppl.):39–55

41. Gulaid JA, Sattin RW. 1988. Drownings in the United States, 1978-1984. *Morbid. Mortal Wkly. Rep. CDC Surveill. Summ.* 37:27–33

42. Gunn WJ, Pinsky PF, Sacks JJ, Schonberger LB. 1991. Injuries and poisonings in out-of-home child care and home care. *Am. J. Dis. Child.* 145:779–81

43. Haddon W Jr, Valien P, McCarroll JR, Umberger CJ. 1961. A controlled investigation of the characteristics of adult pedestrians fatally injured by motor vehicles in Manhattan. *J. Chron. Dis.* 14:655–78

44. Hale WA, Delaney MJ, Cable T. 1993. Accuracy of patient recall and chart documentation of falls. *J. Am. Board. Fam. Pract.* 6:239–42

45. Hansotia P, Broste SK. 1991. The effect of epilepsy or diabetes mellitus on the risk of automobile accidents. *New Engl. J. Med.* 324:22–26

46. Harchelroad F, Clark RF, Dean B, Krenzelok EP. 1990. Treated vs reported toxic exposures: discrepancies between a poison control center and a member hospital. *Vet. Hum. Toxicol.* 32:156–59

47. Hassall C, Trethowan WH. 1972. Suicide in Birmingham. *Br. Med. J.* 1:717–18

48. Insurance Inst. Highway Safety. 1992. *Status Rep.* 27:1–7

49. Jacobs D, Blackburn H, Higgins M, Reed D, Iso H, et al. 1992. Report of the Conference on Low Blood Cholesterol: mortality associations. *Circulation* 86:1046–60

50. Jason J, Carpenter MM, Tyler CW Jr. 1983. Underrecording of infant homicide in the United States. *Am. J. Public Health* 73:195–97

51. Jobes DA, Berman AL, Josselson AR. 1986. The impact of psychological autopsy on medical examiners' determination of manner of death. *J. Foren. Sci.* 31:177–89

52. Jones CP, LaVeist TA, Lillie-Blanton M. 1991. "Race" in the epidemiologic literature: an examination of the American Journal of Epidemiology, 1921–1990. *Am. J. Epidemiol.* 134:1079–1084

53. Kellermann AL, Rivara FP, Rushforth NB, Banton JG, Reay DT, et al. 1993. Gun ownership as a risk factor for homicide in the home. *New Engl. J. Med.* 329:1084–91

54. Kellermann AL, Rivara FP, Somes G, Reay DT, Francisco J, et al. 1992. Suicide in the home in relation to gun ownership. *New Engl. J. Med.* 327:467–72

55. Kemp AM, Sibert JR. 1991. Outcome in children who nearly drown: a British Isles study. *Br. Med. J.* 302:931–33

56. Kerner JF, Dusenbury L, Mandelblatt JS. 1993. Poverty and cultural diversity: challenges for health promotion among the medically underserved. *Annu. Rev. Public Health* 14:355–77

57. Klein D, Reizen MS, Van Amburg GH, Walker SA. 1977. Some social characteristics of young gunshot fatalities. *Accid. Anal. Prev.* 9:177–82

58. Kreitman N, Platt S. 1984. Suicide, unemployment, and domestic gas detoxification in Britain. *J. Epidemiol. Community Health* 38:1–6

59. Landman PF, Landman GB. 1987. Accidental injuries in children in day-care centers. *Am. J. Dis. Child.* 141:292–93

60. Lapidus GD, Gregorio DI, Hansen H. 1990. Misclassification of childhood homicide on death certificates. *Am. J. Public Health* 80:213–14

61. Leland NL, Garrard J, Smith DK. 1993. Injuries to preschool-age children in

day-care centers. A retrospective record review. *Am. J. Dis. Child.* 147:826–31

62. Lestina DC, Williams AF, Lund AK, Zador P, Kuhlmann TP. 1991. Motor vehicle crash injury patterns and the Virginia seat belt law. *J. Am. Med. Assoc.* 265:1409–13

63. Levin DL, Morriss FC, Toro LO, Brink LW, Turner GR. 1993. Drowning and near-drowning. *Pediatr. Clin. North Am.* 40:321–36

64. Liang K-Y, Zeger SL. 1993. Regression analysis for correlated data. *Annu. Rev. Public Health* 14:43–68

65. Libber SM, Stayton DJ. 1984. Childhood burns reconsidered: the child, the family and the burn injury. *J. Trauma* 24:245–52

66. Liberatos P, Link BG, Kelsey JL. 1988. The measurement of social class in epidemiology. *Epidemiol. Rev.* 10:87–121

67. Lillie-Blanton M, Anthony JC, Schuster CR. 1993. Probing the meaning of racial/ethnic group comparisons in crack cocaine smoking. *J. Am. Med. Assoc.* 269:993–97

68. Linakis JG, Frederick KA. 1993. Poisoning deaths not reported to the regional poison control center. *Ann. Emerg. Med.* 22:1822–28

69. Litovitz TL, Clark LR, Soloway RA. 1994. 1993 Annual report of the American Association of Poison Control Centers toxic exposure surveillance system. *Am. J. Emerg. Med.* 12:546–84

70. Mack TM, Yu MC, Hanisch R, Henderson BE. 1986. Pancreas cancer and smoking, beverage consumption, and past medical history. *J. Natl. Cancer Inst.* 76:49–60

71. MacKenzie EJ. 1984. Injury severity scales: overview and directions for future research. *Am. J. Emerg. Med.* 2:537–49

72. Marion DW, Carlier PM. 1994. Problems with initial Glasgow Coma Scale assessment caused by prehospital treatment of patients with head injuries: results of a national survey. *J. Trauma* 36:89–95

73. Marmot MG, Kogevinas M, Elston MA. 1987. Social/economic status and disease. *Annu. Rev. Public Health* 8:111–35

74. Mass. Dep. Public Health. 1993. *Weapon Injury Report.* Boston

75. McClain PW, Sacks JJ, Froehlke RG, Ewigman BG. 1993. Estimates of fatal child abuse and neglect, United States, 1979 through 1988. *Pediatrics* 91:338–43

76. McKenzie KJ, Crowcroft NS. 1994. Race, ethnicity, culture, and science. *Br. Med. J.* 309:286–87

77. McLeer SV, Anwar R. 1989. A study of battered women presenting in an emergency department. *Am. J. Public Health* 79:65–66

78. McLeer SV, Anwar RAH, Herman S, Maquiling K. 1989. Education is not enough: a systems failure in protecting battered women. *Ann. Emerg. Med.* 18:651–53

79. Michaud LJ, Rivara FP, Longstreth WT, Grady MS. 1991. Elevated initial blood glucose levels and poor outcome following severe brain injuries in children. *J. Trauma* 31:1356–62

80. Modell JH, Graves SA, Ketover A. 1976. Clinical course of 91 consecutive near-drowning victims. *Chest* 70:231–38

81. Mueller BA, Rivara FP, Lii SM, Weiss NS. 1990. Environmental factors and the risk for childhood pedestrian-motor vehicle collision occurrence. *Am. J. Epidemiol.* 132:550–60

82. Muscat JE. 1988. Characteristics of childhood homicide in Ohio, 1974–84. *Am. J. Public Health* 78:822–24

83. Natl. Cent. Health Stat. 1967. *International Classification of Diseases.* Washington, DC: PHS Publ. No. 1693, GPO. 8th rev.

84. Natl. Cent. Health Stat. 1991. *International Classification of Diseases. Clinical Modification (ICD-9-CM).* Washington, DC: DHHS Publ. No. (PHS) 91-1260. 9th rev.

85. Natl. Cent. Health Stat. 1992. *Health, United States, 1991.* DHHS Publ. No. (PHS) 92–1232. Hyattsville, MD: Public Health Serv.

86. Natl. Comm. Injury Prev. Control. 1989. *Injury Prevention: Meeting the Challenge.* New York: Oxford Univ. Press

87. Neaton JD, Blackburn H, Jacobs D, Kuller L, Lee D, Sherwin R. 1992. Serum cholesterol level and mortality findings for men screened in the Multiple Risk Factor Intervention Trial. *Arch. Intern. Med.* 152:1490–1500

88. Nelson LM, Longstreth WT Jr, Koepsell TD, van Belle G. 1990. Proxy respondents in epidemiologic research. *Epidemiol. Rev.* 12:71–86

89. Nersesian WS, Petit MR, Shaper R, Lemieux D, Naor E. 1985. Childhood death and poverty: a study of all childhood deaths in Maine, 1976 to 1980. *Pediatrics* 75:41–50

90. O'Carroll PW, Alkon E, Weiss B. 1988. Drowning mortality in Los Angeles County, 1976 to 1984. *J. Am. Med. Assoc.* 260:380–83

91. Orlowski JP. 1979. Prognostic factors

in pediatric cases of drowning and near-drowning. *JACEP* 8:176–79

92. Osborne NG, Feit MD. 1992. The use of race in medical research. *J. Am. Med. Assoc.* 267:275–79

93. Payne SR, Waller JA. 1989. Trauma registry and trauma center biases in injury research. *J. Trauma* 29:424–29

94. Polednak AP. 1989. *Racial and Ethnic Differences in Disease.* New York: Oxford Univ. Press

95. Pollock DA, McClain PW. 1989. Trauma registries. Current status and future prospects. *J. Am. Med. Assoc.* 262:2280–83

96. Quan L, Gore EJ, Wentz K, Allen J, Novack AH. 1989. Ten-year study of pediatric drownings and near-drownings in King County, Washington: lessons in injury prevention. *Pediatrics* 83:1035–40

96a. Quan L, Kinder D. 1992. Pediatric submersions: prehospital predictors of outcome. *Pediatrics* 80:909–13

96b. Quan L, Wentz KR, Gore EJ, Copass MK. 1990. Outcome and predictors of outcome in pediatric submersion victims receiving prehospital care in Kings County, Washington. *Pediatrics* 86:586–93

97. Ray WA, Griffin MR, Schaffner W, Baugh DK. 1987. Psychotropic drug use and the risk of hip fracture. *New Engl. J. Med.* 316:363–69

98. Rivara FP, DiGuiseppi C, Thompson RS, Calonge N. 1989. Risk of injury to children less than 5 years of age in day care versus home care settings. *Pediatrics* 84:1011–16

99. Rivara FP, Morgan P, Bergman AB, Maier RA. 1990. Cost estimates for statewide reporting of injuries by E coding hospital discharge abstract data base systems. *Public Health Rep.* 105:635–38

100. Ropp L, Visintainer P, Uman J, Treloar D. 1992. Death in a city: an American childhood tragedy. *J. Am. Med. Assoc.* 267:2905–10

101. Rosenberg ML, Smith JC, Davidson LE, Conn JM. 1987. The emergence of youth suicide: an epidemiologic analysis and public health perspective. *Annu. Rev. Public Health* 8:417–40

102. Sacks JJ, Smith JD, Kaplan KM, Lambert DA, Sattin RW, Sikes K. 1989. The epidemiology of injuries in Atlanta daycare centers. *J. Am. Med. Assoc.* 262:1641–45

103. Samkoff JS, Baker SP. 1982. Recent trends in fatal poisoning by opiates in the United States. *Am. J. Public Health* 72:1251–56

104. Sniezek JE, Finklea JF, Graitcer PL.

1989. Injury coding and hospital discharge data. *J. Am. Med. Assoc.* 262:2270–72

105. Solomons HC, Lakin JA, Paredes-Rojas RR. 1982. Is day care safe for children? Accident records reviewed. *Child Health Care* 10:90–93

106. Sorenson SB, Richardson BA, Peterson JG. 1993. Race/ethnicity patterns in the homicide of children in Los Angeles, 1980 through 1989. *Am. J. Public Health* 83:725–27

107. Soslow AR, Woolf AD. 1992. Reliability of data sources for poisoning deaths in Massachusetts. *Am. J. Emerg. Med.* 10:124–27

108. Stoneburner RL, Des Jarlais DC, Benezra D, Gorelkin L, Sotheran JL, et al. 1988. A larger spectrum of severe HIV-1 related disease in intravenous drug users in New York City. *Science* 242:916–19

109. Stout N, Bell C. 1991. Effectiveness of source documents for identifying fatal occupational injuries: a synthesis of studies. *Am. J. Public Health* 81:725–28

110. Streff FM, Wagenaar AC, Schultz RH. 1990. Reductions in police-reported injuries associated with Michigan's safety belt law. *J. Safety Res.* 21:9–18

111. Teasdale G, Jennett B. 1974. Assessment of coma and impaired consciousness. *Lancet* 2:81–84

111a. Thach BT. 1986. Sudden infant death syndrome. Old causes rediscovered? *New Engl. J. Med.* 315:126–28

112. US Dep. Health Hum Serv. 1992. Setting the National Agenda for Injury Control in the 1990's. *Natl. Injury Control Conf., 3rd.* Washington, DC: DHHS

113. Veltri JC, McElwee NE, Schumacher MC. 1987. Interpretation and uses of data collected in poison control centres of the United States. *Med. Toxicol.* 2:389–97

114. Walker AM, Velema JP, Robins JM. 1988. Analysis of case-control data derived in part from proxy respondents. *Am. J. Epidemiol.* 127:905–14

115. Waller JA. 1987. Injury: conceptual shifts and preventive medicine. *Annu. Rev. Public Health* 8:21–49

116. Waller JA. 1989. Methodologic issues in hospital-based injury research. *J. Trauma* 28:1632–36

117. Washington State Department of Health. 1992. *Injury Prevention Program.* Olympia, WA

118. Weiss NS. 1991. Epidemiologic studies of diseases in which a necessary cause is known. *Epidemiology* 2:153–54

119. Wingo PA, Ory HW, Layde PM, Lee NC. 1988. The Cancer and Steroid Hor-

mone Study Group. The evaluation of the data collection process for a multi-center, population-based, case-control design. *Am. J. Epidemiol.* 128:206–17

120. Wintemute GJ, Kraus JF, Teret SP, Wright MA. 1988. The epidemiology of drowning in adulthood: implications for prevention. *Am. J. Prev. Med.* 4: 343–48

121. Wysowski DK, Schober SE, Wise RP, Kopstein A. 1993. Mortality attributed to misuse of psychoactive drugs,

1979–88. *Public Health Rep.* 108:565–70

122. Yu MC, Mack TM, Hanisch R, Peters RL, Henderson BE, Pike MC. 1983. Hepatitis, alcohol consumption, cigarette smoking, and hepatocellular carcinoma in Los Angeles. *Cancer Res.* 43: 6077–79

123. Zoltie N, de Dombal FT. 1993. The hit or miss of ISS and TRISS. Yorkshire Trauma Audit Group. *Br. Med. J.* 307: 906–9

Annu. Rev. Public Health. 1995. 16:401–30

RISK ADJUSTING COMMUNITY RATED HEALTH PLAN PREMIUMS: A Survey of Risk Assessment Literature and Policy Applications

Mita Giacomini

Center for Health Economics and Policy Analysis, Department of Clinical Epidemiology and Biostatistics, HSC-3H25, McMaster University, Hamilton, Ontario L8N 3Z5, Canada

Harold S. Luft

Institute for Health Policy Studies, University of California, San Francisco, California 94109

James C. Robinson

School of Public Health, University of California, Berkeley, California 94720

KEY WORDS: capitation fee, insurance selection bias, risk factors, reimbursement, actuarial analysis

ABSTRACT

This paper surveys recent health care reform debates and empirical evidence regarding the potential role for risk adjusters in addressing the problem of competitive risk segmentation under capitated financing. We discuss features of health plan markets affecting risk selection, methodological considerations in measuring it, and alternative approaches to financial correction for risk differentials. The appropriate approach to assessing risk differences between health plans depends upon the nature of market risk selection allowed under a given reform scenario. Because per capita costs depend on a health plan's population risk, efficiency, and quality of service, risk adjustment will most

401

0163-7525/95/0510-0401$05.00

strongly promote efficiency in environments with commensurately strong incentives for quality care.

INTRODUCTION

Capitated prospective financing is an increasingly popular approach to controlling health care expenditures. Capitation fixes health plan or provider revenues at levels based on the average anticipated health resource needs of members of a population, with the expectation that the program will supply necessary care prudently under the fixed budget. This principle is fundamental to community rated health plan premiums, but also applies to other health care financing mechanisms such as global budgeting at a regional level and capitated payments to physicians. The recipient of capitated payment faces a strong incentive to maintain costs below the prespecified reimbursement level. This can be accomplished in three ways: (*a*) by providing services more *efficiently*, either fewer in number or less resource intensive by unit for a given health outcome; (*b*) by undertreating selected individuals or *lowering quality* of services overall; or (*c*) by serving a population with health care requirements below the expected needs on which the payment rate was set, through *risk selection*.

Prospective payment is intended to motivate the first of these three organizational responses, improved efficiency. However, it must be applied within a context that inhibits the two alternative strategies of poor quality care and risk selection. Good quality measures and control mechanisms remain in the early stages of development; their improvement will become increasingly crucial to purchasers responding to health plan performance under competitive, capitated conditions. This paper focuses on policy approaches to redressing the second "pathological" response to capitation, risk selection. Risk adjustment corrects financially for risk selection, to make it a less profitable strategy than improving efficiency, given adequate quality control.

Health plans with sicker enrollees must charge higher premiums than plans with healthier members to cover their costs. *Adverse selection*, or enrolling a disproportionate share of unhealthy members, makes plans less price competitive to potential customers. Eventually it leads to plans either avoiding sick persons or offering them high premiums, which can become unaffordable. Plans successful at enrolling low-risk members should not be rewarded with market advantage for doing so. The purpose of risk adjustment is to reallocate revenues, or alternatively, from low-risk plans to high-risk plans. In either case, the redistribution goes only to the extent that the high-risk plans are equitably compensated for assuming more than their fair share of the sick in the market. Risk adjustment of community rated premiums financially pools underlying population health risk across all plans in a market. Ideally, it also leaves the competing plans financially at risk for their own efficient operation, as well as the insurance of random or preventable changes in members' health.

The purpose of this paper is to highlight the issues that arise in applying the evolving empirical tool of risk assessment in the context of market reforms. Risk assessment and adjustment have promise, as well as important contextual and technical limitations, for combating the deleterious effects of biased selection among competing health plans. This paper reviews risk assessment models for application to risk adjusting community-rated health plan premiums under managed competition through a survey of the empirical literature and recent policy debates regarding the potential role for risk adjusters. First we present theories regarding the nature of risk selection in competitive health plan markets and introduce basic principles for adjusting capitated rates to correct for risk differences among competing plans. We then survey the empirical literature on risk assessment, which is the statistical method for measuring biased selection. We close with a critical analysis of how risk assessment approaches relate to risk adjustment and other market or regulatory controls on risk selection.

BIASED SELECTION IN HEALTH PLAN MARKETS

Risk selection occurs as the result of various actions by consumers, employers, and health plans, which can actively or passively segment risks. Risk segmentation can be the result of active efforts by health plans to attract low-risk enrollees or avoid high-risk enrollees; it can be the result of passive factors such as the location of facilities or the actions of other health plans; or it may result from the level and structure of employer-paid health benefits. The mechanisms and effects vary depending on the regulatory and competitive structure of the market. Unfortunately, most empirical literature to date on risk selection has treated the *criteria* for choosing a particular plan as a black box. Studies instead have focused primarily on which types of consumers pick which general type of plan (usually HMO vs FFS). Relatively few studies have ventured further to examine the role of generic plan features in repelling or attracting particular risks.

Discussions of biased risk selection provide a number of credible (although largely unproven) hypotheses about both plan and market features that might affect biased selection. First, a number of factors could determine whether a particular plan itself is susceptible to adverse selection. Health plans may affect their risk through a number of mechanisms; these are summarized in Table 1. Currently, health plans can select risks on two levels: through the employers or groups they contract with, and through the subscribers within each group who might select the plan over others offered (23). A plan may design and package its product specifically to attract low risks and discourage high risks (19). High-quality benefits for the typical complaints of the healthy (e.g. maternity care, sports medicine, short-term psychotherapy) and spottier benefits for chronic health care conditions (e.g. restricted access to specialists, maximum coverage limits, etc) tend to attract better risks (17, 22). Bonus preventive services may appeal more to the healthy than to the ill (22). Inconvenient care for chronic diseases might be used to discourage low risks (17, 25, 27). Targeted advertising can appeal to healthy lifestyles, and enrollment procedures can require education or mobility correlated with better health (17). Sicker persons tend to be more attracted to low-cost sharing in exchange for high but predictable premiums, wider selection of physicians, and access to prestigious specialists. They are more likely to be in older plans (typically, but not necessarily, non-HMOs) because of long-term relationships with their plan's contracting providers (18, 19); these relationships make them less willing to switch plans (12, 22, 38). Because sick persons visit physicians more frequently, plans with geographically centralized providers may appeal to a smaller proportion of the sick in a region than plans with well-dispersed providers.

Alternatively, the plan may explicitly try to exclude high risks, for example through underwriting for preexisting conditions or risk factors. Plans may avoid epidemiologically risky communities by contracting only with providers in certain geographic locations (i.e. wealthier and healthier neighborhoods) or by redlining (or refusing to sell to) certain neighborhoods (e.g. gay communities to

Table 1 Health plan attributes potentially affecting biased selection

Mechanisms	Brings in higher risks (Adverse selection)	Brings in lower risks (Favorable selection)
Copayment/premium tradeoff	Low copayment/high premium	High copayment/low premium
Covered services	More comprehensive Conventional medicine . . .	Less comprehensive . . . with preventive emphasis
Geographic location of contracting providers	Less healthy, poorer areas	Healthier, wealthier areas
Geographic area covered by providers	Broadly distributed within region	Concentrated within region
Specialists, tertiary care	High quality, accessible	Low quality, inaccessible
Age of plan	Older, established plan	Newer, less familiar plan
Choice of providers	Free choice of provider	Restricted networks
Medical screening, underwriting	Prohibited	Allowed
	No preexisting exclusion	Exclusion of preexisting conditions
Rating method	Community rating	Experience rating

avoid persons with HIV) (22). Geographically concentrated providers may selectively inconvenience those frequently ill who are dispersed through a region (23). Finally, plans that historically have differentiated their prices across employer groups on the basis of risk or past claims (e.g. indemnity plans) may be less likely to have established relationships with high-risk employer groups (22).

A number of market and regulatory features also potentially affect plans' more passive susceptibility to selection resulting from information asymmetries between plans and consumers, sometimes referred to as consumer self-selection. Various health care reform proposals may modify these features to control the degree of risk segmentation, or to achieve other policy aims. First, some reforms aim at mandated universal coverage, whereas others aim more modestly at universal opportunities to buy coverage. The latter type of reform particularly invites adverse selection by persons who buy health insurance only on the occasion of becoming ill. Guaranteed issue of coverage and requirements for plans to cover preexisting conditions would further compound consumers' incentives to do so; together such reforms could result in higher premiums across the market if the healthy can avoid subsidizing the sick by staying out of the health insurance market entirely. Open enrollment and lock-in periods control the frequency with which consumers may change plans; shorter periods between plan choices generally encourage risk segmentation as consumers respond opportunistically to changes in their own health (22, 29). One-year lock-in, for example, may lower the incidence of risk-motivated plan switching compared to the one-month HMO lock-in currently used by the Medicare Risk program (22). Even longer lock-in periods could further decrease risk selection as fixed memberships' risk differences regress to the mean (37, 38). Requiring purchasing alliances or employer groups to offer their members a number of diverse plan choices also naturally increases opportunities for consumers to self-select according to risk, but encouraging continuity of coverage, rather than tying coverage options to the vagaries of employment options, may reduce selection.

Employer contribution strategies also affect employee price sensitivity and consequent self-selection among plans; reforms requiring employers or alliances to contribute only a flat amount approximating the lowest-cost plan toward premiums would raise price consciousness the most (6, 10, 21, 28). Because healthy persons are more price sensitive, more risk selection might ensue. Employers who pay a large percentage of all employees' premiums have good reason to encourage high utilizers to select the low-cost plan. Employers may also resist joining group purchasing arrangements (e.g. health alliances) if such pooling with alliance members might increase their premiums; plans in turn may avoid high-risk members by selectively contracting with low-risk employers or private, limited alliances. Some risk selection will also inevitably occur at random; this factor may impair the market entry and survival of smaller plans, and could inhibit efficient pricing in all plans. Random risk fluctuations may become less important if the market consolidates into a few large plans under the increased competitive pressures and risk is spread across larger numbers within plans. The evolution over time of markets under proposed reforms will also affect likely risk segmentation patterns. Early in the process of implementing managed competition reforms, consumers may suddenly face more choices among health plans with standard benefits, and there could be large swings in enrollment. Traditionally, the more price-sensitive low risks move to less expensive plans, but their price sensitivity may be largely a function of willingness to switch providers, not of illness per se (5). If high-risk persons are able to change health plans without changing providers, their price sensitivity may increase. This may be expected in metropolitan markets where plans have overlapping provider networks, as well as wherever point-of-service options are mandated for HMOs. Stability of the supply side of the market will also affect risk selection. There is a "regression to the mean" effect as members age in their chosen plan (37), so fewer occasions of plan entry and exit from the market could mean more moderate biased selection. Finally, if the reform ensures universal coverage, an influx of price-sensitive, low-income persons who had been previously uninsured or publicly insured (and largely underserved) could also affect risk distributions.

Many risk-selection mechanisms may be amenable to regulatory control. Reform proposals commonly limit opportunities for health plans to select risks actively, by requiring a standard package of covered services, limiting cost-sharing options, prohibiting selective underwriting practices, requiring fair and uniform advertising practices, enforcing quality standards in care for the chronically ill, and prescribing community rating of premiums. Nevertheless, risk selection could not be eliminated entirely. To the extent that a reform allows health plans to differentiate their products *at all* on the basis of cost sharing, price, or contracting providers, they will attract different risks. Risk selection would also continue because employers and consumers have their own motives and methods for self-selection, and these practices are generally less appropriate to regulate because they are the same ones that drive market choices on the basis of efficiency, price, and quality. It is unlikely that any set of reforms will eliminate risk differences among health plans, so specific methods to assess and adjust for remaining differences will be necessary.

RISK AND RISK ADJUSTMENT

Risk adjustment policy is based on the simple idea that epidemiological factors partly determine health care utilization, which in turn partly determines health care expenditures. Given standardized benefits, variations in expenditures between health plans which are not due to these underlying health needs could be attributed to efficiency differences in care delivery or administration. Risk, for risk-adjustment purposes, is a population's innate need for and propensity to use health care, independent of utilization (in)efficiencies. It is operationalized as essential health care expenditures. Hornbrook & Goodman (14) accordingly have defined risk as, "... the expected value of the distribution of per capita costs of efficiently provided preventive, diagnostic, and therapeutic health care services delivered to a defined group of enrollees for a specific future period."

Risk assessment models use a set of independent variables, risk factors, or risk adjusters, to predict necessary expenditures. For a study population, each risk factor is statistically associated with the dollar amount by which it typically increases or decreases the expected annual health care costs of an individual. Usually multiple regression or analysis of variance techniques are used. The resulting parameters, or cost weights, can then be applied to the members of another group to predict its total expected costs, or absolute risk. The group's risk is estimated by summing the expected expenditures of its members as predicted by the model. Relative risks are the ratios of these estimated total costs (absolute risks) between groups. To generate standardized relative risks, several groups are compared to a standard average-risk group, usually the potential market. For example, a health plan with a standardized relative risk of 1.1 would have 10% above average-risk members, compared to other plans serving the same market. It might legitimately require revenue 10% higher than the revenues of competing plans, due to its case mix and not its relative inefficiency.

There are two policy goals of risk adjustment: (*a*) to allow consumers to compare premium price differences that are not distorted by the health risk differences between the plans' memberships, but rather vary with the plans' value and efficiency, and (*b*) to reimburse each plan fairly for the proportion of population health risk that the plan assumes. The population is simply the market of all potential consumers who are choosing between a set of competing plans. Successful risk-adjustment policy means that if an efficient plan happens to enroll the sickest people in the market, it will be still be able to market at a competitive premium without this low premium translating into inadequate revenues to care for its needier members.

The financial transfers based on risk differences between plans may be approached in a number of ways. The first is to adjust community-rated premiums according to plans' relative risks. If plans rate prospectively on the basis of the market (e.g. alliance) population, then consumer prices automatically would be risk neutral, but plan revenues would have to be adjusted for risk segmentation. Higher-risk plans would receive more per capita than their quoted premium, and lower-risk plans would receive less. Alternatively, if plans adopt the community rate based on expected costs of current membership, premium prices will be distorted by the plans' relative risk advantages or disadvantages in the market. Low-risk plans with lower per member per month expenses will naturally be able to offer lower rates. In this case, risk adjustment of market prices is required to raise the effective consumer price of low-risk plans, and lower that of high-risk plans. This may be done simply by adjusting the enrollee's premium contribution. If risk-selection patterns do not change after open enrollment, plans may be paid fairly at their quoted (not marketed) rates. If further risk segmentation changes as a result of open enrollment, a second adjustment of revenues might be in order.

There are alternatives to this standard approach to risk adjusting community-rated premiums. In a less price competitive environment, a large payer might use risk assessment information to formulate fair fixed rates that all health plans must accept as payment. This process is analogous to the "Adjusted Average Per Capita Cost" (AAPCC) concept used by the Health Care Financing Administration (HCFA) to determine reimbursement rates for Medicare risk contracting. The formula may rely on absolute risk calculations (actual expected costs produced by a risk assessment model), or apply relative risk estimates to modify some standard premium.

An alternative to community rating is to allow health plans to quote different rates for different risk categories. This can undermine the social insurance objective of reforms mandating community rating, but, like risk-adjusted community rating, helps enhance price competition based on efficiency rather than risk selection. A version of this method is being implemented in California's new purchasing pool for small groups. The risk-specific rates can be charged directly to members, such that high-risk consumers pay more than low-risk, or they can be composited by the purchasing group(s) to have low-risk members subsidize high-risk members. The latter method is somewhat analogous to community rating by class (CRC) practiced by some HMOs, except that the health plan quotes and receives class-specific payments rather than the group's average-risk class rate. Another key difference is that if the rate is composited, the purchasing group becomes financially at risk for added premium costs if high-risk members tend to choose less efficient plans. Unlike CRC, the individual plan is not vulnerable to inadequate payment if it experiences adverse risk selection from that particular purchasing group.

A final alternative is the high-cost condition pool, a form of prospectively priced reimbursement for unusually expensive, clinically specific conditions or condition-treatment pairs. The purpose is to reimburse plans fairly for disproportionate adverse selection by extreme cost outlier cases, to the extent the high costs are due to inevitable health care needs and not extravagant overutilization (classic stop-loss reinsurance can indiscriminately reward overtreatment as well, and thus deter efficiency). This method can be used to supplement other types of risk adjusted community rating and has recently been implemented in New York State's small group purchasing pool. The condition pool approach estimates expected expenditures for selected health problems and pays plans either a lump or capitated monthly sum based directly on this. In the New York model, reimbursements are set at slightly below expected cost to create a disincentive to draw on the pool. Conditions covered in this manner include transplants for certain end-stage organ diseases, very low birthweight, advanced HIV disease, and ventilator dependency for ALS, severe trauma, or muscular dystrophy (33).

RISK ASSESSMENT

The following discussion of risk assessment modeling focuses on the problem of adjusting comprehensive community-rated premiums according to relative risk differences between competing health plans. However, many of the technical and conceptual issues generalize to all applications of risk information to determining appropriate prospective reimbursement rates.

The Dependent Variable: Health Expenditures

There are several ways to define the risk assessment model's dependent variable, future per capita health care expenditures. The most common is to use the dollar claims from a fee-for-service (FFS) plan. Studies based on group practice model HMO populations simulate FFS charges by imputing resource costs (11, 13, 15, 16, 35). Actual claims based on providers' comparable charges to non-HMO customers may be available for network model HMOs. Imputation is required in data systems that only measure utilization, rather than expenditures or resource use. It typically involves applying an average value (absolute or relative) to particular services, such as physician office visits or hospital admissions. Imputed costs tend to vary less than actual claims, and the restricted range can erroneously inflate the explanatory power of the model.

Another problem is the notorious skewness of per capita health care expenditures. Most people incur low annual expenditures while very few incur extremely high expenses. Linear risk assessment models can be quite sensitive to outliers (11, 16); models using log transformations or multiple equations provide a more accurate fit (26, 27). Estimating annual costs for persons who die or disenroll from a group during the year can compound the skewness problem. For example, when the costs of a "million dollar baby" who dies after a three-month life under neonatal intensive care are annualized, the result is not only an outlier, but an outlier of a magnitude beyond financial possibility. On the other hand, removing persons who die from the analysis introduces bias because mortality is systematically correlated with both risk factors and expenditures. Researchers often log or truncate expenditures, and sometimes use mortality or part-year enrollment as a control variable or selection criterion to deal with these problems. However, while investigators must often use such methods to deal with limited data and analytic constraints, health plans are liable for real, not log expenditures and cannot ignore outlier cases.

The dependent variable becomes further complicated when health care is conceptualized as more than medical care. This issue arises, for example, in comparative risk analyses of Medicare risk contracting, where HMO enrollees receive more preventive and supplementary services at low out-of-pocket cost than do their FFS counterparts. Similarly, some large employers argue that reforms should not force them to pool risk with other groups, because their health promotion programs actively invest in employee health and so they should reap the rewards in terms of lower medical insurance expenses. Benefits such as covered services and cost-sharing arrangements must be well defined, and preferably standardized between any populations whose risk is being compared. Supplemental care and spending on health promotion ideally should be included in a risk assessment model if it has potential impact on externalized health care costs or benefits, utilization of covered services, and longer term health risk. Whether payers, patients, or others should be able to recapture the difference in expected costs attributable to their health-promoting or risk-taking behavior is a question for another paper.

A critical and difficult risk-modeling task involves differentiating efficient and necessary care from superfluous care. Efficient means having a high ratio of benefits to costs. Quality of care, supplier-induced demand, moral hazard, and nonmedical aspects of consumer demand all confound risk assessment's assumption that historical correlates of expenditures can be used as meaningful proxies for health care needs. Risk assessment models can be judged in part by how cleverly they control for the effects of costs potentially containable through efficiency improvements, and focus instead on those driven by epidemiological and demand characteristics beyond the control of the plans or the providers.

The Independent Variables: Risk Factors

Risk assessment models are characterized by their independent variables, or risk factors. The major variables are: (a) those epidemiologically associated with populations' morbidity or demand patterns (demographic factors); (b) those that are more direct proxies for individuals' health conditions (health status factors); and (c) those that measure clinical precursors of health problems (clinical factors). Table 2 offers a fairly exhaustive list of the types of variables that have been proposed as risk adjusters. Several features determine whether a particular variable is appropriate to use for risk assessment: its conceptual relationship to health risk, the ability to measure it accurately from available data, its statistical contribution to accurate predictions of expense, its social acceptability for application to health care financing, and its susceptibility to gaming by financially interested parties.

Table 2 Variables proposed or used for risk assessment models based on individual or family unit of analysis

Independent variables

Demographics, Socioeconomic Status, or Local Market Characteristics

Age	Job classification
Gender	Education level
Family size	Geographic location
Family composition	Industry of employment
Marital status	Institutional status
Ethnicity	Transportation access
Primary language	Supply of providers, facilities
Welfare status	Urban residence
Welfare eligibility	Familiarity with services
Poverty	Supplementary insurance
Body weight relative to height	coverage
Income	
Employment status	

Health status

Self-reported health status	Diagnosis based on prior use of:
Mental health	Hospital services
Prior expenditures	Outpatient services
Quantity of inpatient services	Prescription drugs
Quantity of outpatient services	Use of ancillary/support services
Quantity of drugs	Disability status
Mortality (population rates)	Functional impairment

Health risk

Clinical values:	Behaviors predisposing disease:
Laboratory values	Social support
Genetic screening	Nutrition, weight
Physical exam findings	Smoking

Dependent variables

  Claims based, e.g. FFS claims

  Resource value based, e.g. HMO costs imputed from encounter
    data

  Total health care costs, including consumer out-of-pocket costs

  Costs for covered benefits only

Risk factors should relate closely to the health status of individuals or to the epidemiology of communities. Demographics such as age, gender, ethnicity, marital status, and family size correspond to population determinants of health relating to genetics, aging, and fertility, as well as to economic status and social support. Welfare status and employment data can be proxies for socioeconomic status and lifestyle factors associated with health risk. Some demographic risk factors pertain to demand characteristics as well as epidemiology, for example, geographic proximity of providers, familiarity with services, and transportation access. There is some controversy as to whether these demand or taste factors are appropriate risk adjusters. If their effect on utilization were truly exogenous to the delivery system (that is, members could not be convinced to utilize services more efficiently), they would be acceptable adjusters (14).

Direct measures of health status may come from a variety of sources. The most common are utilization data. However, all measures of utilization tend to be confounded to varying degrees by practice style or efficiency differences among the plans. Prior health expenditures and crude utilization data (e.g. quantity or incidence of services) are most susceptible to this bias. Utilization data that yield specific morbidity information by diagnosis allow for discriminating risk factors on the basis of whether they are chronic or acute, severe or not, and in some cases, more amenable to managed care or not. Mortality rates may be useful predictors of risks in groups. Surveys that question people directly about their health bypass confounding interactions with the health care system. However, like demographic factors, perceptions can reflect culture or taste factors as much as physical health determinants of demand.

In addition to conceptual appropriateness, accurate measurements of the variables should be available both to generate good estimates and to deter gaming. For adjustment of per capita premium rates, the adjuster should be measurable on an individual or family unit level. This is most easily done through administrative databases generated for other purposes in the health care market, such as medical records, claims, or personnel files. It may also be possible to collect data specifically for risk assessment (e.g. through special population surveys) if the information will improve risk prediction substantially over more easily available data and if it is worth the additional cost. Age and gender are available from almost all potential data sources. Personnel file variables such as job classification, marital status, family composition, salary, and education can be used to improve demographic models. Administrative files maintained by public agencies also yield useful risk information; Medicare, for example, uses age, gender, welfare status, institutional status, and residence county expenditure levels to determine the AAPCC that it pays HMOs under risk contracts. Finally, medical utilization and clinical data contained in automated medical records can be used for risk assessment based on direct health status measures. Databases vary in accuracy and in quality of information. Data used for financial purposes (e.g. claims) tend to be audited more carefully than data used for other administrative or bureaucratic purposes (e.g. encounters).

The risk adjuster must contribute substantially and significantly to explaining expenditures. This contribution is not an immutable statistical fact, but will be affected by the particular incentives, opportunities, and information driving the risk-selection process. Statistical power may be sacrificed to meet other criteria for a good risk assessment model. For example, limiting past hospital diagnoses used to predict next year's costs to those that are relatively non-discretionary mitigates providers' incentives to hospitalize inefficiently, but also decreases statistical power because many meaningful diagnoses cannot be used (2).

Regardless of how accessible, measurable, or powerful a predictor may be, other social values might interfere with its measurement or application. For instance, privacy considerations may limit access to information such as individuals' income, self-reported health, functioning, mental health, genetics, ethnicity, or health-related behaviors. Potentially conflicting interests on the part of the organization administering the risk assessment, for example, government agencies or employers, naturally compound privacy concerns. Some critics also worry that explicitly associating cost factors with risk characteristics such as race, language, disability, or economic class might reinforce social stigmas. Conversely, however, these risk factors could improve medical access for disadvantaged groups if they result in higher financial rewards for members' enrollment or treatment. The Clinton Health Security Act, for example, specified risk adjusting premiums according to socioeconomic status and mental health (although these factors have been little studied as risk assessment variables).

Finally, measurements of the adjuster should not be easily gameable, that is, distorted by market participants trying to enhance their profit from the financial transfers based on the assessed risk differences. Gaming could occur in a number of ways: Data could be falsified or, probably more likely, assignment of individuals to ambiguous risk categories could be distorted. This is most likely with utilization-based health measures (e.g. diagnoses), and less feasible with self-reported health status or demographic statistics. An example has been seen in the case of DRG creep under prospective payment for hospital care: Patterns of disease incidence appeared to shift as patients were classified into higher-profit diagnosis categories (7, 8, 32). Finally, utilization-based measures of health status such as diagnosis at hospitalization can create incentives for providers to overutilize services on which lucrative flags are based.

Study Population

The study population used to estimate the parameters can determine how well the cost weights generalize to other populations. Artifacts of cost data, such as imputing incomplete costs or truncating very high costs, can affect the estimated impact of risk factors on expenditures. The study group's benefit coverage will also influence the pattern of expenditures. Although differing benefit packages can be partially controlled for by removing services from the analysis to simulate a standard package, the influence of omitted services on the use of covered services is lost. Dual coverage and supplementary benefits patterns can also distort a risk assessment model because (*a*) some costs may not appear in the data set, and (*b*) the cost-containing impact of copayment is lessened. Mortality and migration (between health plans as well as regions) introduce sampling and measurement problems.

The association of risk factors with individuals' expected expenditures may also be biased wherever unmeasured population-specific social and epidemiological determinants of need interact with the risk factors included in the model. For example, a risk assessment model may yield different cost weights for age and gender if it is estimated on data from a privately insured population than it might on data from a Medicaid-insured population.

Different risk factors predict well in different populations. In the elderly, for example, hospitalizations are both more frequent and more likely to be for chronic conditions; their measurement contributes important information to risk assessment. In the frail elderly, physical functioning may predict resource needs better than clinical diagnoses, which become numerous and interactive in very old age (M Hornbrook, personal communication). In contrast, the nonelderly are rarely hospitalized; when they are, it is most typically for acute conditions that do not affect next year's resource needs (15, 27). Consequently, hospital-based diagnoses are less useful predictors in this population; demographics and family composition may be better proxies for health care needs. Identification of the relatively few young individuals with chronic illnesses would of course improve any model. Indicators based on ambulatory diagnoses or sentinel drug prescriptions may detect more high-risk diagnoses than hospital discharge diagnoses would in the nonelderly.

Problems of empirical bias are compounded when generalizing risk models from one population to another. The best solution is to calibrate the model on a study population as representative as possible of the actual population across which financial risk adjustments will be made. For example, if risk adjustments will be made between health plan enrollees in a regional alliance, the model should be calibrated on a regionally representative population. Even so, there will be difficulty generalizing any model calibrated under today's financing environment to populations experiencing profound improvements in coverage and access under universal coverage and health care reforms. Risk forecasts for the uninsured, underinsured, or Medicaid-insured may be particularly underestimated owing to pent-up demand.

Accuracy

A number of empirical studies of potential risk assessment models have been published in recent years. For this review, we selected only studies using risk factors to predict or explain population *expenditures* for health care (and not merely service utilization). The study designs for these 17 papers are summarized in the Appendix. Six research teams studied Medicare populations; 11 studied nonelderly populations. Five studies addressed HMO populations, and the rest used subjects covered by variants of FFS plans. Most investigators formulated models using risk information from one year to predict the following year's expenses, but several modeled expenditures instead as a function of concurrent risk status. The risk factors in the latter models would appear more powerful than they would be if applied to prospective financing. The remainder of our review focuses on how the various risk factors appear to perform across this diverse body of literature.

Several measures are currently available for evaluating risk assessment models for accuracy. Each addresses somewhat different aspects of a model's performance. The most intuitive are measures of correlation. These represent how tightly actual expenditures match predicted expenditures, both at the individual and at the group levels. A related question is how far group predictions tend to be off on average, in dollar or relative terms. Bias is another issue: To the extent that a model predicts imperfectly, in what identifiable individuals or groups does it systematically overpredict or underpredict? This bias is especially important for subpopulations, such as the chronically ill, who could suffer discrimination as a result of cost underestimation.

The first criterion is how closely the model predicts expenditures at the level of the *unit of analysis* used to develop the model, i.e. the individual plan member or subscriber unit (subscriber and covered family members). For regression models, the R^2 statistic represents the fraction of the variation in expenditures *across individuals* that can be explained by the risk factors. This R^2 is useful for refining the statistical models; the higher the R^2, the better the model is at predicting individuals' health care costs. However, health care expenses for individuals are notoriously variable and unpredictable. A few studies have estimated that a risk assessment model accounting for all predictable expenditures might at best achieve an R^2 of only 0.15 for adults (26, 35) and 0.37 for children (27). This maximum R^2 statistic is specific to the population being studied; some published risk assessment models have achieved individual R^2s well above these limits (9, 16, 36).

Table 3 summarizes published risk assessment models calibrated on non-Medicare populations. It is important to note that these studies use varying population samples and analytic approaches. Because of this, the explained variance (e.g. R^2) of the models should not be compared directly between studies. In other words, a model showing a higher R^2 in one study is not necessarily better than a different model with a lower R^2 in another study. Within each class of adjusters, the relatively wide variation in R^2s demonstrates that model accuracy is clearly sensitive to a number of technical issues beyond whether *demographic* or *health status* adjusters are used: sampling approach, study population, modeling techniques (multi- or single-equation, functional

Table 3 Risk assessment models estimated on non-Medicare populations

Risk factors	Approximate R^2	Model	Population	1st author	Notes
DEMOGRAPHIC MODELS					
Age, gender	0.01	Predict	HMO Oregon adults	Hornbrook (13)	
Age, gender	0.02	Predict	HMO Oregon adults	Hornbrook (15, 16)	
Age, gender	0.03	Predict	HMO California adults	Hayes (11)	
Age, gender	0.04	Explain	HMO Minnesota adults	Weiner (36)	
AAPCC	0.02	Predict	FFS US adults	Newhouse (26)	4-equation model
Age, gender, site, AFDC	0.02	Predict	RAND except children	Newhouse (27)	2-equation model
Age, gender, employment variables	0.02	Predict	HMO Oregon adults	Hornbrook (16)	
Age, gender, supplement insurance, region	0.02	Predict	Insured Netherlands	van Vliet (35)	2-equation model
Age, gender, step	0.03	Explain	Bank FFS N California	Rosencranz*	Log costs
Demographics, socioeconomic variables	0.03	Predict	Insured Netherlands	van Vliet (35)	2-equation model
Age, gender, supplemental insurance, region	0.03	Predict	Random Netherlands	van Vliet (35)	4-equation model
Age, gender, step, employment variables	0.04	Explain	Bank FFS N California	Rosencranz*	Log costs
Demographics, socioeconomic variables	0.04	Predict	Random Netherlands	van Vliet (35)	4-equation model
CRC–age, gender, employment variables	0.21	Predict	HMO California	Cave (9)	Log costs
SELF-REPORTED HEALTH STATUS MODELS					
AAPCC, subjective health	0.03	Predict	FFS US adults	Newhouse (26)	4-equation model
Self-reported health status	0.04	Predict	HMO Oregon adults	Hornbrook (13)	
Demographics, subjective health	0.05	Predict	RAND experiment children	Newhouse (27)	2-equation model
Self-reported by parent	0.05	Predict	FFS US children	Newhouse (27)	2-equation model
Age, gender, self-reported health	0.06	Predict	HMO Oregon adults	Hornbrook (13)	
Self-reported health	0.18	Predict	HMO Oregon adults	Hornbrook (16)	
PHYSIOLOGICAL MEASURES					
AAPCC, physiological health (claims)	0.05	Predict	FFS US adults	Newhouse (26)	4-equation model
Demographic, physiological health	0.11	Predict	RAND experiment children	Newhouse (27)	2-equation model
Physiologic measures	0.11	Predict	FFS US children	Newhouse (27)	

PRIOR UTILIZATION

Inpatient diagnosis	0.04	Predict	HMO California adults	Hayes (11)	
Prescription drugs	0.05	Predict	HMO Oregon	Hornbrook (15)	
Demographics, prior in/out use	0.07	Predict	Insured Netherlands	van Vliet (35)	2-equation model
Drugs, outpatient diagnosis	0.07	Predict	HMO Oregon	Hornbrook (15)	
ACGs−outpatient diagnosis cost groups	0.15	Explain	HMO Minnesota adults	Weiner (36)	
Age, gender, ADGs−outpatient diagnosis groups	0.19	Explain	HMO Minnesota adults	Weiner (36)	
Demographics, prior in/outpatient utilization	0.21	Predict	RAND except children	Newhouse (27)	2-equation model

PRIOR EXPENDITURES

AAPCC, prior cost	0.06	Predict	FFS US adults	Newhouse (26)	4-equation model
Demographics, prior cost	0.07	Predict	Insured Netherlands	van Vliet (35)	2-equation model

MIXED MODELS

Demographics, chronic condition, impair	0.08	Predict	Random Netherlands	van Vliet (35)	4-equation model
AAPCC, physiologic health, subjective health, prior use	0.09	Predict	FFS US adults	Newhouse (26)	4-equation model
Demographics, physiologic health, subjective health	0.11	Predict	RAND except children	Newhouse (27)	2-equation model
Demographics, chronic disease, functioning, self-reported health	0.11	Predict	Random Netherlands	van Vliet (35)	4-equation model
Demographics, physiological, subjective health, prior use	0.24	Predict	RAND except children	Newhouse (27)	2-equation model
In/outpatient utilization, expenditures	0.33	Predict	HMO California	Cave (9)	Log costs
CRC, prior in/outpatient utilization, expenditures	0.38	Predict	HMO California	Cave (9)	Log costs

Key: Predict = predictive model; Explain = explanatory models (contemporaneous)

*Rosencranz SL, Luft HS. 1993. Changing the focus: evaluating health care expenditure models on risk-stratified groups of enrollees. (Unpublished manuscript; 30a).

form, explanatory or predictive), data sources, measurement of the variables, and data modifications (cleaning, imputation of missing information, functional transformations, etc).

Simple age and gender models appear to explain 1–4% of cost variations among subscribers or individuals. Demographic models that add more detailed information regarding employment and welfare still explain only 2–4%. One model using *community rating by class* variables and HMO data explained an unusual 21%; imputed cost data and logarithmically transformed expenditures may have contributed to this unusual goodness-of-fit. More complex health status models usually include age and gender; these variables contribute independently to risk estimates and help minimize potential model bias and cross subsidization between old and young or male and female (15, 16). Self-reported health status measures in addition to age and gender perform slightly better, typically explaining 3–6% of the variance, and in one study up to 18%. Physiological measures based on physical examination explained 5–11%. Prior utilization models relying on the incidence, volume, or diagnosis recorded from either inpatient or outpatient episodes vary substantially in their predictive power, and explain 4–21% of individual differences in expenditures. Models incorporating diagnosis information seem to perform better than pure utilization models in adults. Prior utilization with demographics appeared relatively accurate in the one model calibrated on children. Individuals' prior health care costs plus simple demographics achieved relatively low R^2s of 6–7% in the two studies reviewing these types of models for comparative purposes. In contrast, another study combining prior spending with utilization information reported R^2s of over 0.3. Finally, models combining data from disparate sources (i.e. demographic, personnel, financial, medical records) reported R^2s ranging from 0.08 to 0.29. These models are probably the least administratively feasible to apply because of the extensive data required.

Table 4 surveys published risk assessment models calibrated on Medicare populations. As in non-Medicare populations, demographic AAPCC factors explained little of the cost variations between population members, from less than 1% to 3%. Models relying on direct measures of well being, such as disability, activities of daily living, or self-reported health status, achieved R^2s of 0.02 to 0.07. Similarly, prior utilization models not incorporating diagnosis information also yielded R^2s ranging from 0.02 to 0.07; utilization-based diagnosis models performed somewhat better, explaining 4–16% of the variance in expenditures. The two prior expenditure models explained 6–9% of individual variance. A model combining physiological measures of clinical risk, disability, and prior utilization in a small regional population produced an R^2 of 0.10.

In summary, models vary in their ability to predict (or in some cases, contemporaneously explain) expenditure differences between individuals. In

Table 4 Risk assessment models estimated on Medicare populations

Risk factors	Approximate R^2	Model	Population	1st author	Notes
DEMOGRAPHIC MODELS					
AAPCC	0.00	Predict	MC FFS Michigan	Lubitz (20)	
AAPCC	0.01	Predict	MC FFS National	Ash (3)	
Age, gender, welfare	0.01	Predict	MC FFS National	Beebe (4)	
AAPCC	0.03	Explain	MC S Carolina	Manton (24)	
AAPCC	0.03	Predict	MC Framingham	Schauffler (31)	Log costs
NON-UTILIZATION MEASURES OF HEALTH					
Perceived health status	0.02	Predict	MC FFS Michigan	Lubitz (20)	
IADL	0.03	Predict	MC FFS Michigan	Lubitz (20)	
PHYSIOLOGICAL MEASURES					
AAPCC, clinical risk factors	0.05	Predict	MC Framingham	Schauffler (31)	Log costs
AAPCC, disability	0.07	Predict	MC Framingham	Schauffler (31)	Log costs
PRIOR UTILIZATION MEASURES					
Demographics, any inpatient use	0.02	Predict	MC FFS National	Beebe (4)	
Demographics, any inpatient use	0.03	Predict	MC FFS National	Ash (3)	
Chronic conditions	0.04	Predict	MC FFS Michigan	Lubitz (20)	
Demographics, days inpatient	0.04	Predict	MC FFS National	Beebe (4)	
Demographics, DCG	0.05	Predict	MC FFS National	Ash (3)	
Demographics, inpatient days, any outpatient	0.05	Predict	MC FFS National	Ash (3)	
AAPCC, prior inpatient/outpatient use	0.06	Predict	MC Framingham	Schauffler (31)	Log costs
Prior inpatient/outpatient utilization	0.07	Predict	MC FFS Michigan	Lubitz (20)	
AAPCC, in/outpatient diagnosis	0.12	Explain	MC S Carolina	Manton (24)	
AAPCC, in/outpatient, mortality	0.16	Explain	MC S Carolina	Manton (24)	
PRIOR EXPENDITURES					
Prior expenditures	0.06	Predict	MC FFS Michigan	Lubitz (20)	
Part B expenditures only	0.09	Predict	MC FFS National	Ash (3)	
MIXED MODELS					
AAPCC, prior use, clinical risk	0.08	Predict	MC Framingham	Schauffler (31)	Log costs
AAPCC, prior use, clinical risk, disability	0.10	Predict	MC Framingham	Schauffler (31)	Log costs

Key: Predict = predictive model; Explain - explanatory models (contemporaneous)

addition, the wide variation in R^2s among models using similar variables illustrates the sensitivity of risk assessment model performance to research design. Some models produced high R^2s in part by using multiple or nonlinear equations. In general, demographic models, even fairly sophisticated versions, explain the least at the individual level. Not surprisingly, more direct measures of health status do better at predicting individuals' health care spending next year.

Ability to explain *individuals'* variations in expected costs is not the only measure of a good risk assessment model. The assessment of biased selection across health plans in a market requires that models be accurate when applied to *groups* of health plan enrollees; consequently, a fundamental issue is how well the model predicts expenditures within, and expenditure differences across, large groups. A statistic sometimes used to demonstrate this dimension of accuracy is the prediction error, or the related predictive ratio. Predictive error statistics compare predicted costs with actual costs (either the difference or the ratio) for selected groups or individuals. The mean prediction error is the average dollar amount by which estimates deviate from the real cost. To validate models, this statistic is commonly applied to random samples from the population on which the model was calibrated. Predictive errors appeal to policymakers because they can be used to assign a dollar value to a model's potential inaccuracy at the group or individual level. However, a major drawback of the statistic is that the dollar value is highly specific to the study population and may not be generalized with confidence to actual, risk-stratified groups. It is typically generated by estimating risks based on *random* samples, which, by definition, approximate average risk of the population from which they are drawn. Due to the law of large numbers, it is not surprising that, as larger samples are drawn, the predictive error improves; this relationship holds regardless of the how poorly a model's risk factors predict expenditures at the individual level. Even demographic models with relatively small individual level R^2s can yield highly accurate and reliable expenditure predictions when applied to large groups; demographic models, for instance, are highly accurate in randomly drawn groups of 1000 or more (30).

Most policy relevant are measures of a model's accuracy in groups that are *different from the sample* used to calibrate the model, and for comparing groups that *differ from each other* in their risk composition. Useful metrics include group-level prediction errors and group R^2. Group-level predictive error statistics have been used to test for bias in subpopulations of high- or low-risk individuals (rather than random samples) as defined either by the model's dependent or independent variables, such as women, persons with cancer or heart disease, persons with no prior costs, or those with a recent history of low or high hospital utilization (3, 4, 15, 16, 31). A group R^2 measures correlation between actual and expected costs across risk-segmented groups. The group R^2 is generated by arranging a population into risk-stratified groups as defined by the expected value of the dependent variable (predicted cost), and then measuring the correlation between expected and actual expenditures by group. This measure has been used on fully risk-stratified groups (i.e. the 50 highest-risk persons in one group, the 50 next most expensive persons in the next group, and so forth) (SL Rosenkranz & HS Luft, unpublished manuscript). The simulations in an employed population yield a group R^2 of 58% for a simple demographic model and 63% for a model based on personnel data even though these models yielded R^2s of less than 0.04 at the subscriber unit level.

However, neither randomly selected nor fully risk-segmented groups occur in health care markets. One study has looked at naturally occurring risk selection, using 542 employer groups within a single health plan (11). Using the *group* as the unit of analysis, regression modeling yielded an R^2 of 0.51 for a demographic model, 0.52 for a model with inpatient admission data. In this study, the demographic model's predictive power at the *subscriber* level was approximately half that of a model incorporating hospitalization diagnoses, but not much less accurate at predicting actual costs of the 542 employer *groups*. Further research is needed to assess various models' performance under conditions of realistic risk segmentation, especially between health plans or providers rather than between employer groups within a single delivery system.

A risk assessment model should be unbiased, that is, it must not systematically under- or overestimate the expenditures of identifiable subpopulations (e.g. male vs female, young vs old, members of one plan vs another). The last criterion is particularly important: risk assessment models should not systematically reward low quality delivery systems by confusing the process or consequences of poor care with members' innate health risk. Models relying on prior utilization measures, for example, may favor *inefficient* health plans that indulge in more unnecessary utilization. Health surveys as well as utilization measures of diagnoses could favor *ineffective* health plans if bad health reflects a history of inadequate treatment or prevention in addition to exogenous influences (22).

Biases that erroneously favor particular demographic groups could create unfair financial subsidies (15, 16), as well as opportunities for competitive risk selection. The inclusion of a risk factor in the model (e.g. gender) tends to decrease bias (15), but unfortunately this does not necessarily ensure that the model will predict well for groups in one particular risk category (e.g. females). Higher predictive accuracy at the individual level has also been associated with lower age and gender bias at the group level (15). Wherever a model regularly overpredicts for one easily identified group and underpredicts for another, capitated health plans or providers can profit by pursuing the first and avoiding the second. The problem of bias directly relates to the problem of assessing goodness-of-fit at the level of group estimates under conditions of strategic risk selection. A model that appears unbiased and accurate in random populations may be very biased or inaccurate in risk-segmented populations if the risk segmentation occurs on the basis of (or correlated with) risk factors that interact with other determinants in the model.

The Problem of Selection Within Risk Classes

Risk assessment models that appear powerful at the group level but weak at the individual level could, in theory, be defeated by sophisticated selection of risks on a case-by-case basis, using information not captured by the model (25). Health care spending is skewed and difficult to predict in general. Even within tightly defined risk categories (e.g. women aged 40–50 with cancer), expected expenditures will still vary widely between individuals. Because health plans and providers possess information that allows them to discern high-risk from low-risk individuals *within* most risk-adjuster classes, they could, in theory, game the system by catering to low risks and repelling high risks within defined risk classes. However, there could be several remedies to the potential problem of selective disenrollment.

Perhaps least effectively, sophisticated risk selection could be detected and corrected for with a model that is maximally accurate at the individual level. A perfect model would be prohibitively expensive to administer, and imperfect models fail to eliminate substantial profitability to health plans of aggressive disenrollment of high risks (26). Another approach involves enforcing high-quality standards or relying on professional norms to inhibit the plans' administrators or providers from actively discouraging targeted members. Probably the most compelling deterrent would be market reputation. Selective disenrollment means that one plan's sick members are systematically unloaded onto competitors (the Queen of Spades phenomenon in the game of Hearts). Especially under universal coverage where one plan's dump automatically becomes another plan's new member, any plan successful at selective disenrollment would be easily identified and exposed by its competitors. Unsatisfactory services for the chronically ill may also appear as lower quality and may be unattractive to healthy prospective customers, jeopardizing the plan's market share. In short, under competitive conditions it may be more profitable for plans and providers to care for their high-risk patients than to have their reputation—and market share—endangered by aggressive selective disenrollment strategies. Failing that, side payments from a patient's old plan to the newly selected plan may be a direct way of discouraging the practice (22).

DISCUSSION

Financially risk adjusting capitated premiums mitigate health plans' incentive to select risks, but this is not its primary purpose (22). Uneven risk between health plans does not itself threaten effective competition. For example, it may be socially desirable for health plans to specialize in the efficient care of particular diseases or populations. Rather, risk adjustment reverses the undesirable results of risk segmentation, without seeking to undo all of the *processes* that create it. Adjustments must accomplish health risk pooling in spite of the emergence of risk-biased associations between consumers, employers, and health plans from a competitive market.

This raises two important points about designing risk-adjustment systems. First, risk adjustment achieves financial subsidization of the sick by the healthy. It supports a solidarity perspective of social health insurance rather than one based on actuarial fairness (34) because it requires all health plans in a market to contribute equitably to caring for the net burden of illness in the market population. The level at which risk is pooled, and consequently the means by which risk is adjusted, depend upon what subsidies are intended as well as allowed under health care reforms.

Second, the factors used for assessing risk must accurately detect the particular type of risk segmentation one expects to find in the reformed market. The risk factors must relate to the information asymmetries and strategic practices driving selection. As a rule, the less random and more opportunistic the risk selection, the more sophisticated the risk assessment model will need to be to estimate the risk differences correctly. For example, if consumers were randomly allocated to large plans, the resulting expected cost differences could be measured accurately by using very simple demographics. If, at the other extreme, plans were allowed to examine and exclude members on a case-by-case basis, risk assessment likewise must be based on more clinically detailed measures of group members' epidemiology.

As market reforms are implemented, any reasonable risk adjustment would be an improvement over unadjusted capitated financing. However, assessment methods and models will need to continually evolve in sophistication to keep up with strategic responses to reformed market conditions and risk-adjustment policy. There are several reasons for this. First, if reforms achieve their goal and all plans and providers become more efficient, the profitability of marginal improvements in efficiency will drop and the relative profitability of risk selection will rise. Second, with time and familiarity, payers and providers may develop new ways of gaming the adjustment process (25). More sensitive risk assessment models will be needed to detect potentially more devious risk selection. Third, part of the managed care philosophy is for the capitated health plan to take some responsibility for preventing disease and maintaining members' health. Although health care systems should not be penalized for the morbidity of cases they assume, they should not be rewarded for morbidity they cause, or fail to prevent. Dynamic risk adjustment models should be developed that appropriately consider risk as an output as well as an input of health care. Quality management and risk adjustment can become a more continuous process if the health risk of inputs can be differentiated from the health risk of outputs. For example, in risk adjusting premiums between health plans, plans could be more generously rewarded for very sick persons who join than they are for members who become sicker with preventable diseases, or for very sick members who leave the plan.

Finally, risk assessment models will require regular re-estimation and calibration to keep pace with changes in epidemiology and medical practice. Technological improvements, clinical guidelines, and organizational efficiencies should be expected to—indeed, should be *designed to*—alter the relationship of risk factors to health care costs over time. If medical science and delivery systems truly progress over the years, high-risk categories should regress to the mean, while low-risk categories do not.

Health plan premiums are determined by a basic triad of risk, efficiency, and quality. Risk adjustment forces health plans to pursue efficiency and quality to achieve an attractive product and competitive pricing. Many discussions of risk adjustment policy focus on encouraging efficiency while leaving quality as a concern for other areas of health care reform. However, these three elements form a true system of incentives. Strong incentives toward one put pressure on the others, which in turn require commensurate support through appropriate regulatory and market incentives. Successful risk adjustment imposes burdens particularly on policy reforms in quality management. Pressures and means to demonstrate quality must rise in concert with disincentives to risk select in order to ensure that efficiency improvements rather than quality erosion become the most profitable enterprise for health plans.

APPENDIX Summary of empirical risk assessment studies surveyed

First author	Sample	N	Risk factors	Dependent variable
Anderson (1)	1983–84 FFS aged Medicare beneficiaries, 2.5% national sample	213,844	AAPCC CRCs: "Cost Related Groups" based on less discretionary inpatient diagnosis, demographics DCGs: "Diagnostic Cost Groups" based on less discretionary inpatient diagnosis + AAPCC variables PACs: "Payment Amount for Capitated Systems": inpatient MDC, chronicity, outpatient use, + demographics, disability	Parts A & B Medicare expenditures Truncated at 99th percentile
Ash (3)	1974–80 FFS aged Medicare beneficiaries; 5% national sample	18,677 for 1975–77 20,263 for 1978–80	AAPCC DCGs: "Diagnostic Cost Groups" based on less discretionary inpatient diagnosis + AAPCC variable	Medicare expenditures
Beebe (4)	1975–78 FFS aged Medicare beneficiaries; 5% national sample	20,773	Age, gender, Medicaid/welfare proxy Demographics + any inpatient Demographics + days inpatient	Total Medicare reimbursement
Cave (9)	1984–85 Staff HMO, families, ages 1–64 yrs, Southern California	24,330	CRC: "Community rating by class" age, gender, marital status, family size, family composition, industry Prior utilization and expenditures Combined CRC and prior expenditures	Inputed from HMO encounters, + contracting provider claims Log transformed

APPENDIX *(Continued)*

First author	Sample	N	Risk factors	Dependent variable
Hayes (11)	1984–88 PGP HMO subscriber units, subscriber under 65, employed, non-Medicaid, non-Medicare; Northern California	587,659	Age, gender, step Length of enrollment Nondiscretionary hospital admissions 2 yrs prior (consult w/MDs, 14 categories)	Imputed from HMO utilization records, no trans (truncated for comparison only)
Hornbrook (15)	1980–87 PGP HMO individual members under 65, employed, non-Medicaid, non-Medicare; Oregon	51,633 pooled time series cross section	Age, gender "Clinical-behavioral classes" of diagnoses (medical chart); Drug orders (medical chart) Prior year utilization expense	Imputed from HMO utilization records
Hornbrook (16)	1980–81; 1985–86 PGP HMO subscriber units, subscriber under 65, employed, non-Medicaid, non-Medicare; Oregon	1545 for 1980–81; 842 for 1985–86	Age, gender Education, occupation, marital status Self-reported health status Self-reported N outpatient visits Self-reported medical conditions	Imputed from HMO encounters
Hornbrook (13)	1990–91 PGP HMO individual members under 65, employed, non-Medicaid, non-Medicare; Oregon	8265	Age, gender Self-reported health status	Imputed from HMO encounters
Lubitz (20)	1982–83 FFS Medicare enrollees, Michigan	2000	AAPCC Perceived health status IADL Chronic conditions Prior expenditures Prior in/outpatient utilization	Medicare charges

Manton (24)	1981 FFS Medicare Southern Carolina	4000	AAPCC In/outpatient diagnosis Mortality	Medicare charges
Newhouse (26)	1974–82 individuals over age 14 participating in Rand Experiment	3958 (7690 person-years)	AAPCC: age, gender, site, AFDC status Physiologic health Subjective health Prior year inpatient/outpatient use	Claims
Newhouse (27)	Children *under* age 14 participating in Rand Experiment	1844 2185 person-years	AAPCC: age, gender, site, AFDC status Physiologic health Subjective health (parent's perception) Prior year inpatient/outpatient use	Claims
Robinson (30)	1981–84 FFS bank employee subscriber units; Northern California	31,849	Age, gender, personnel variables: step, educ, salary, occup level, marital, length employ, coverage eligibility full/part year	Log $ claims; truncated at $25K Part-year eligibility controlled with independent variables
Rosencranz*	1989 FFS bank employee subscriber units; Northern California	5000	Age, gender, step Marital status, salary, state of residence, length employ	Log $ claims Truncated at $50K
Schauffler (31)	1982–85 FFS aged Medicare beneficiaries; Framingham, Mass.	1162	AAPCC inpt/outpt use disability index clinical risk factors	Log $ payments

APPENDIX (*Continued*)

First author	Sample	N	Risk factors	Dependent variable
Van Vliet (35)	1976–80 individuals in large private insurance company, Netherlands	~35,000	Age, gender Supplementary insurance, geographic region	Claims
	1976 same as above	~14,000	Same as above, + family size, employment, income, education, urbanization Prior utilization Prior costs	Claims
	1981–82 individuals, national health survey data, Netherlands	~20,000	Age, gender, supplementary insurance, region Family size, "socioeconomic status:" body weight, urbanization, facilities supply Self-reported health status Chronic conditions, physical impairment	Imputed from utilization information
Wiener (36)	1980 or 1981; Network HMO individual members; Minnesota	Approx 35,000–40,000	Age, gender ADG—ambulatory diagnostic groups ACG—ambulatory cost groups	"Claims"—would be charges if FFS

* Rosencranz SL, Luft HS. 1993. Changing the focus: evaluating health care expenditure models on risk-stratified groups of enrollees. Unpublished manuscript. Earlier version presented at the annual meeting of the Association for Health Services Research, June 1993.

Literature Cited

1. Anderson GF, Steinberg EP, Powe NR, Antebi S, Whittle J, et al. 1990. Setting payment rates for capitated systems: a comparison of various alternatives. *Inquiry* 27:225–33
2. Ash A. 1994. Presented at Natl. Health Policy Forum, Washington, DC, Feb. 23
3. Ash A, Porell F, Gruenberg L, Sawitz E, Beiser A. 1989. Adjusting Medicare capitation payments using prior utilization data. *Health Care Fin. Rev.* 10:17–29
4. Beebe J, Lubitz J, Eggers P. 1985. Using prior utilization to determine payments for Medicare enrollees in health maintenance organizations. *Health Care Fin. Rev.* 6:27–38
5. Berki SE, Ashcraft MLF. 1980. HMO enrollment: who joins and why: a review of the literature. *Milbank Q.* 58:588–632
6. Bowen BD, Slavin EL. 1991. Adjusting contributions to address selection bias: three models for employers. *Adv. Health Econ. Health Serv. Res.* 12:77–96
7. Carter GM, Ginsburg PB. 1985. The Medicare case mix index increase, RAND (Santa Monica, CA), R-3292-HCFA
8. Carter GM, Newhouse JP, Relles DA. 1990. How much change in the case mix index is DRG creep?, RAND (Santa Monica, CA), R-3826-HCFA
9. Cave DG, Schweitzer SO, Lachenbruch PA. 1989. Adjusting employer group capitation premiums by community rating by class factors. *Med. Care* 27:887–99
10. Enthoven A. 1989. Effective management of competition in the FEHBP (Federal Employees Health Benefits Program). *Health Aff.* 8:33–50
11. Hayes ST. 1991. Demographic risk factors derived from HMO data. *Adv. Health Econ. Health Serv. Res.* 12:177–96
12. Hellinger FJ. 1987. Selection bias in health maintenance organizations: analysis of recent evidence. *Health Care Fin. Rev.* 9:55–63
13. Hornbrook MC, Goodman MJ. 1993. *Assessing relative health plan risk with the Rand-36 health survey.* Presented at Annu. Meet. Assoc. Health Serv. Res., June
14. Hornbrook MC, Goodman MJ. 1991. Health plan case mix: definition, measurement, and use. *Adv. Health Econ. Health Serv. Res.* 12:111–48
15. Hornbrook MC, Goodman MJ, Bennett MD. 1991. Assessing health plan case mix in employed population: ambulatory morbidity and prescribed drug models. *Adv. Health Econ. Health Serv. Res.* 12:197–232
16. Hornbrook MC, Goodman MJ, Bennett MD, Greenlick MR. 1991. Assessing health plan case mix in employed population: self-reported health status models. *Adv. Health Econ. Health Serv. Res.* 12:233–72
17. Jones SB. 1993. *Health plans, risk adjusters, and corporate alliances.* Testimony submitted to Subcomm. Health Environ., US House Represent. Comm. Energy Commer., Dec. 9
18. Jones SB. 1990. Multiple choice health insurance: the lessons and challenge to private insurers. *Inquiry* 27:161–66
19. Juba DA, Lave JR, Shaddy J. 1980. An analysis of the choice of health benefits plans. *Inquiry* 17:62–71
20. Lubitz J. 1987. Health status adjustments for Medicare capitation. *Inquiry* 24:362–75
21. Luft HS. 1986. Compensating for biased selection in health insurance. *Milbank Q.* 64:566–91
22. Luft HS, Miller RH. 1988. Patient selection in a competitive health care system. *Health Aff.* 7:97–119
23. Luft HS, Trauner JB, Maerki SC. 1985. Adverse selection in a large, multiple option health benefits program: a case study of the California Public Employees' Retirement System. *Adv. Health Econ. Health Serv. Res.* 6:197–229
24. Manton KG, Tolley HD, Vertrees JC. 1989. Controlling risk in capitation payment. Multivariate definitions of risk groups. *Med. Care* 27:259–72
25. Newhouse JP. 1994. Patients at risk: health reform and risk adjustment. *Health Aff.* 13:132–46
26. Newhouse JP, Manning WP, Keeler EB, Sloss EM. 1989. Adjusting capitation rates using objective health measures and prior utilization. *Health Care Fin. Rev.* 10:41–54

27. Newhouse JP, Manning WP, Keeler EB, Sloss EM. 1993. *Risk adjustment for a children's capitation rate.* Presented at Annu. Meet. Assoc. Health Serv. Res., Washington, DC, June 29

28. Robinson JC. 1993. A payment method for health insurance purchasing cooperatives. *Health Aff.* Suppl:65–75

29. Robinson JC, Gardner LB, Luft HS. 1991. Health plan switching in anticipation of increased medical care. *Med. Care* 31:43–51

30. Robinson JC, Luft HS, Gardner LB, Morrison EM. 1991. A method for risk adjusting employer contributions to competing health insurance plans. *Inquiry* 28:107–16

30a. Rosencranz SL, Luft HS. 1993. *Changing the focus: evaluating health care expenditure models on risk-stratified groups of enrollees.* Presented at Annu. Meet. Assoc. Health Serv. Res., Washington, DC, June

31. Schauffler HH, Howland J, Cobb J. 1992. Using chronic disease risk factors to adjust Medicare capitation payments. *Health Care Fin. Rev.* 14: 79–90

32. Simborg D. 1981. DRG Creep—A new hospital acquired disease. *New Engl. J. Med.* 304:1602–04

33. State of New York, Insurance Department. 1993. Regulation No. 146 (11 NYCRR 361): Establishment and Operation of Market Stabilization Mechanisms for Individual and Small Group Health Insurance and Medicare Supplement Insurance

34. Stone D. 1993. The struggle for the soul of health insurance. *J. Health Polit. Policy Law* 18:287–317

35. van Vliet RC, van de Ven WP. 1992. Towards a capitation formula for competing health insurers: an empirical analysis. *Soc. Sci. Med.* 34:1035–48

36. Weiner JP, Starfield BH, Steinwachs DM, Mumford LM. 1991. Development and application of a population-oriented measure of ambulatory care case-mix. *Med. Care* 29:452–472

37. Welch WP. 1985. Regression toward the mean in medical care costs, implications for biased selection in Health Maintenance Organization. *Med. Care* 23: 1234–41

38. Wilensky GR, Rossiter LF. 1986. Patient self-selection in HMOs. *Health Aff.* 5:66–80

Annu. Rev. Public Health. 1995. 16:431–45

VARIATIONS IN RESOURCE UTILIZATION AMONG MEDICAL SPECIALTIES AND SYSTEMS OF CARE

Richard L. Kravitz

University of California, Davis, Department of Internal Medicine, 2221 Stockton Boulevard, Sacramento, California 95817

Sheldon Greenfield

The Health Institute, New England Medical Center, Tufts University, Boston, Massachusetts 02111

KEY WORDS: utilization, health care resources, comparative study, managed care, medical specialties

ABSTRACT

As sweeping changes in the organization and delivery of health care are implemented, it is important to examine the relationship between various types of cost-containment efforts, health care costs, and quality of care. This article reviews the evidence that physician specialty training, the organization of physicians, and the method of physician payment are significant influences upon the utilization of health care services. Data from before the late 1980s raised the possibility that family practitioners employed fewer resources than general internists and that health maintenance organizations used fewer resources than solo practitioners. However, the studies from which these data were derived were marred by insufficient attention to patient mix, failure to account for interactions between specialty and system, and inadequate regard for the complexities of modern practice structures. More recent data from the Medical Outcomes Study (MOS) overcomes some but not all of these problems. In general, it can be safely concluded that primary care specialty training, group practice, and prepaid care are associated with less utilization. Nevertheless, much more research is needed to address remaining methodologic prob-

431

0163-7525/95/0510-0431$05.00

lems and to obtain data that are generalizable to the wide array of modern practice settings.

INTRODUCTION

Health care costs in the U.S. continue to grow rapidly, causing alarm and dismay among policy makers. Several factors have contributed to these increases, including the aging population, development of new technologies, and diminished tolerance of uncertainty among patients, physicians, and malpractice lawyers (25). Amidst concerns that current trends cannot be sustained for long, the marked geographic variations in utilization of selected services noted in several studies (4) reinforces the perception that medical practice is out of control. Demands from politicians, business interests, and the public that "something be done" has led to the proliferation of "managed care" and has prompted suggestions to radically restructure the physician workforce (34). As changes in the organization and delivery of care are implemented, it is critical to examine the relationship between various types of cost-containment efforts, health care costs, and quality of care. If we can discriminate between features of the health care system and specific health services that contribute either substantially or very little to better patient outcomes, then cost-containment efforts can be targeted effectively to achieve the most health care benefit at the lowest cost.

Research spanning several decades has identified several potentially mutable factors that influence health care costs, including provider specialty training and professional socialization, the organization of physician services, and the method of physician payment. However, several problems have plagued past studies relating these factors to health care utilization. One problem is the difficulty in isolating the effects of these factors as they are not independent of each other. Certain forms of medical practice may have specialists working in different ways than they would in other forms of care. Certain systems of care may attract different kinds of patients. Different kinds of provider organizations may receive income through multiple forms of payment, including, as a fairly recent development, the incorporation of capitation patients into solo or single-specialty group practices. A related issue, recently highlighted by Miller & Luft (23), is the shifting and evolving nature of organizational structures, particularly as they relate to managed care.

A second major problem is the difficulty in taking into account "selection bias" (18, 36). This term refers to the tendency of patients with differing levels of health to be drawn into different kinds of medical practices. Selection bias can lead to faulty comparisons of specialties and systems of care. Optimally, fair comparisons can be made by randomizing patients, or alternatively, by controlling for disease-specific severity, health status, and sociodemographic factors that are potentially related to utilization.

In this article, we review the evidence that physician specialty training, the organization of physicians, and the method of physician payment are important influences upon the utilization of health care resources. A common theme throughout is the constant threat of selection bias and the importance of careful adjustment for patient mix. Our general approach is to review the relevant literature from before the late 1980s, first with respect to specialty and then with respect to system of care. Then we discuss some results from the Medical Outcomes Study (MOS), a recent multicenter longitudinal study providing the most detailed information available on the simultaneous effects of case mix, specialty, and system of care on utilization. Finally, we identify remaining gaps and identify directions for future research.

VARIATIONS IN RESOURCE USE AMONG SPECIALTIES

The relationship of specialty to resource use has received relatively little attention from researchers and policy makers. Part of the reason may relate to the misperception that each specialty has a unique scope of practice. While it is true that heart bypass surgery is performed only by cardiac surgeons and computed tomographic scan interpretation primarily by radiologists, the range of services provided by generalists and by many subspecialists is in fact fairly similar. Even as specialists develop new technologies, the amount of overlap may be increasing; for example, primary care practitioners have joined urologists in treating prostatism; and cardiologists and radiologists as well as vascular surgeons now treat peripheral vascular disease. A second (and related) reason for the paucity of research in this area is competition over turf: Specialists have not encouraged research that compares specialties to one another. The existing literature tends to focus on comparisons among general practitioners, family practitioners, and general internists, and to a lesser extent, pediatricians, obstetrician-gynecologists, and selected internal medicine subspecialists. The most studied specialties have tended to share patient populations (e.g. healthy middle-aged adults), disease conditions (e.g. hypertension), or procedures (e.g. newborn delivery). The results of these comparisons have assumed new policy relevance as managed care organizations and policy makers seek to identify the medical practitioners who are best prepared to assume the role of primary care physician.

Family Practitioners and General Internists

As general physicians for the adult population, family practitioners and general internists have been the focus of the largest number of comparative studies. While several small studies focusing on the inpatient setting furnished conflicting results (3, 8), three large and much-cited studies identified consistently higher resource use by internists. In 1980, Noren et al published data from the National Ambulatory Medical Care Survey showing that compared to family-general practitioners, internists spent more time with patients (mean 18.4 vs 13.0 min), provided more health education (18% vs 12% of visits), and ordered more than twice as many tests and x-rays per visit (26). In 1984, Greenwald et al used a national data set to show that family practitioners used specific components of care less often than internists in almost all instances studied (12). Then, in a detailed survey of physicians from seven states, Cherkin et al concluded that internists hospitalized patients slightly more often than family practitioners and incurred nearly twice the diagnostic charges per visit, primarily by ordering twice as many diagnostic tests (5).

As to why these differences should occur, the literature speaks almost with one voice. Several studies using clinical scenarios indicate that in solving clinical problems internists select more history and physical examination items, order more laboratory tests, and generate more diagnostic hypotheses than family practitioners (29–31). Although a single study focusing on psychosocial problems came to different conclusions (37, 38), scenario-based research generally supports the idea that internists are "more thorough" or "less focused" than family practitioners, depending on one's point of view. It is important to recognize that no study reviewed so far measured patient outcomes as a function of differing practice styles.

Outcomes aside, the major limitation of most past studies comparing utilization among specialties is limited control for potential differences in patient mix. For example, the study by Noren et al did not consider patient mix, Greenwald et al used only simple diagnostic categories, and Cherkin et al used physicians' subjective ratings of the seriousness of patients' conditions. These measures may not adequately represent real differences in the average "sickness" of patients seen by different specialties, which may vary widely even among patients with the same diagnosis. For example, one recent study indicated that outpatients with diabetes may be as well as patients with no disease or as sick as those with near-terminal illness, as judged by measures of generic health status, depending on the presence of various diabetic complications and comorbidities (11). In addition, some past studies did not make a clear distinction between general internists and internists with subspecialty certification (12, 26). Finally, the several studies based on inpatient care must be interpreted cautiously because of the involvement of multiple providers (including both formal and informal consultants) in the hospital setting. More recently, the Medical Outcomes Study has begun to clarify some of these issues.

Primary Care Specialists and Medical/Surgical Subspecialists

Despite the importance of these comparisons for the formulation of health manpower policy, there has been relatively little work addressing them. In one recent article, Welch, Miller & Welch analyzed inpatient practice profiles of generalist and specialty physicians in Florida and Oregon (35). After using modified-Diagnostic Related Groups (DRGs) to adjust for case mix, they found that Oregon generalists used marginally fewer resources than subspecialists, but this relationship failed to hold in Florida. Furthermore, variations in practice patterns between states were much more pronounced than among specialties. Other studies have compared specialties with respect to their treatment of specific conditions, using either clinical scenarios (20, 37, 38) or clinical data (2, 21), but these have been neither large nor comprehensive. Among these is a provocative but preliminary study showing decreased knowledge and self-reported use of indicated therapies for acute myocardial infarction among generalists as opposed to cardiologists (1). Thus, at least until the MOS, few data were available to support any conclusion one way or the other.

VARIATIONS IN RESOURCE USE BY SYSTEM

Numerous studies, including a recent comprehensive meta-analysis by long-term observers (23), have documented variations in resource utilization by system. However, there is considerable confusion as to what constitutes a "system." System of care can be viewed at three levels: (a) the distribution, accessibility, and integration of health care capacity (hospitals, physicians, laboratories, etc) within a nation, state, or community; (b) the way in which physicians and other health care providers relate to each other within a local organizational framework; and (c) the way in which physicians are paid (e.g. capitated vs fee-for-service). Limited data suggest that all three levels are important. At the macro level, health care utilization has been linked to hospital bed supply (28), competition for patients (22), and the availability of specialized equipment or care units (6).

At the level of the local organizational framework, many studies have compared staff- or group-model Health Maintenance Organizations (HMOs) to more traditional forms of practice. In the largest such effort (and the only randomized controlled trial), the RAND Health Insurance Experiment evaluated the performance of one staff model HMO (Group Health Cooperative of Puget Sound in Seattle) against various indemnity plans using 1976–1981 data (19). Rand investigators concluded that the HMO reduced resource consumption by 25%. Some increase in the use of ambulatory and preventive services in the HMO was offset by a 40% reduction in hospitalizations. Results emerging from other studies during the 1970s and 80s are difficult to interpret because of selection bias, the tendency of HMOs to attract healthier patients (13, 18).[1] In addition, none of these studies attempted to sort out the independent effects

[1]This selection effect appears to have persisted at least into the late 1980s. Medical Outcome Study baseline data documented important differences in patient severity and health status between HMOs and fee-for-service practice (16).

of organizational structure (e.g. gate-keeping requirements) and payment scheme.

Two more recent studies are worth noting. In their 1989 comparison of hospitalized HMO and fee-for-service patients, Stern et al found that HMO patients had shorter lengths of stay but comparable costs (32a). This study used fairly sophisticated case mix controls (Horn's Severity of Illness Index in addition to subjective physician ratings), and it isolated the effect of payment mechanism because all patients were admitted to the same hospital and cared for by the same team of physicians.

In the Medicare TEFRA (Tax Equity and Fiscal Responsibility Act) Evaluation (3a), HMO plans had 15% to 20% fewer hospital days per enrollee and 6% to 19% shorter lengths of stay compared to standard Medicare coverage; physician visit rates were decreased among patients in staff model HMOs and prepaid group plans but not in IPAs (independent practice associations).

In their recent meta-analysis, Miller & Luft (23) found that compared with indemnity plans, HMOs had lower hospital admission rates, shorter hospital lengths of stay, the same or more physician visits per enrollee, less use of expensive procedures and tests, and greater use of preventive services. They concluded, however, that because of unmeasured selection bias, the diversity of health plan types, and the rapidity with which plans and local market conditions are changing, making generalizations is hazardous.

Another aspect of local organizational structure is the size of physician group. Although there is reason to believe that even outside of HMOs, solo practitioners practice differently than physicians in multispecialty groups, to our knowledge no study prior to the MOS addressed this issue directly.

Finally, a number of studies have examined the relationship between utilization and physician payment mechanism. Prepaid and fee-for-service systems operate under overarching financial incentives that are different and likely to influence utilization of services in opposite ways (14, 15). In theory, clinicians in prepaid systems will tend to recommend less care—to "conserve" valuable resources—whereas practitioners in fee-for-service systems will tend to recommend more tests and procedures. One small study of hypertensive patients in an academic teaching center found that the same physicians used fewer resources (diagnostic tests, referrals, etc) for their prepaid patients than for their fee-for-service patients, providing unambiguous but nongeneralizable support for this assertion (24). However, in the real world, the relationships are often more complex. For example, Stearns et al (32) showed that switching from strict fee-for-service reimbursement to a mixed plan employing capitation for primary care physicians and a reduced fee schedule for specialists resulted in fewer hospitalizations but an increase in hospital length of stay and ambulatory visits. The authors posited that the mixed reimbursement plan may have led to a greater number or referrals with no incentives in place for reductions in length of stay for specialty admissions.

In summary, most studies to date looking at the effects of specialty and system of care on utilization of resources have been less than definitive. Among the principal problems hindering these studies (apart from lack of generalizability) are: (*a*) insufficient attention to patient mix; (*b*) failure to account for interactions between specialty and system; and (*c*) inadequate regard for the complexities of modern practice structures (especially the separation between organizational system of care and payment mechanism). Because it addresses several of these issues, the Medical Outcomes Study deserves more detailed discussion.

THE MEDICAL OUTCOMES STUDY

This large study compared a wide variety of resource utilization and outcome dimensions among patients of five kinds of specialists (family physicians, general internists, endocrinologists, cardiologists, and mental health professionals) in three systems of care. Several features of its design provided advantages over past studies: (*a*) use of a comprehensive set of variables to control for selection bias and patient mix; (*b*) replication of the study in three diverse geographic locations; and (*c*) inclusion of a large cross-sectional population sampled heavily from patients with multiple chronic diseases. Despite the limited number and type of medical subspecialists (endocrinologists and cardiologists) participating in the study, the MOS provides what are perhaps the best data available regarding the effects of specialty training and system on resource use. For this reason, we summarize its methods and main results in some detail [for further information see (9, 16, 33)].

DESIGN, SAMPLING, AND DATA   The MOS sampled physicians and patients in different systems of care in three geographic sites—Boston, Chicago, and Los Angeles. Data describing the patients, the clinicians, treatment processes, utilization of resources, and health outcomes were gathered from multiple sources including clinician reports, patient reports, and independent clinical examinations. A subset of patients was followed up longitudinally (see 33).

A four-step process was used to select geographic sites, systems of care, clinicians, and patients. First, three MOS cities were selected. Second, one large HMO, several multispecialty groups, and physicians practicing within solo or single-specialty small group practices were selected within each city. Third, board-eligible physicians aged 31–55 were asked to participate. In the analysis of non-psychiatric conditions, the final sample included 362 providers (349 non-psychiatric physicians and 12 nurse practitioners); 114 (31%) were in HMOs, 76 (21%) in large multispecialty groups, and 172 (48%) in solo or small single-specialty group practices. Among the physicians, 194 (56%) practiced general internal medicine, 91 (26%) family medicine, 40 (12%) cardiology, and 24 (7%) endocrinology. The fourth step was to sample English-speaking adults among patients visiting the study clinicians during nine-day screening periods from February through October 1986. For the cross-sectional portion of the MOS, 21,158 patients of medical providers were available for analysis. Of these, just over 2000 patients with one or more chronic tracer conditions (diabetes mellitus, hypertension, recent myocardial infarction, congestive heart failure and/or depression) were followed closely for two years; data on mortality are available for an additional five years.

Data were collected from both physicians and patients. For the cross-sectional study, patients and physicians completed screening questionnaires containing information about patient demographics, clinical illness, health status, and process of care. Patients enrolled in the longitudinal study were surveyed every six months and also underwent periodic physical examinations and laboratory testing.

PATIENT MIX ADJUSTMENT   The MOS considered patient mix to consist of four components: sociodemographic characteristics, prevalence of both the primary tracer condition and comorbidities, disease-specific severity as measured using conventional biomedical parameters, and functional status and well-being. Comparisons of patient mix across specialty and system were approached in four ways. First, the sociodemographic characteristics of patients in the different practices were compared. Second, information was obtained directly from patients on their functional status and well-being (including general health perceptions, physical functioning, and role functioning), using the MOS short-form health status measures as previously described. Third, the prevalence of the four medical MOS tracer conditions (hypertension, diabetes, recent myocardial infarction, and congestive heart failure) was estimated using information from the physician-completed encounter form. Patient-derived information was used to determine the prevalence of chronic conditions other than the MOS tracer conditions and to verify that all specialists were equally likely to be aware of, and report, each disease. Fourth, for each of the four MOS tracer conditions, disease-specific severity was measured using information from the physicians. This approach represented a departure from traditional models of case-mix measurement developed for the inpatient setting (10).

DEFINITION OF SYSTEM OF CARE   In the MOS, "system of care" was defined to incorporate the type of practice organization (i.e. group vs solo), the physician specialty mix within a group (i.e. single vs multispecialty) and the method of payment (i.e. prepaid vs fee-for-service). Patients were classified into five systems: (*a*) prepaid group practice form of health maintenance organization (HMO), (*b*) large multispecialty group practice-prepaid, (*c*) large multispecialty group-fee-for-service, (*d*) solo or small single-specialty group practice-prepaid, or (*e*) solo or small single-specialty group practice-fee-for-service.

Table 1 shows utilization indicator profiles of the four physician specialties. The top panel summarizes patient mix. In the middle panel for the unadjusted rates, the specialties are arrayed in relation to family medicine. The numbers in the middle panel represent the unadjusted, actual rates of utilization of the six utilization indicators, and the numbers in parentheses represent the ratio of each specialty to family practice, which was set to 100. The use rates for these six indicators of utilization generally run parallel to the mix of patients.

The third panel shows the results after adjustment. Overall, family practitioners and internists had only small differences in utilization profiles, while cardiologists and endocrinologists remained considerably higher utilizers than the primary care specialists. This pattern held for all indicators except for office visits, for which only endocrinologists had higher rates than the primary care specialties. The results were similar after excluding HMO patients from the analysis.

The effects of system of care on utilization are shown in Table 2, with the top panel summarizing the mix of patients across the five systems, the middle panel indicating the unadjusted utilization rates, and the bottom, the adjusted rates.

In the middle panel, unadjusted utilization rates for four different systems are shown in relation to the HMO, with the ratio of the rates of the other systems to the HMO noted in parentheses. The bottom panel shows the utilization rates adjusted for sociodemographic status, MOS tracer disease presence, MOS tracer disease severity, chronic comorbid conditions, general health perceptions, and the season in which sampling occurred. The results are not adjusted for specialty because the mix of specialists hired may be one method of resource allocation used by different systems. The middle and bottom panels differ because of the differences in patient mix as seen in the top panel. The differences in patient mix explain a large part, but not all, of the differences between systems.

The adjusted findings showed that fee-for-service patients had significantly higher probabilities of hospitalization than did prepaid patients, independent of the type of physician organization. Solo practice/single-specialty group patients had significantly higher rates of hospitalization than multispecialty group patients, independent of the payment system.

More recent, unpublished results from the MOS suggest that, among diabetic patients, the increased levels of utilization noted among subspecialists and in

Table 1 Comparison of patient mix and unadjusted and adjusted utilization rates for six indicators among the four specialties*

	Family physicians	General internists	Endocrinologists	Cardiologists	P
		Patient Mix Indicators			
Mean age, y	40.0	46.9	44.2	55.5	<.0001
Educational level, y	13.6	13.5	14.0	13.1	<.01
No. of chronic diseases per patient	0.70	1.02	1.05	1.32	<.0001
General health perception (0–100 scale)	72.8	67.0	67.9	63.0	<.0001
		Unadjusted Utilization Rates			
% Hospitalized	4.30	5.43 (126)†	8.18 (190)†	15.64 (364)†	<.001
Office visits per patient per y	4.53	4.37 (96)	5.57 (123)†	5.19 (115)†	<.001
Prescription drugs per patient	1.18	1.47 (125)†	1.67 (142)†	2.30 (195)†	<.001
% Patients having tests per visit‡	38.8	43.7 (113)†	62.7 (162)†	47.2 (122)†	<.001
Mean value of tests per visit‡	22.00	26.90 (122)†	22.70 (103)	33.80 (154)†	<.001
Mean value of tests per patient per y‡	85.30	109.80 (129)†	112.00 (131)†	158.00 (185)†	<.001
		Adjusted Utilization Rates			
% Hospitalized	4.77	5.59 (117)	7.15 (150)†	10.55 (221)§	≤.001
Office visits per patient per y	4.64	4.42 (95)	5.22 (113)†	4.53 (98)	≤.001
Prescription drugs per patient	1.40	1.46 (104)	1.54 (110)§	1.74 (124)†	≤.001
% Patients having tests per visit‡	40.0	44.2 (111)†	55.9 (148)†	47.7 (119)†	≤.001
Mean value of tests per visit‡	23.10	26.40 (114)†	24.00 (104)	34.10 (148)†	≤.001
Mean value of tests per patient per y‡	104.30	110.10 (106)	132.10 (127)†	150.50 (144)†	≤.001

* Numbers in parentheses are the ratios of that specialty's utilization rate to that of family medicine, which was set to 100. Sample size varies by type of utilization: for hospitalizations, 9020; for office visits, 17,580; for prescription drugs, 17,780; for tests and procedures, 17,498. Of the total number of patients studied, 28% were seen by family physicians, 59% by general internists, 6% by endocrinologists, and 7% by cardiologists.

† P ≤ .01.

‡ Mean value of tests *or* procedures.

§ P ≤ 0.5.

Reproduced from *J. Am. Med. Assoc.* 1992, 267: 1626, with permission.

Table 2 Comparison of patient mix and unadjusted and adjusted utilization rates for six indicators among the five systems*

	HMO	MSG-PP	Solo/SSG-PP	MSG-FFS	Solo/SSG-FFS	P
			Patient Mix Indicators			
Mean age, y	45.0	38.6	42.4	48.8	49.2	<.0001
Educational level, y	13.6	13.6	13.9	13.1	13.6	.001
No. of chronic diseases per patient	0.93	0.69	0.81	0.93	1.10	<.0001
General health perception (0–100 scale)	68.2	71.1	69.0	67.1	67.6	.02
			Unadjusted Utilization Rates			
% Hospitalized	4.43	3.60 (81)	4.35 (98)	5.98 (135)	8.01 (181)†	<.01
Office visits per patient per y	4.35	4.35 (100)	4.21 (97)	4.29 (99)	4.70 (108)	<.001
Prescription drugs per patient	1.31	1.18 (90)	1.21 (92)	1.49 (114)	1.69 (129)†	<.05
% Patients having tests per visit‡	43.9	37.4 (85)§	47.7 (109)	41.3 (94)	47.4 (108)	<.05
Mean value of tests per visit‡	26.30	20.50 (78)§	25.70 (98)	23.30 (89)	28.50 (108)†	<.05
Mean value of tests per patient per y‡	105.70	82.40 (78)	94.90 (90)	91.10 (86)	122.20 (116)	<.01
			Adjusted Utilization Rates			
% Hospitalized	4.93	4.24 (86)	4.92 (100)	5.58 (113)	6.94 (141)§	<.05
Office visits per patient per y	4.68	4.73 (101)	4.33 (93)	4.17 (89)†	4.30 (92)§	<.001
Prescription drugs per patient	1.37	1.45 (106)	1.32 (96)	1.46 (107)§	1.53 (112)†	<.01
% Patients having tests per visit‡	43.8	38.4 (88)	48.0 (110)	42.1 (96)	47.0 (107)	.06
Mean value of tests per visit‡	26.10	22.40 (86)	26.50 (102)	24.50 (94)	27.40 (105)	<.01
Mean value of tests per patient per y‡	116.40	103.70 (89)	110.00 (95)	91.70 (79)†	113.80 (98)	<.05

*HMO indicates health maintenance organization; MSG-PP, multispecialty group — prepaid; Solo/SSG-PP, solo practice/single-specialty group — prepaid; MSG-FFS, multispecialty group — fee-for-service; and Solo/SSG-FFS, solo practice/single-specialty group — fee-for-service. Numbers in parentheses are the ratios of that system's utilization rate to that of the HMO, which equals 100. Sample size varies by type of utilization: for hospitalizations, 9435; for office visits, 18,353; for prescription drugs, 18,573; for tests and procedures, 18,269. Of the total number of patients studied, 37% were in HMOs, 10% MSG-PP, 12% Solo/SSG-PP, 6% MSG-FFS, and 34% Solo/SSG-FFS.

† $P \leq .01$.

‡ Mean value of tests or procedures.

§ $P \leq 0.5$.

Reproduced from *J. Am. Med. Assoc.* 1992, 267: 1627, with permission.

the fee-for-service system were not associated with significantly better phys-iological, functional, or mortality outcomes. Among hypertensive patients, system differences were again small, but patients of subspecialists had some-what better blood pressure control, possibly at the expense of some decreases in functional health (W Rogers, personal communication). The failure of the MOS to detect substantial differences in clinical outcomes between specialties or systems mirrors results recently reported for the Medicare population (27).

In summary, the Medical Outcomes Study provides fairly convincing evi-dence that subspecialty care, solo-practice, and fee-for-service payment mech-anisms are associated with greater use of medical resources. However, the results should probably not be generalized beyond the specific types of systems of care examined in the study or the three MOS cities. Furthermore, although preliminary analyses suggest little outcomes "bang" for the utilization "buck" of more subspecialty and fee-for-service care, the relatively small sample of patients limits precision and precludes important subgroup analyses. Never-theless, the methodologic and conceptual advances provided by the MOS and other recent studies should pave the way for increasingly productive research in the future.

PROBLEMS WITH THE EXISTING RESEARCH BASE

Despite the advances represented by the MOS, major gaps in the current literature make it difficult to reach final conclusions about the effect of spe-cialty and system on utilization. Three problems need researchers' attention: (a) frequently inadequate case-mix control, (b) the paucity of comparisons between generalists and specialists, and (c) rapidly changing definitions of managed care. In addition, recent concerns over the meaning of variations in resource use, and more pointedly, whether stringent cost-containment efforts will be associated with sacrifices in quality of care, have highlighted a fourth problem: lack of data relating resource utilization to quality (process and outcomes of care).

The MOS developed and applied what are perhaps the most comprehensive set of case-mix measures used in policy-relevant health care research. Never-theless, like other observational studies attempting to relate physician specialty training and system of care to health care utilization and outcomes, the MOS is vulnerable to charges of insufficient case mix control leading to bias (17). While randomized clinical trials comparing different specialties and systems would appear desirable, such studies are enormously difficult and expensive to conduct in broad-based patient populations. The case mix approaches in the MOS and other recent studies, therefore, represent a necessary compromise between the experimental ideal and logistical realities. Clearly, these measures can be improved, and more refined approaches are under development (11).

Another objection relating specifically to the MOS involves the generalizability of the interspecialty comparisons. Results from the MOS were consistent with prior studies in showing somewhat increased case-mix adjusted utilization for internists as compared to family practitioners. However, MOS data comparing generalists to subspecialists were derived from 285 family practitioners and general internists, but only 40 cardiologists and 24 endocrinologists. Although the generalist-subspecialty differences were statistically significant and clinically believable (endocrinologists used the most lab tests whereas cardiologists had the greatest propensity to hospitalize), the sample of subspecialty physicians was too small to allow facile generalization.

An equally important problem for researchers in the field is the changing nature of health care organizations. As described by Miller & Luft (23), managed care organizations currently consist of at least five types: (a) staff model HMOs, (b) group-model HMOs, (c) network (IPA) model HMOs, (d) PPOs, and (e) "point-of-service" HMOs. Some clarity is obtained by heeding Miller & Luft's advisement that in managed care, physician behavior is what is managed. Thus, attention should focus on how health care systems attempt to influence physician behavior, and how physicians respond to these attempts.

Managed care organizations, especially group and IPA-model HMOs and PPOs (which are likely to be the dominant form in the near future), may try to shape physician behavior by restructuring financial incentives, maintaining provider utilization profiles, or imposing various elements of utilization management and/or quality assurance requirements. However, the organizational signal will have a differing effect on physician behavior depending on physicians' attentiveness to the signal. This may depend on a number of factors, including the percentage of patients in a practice covered by that managed care plan. Any comprehensive study of the effect of "system" on utilization must account for these variables.

A final problem with the state of the literature is its cursory treatment of quality-of-care differences among specialists and systems, measured either in terms of validated processes of care or case mix–adjusted outcomes. Consideration of costs/utilization without concomitant measurement of quality gives an incomplete picture of value received.

CONCLUSIONS

In summary, the available evidence supports the view that physician specialty and system of care both have substantial, independent effects on utilization of health care resources. In general, primary care specialty training, group practice, and prepaid care seem to be associated with less use. However, information on the relationship of utilization to quality of care is currently lacking. Further, very few of the myriad permutations of specialty and system have been explicitly examined in controlled studies. As the political bandwagon moves inexorably toward primary care and managed care, research is needed to identify more precisely those aspects of physician training and health care organization that reduce resource use without hurting quality.

Literature Cited

1. Bernard AM, Shapiro LR, McMahon LF. 1990. The influence of attending physician subspecialization on hospital length of stay. *Med. Care* 28:170–74
2. Bertakis KD, Robbins JA. 1988. Utilization of hospital services: a comparison of internal medicine and family practice. *J. Fam. Pract.* 28:91–96
3. Deleted in proof
4. Chassin MR, Brook RH, Park RE, Keesey J, Fink A, et al. 1986. Variations in the use of medical and surgical services by the Medicare population. *New Engl. J. Med.* 314:285–90
5. Cherkin DC, Rosenblatt RA, Hart LG, Schneeweiss R, Lo Gerfo J. 1987. The use of medical resources by residency-trained family physicians and general internists: is there a difference? *Med. Care* 25:455–69
6. Every NR, Larson EB, Litwin PE, Maynard C, Fihn SD, et al. 1993. The association between on-site cardiac catheterization facilities and the use of coronary angiography after acute myocardial infarction. *New Engl. J. Med.* 329:546–51
7. Deleted in proof
8. Franks P, Dickinson JC. 1986. Comparison of family physicians and internists. Process and outcome of adult patients at a community hospital. *Med. Care* 24:941–48
9. Greenfield S, Nelson EC, Zubkoff M, Manning W, Rogers W, et al. 1992. Variations in resource utilization among medical specialties and systems of care. *J. Am. Med. Assoc.* 267:1624–30
10. Greenfield S, Sullivan L, Silliman RA, Dukes K, Kaplan SH. 1994. Principles and practice of case mix adjustment: applications to end-stage renal disease. *Am. J. Kidney Dis.* In press
11. Greenfield S, Sullivan L, Dukes KA, Silliman R, D'Agostino R, Kaplan SH. 1994. Development and testing of a new measure of case mix for use in office practice. *Med. Care.* In press
12. Greenwald H, Peteson ML, Garrison LP, Hart LG, Moscovic IS, et al. 1984. Interspecialty variation in office-based care. *Med. Care* 22:14–29
13. Hellinger FJ. 1987. Selection bias in health maintenance organizations: analysis of recent evidence. *Health Care Fin. Rev.* 9:55–63
14. Hillman AL. 1990. Health maintenance organizations, financial incentives, and physicians' judgements. *Ann. Intern. Med.* 112:891–93
15. Hillman AL, Pauly MV, Kerstein JJ. 1989. How do financial incentives affect physicians' clinical decisions and the financial performance of health maintenance organizations? *New Engl. J. Med.* 321:86–92
16. Kravitz RL, Greenfield S, Rogers W, Manning WG, Zubkoff M, et al. 1992. Differences in the mix of patients among medical specialties and systems of care: results from the Medical Outcomes Study. *J. Am. Med. Assoc.* 267:1617–23
17. Lasker RD, Shapiro DW. 1992. Specialists or generalists? The Medical Outcomes Study. *J. Am. Med. Assoc.* 268:1537–38
18. Luft H. 1981. *The operations and performance of health maintenance organization.* Washington, DC: US Gov. Print. Off.
19. Manning WG, Leibowitz A, Goldberg GA, Rogers WH, Newhouse JP. 1984. A controlled trial of the effect of a prepaid group practice on use of services. *New Engl. J. Med.* 310:1505–10
20. McFall SL, Warnecke RB, Kalvzny AD, Aitken M, Ford L. 1994. Physician and practice characteristics associated with judgements about breast cancer treatment. *Med. Care* 32:106–17
21. McGillivray DL, Roberts-Brauer MA, Kramer MS. 1993. Diagnostic test or-

dering in the evaluation of febrile children. *Am. J. Dis. Child.* 147:870–74

22. Melnick GA, Zwanziger J. 1988. Hospital behavior under competition and cost-containment policies. The California experience. *J. Am. Med. Assoc.* 260: 2669–75

23. Miller RH, Luft HS. 1994. Managed care plan performance since 1980. A literature analysis. *J. Am. Med. Assoc.* 271:1512–19

24. Murray JP, Greenfield S, Kaplan SH, Yano EM. 1992. Ambulatory testing for capitation and fee for service patients in the same practice setting: relationship to outcomes. *Med. Care* 30: 252–61

25. Newhouse J. 1993. An iconoclastic view of health cost containment. *Health Aff.* (Suppl.):152–171

26. Noren J, Frazier T, Altman I, DeLozier J. 1980. Ambulatory medical care a comparison of internists and family-general practitioners. *New Engl. J. Med.* 302:11–16

27. Retchin SM, Clement DG, Rossiter LF, Brown B, Brown R, Nelson L. 1992. How the elderly fare in HMOs: outcomes from the Medicare competition demonstrations. *Health Serv. Res.* 27: 651–69

27a. Robbins JA, Bertakis KD. 1983. Costs of care provided by trainees in internal medicine and family practice. *Western J. Med.* 138:118–19

28. Roemer MI. 1961. Bed supply and hospital utilization. *J. Am. Med. Assoc.* 35: 36–42

29. Scherger JE, Gordon MJ, Phillips TJ, LoGerfo JP. 1980. Comparison of diagnostic methods of family practice and internal medicine residents. *J. Fam. Pract.* 10:95–101

30. Simpson DE, Rich EC, Dalgaard KA, et al. 1987. The diagnostic process in primary care: a comparison of general internists and family practitioners. *Soc. Sci. Med.* 25:861–66

31. Smith DH, McWhinney IR. 1975. Comparison of the diagnostic methods of family physicians and internists. *J. Med. Educ.* 50:264–70

32. Stearns SC, Wolfe BL, Kindig DA. 1992. Physician responses to fee-for-service and capitation payment. *Inquiry* 29:416–25

33. Tarlov AR, Ware JE, Greenfield S, Nelson EC, Perrin E, Zubkoff M. 1989. The Medical Outcomes Study: an application of methods for monitoring the results of medical care. *J. Am. Med. Assoc.* 262: 925–30

34. Wartman SA, Wilson M, Kahn N. 1994. The generalist health care workforce: issues and goals. *J. Gen. Intern. Med.* 9 (Suppl. 1):S7–13

35. Welch HG, Miller ME, Welch WP. 1994. Physician profiling: an analysis of inpatient practice patterns in Florida and Oregon. *New Engl. J. Med.* 330: 607–12

36. Wilensky GR, Rossiter LF. 1986. Patient self selection in HMOs. *Health Aff.* 5: 66–80

37. Yager J, Linn LS, Leake B, Gastaldo G, Palkowski C. 1986. Initial clinical judgments by internists, family physicians, and psychiatrists in response to patient vignettes: I. assessment of problems and diagnostic possibilities. *Gen. Hosp. Psychiatry* 8:141–51

38. Yager J, Linn LS, Leake B, Gastaldo G, Palkowski C. 1986. Initial clinical judgements by internists, family physicians and psychiatrists in response to patient vignettes: II. ordering of laboratory tests, consultations, and treatments. *Gen. Hosp. Psychiatry* 8:152–57

Annu. Rev. Public Health. 1995. 16:447–72

NONFINANCIAL BARRIERS TO CARE FOR CHILDREN AND YOUTH

Neal Halfon[1,2,4], *Moira Inkelas*[1,3], *and David Wood*[1,2,3,4]

[1]Child and Family Health Program, School of Public Health, [2]Department of Pediatrics, School of Medicine, University of California Los Angeles, Los Angeles, California 90024-1772; [3]Ahmanson Department of Pediatrics, Cedars-Sinai Medical Center, Los Angeles, California 90048, and [4]RAND Corporation, 1700 Main Street, Santa Monica, California 90047

KEY WORDS: access, managed care, delivery system, children's health care, health system reform

ABSTRACT

Public health and medical care interventions have produced dramatic changes in the health of children in the United States. Emerging new morbidities such as behavioral and learning disorders, and child abuse and neglect, highlight the lack of an integrated system of health. Children's developmental vulnerability, dependency, and unique morbidities have been underemphasized in the organization and delivery of health care. The Andersen and Aday model of health care utilization is used to describe financial and nonfinancial barriers to care for children that include family characteristics and organizational characteristics of the health system. Case studies of immunization delivery, children with chronic illness, and mobile populations of children reveal the mismatch between the health care system and children's basic health needs. Integrated service models for high-risk populations of children represent an essential mechanism for coordinating the delivery of medical, developmental, educational, and social services needed by children and families. Universal, coordinated public health and medical services of adequate scope and quality should be assured for children through market and health system reform.

INTRODUCTION

The health of children in the United States has changed dramatically over the past century. Public health interventions and medical care innovations have

447

greatly reduced morbidity and mortality associated with poor living conditions and sanitation, and nutritional and infectious disease. However, as many traditional threats to children's health were addressed, an entirely new set of threats emerged that includes family violence and drug use, child abuse and neglect, and learning and behavioral problems. These new morbidities pose new challenges to a nation that lacks a coherent, integrated system of care and that traditionally has undervalued disease prevention and health promotion activities.

Comparison of the US with other industrialized countries across many indicators of child health such as infant mortality, child mortality, and age-appropriate immunization rates reflects the inadequacies in our health delivery system (33, 98). Evidence for substantial ethnic and income-related disparities in child health indicators and patterns of care (Table 1) suggests that effective health services are not reaching all children. The resulting human and economic toll can be measured in preventable deaths, disease, and unrealized potential, as well as unnecessary economic expenditures. The economic costs include hospital expenditures for premature and low-birthweight infants, preventable hospitalizations for children with asthma and other conditions who do not receive appropriate ambulatory care, and special education and mental health services for children with unmet developmental needs. Continued failure of our health system to adequately and equitably serve children's health needs will compound the social and economic costs.

Children's underservice in the United States can best be explained through

Table 1   Health indicators, health problems, and health services for children, 1991

Indicator of child health status	Rate	Reference
US infant mortality	8.9 per 1000	95
Black-white ratio	2.4	
International ranking	#22	
US low birthweight	7.1 per 100	95
Black-white ratio	2.3	
US mortality from prematurity and low birthweight	10.1 per 10,000	95
Black-white ratio	4.4	
Age-appropriate immunization for 2-year-old children in selected US cities	10–42%	15
Age-appropriate immunization rate for 2-year-old children in the U.S.	57%	33
Likelihood of >1 hospitalization for asthma among US children with asthma: poor–non-poor ratio	1.77	43
Proportion of children with mental disorder(s)	12%	73
Adolescents with mental disorders	18–22%	
Number of children in foster care	429,000	34

the structure of the child health system and the organization of specific types of services. Three distinct yet interrelated components of the child health service system include:

1. The personal medical care service sector,
2. The community- and population-based service sector, and
3. The health-related support and developmental and educational service sector.

Personal medical services within the health care system include services for traditional pediatric illnesses—from prematurity to ear infections. Within this sector the vast majority of children receive care through private physicians and hospitals, although public health and community clinics also provide personal medical services. Although most medical services for children are delivered privately, many are publicly financed through Medicaid or, for the 9 million uninsured children, financed and delivered by local (public) health clinics.

Community- and population-based services encompass traditional public health programs such as lead screening and abatement programs, perinatal outreach programs, immunization monitoring programs, and the like. In many other industrialized countries, this sector plays a pivotal role in ensuring that all children receive appropriate disease prevention and health promotion services. However, in the United States these programs have been increasingly underfunded as more public dollars are reallocated for provision of personal medical services to the uninsured (56a).

The third essential component of the children's health system distinguishes children's health care from that of most adults, and is comprised of health-related support and developmental services. These services include developmental services for premature infants, special education and mental health services provided in the schools, child abuse and neglect services, and programs for children at risk for developmental delay due to biological or environmental risk. These "wrap-around" services play an increasingly important role in promoting and maintaining a child's functional status by focusing on the child in the family and community context. Federal recognition of the essential role of these services includes Part H of the Individuals with Disabilities Education Act (IDEA), which mandates coordination between medical, developmental, and educational services to intervene early with children at risk for developmental delay.

While all children require access to appropriate medical care services when sick, many children who are uninsured or living in particularly poor environments face numerous barriers to receiving essential care. In contrast to most other industrialized countries, the US has chosen not to develop a well organized and comprehensive set of child disease prevention and health promotion services and instead provides a patchwork safety net of services composed of underfunded and disconnected programs. A growing number of children living in poverty or with multiple risks make the need for adequate health-related support and developmental services even more acute. However, the three components of the child health system each possess unique financial and nonfinancial barriers to care. Moreover, because each sector is independently financed and organized, additional barriers arise through the lack of integrated structure, causing families to face substantial difficulty in negotiating the different service sectors. We contend that the combined structural and financial barriers to care that exist for many children reflect a fundamental mismatch between the composition and distribution of health services and the health needs of these children. New and emerging health problems further exacerbate this mismatch and challenge the system to appropriately address the complex determinants of children's health.

How can the health services for children be improved in the context of health system reform? Two guiding tenets of the current focus on health care reform include extending health insurance to all Americans, and rationalizing the delivery of health services through managed care and other organizational techniques. Extending health insurance coverage to the 9 million currently uninsured children would greatly reduce financial constraints that impede children's access to basic medical care. However, without broader reform to address the unique characteristics of children and to assure access to appropriate community-based health promotion and disease prevention services, many barriers to care will remain unresolved. Moreover, while access to conventional, personal medical care services is necessary, it is insufficient to protect and promote children's health. Population- and community-based preventive health promotion services and a spectrum of health-related support services are also essential.

This paper examines key issues underlying the mismatch between child health needs and the organization of health services. We describe children's unique health risks, conditions, and service needs, and detail the nonfinancial barriers to children's access to medical care. We offer case studies of services (child immunizations), conditions (asthma), and high-risk populations (homeless and foster children) in order to elucidate the nature of this mismatch. By presenting alternative models and approaches to delivering children's health services, we hope to illustrate how health system reform can be made more responsive to their unique health needs.

UNIQUE CHARACTERISTICS OF CHILDREN

Children's health needs and capacity to respond to health risks are quite different from those of adults and require special consideration in the structure, organization, and delivery of health care. Children differ from adults in three clinically important ways: (*a*) developmental vulnerability; (*b*) dependency; and (*c*) different morbidity (49).

The continual process of development in childhood is characterized by rapid, cumulative, and interdependent physical, emotional, and cognitive changes. Interrupting or altering the developmental trajectory can permanently undermine the child's developing capacities. Ecologically focused models of human development and morbidity emphasize the contribution of children's environments to their health status and longitudinal development (31a, 81a). Biologic threats to normal development (e.g. low birthweight) and social threats to children's well-being (e.g. family dysfunction and instability) can act synergistically in delaying children's development and function. Overcoming these risks requires timely, developmentally appropriate and comprehensive primary health care services responsive to physiologic, environmental, and social conditions. However, maintaining continuity, periodicity, and timeliness of children's health services is difficult in a system in which care is episodic and frequently inaccessible. Community-based and health-related services that attempt to support and integrate health and child developmental services, such as the Head Start program, often do not reach all children who need services and are not sufficient in scope and duration to provide the level of support that many families need.

The dependency that characterizes childhood is captured in the African adage that "it takes a village to raise a child." Children depend upon their parents or other adult caregivers to seek, consent to, and pay for health care, and rely further upon a range of medical, educational, and social institutions to promote optimal development. The extent of children's dependency fluctuates with changes in life and social circumstances and diminishes with age. As a result, children living in economically deprived, violent inner-cities may have different health needs and dependency characteristics than suburban children, and thus require quite different health-promotion and disease-prevention services.

Finally, the patterns, prevalence, and manifestation of health conditions are different in children than in adults. While adults suffer from their share of rare as well as self-limited conditions, adult health services focus upon common and severe degenerative conditions that often require technologically intensive services. Fewer children suffer from such serious degenerative conditions. However, many children have relatively low morbidity conditions such as asthma, otitis media, and learning disabilities. The combined and cumulative impact of these conditions can be functionally disabling. Dramatic changes in threats to children's health over recent decades (92) further underscore children's unique health care needs. Behavioral and emotional problems, child abuse and neglect, and exposure to drugs, alcohol, and violence are increasingly important determinants of children's health and well-being. The complex, socioeconomic origins of these and other conditions are not easily resolved through conventional, personal medical care services, and community-based prevention strategies are likely to provide better outcomes.

In sum, the nature of children's health problems, their dependency, and their developmental vulnerability require readily accessible, coordinated, multidisciplinary health services (2). Essential features of appropriate care for children include primary care with a strong preventive focus, and targeted population-based health-promotion services. Appropriately constituted continuums of primary care services are particularly important given the changing prevalence and impact of morbidities in children. Because the health care system has not been organized, structured, or financed to address the unique clinical characteristics of children, or even to emphasize preventive care, the system is inadequately positioned to resolve children's health risks and conditions, particularly for children whose health care needs cannot be telescoped into brief, intermittent office visits. The mismatch has become more striking as the number of children from high-risk environments, with multiple or chronic health conditions, continues to grow.

MODELS OF ACCESS TO CARE

The analytic framework developed by Andersen & Aday (4) to examine utilization of care is useful in assessing the relationship between children's health needs, service availability, and realized access. The concept of access to care has been used to capture the complex relationship between the need for health services and the response of the health system to identified needs. Andersen and colleagues have defined access as potential and realized entry to the health system, and further defined equity of access as the distribution of services according to need (5). Reflecting emerging notions of appropriateness, Weissman & Epstein elaborate the concept of access as "the attainment of timely, sufficient, and appropriate health care of adequate quality such that health outcomes are maximized" (96).

Access to some child health services (e.g. immunization) can be assessed easily in terms of timeliness, sufficiency, and appropriateness. However, for other health needs related to emerging patterns of risk, quantifying the relationship between need and utilization in the context of children's developmental vulnerability and dependency is a complex process. Newer health risks and conditions in children have not yielded standard and universally applicable interventions or quantifiable effectiveness measures. For example, while early intervention programs have effectively reduced the risk of developmental delay in biologically or environmentally vulnerable children, no standardized set of early interventions have been specified for these high-risk children. As a consequence, our review of children's access to care is focused on basic measures of medical service utilization such as the number of physician visits reported in a year.

Empirical studies have identified the individual characteristics of children and families and system characteristics that pose important barriers to obtaining this basic medical care. Barriers to medical care traditionally have been classified as financial (i.e. insurance-based) or nonfinancial (e.g. family characteristics, the structure and organization of the health service delivery system). Diminished access has most frequently been inferred from utilization patterns for specific medical services (e.g. number of annual physician visits), designated populations (e.g. adolescents, children in foster care), groups with specific conditions (e.g. children with asthma), or specific services (e.g. immunization, prenatal care). Such analyses have produced extensive inventories of barriers and have accounted for relative differences in utilization rates by factors such as ethnicity, income, and residence, in consideration of health need as measured by health status indicators, activity limitations, and number and type of conditions (see Table 2) (1, 22, 37, 67, 68, 101, 102). Unfortunately, because many studies are based upon national household surveys, researchers have rarely been able to empirically describe the interface between system and personal factors by linking individual characteristics and outcomes with organizational and financial characteristics of the delivery system.

EMPIRICAL STUDIES OF NONFINANCIAL BARRIERS

Individual, Predisposing, and Enabling Factors

The relative visibility of nonfinancial barriers to care for children has increased as policies geared toward expanded financial access to care are pursued at the national level and in certain states. Mounting evidence suggests that many children, and particularly those who are poor or with multiple risks or special needs, would continue to experience difficulty in accessing appropriate and timely care if universal health insurance were enacted without changes in the delivery system. Substantial barriers that exist independent of insurance-related factors must be resolved to improve the allocation and scope of health services for children and families.

Because of the strong correlation between insurance and socioeconomic status, we focus our review on studies of nonfinancial characteristics that also account for potential financial barriers. Recent empirical studies that examine nonfinancial barriers to care for children in the context of children's health insurance coverage are presented in Table 3.

Table 2 Indicators and components of health care access

HEALTH POLICY		
Indicators of potential access to care		
Predisposing		Age
		Gender
		Ethnicity
		Education
		Occupation
		Family structure
Health need		Perceived need
		Health risk
		Health status measures
	FAMILY	SYSTEM
Enabling	CHARACTERISTICS	CHARACTERISTICS
		Personal medical care
		Delivery system
		Organizational structure
	Insurance coverage	Benefits, funding sources
	Income	
	Attitudes and beliefs	Cultural competence
	Regular provider, source of care	Provider type, training, attitudes
		Location and sites of care
	Residential location	Geographic distribution and location
	Transportation	Service capacity
	Time to appointment	Models of care
	Convenience of services	System and service integration
		Co-location and collaboration
Indicators of realized access to care		
Utilization	Entry to care	Patterns of utilization
	Volume of services	Expenditures
	Type of services	
Outcomes	Satisfaction	Preventable morbidity and mortality
	Health outcomes	Population mortality and morbidity

Source: Adapted and modified from Andersen, McCutcheon, Aday, Chiu, & Bell 1983 (5), Penchansky & Thomas, 1981 (76), and Weissman & Epstein, 1993 (96).

Table 3 Empirical multivariate studies of noninsurance barriers to care for children

Author	Age group	Dataset	Noninsurance factor	Outcome measure
Short & Lefkowitz[a,c] 1992 (87)	0–4 years	1987 National Medical Expenditure Survey (NMES)	Poverty Ethnicity Birth order Mother's age Mother's education Family structure Residential location Physician supply	Well-child visit past year Compliance with AAP well-child schedule Any sick visit Number of sick visits
Newacheck[a,c] 1992 (67)	0–17 years	1988 National Health Interview Survey on Child Health (NHIS)	Poverty Ethnicity Maternal education Family size Family structure Maternal use of health care Residential location	Number of physician visits (no physician visits vs >10 visits in past year)
Wood et al[a] 1990 (104)	0–17 years	RWJ national telephone survey of 2182 families	Poverty Ethnicity	Regular source of care Site of care Physician visit in past year Up-to-date on immunizations
Newacheck & Halfon[d] 1988 (70)	5–16 years	1982 National Health Interview Survey (NHIS) Preventive Care Supplement	Poverty/Income	Utilization of preventive care services Utilization of dental, medical, vision care

Table 3 (*Continued*)

Author	Age group	Dataset	Noninsurance factor	Outcome measure
Newacheck & Halfon[a,c] 1986 (68)	2–16 years	1978 National Health Interview Survey (NHIS)	Income Ethnicity Maternal education Maternal occupation Residence Travel time to care Family structure Maternal use of care	Physician visit in past year Number of physician visits
Guendelman & Schwalbe[b,c] 1986 (38)	0–16 years	1979 National Health Interview Survey (NHIS)	Poverty Ethnicity Education level of household head Family size Family structure Residence	Any physician contact in past year
Wolfe[a,c] 1980 (101)	1–11 years	1975 Rochester Community Child Health Survey (814 children)	Income Community median income Ethnicity Maternal education Maternal occupation Family structure Family size Parental use of care	Physician visit in past year Number of physician visits Site of care

[a] denotes analysis controlled for health insurance status
[b] denotes analysis controlled for Medicaid vs non-Medicaid insurance status
[c] denotes analysis controlled for child health status
[d] denotes bivariate analysis

ETHNICITY AND CULTURE   Ethnic disparities in access to care for children cannot be fully attributed to financial barriers or explained by differential health status (67, 68, 70, 75, 87, 104). Findings from the 1987 National Medical Expenditures Survey (NMES) and 1978 National Health Interview Survey (NHIS) show that nonwhite children are less likely to have a physician visit and have fewer total physician visits than white children (68, 87). The Robert Wood Johnson Foundation (RWJF) access to care surveys revealed that nonwhite children age 1 to 5 were more than three times *less* likely to have a physician visit in the past year (104). A study of children in a health maintenance organization found that minority status was associated with lower utilization of health care, independent of health need and maternal utilization of care (79). In a national survey that controlled for different types of insurance coverage, minority adolescents had fewer visits with physicians, were less likely to have a regular source of care, and lacked continuity of care as compared to nonminority adolescents (58). Poor access to appropriate care may explain RWJF survey findings that Hispanic and African-American families are less likely than white families to report satisfaction with their children's medical care (103).

Although there is substantial evidence that nonwhite children face barriers to obtaining basic medical care, the unique contribution of ethnicity to access barriers stems from social correlates and may be largely mutable. Studies of African-American families with diminished financial and accommodation barriers (e.g. waiting and appointment times) demonstrate that lower utilization and poorer health outcomes for African-American children can be minimized by organizational interventions (75). This is further supported by a study of African-American women receiving prenatal care in an environment of equalized family access to care (a US army base) (77). The infant mortality rate for these mothers was 11.1 per 1000 live births, as compared to the national average for all women (9.9) and for African-American women in nonmilitary settings (17.9).

Differential patterns of health care utilization across ethnic groups have been attributed partly to cultural beliefs and values that influence care-seeking behavior (62). For Latino families, poor access to care is associated with lower income, lack of citizenship documentation, holding traditional rather than dominant-culture health beliefs, and inadequate cultural competency of providers (17, 23, 34). Communication difficulties between families and providers have been shown to inhibit care-seeking and to reduce parental satisfaction with the child's care (59, 94). Greater acculturation has been associated with improved access to care for families with children, irrespective of socioeconomic status (91, 97).

EDUCATION   Low parental (particularly maternal) educational levels predict children's delayed entry into care (37, 38, 67, 69, 87), lower preventive care utilization for children (11, 23), and lack of compliance with the recommended well-child visit schedule (87). Studies of children's utilization of ambulatory care in Canada suggest a continued negative impact of lower maternal education levels upon appropriate utilization, in spite of comprehensive, universal coverage (106). A mother's own health care utilization pattern exerts an effect upon her child's utilization of care independent of the child's health needs. Similar patterns of utilization for mothers and their children have been found both for use of preventive health care and for the total number of physician visits (67, 69, 79). These findings underscore the significance of children's dependence upon the care-seeking behavior of others for receipt of their own care.

FAMILY STRUCTURE AND FAMILY SOCIAL SUPPORT   Characteristics of family structure appear to influence children's access to care through several mechanisms. Children's utilization of care decreases with larger family size (18, 38, 53, 67). Children in single-parent families have more physician visits than other children when other factors including need, insurance status, and other demographic characteristics are held constant (69). Young teenage mothers living with their own mothers report that their children received fewer than the appropriate number of well-child visits (87). Healthy children whose mothers work outside of the home are likely to have fewer ambulatory physician visits (13, 69).

The level of social support experienced by the mother, who is usually the primary caretaker of the child, is closely related to family structure. Social support and social networks have important but complex implications for caregivers' care-seeking behavior for their children (44). In one prepaid plan, families with larger social networks available to them had lower pediatric utilization rates for illness or injury (45). In another study, African-American and Mexican-American families who were socially isolated were less likely to have a regular source of care for their children, irrespective of health insurance status (57).

INCOME   Children living in poverty have substantially greater health risks and generally poorer health status in addition to having limited access to care (99, 104). Poverty exerts complex and multidimensional effects upon access to care that includes barriers to obtaining health insurance and proximity to appropriate care, among other factors. Poor children generally have fewer physician visits, are under-immunized, and experience delayed entry to care (56, 70, 104). This differential access to care is even more substantial for those low-income children who are identified with one or more health problems or reported to be in fair or poor health by their parents (56, 68, 72).

The quality and appropriateness of care obtained for poor children are not optimal, as evidenced by both satisfaction and utilization indicators. Poor families are twice as likely as nonpoor families to be dissatisfied with the medical care delivered to their children, irrespective of insurance status, health need, or other factors (102), and are more likely than nonpoor families to resort to emergency rooms for their children's routine sick care (81; N Halfon, PW Newacheck, D Wood, RF St. Peter, unpublished data). Basic measures of access to care that have been associated with poverty (e.g. provider availability) provide only part of the story. Economically disadvantaged families may be disinclined to seek and utilize health services appropriately because other severe and complex social problems associated with poverty act as additional obstacles. Many poor families live in communities that are plagued with other environmental and access barriers including transportation difficulties and safety concerns. For example, homeless children and families have multiple health problems and poor access to care that stem from their unhealthy environments, mobility, and instability (10a, 105).

System Level Factors

Personal medical services have generally not been organized to respond adequately to the full scope of children's health needs. Structural characteristics of the health system that pose barriers to care for children include insufficient numbers of appropriately trained and located providers, lack of regular sources of primary care, and the manner in which services are organized that negatively affect child health care delivery. The delivery of personal medical care service is currently being transformed by managed care frameworks that promise to allocate costly health resources more efficiently. At the same time, although on a much smaller scale, alternative delivery models are being developed to more effectively serve high-risk populations and children with special health needs who require a range of services currently provided in a fragmented array of separately funded and administered programs, largely outside of the traditional medical delivery system. The extent to which market-driven changes in health care incorporate and integrate more appropriate models of service delivery will be critical to meet the full range of children's health needs.

PROVIDER TRAINING   Because of the complexity involved in detecting new morbidities and psychosocial pathologies in children, inadequate identification of conditions requiring treatment constitutes an important barrier to effective care. Current clinical training insufficiently prepares providers to diagnose and treat the increasingly complex, interdependent problems of children, families, and adolescents (7, 9, 93). National surveys of health professionals who provide care to adolescents, including nurses, physicians, social workers, nutritionists, and psychologists, reveal substantial self-reported inadequacies in competency and training in a number of essential health care concerns of adolescents, such as psychosocial morbidities of adolescents (7, 9). Several surveys and anecdotal reports document similar inadequacies in the preparation of health professionals to identify, treat, or refer children at risk for mental disorders, developmental problems, complex psychosocial problems, and abuse and neglect (31, 36, 90). For example, in a study of provider screening and assessment, providers identified less than 50% of the emotional problems in the children they examined (20). These findings reveal patterns of care that are not exclusively a function of inadequate provider training and knowledge, but are related to other constraints such as patient attitudes, the time-consuming nature of assessment for these problems, and dearth of treatment resources in the community (51, 73, 90). In combination, these factors result in the failure of the health system, in a number of dimensions, to adequately detect and treat psychosocial problems in children.

GEOGRAPHIC AVAILABILITY OF PROVIDERS   Geographic access barriers pose problems for both insured and uninsured poor families. Travel time for families in underserved urban areas or rural locations may be substantial (47) and results in reduced utilization of care (24), particularly for children's preventive services (23). Short & Lefkowitz' analysis of the NMES revealed that local physician supply predicts children's compliance with preventive care schedules for children with family incomes of less than 200% of the federal poverty level (87). The general availability of providers to care for poor children has been further compromised in recent years; the number of office-based physicians delivering primary care services in low-income areas declined by 45 percent between 1963 and 1980 (55). Shortages of local primary care and mental health providers for children exist in both urban and rural areas (27, 55). Pediatricians nationwide reported limiting their acceptance of children with Medicaid, further reducing access to children in poor, inner-city areas (107). One consequence of the shortage of office-based primary care providers has been a high rate of inappropriate emergency department utilization (53, 75; N Halfon, PW Newacheck, D Wood, RF St. Peter, unpublished data), which affects the adequacy and scope of care that these children receive. Lower levels of provider availability also lead to depressed utilization (91) and to lower satisfaction of mothers with their child's care (25).

HAVING A REGULAR PROVIDER OF CARE   The benefits of having a regular provider of care are particularly significant for children. Families who identify a regular provider for their child are more likely to have obtained medical services for the child (53) and to report satisfaction with that care (8). A study of low-income children found that having a regular provider is associated with a greater total number of immunizations received by the child by age 6, and with the child having had a preventive visit in the past year (87). The location, setting, and provider type substantially affect children's continuity of care (19). Persons who identify their regular provider of care as a hospital outpatient department, rather than a medical office, are significantly less likely to see the same provider on a subsequent visit (12), and young children receive less preventive care, including immunizations, in these settings (53). Physician continuity increases family satisfaction with the care provided to chronically ill children (10, 54), and is associated with quality of care and more consistent utilization patterns for preventive care. Overall, parental satisfaction with the parent-physician interaction surrounding the care of their children is three times greater among office-based physicians than for physicians in public clinics (32).

Despite differential patterns of utilization and satisfaction, outpatient departments of hospitals have increasingly replaced offices of private physicians as the site of the regular source of care for poor children (82). In 1990, more than 50 percent of children on Medicaid received care from public, nonoffice-based providers (104). Children whose regular site for well-childcare is a community health center are more likely to have different providers for well and sick care, and to frequent emergency departments for nonemergent acute care (43, 81).

MANAGED CARE   In 1980, the Select Panel for the Promotion of Children's Health issued a series of recommendations aimed at enhancing delivery of health services for children (86). The Panel looked toward managed care models to resolve system and service fragmentation by providing an essential mechanism for increased access, coordination, and accountability in children's health care that is often lacking in fee-for-service arrangements. Since the time of that report, managed care is increasingly being used to rationalize the health care marketplace, primarily as a means to control costs. A number of studies have examined the potential benefits and pitfalls of such arrangements for children (29, 30). Health maintenance organizations (HMOs) have demonstrated marginally higher preventive care utilization and immunization rates, and some reduction in emergency room use as compared to indemnity financing systems (29, 60). However, the allocative efficiencies that HMOs extract may come at the expense of care that is most effective and appropriate for children. Pediatricians participating in managed care plans revealed higher rates of denied referrals to specialists and inpatient services for children, reporting twice as many referral barriers as for traditionally reimbursed referrals, and indicating that a third of these denied referrals compromised the child's health (14).

Current managed care models may inadequately serve the needs of children with chronic illness due to lack of organizational experience with comprehensive delivery systems of care for children, and the tendency to control, rather than coordinate, service utilization (46, 71). Analyses of HMO management of children with special health care needs suggest that HMOs often provide specialty services only when the child's health is expected to immediately improve, and limit mental health and related services as well as limit access to specialists (28).

The evidence of a positive impact of managed care arrangements for poor children covered by Medicaid is even less clear. The Medicaid Competition Demonstration showed improved preventive care and immunization rates for children (29, 35), whereas a randomized study of Medicaid managed care and fee-for-service arrangements found equivalent utilization of preventive care across groups (61). Acute visits for children without health problems at the study's outset were reduced in the managed care plan, but not in the fee-for-service plan, which the authors attribute to appropriate rationalizing of care.

However, a number of anecdotal reports and localized studies suggest that at least some Medicaid HMOs inadequately serve children's most basic health needs. A study of immunization coverage of inner-city children found that children in Medicaid HMOs were less likely to be age-appropriately immunized than children cared for by private physicians or by public health clinics (103). A health department survey following the 1989–90 measles epidemic in Milwaukee revealed that, of the confirmed measles cases among children 1–4 years, 83% were enrolled in Medicaid HMOs. Of those children, two thirds were inadequately immunized, and 30% were using emergency departments for primary care (65). Finally, HMOs that serve Medicaid patients may restrict access to EPSDT (Early Periodic Screening Diagnosis and Treatment) benefits, referrals, and other services for children with special health care needs (80). The poor performance of managed care in Medicaid arrangements may result from several factors including a less developed market place, excessive transfer of financial risk to providers, and inadequate capitation rates coupled with incentives to underserve.

CASE STUDIES OF BARRIERS TO CARE

The following case studies highlight the unique needs of children with special living situations and health conditions and the problems that result from inadequate health service delivery.

Mobile Populations: Homeless Children and Children in Foster Care

Children who are homeless or in foster care represent a growing population of children with special health needs who rely upon coordinated delivery systems for timely, sufficient, and appropriate health services. The mobility that characterizes these children's environments creates unique challenges to a health care system grounded in the assumption that children live in stable, sedentary families. Studies of both populations have documented very high rates of emotional, developmental, and behavioral problems as well as chronic medical conditions (6, 16, 105).

For foster children, removal from their homes not only accentuates their developmental vulnerability but also renders them completely dependent upon the state to fulfill their health and human needs. Despite high prevalence of physical and mental health problems, children in foster care are frequently not provided with comprehensive health assessments, follow-up, and appropriate patterns of care (41, 42). Accountability, continuity of care, and provider relationships are jeopardized when children experience several different placements. The current health system lacks the ability to systematically monitor and serve the health needs of foster children, despite their increased medical and social risks (88).

The mismatch between needs of this special population and traditional models of care has prompted the development of guidelines for appropriate care by programs and organizations, and the design of special health programs in several urban areas for children in foster care (88, 89). These programs are characterized by their focus upon serving physical, emotional, and cognitive health needs, and integrating the provision of health and social services. For example, the County of Los Angeles is developing the Protective Services Child Health System. This system is designed to provide comprehensive care through a series of regionalized multidisciplinary assessment centers, each with its own geographically defined provider network to guarantee availability of a full continuum of needed services. In addition, public health nurse-health care case managers are employed to link the delivery of services between the health and public social services agencies into a more integrated set of services. In order to integrate services into a coherent delivery system, several federal funding streams (Medicaid, EPSDT, and Title IV-E) are combined to form a composite funding base.

The mobility and instability of homeless families creates similar barriers to care for homeless children. These barriers are particularly harmful given the substantial physical and developmental problems often identified in homeless children (108). Poor access to care for homeless children (3, 78) contributes to under-immunization, lack of a regular provider, and dependence upon emergency room care (64). The discontinuous health care and delayed identification and treatment of conditions experienced by homeless children increase the health risks within this population. Special clinical systems have also been developed for these children and families to meet their unique unmet needs (78). Unfortunately, for both homeless children and those in foster care, these specialized delivery formats are the exception rather than the rule.

Childhood Immunizations

The delivery of immunizations in the U.S. provides an especially informative view of the effects of nonfinancial and systemic barriers to access to care for children. Immunizations are unique among children's health services as unquestionably cost-effective, universally indicated services with a prescribed schedule. Immunizations are relatively inexpensive to administer and easily delivered by a range of health professionals. However, only 10 to 42 percent of 2-year-old children in major cities surveyed by the CDC are adequately immunized (15). Despite the relative simplicity of the service, immunization delivery has become highly complex due to the disjointed structure of the US health care system for children.

Substantial provider and system-related barriers impede delivery. Interventions need to be targeted at infrastructural improvement and greater accountability (21, 66). Children who receive inadequate preventive services or who have multiple providers of care are more frequently under-immunized (39). Further, many children receive ambulatory care in sites such as emergency and outpatient departments that are not conducive to continuity of care, and lack a monitoring or follow-up role for children who receive one or more immunizations at these sites (104).

Many low-income parents must negotiate both private and public sectors to obtain immunization services. Financial barriers and provider practices frequently divert even insured children from their regular providers of care to public clinics for immunizations (85). One implication of this trend is that accountability for children's age-appropriate immunization status is divided between the public and private sectors and does not rest with one regular primary care provider. A second implication is that many public health systems have expanded their personal medical service delivery to meet the demand for immunizations. As public health financing has eroded over the past twenty years, the essential public health role in monitoring children's immunization status, and assuring age-appropriate immunization levels, has been significantly compromised.

Asthma

Asthma is the most common chronic illness in children and has been studied frequently as an indicator of the adequacy and appropriateness of care delivered to children. Preventable hospitalizations and morbidity have been associated with inadequate access of poor and nonwhite children to regular preventive care (43, 100). The comprehensive care and range of services required for children with asthma (e.g. patient education, after-hours care) are frequently unavailable in community clinics, which are increasingly the regular providers of care for poor children. Moreover, studies show that when children receive comprehensive and coordinated ambulatory services, expensive hospitalizations are reduced, and fewer schooldays are lost. The separation of well- and sick-child care frequently experienced by poor families fragments the care delivered to asthmatic children and has potentially significant clinical consequences for these children. Adequate care for many poor children requires improving access to timely medical care and a broader range of services designed to mitigate the social and environmental risks that these children experience (43, 99).

EMERGING INTEGRATED SERVICE MODELS FOR HIGH-RISK POPULATIONS

The emerging model of managed care, as exemplified by the staff model HMO, represents a market-driven, vertically integrated system designed to rationalize service delivery and improve allocative efficiency. Alternate models of care tailored to high-risk children and their families also have emerged in response to perceived and well-documented deficits within the health system that have remained unaddressed within the commercial health care market. Each of these developing models seeks to customize the service delivery system to children's needs by improving the comprehensiveness, availability, and coordination of health services and integrating services across the health and human service systems (40).

Organizational and personal barriers to care are particularly important for the child with multiple or severe needs, who must negotiate a number of health care providers and health service systems to obtain care. Many children currently receive health and health-related care in the medical, educational, and social sectors. Moreover, the early intervention, family preservation, and violence prevention programs that are increasingly important supplements to traditional medical and community-based health services require even broader multidisciplinary approaches. For the most part, services currently delivered by professionals in health, mental health, social service, and educational fields are not coordinated at an agency level, and have conflicting eligibility and administrative requirements that are difficult for many families to negotiate (50, 83). The lack of referral systems, agency and client-level service integration, and collaborative mechanisms represents an extremely important barrier to access for children and families (26, 50, 92).

There are many examples of multidisciplinary model programs successfully addressing systems barriers to care. A New York City model, The Door, provides a customized continuum of services to adolescents that coordinates traditional medical and mental health diagnostic and treatment services with social and counseling services delivered by providers who have special training and interest in this population (73). Emerging school-linked health centers for hard-to-reach adolescents provide another example of accessible, tailored delivery sites that fill acknowledged service delivery gaps (26). The Protective Services Child Health System being developed in Los Angeles (see above) is another example of a ground-up approach to customizing the management of care. Despite their potential to provide an effective continuum of care, innovative and ecologically relevant models of care that are multidisciplinary, comprehensive, and community based are few in number (40, 84).

So-called "one-stop shopping" programs developed for young mothers and pregnant women seek to provide in one facility all of the health and human services that these women may need (10a). These services include traditional medical services, family planning, nutrition and health counseling, case management, social services such as housing assistance and income support, and therapeutic programs such as mental health and drug and alcohol counseling. The Ventura model of mental health care delivery provides another example of an initiative that explicitly and effectively addresses the unique needs of children and the barriers to their care (63). This innovative model is characterized by its collaborative approach and targeting of services. Interagency agreements enable mental health workers to promote and coordinate the delivery of mental health services within the sectors of juvenile justice, child welfare, and special education. This system incorporates explicit mandates to target the most vulnerable children, to identify the most appropriate venue for service delivery, and to create multidisciplinary teams that assess the child's needs and develop treatment plans. These initiatives are grounded in models of care that seek to modify the mismatch we have described, rationalizing the delivery of care to children by customizing the delivery system.

SUMMARY

In this review, we have focused the relationships between individual and delivery system characteristics and diminished access to children's health services. Several limitations of the literature indicate directions that should be pursued in future child health service research. Much of the data and analyses currently available on access to care has examined utilization of physician services without reference to physician type or site of care. These studies have not accounted for nonphysician providers or other types of nonmedical health services important to children, and also do not usually distinguish between the acute or preventive nature of care delivered. Further, because the national surveys and many other studies rely upon cross-sectional data, causality for certain enabling factors cannot be inferred, and the relationship between utilization of care and health outcomes cannot be reliably assessed. Finally, quality of care and effectiveness measures for emerging service systems for children are only in the early stages of development and require further elaboration (61a).

In spite of these shortcomings, the catalog of individual and system-level barriers provides substantial evidence of a mismatch between children's needs and the current organization of the health system. Even if the United States were to radically reform payment for basic medical services by assuring universal coverage, differential access and nonfinancial barriers would persist. The episodic, acute-care orientation of the health system would continue to result in inadequate access and inappropriate service delivery format for many children.

Our case studies further elucidate the systemic structural barriers to appropriate, timely, and sufficient care for children. These barriers include fragmented public and private delivery systems, lack of comprehensive, developmentally appropriate services, and shortages of accessible sites, delivery systems, and appropriately trained providers.

Federal and state governments have created a variety of publicly financed and administered programs that are designed to bridge many of the service gaps and to overcome barriers to care. The Part H legislation of the Individuals with Disabilities Education Act (IDEA) requires that states develop effective interagency approaches for children with developmental disabilities by mandating interagency collaborations and providing methodologies for pooling funds in order to provide a comprehensive set of developmentally appropriate health and education services. Part H requires that children and families receive multidisciplinary evaluations, family assessments, and coordinated care as well as a variety of other services. It also mandates that public and private delivery systems be used to facilitate the delivery of care. The Head Start program represents an earlier federal effort to combine health education and early childhood development services. While these two major federal efforts represent expansive and integrative approaches to the health and development problems in early childhood, a recent GAO report identifies over 111 different federal programs targeted at the health and developmental needs in early childhood (35a). Federal and state "wrap-around" programs that were intended to fill in many important service gaps also contribute to an irregular network of fragmented services.

A major conundrum faced in the evolving health care system is how diverse public programs with categorical eligibility criteria and separate funding streams can be integrated into the managed care marketplace. Systems of managed care that vertically integrate traditional medical services (physician and hospital services) may find it very difficult to also integrate or coordinate the delivery of this diverse set of so-called wrap-around services.

CONCLUSION

Improving access to care for children and youth will require substantial restructuring and refinancing of current delivery systems. Customizing delivery systems for children will only be possible if their unique needs are acknowledged as a primary focus and priority for health care reform. Greater emphasis on preventive services and population-based approaches is fundamental to improving the delivery of appropriate health services to children and young families. Market-driven reforms that curtail costly services and overutilized, marginally efficacious expensive procedures rely on managed care and vertically integrated provider networks to improve allocative and productive efficiencies. Although the underlying principles are sound, the current models of managed care must also be customized so that health concerns of children are not ignored or minimized by organizations that cannot provide essential continuums of care. Universal access to appropriate care for children requires affordable, available continuums of care that integrate personal medical services, community-based health services with education and social programs and agencies from both public and private sectors.

As market reform proceeds, the accountability of managed and integrated health systems for improving health outcomes must be assured, not only for individual clients but for populations. New measures essential to assure such accountability and performance will be possible only with the collection of adequate data on the health needs of the child population and linkage with utilization and outcome data. The Annie B Casey Foundation's Kids Count Program and the Robert Wood Johnson Children's Health Initiative are the first steps in that direction. Such performance measures will serve an important role in identifying service gaps as well as effective models of care as market transformations take place.

Can these objectives be achieved? Universally available integrated child health services are the norm in most industrialized countries (98). Most European countries provide a broad range of health, developmental, and social services to children, beginning at conception and continuing through majority. These systems are grounded in a national health insurance policy and include maternity leave and support, and childcare and development programs, which are linked and integrated into coherent systems (33, 98). Providing comprehensive preventive care to all children through integrated systems of public and private sources can assure timely care and measurable results across a variety of health status indicators.

The essential challenge is not obtaining the knowledge or tools necessary to achieve these objectives, but developing policies and the political will that can accomplish the task. Creating a child health system that works for all children should be a major, if not the first, priority of national health care reform.

Literature Cited

1. Aday LA, Andersen RM. 1974. A framework for the study of access to medical care. *Health Serv. Res.* 9:208–20
2. Aday LA, Begley CE, Lairson DR, Slater CH. 1993. *Evaluating the Medical Care System: Effectiveness, Efficiency, and Equity.* Ann Arbor, MI: Health Admin. Press
3. Alperstein G, Rappaport C, Flanigan JM. 1988. Health problems of homeless

children in New York City. *Am. J. Public Health* 78:1232–33

4. Andersen RM, Aday LA, Lyttle CS, Cornelius LJ, Chen MS. 1987. *Ambulatory Care and Insurance Coverage in an Era of Constraint.* Chicago: Pluribus Press

5. Andersen RM, McCutcheon A, Aday LA, Chiu GY, Bell R. 1983. Exploring dimensions of access to medical care. *Health Serv. Res.* 18:49–74

6. Bassuk EL, Rosenberg, L. 1990. Pediatrics. Psychosocial characteristics of homeless children and children with homes. *Pediatrics* 85:257–61

7. Bearinger LH, Wildey L, Gephart J, Blum, RW. 1992. Nursing competence in adolescent health: Anticipating the future needs of youth. *J. Prof. Nursing.* 8:80–86

8. Becker MH, Maiman LA. 1975. Sociobehavioral determinants of compliance with health and medical care recommendations. *Med. Care* 13:10–24

9. Blum RW, Bearinger LH. 1990. Knowledge and attitudes of health professionals toward adolescent health care. *J. Adol. Health Care* 11:289–94

10. Breslau N, Mortimer EA. 1981. Seeing the same doctor: determinants of satisfaction with specialty care for disabled children. *Med. Care* 19:741–58

10a. Brown SS, ed. 1988. *Prenatal Care: Reaching Mothers, Reaching Infants.* Washington, DC: Inst. Med./Natl. Acad. Press

11. Bullough B. 1972. Poverty, ethnic identity and preventive health care. *J. Health Soc. Behav.* 13:347–59

12. Butler JA, Winter WD, Singer JD, Wenger M. 1985. Medical care use and expenditure among children and youth in the United States: analysis of a national probability sample. *Pediatrics* 76:495–507

13. Cafferata GL, Kasper JD. 1985. Family structure and children's use of ambulatory physician services. *Med. Care* 23:350–60

14. Cartland JDC, Yudkowsky BK. 1992. Barriers to pediatric referral in managed care systems. *Pediatrics* 89:183–92

15. Centers for Disease Control and Prevention. 1992. Retrospective assessment of vaccination coverage among school-aged children. Selected cities 1991. *Morbid. Mortal. Wkly. Rep,* Feb. 14

16. Chernoff R, Combs-Orme T, Risley-Curtis C, Heisler A. 1994. Assessing the health status of children entering foster care. *Pediatrics* 93:594–601

17. Chesney AP, Chavira JA, Hall RP, Gary HE. 1982. Barriers to medical care of Mexican-Americans: the role of social class, acculturation, and social isolation. *Med. Care* 20:883–91

18. Colle AD, Grossman M. 1978. Determinants of pediatric care utilization. *J. Hum. Resourc.* 13:115–58 (Suppl.)

19. Cornelius LJ. 1993. Barriers to medical care for white, black, and Hispanic American children. *J. Natl. Med. Assoc.* 85:281–88

20. Costello EJ. 1986. Primary care pediatrics and child psychopathology: a review of diagnostic, treatment, and referral practices. *Pediatrics* 78:1044–51

21. Cutts FT, Orenstein WA, Bernier RH. 1990. Causes of low preschool immunization coverage in the U.S. Atlanta. Cent. Dis. Control Prevent.

22. Dutton DB. 1978. Explaining the low use of health services by the poor: costs, attitudes, or delivery systems? *Am. Soc. Rev.* 43:348–68

23. Dutton DB. 1981. Children's health care: the myth of equal access. In *Better Health for Our Children: A National Strategy.* Rep. Sel. Panel Promot. Child Health, Vol. 4. US HHS

24. Dutton DB. 1986. Financial, organizational, and professional factors affecting health care utilization. *Soc. Sci. Med.* 23:721–35

25. Dutton DB, Gomby D, Fowles J. 1985. Satisfaction with children's medical care in six different ambulatory settings. *Med. Care* 23:894–912

26. Farrow F, Joe T. 1992. Financing school-linked, integrated services. *Futur. Child.* 2:56–67

27. Fossett JW, Peterson JD, Kletke PR, Peterson JA. 1992. Medicaid and access to child health care in Chicago. *J. Health Polit. Pol. Law* 17:273–98

28. Fox HB, Wicks LB, Newacheck PW. 1993. Health maintenance organizations and children with special health needs. A suitable match? *Am. J. Dis. Child.* 147:546–52

29. Freund DA, Rossiter LF, Fox PD, Meyer JA, Hurley RE, et al. 1989. Evaluation of the Medicaid Competition Demonstrations. *Health Care Financ. Rev.* 11:81–97

30. Freund DA, Lewit EM. 1993. Managed care for children and pregnant women: promises and pitfalls. *Futur. Child.* 3:92–122

31. Friedman LS, Johnson B, Brett AS. 1990. Evaluation of substance-abusing adolescents by primary care physicians. *J. Adol. Health Care* 11:227–30

31a. Gabarino J. 1990. The human ecology of early risk. Ses Ref. 62a, pp. 78–96

32. Garrison WT, Bailey EN, Garb J, Ecker

B, Spencer P, Sigelman D. 1992. Interactions between parents and pediatric primary care physicians about children's mental health. *Hosp. Commun. Psychol.* 43:489–93

33. General Accounting Office. 1993. Preventive care for children in selected countries. *GAO/HRD-93–62*

34. General Accounting Office. 1993. Foster care: services to prevent out-of-home placement are limited by funding barriers. GAO/HRD-93-76

35. General Accounting Office. 1993. Medicaid: states turn to managed care to improve access and control costs. *GAO/HRD-93–46*

35a. General Accounting Office. 1994. Early childhood programs: multiple programs and overlapping target groups. *GAO/HEHS-95-4FS*

36. Goldberg ID, Roghmann KJ, McInerny TK, Burke JD. 1984. Mental health problems among children seen in pediatric practice: prevalence and management. *Pediatrics* 73:278–93

37. Guendelman S. 1985. The ethnic dilemma in children's health: class versus culture. *Border Health* 1:27–34

38. Guendelman S, Schwalbe J. 1986. Medical care utilization by Hispanic children: how does it differ from black and white peers? *Med. Care* 24:925–40

39. Guyer B, Hughart N, Holt E, Ross A, Stanton B, et al. 1994. Immunization coverage and its relationship to preventive health care visits among inner-city children in Baltimore. *Pediatrics* 94:53–58

40. Halfon N, Berkowitz G. 1993. Health care entitlements for children: providing health services as if children really mattered. In *Visions of Entitlement: The Care and Education of American's Children,* ed. MA Jensen, SG Goffin, pp. 175–212. New York: SUNY Press

41. Halfon N, Klee L. 1987. Health and development services for children with multiple needs: the child in foster care. *Yale Law Pol. Rev.* 9:71–96

42. Halfon N, Klee L. 1987. Health services for foster children in California: current practices and policy recommendations. *Pediatrics* 80:183–91

43. Halfon N, Newacheck PW. 1993. Childhood asthma and poverty: differential impacts and utilization of health services. *Pediatrics* 91:56–61

44. Horwitz A. 1978. Family, kin, and friend networks in psychiatric help-seeking. *Soc. Sci. Med.* 12:297

45. Horwitz SM, Morgenstern H, Berkman LF. 1985. The impact of social stressors

and social networks on pediatric medical care use. *Med. Care* 23:946–59

46. Horwitz SM, Stein REK. 1990. Health maintenance organizations vs. indemnity insurance for children with chronic illness: trading gaps in coverage. *Am. J. Dis. Child.* 144:581–86

47. Hughes D, Rosenbaum S. 1989. An overview of maternal and infant health services in rural America. *J. Rural Health* 5:299–319

48. Deleted in proof

49. Jameson EJ, Wehr E. 1993. Drafting national health care reform legislation to protect the health interests of children. *Stanford Law Pol. Rev.* 5:152–76

50. Kahn AJ, Kamerman SB. 1992. *Integrating Services Integration: An Overview of Initiatives, Issues, and Possibilities.* Natl. Cent. Child. Poverty. Columbia Univ. Sch. Public Health

51. Kamerow D, Pincus H, Macdonald D. 1986. Alcohol abuse, other drug abuse, and mental disorders in medical practice. *J. Am. Med. Assoc.* 255:2054–57

52. Kasper JD. 1975. Physician utilization and family size. In *Equity in Health Services: Empirical Analysis in Social Policy,* ed. R Andersen, J Kravits, OW Anderson, pp. 55–70. Cambridge MA: Ballinger Publ.

53. Kasper JD. 1987. The importance of type of usual source of care for children's physician access and expenditures. *Med. Care* 25:386–98

54. Kelley MA, Alexander CS, Morris NM. 1991. Maternal satisfaction with primary care for children with selected chronic conditions. *J. Commun. Health* 16:213–24

55. Kindig D, Movassaghi H, Dunham N, Zwick D, Taylor C. 1987. Trends in physician availability in 10 urban areas from 1963 to 1980. *Inquiry* 24:136–46

56. Kleinman JC, Gold M, Makuc D. 1981. Use of ambulatory care by the poor: another look at equity. *Med. Care* 19:1011–21

56a. Lasker RD, Lee PR. 1994. Improving health through health system reform. *J. Am. Med. Assoc.* 272:1297–98

57. Lewin-Epstein N. 1991. Determinants of regular source of care in black, Mexican, Puerto Rican, and non-Hispanic white populations. *Med. Care* 29:543–57

58. Lieu TA, Newacheck PW, McManus MA. 1993. Race, ethnicity, and access to ambulatory care among U.S. adolescents. *Am. J. Public Health* 83:960–65

59. Malach RS, Segel N. 1990. Perspectives on health care delivery systems for

American Indian families. *Child. Health Care* 19:219–28

60. Manning WG, Leibowitz A, Goldberg GA, Rogers WJ, Newhouse JP. 1984. A controlled trial of the effect of a prepaid group practice on utilization. *New Engl. J. Med.* 310:1505–10

61. Mauldon J, Leibowitz A, Buchanan JL, Damberg C, McGuigan KA. 1994. Rationing or rationalizing children's medical care: comparison of a Medicaid HMO with fee-for-service care. *Am. J. Public Health* 84:899–904

61a. McGlynn EA, Halfon N, Leibowitz A. 1995. Assessing the quality of care for children: prospects under health reform. *Arch. Pediatr. Adolesc. Med.* In press

62. Mechanic D. 1979. Correlates of physician utilization: why do major multivariate studies of physician utilization find trivial psychosocial and organizational effects? *J. Health Soc. Behav.* 20:387–96

62a. Meisels SJ, Shonkoff JP, eds. 1990. *Handbook of Early Childhood Intervention.* New York: Cambridge Univ. Press

63. Melaville AI, Blank M. 1991. *What It Takes: Structuring Interagency Partnerships to Connect Children and Families with Comprehensive Services.* Washington, DC: Educ. Hum. Serv. Consort.

64. Miller DS, Lin EH. 1988. Children in sheltered homeless families: reported health status and use of health services. *Pediatrics* 81:668–73

65. Nannis P. 1993. *Managed care and MCH in cities: a local perspective.* Strengthening Urban MCH Capacity: Highlights 1992 Urban MCH leadersh. conf. Washington, DC: US HHS

66. National Vaccine Advisory Committee. 1991. The measles epidemic: the problems, barriers, and recommendations. *J. Am. Med. Assoc.* 266:1547–52

67. Newacheck PW 1992. Characteristics of children with high and low usage of physician services. *Med. Care* 30:30–42

68. Newacheck PW, Halfon N. 1986. Access to ambulatory care services for economically disadvantaged children. *Pediatrics* 78:813–19

69. Newacheck PW, Halfon N. 1986. The association between mothers' and children's use of physician services. *Med. Care* 24:30–38

70. Newacheck PW, Halfon N. 1988. Preventive care use by school-aged children: differences by socioeconomic status. *Pediatrics* 82(pt 2):462–68

71. Newacheck PW, Hughes DC, Stoddard JJ, Halfon N. 1994. Children with chronic illness and Medicaid managed care. *Pediatrics* 93:497–500

72. Newacheck PW, Starfield B. 1988. Morbidity and use of ambulatory care services among poor and non-poor children. *Am. J. Public Health* 78:927–33

73. Office of Technology Assessment. 1991. Adolescent Health Vol. III. Cross-cutting issues in the delivery of health and health-related services. *OTA-H-469.* Washington, DC: US GPO

74. Office of Technology Assessment. 1988. Healthy children: investing in the future. *OTA-H-345.* Washington, DC: US GPO

75. Orr ST, Charney E, Straus J. 1988. Use of health services by black children according to payment mechanism. *Med. Care* 26:939–47

76. Penchansky R, Thomas JW. 1981. The concept of access: definition and relationship to consumer satisfaction. *Med. Care* 19:127–40

77. Rawlings JS, Weir MR. 1992. Race- and rank-specific mortality in a U.S. military population. *Am. J. Dis. Child.* 146:313–16

78. Redlener IE. 1988. Caring for homeless children: special challenges for the pediatrician. *Today's Child.* 2

79. Riley AW, Finney JW, Mellits ED, Starfield B, Kidwell S, et al. 1993. Determinants of health care use: an investigation of psychosocial factors. *Med. Care* 31:767–83

80. Rosenbaum S, Hughes DC, Butler E, Howard D. 1988. Incantations in the dark: medicaid, managed care and maternity care. *Milbank Mem. Fund Q.* 66:661–93

81. St. Peter RF, Newacheck PW, Halfon N. 1992. Access to care for poor children: separate and unequal? *J. Am. Med. Assoc.* 267:2760–64

81a. Sameroff AJ, Fiese BH. 1990. Transactional regulation and early intervention. See Ref. 62a, pp119–49

82. Schlesinger M, Eisenberg L. 1990. Little people in a big policy world: lasting questions and new directions in health policy for children. In *Children in a Changing Health System: Assessments and Proposals for Reform,* ed. M Schlesinger, L Eisenberg. Baltimore: Johns Hopkins Univ. Press

83. Schorr LB, Schorr D. 1988. *Within Our Reach: Breaking the Cycle of Disadvantage.* Doubleday: New York

84. Schorr LB, Both D. 1990. *Attributes of effective services for young children: a brief survey of current knowledge and its implications for program and policy development.* Effective services for young children: Rep. Workshop. Washington, DC: Natl. Acad. Press

85. Schulte JM, Brown GR, Zetzman MR, Schwartz B, Green HG, et al. 1991. Changing immunization referral patterns among pediatricians and family practice physicians, Dallas County, Texas. *Pediatrics* 87:204–7

86. Select Panel for the Promotion of Child Health 1981. *Better Health for Our Children: A National Strategy.* Washington, DC: US DHHS

87. Short PF, Lefkowitz DC. 1992. Encouraging preventive services for low-income children: the effect of expanding Medicaid. *Med. Care* 30:766–80

88. Simms MD. 1991. Foster children and the foster care system, Part II: impact on the child. *Curr. Prob. Pediatr.*

89. Simms MD, Halfon N. 1994. The health care needs of children in foster care: a research agenda. *Child Welf.* 78:505–24

90. Singer MI, Petchers MK, Anglin JM. 1987. Detection of adolescent substance abuse in a pediatric outpatient department: a double-blind study. *J. Pedistr.* 111:938–41

91. Solis JM, Marks G, Garcia M, Shelton D. 1990. Acculturation, access to care, and use of preventive services by Hispanics: findings from HHANES 1982–84. *Am. J. Public Health* 80:11–19 (Suppl.)

92. Starfield B. 1992. Child and adolescent health measures. *Futur. Child.* 2:25–39

93. Starfield B, Newacheck P. 1990. Children's health status, health risks, and use of health services. In *Children in a changing health system*, ed. MJ Schlesinger, L Eisenberg. Baltimore: Johns Hopkins Univ. Press

94. Uba L. 1992. Cultural barriers to health care for southeast Asian refugees. *Public Health Rep.* 107:544–48

95. Wegman ME. 1993. Annual summary of vital statistics—1992. *Pediatrics* 92: 743–54

96. Weissman JS, Epstein AM. 1993. The insurance gap: does it make a difference? *Ann. Rev. Public Health* 14:243–70

97. Wells KB, Golding JM, Hough RL, Burnam MA, Karno M. 1989. Acculturation and the probability of use of health services by Mexican Americans. *Health Serv. Res.* 24:237–57

98. Williams BC, Miller CA 1992. Preventive health care for children: findings from a 10-country study and directions for United States policy. *Pediatrics* 89: 983–98 (Suppl.)

99. Wise PH, Meyers A. 1988. Poverty and child health. *Pediatr. Clin. N. Am.* 35: 1169–86

100. Wissow LS, Gittelsohn AM, Szklo M, Starfield B, Mussman M. 1988. Poverty, race, and hospitalization for childhood asthma. *Am. J. Public Health* 78: 777–82

101. Wolfe BL. 1980. Children's utilization of medical care. *Med. Care* 18:1196–207

102. Wood DL, Corey C, Freeman HE, Shapiro M. 1992. Are poor families satisfied with the medical care their children receive? *Pediatrics* 90:66–70

103. Wood DL, Halfon N, Sherbourne C, Grabowsky M. 1994. Access to infant immunization for poor inner-city families: what is the impact of managed care? *J. Health Care Poor Underserv.* 5:112–23

104. Wood DL, Hayward RA, Corey CR, Freeman HE, Shapiro MF. 1990. Access to medical care for children and adolescents in the United States. *Pediatrics* 86:666–73

105. Wood DL, Valdez RB, Hayashi T, Shen A. 1990. Health of homeless children and housed, poor children. *Pediatrics* 86:858–66

106. Woodward CA, Boyle MH, Offord DR, Cadman DT, Links PS, et al. 1988. Ontario Child Health Study: patterns of ambulatory medical care utilization and their correlates. *Pediatrics* 82:425–34

107. Yudkowsky BK, Cartland JDC, Flint SS. 1990. Pediatrician participation in Medicaid: 1978 to 1989. *Pediatrics* 85: 567–77

108. Zima BT, Wells KB, Freeman HE. 1994. Emotional and behavioral problems and severe academic delays among sheltered homeless children in Los Angeles County. *Am. J. Public Health* 84260–264

Annu. Rev. Public Health. 1995. 16:473–95

MEDICAID MANAGED CARE:
Contribution to Issues of Health Reform

Deborah A. Freund

The School of Public and Environmental Affairs and Bowen Research Center, Indiana University, 1100 West Michigan Street, Indianapolis, Indiana 46202

Robert E. Hurley

Department of Health Administration, Medical College of Virginia/Virginia Commonwealth University, Richmond, Virginia 23298

KEY WORDS: Medicaid, managed care, health reform, health maintenance organizations

ABSTRACT

This chapter examines the emergence of managed care in Medicaid from an alternative to the mainstream delivery system for many beneficiaries. It offers a definition that encompasses the broad spectrum of program manifestations, and presents a brief historical perspective on the major eras of managed care in Medicaid. The major program prototypes are described and their contribution to enrollment growth is discussed. Research evidence is examined to address both operational issues and program impacts. Finally, we conclude with an appraisal of contemporary issues of importance and speculation on the next generation of Medicaid managed care programs with an eye to how federal and state health care reform proposals will shape this future.

INTRODUCTION

The number of Medicaid beneficiaries enrolled in managed care arrangements passed 5 million in 1993 and should exceed 10 million by the end of 1995 (19). This enrollment represents a nearly twentyfold increase since 1981 when experimentation with managed care models began in earnest in the Medicaid

473

0163-7525/95/0510-0473$05.00

program with the passage of the Omnibus Budget Reconciliation Act (OBRA). Enrollees now represent more than 15 percent of all Medicaid-eligible persons and nearly 25 percent of AFDC recipients, because most enrollees are in the AFDC-related eligibility categories. Viewed against the backdrop of the early 1980s when the types of models were limited, provider resistance was high, and skepticism about the feasibility of enrolling beneficiaries was extensive, this expansion is remarkable.

The dramatic growth reflects the confluence of three major forces. One is the pervasive proliferation of managed care models in the commercial sector to the point where they now reflect the predominant delivery system for private health benefits (38). The second trend is the extraordinary financial pressure brought on state governments by the growth in Medicaid expenditures over this same period (27, 28, 35, 39). A program that cost $27 billion in 1981 reached $130 billion in 1993. Seeking respite from these pressures, states have increasingly turned to managed care arrangements as a means to control the growth and improve the predictability of expenditure increases. The third force has been the cumulative experience of Medicaid programs with managed care initiatives. This experience has provided a wide range of lessons about development, implementation, and operation that have guided subsequent program expansions in second and third wave states (26). By 1994, more than 40 states were operating or developing managed care programs (19, 20).

This chapter examines the rationales undergirding managed care in Medicaid, offers a definition that encompasses the broad spectrum of program manifestations, and presents a brief historical perspective on the major eras of managed care in Medicaid. The major program prototypes are described and their contribution to enrollment growth is discussed [for an earlier review on this topic, see (26)]. Research evidence, now substantially more abundant, is examined to address both operational issues and program impacts. Finally, we conclude with an appraisal of contemporary issues of importance and speculation on the next generation of Medicaid managed care programs with an eye to how health care reform proposals will shape this future.

MEDICAID'S ROAD TO MANAGED CARE

Medicaid is a health care financing and delivery system for the poor that was developed first with a consuming concern for access (7) and later with cost containment objectives. Almost from the start of the program (37) its costs exceeded estimates, which set in motion a persistent, albeit futile, preoccupation with controlling growth in its expenditures. This growth has been driven by many factors including medical care inflation, expanded benefits, and enormous, though intermittent, increases in the number of beneficiaries covered (9, 27). Moreover, its joint federal-state financing has served to underscore the cost problem, because states are not permitted to finance their Medicaid programs through deficit spending. The flurry of creative matching schemes devised in the late 1980s by the states has been insufficient to give relief from the relentless consumption of limited state resources to meet Medicaid obligations (27, 28, 35). The federal government has now moved to suppress these matching schemes devised by the states to enable them to capture more federal dollars. These initiatives used provider donation programs and intergovernmental transfer of funds to effectively increase the apparent investment of state dollars in Medicaid that could be used to qualify for additional federal matching funds. While these arrangements vied to improve reimbursement for many providers, they nonetheless accounted for a substantial proportion of the increase in Medicaid expenditures during the period (27).

In many respects, Medicaid encountered earlier the choices inherent in meeting what seems like a virtually infinite demand for medical care with limited resources—a confrontation now faced by every other purchaser of care. Medicaid agencies have had to wrestle with the tradeoffs among which beneficiaries to cover, what services to include in the benefit package, and how best to administer the program. They have progressed through the same range of efforts found in the private sector: targeted interventions like access controls (cost sharing and restrictions on choice), creative payment methods (prospective payment for hospitals and nursing homes), and utilization review (preservice authorization). Ultimately, these interventions have been subsumed into more comprehensive approaches under the rubric of "managed care arrangements/systems" that offer public and private purchasers new opportunities to address the basic problems of a freedom-of-choice, fee-for-service delivery system.

The particular appeal of managed care arrangements for Medicaid programs is in addressing the interlocking, reinforcing problems endemic to the program that have not been responsive to single-focus interventions (26). Concerns about escalating program costs contributed to disappointing payment levels and declining provider participation. Limited provider involvement resulted in corresponding diminished access to quality services, especially to mainstream primary care providers and obstetricians and gynecologists. This diminished access led to reliance on inappropriate sites of care that are unnecessarily costly (especially emergency rooms) and lack the capacity to provide continuity and coordination of services, or that are high-volume providers of questionable competence (so-called Medicaid mills). This syndrome of related problems has demanded concerted efforts to interrupt the pathology. A variety of managed care models have been introduced in response.

Managed care in Medicaid represents an attempt to enroll beneficiaries in service delivery arrangements that promote the provision of coordinated services and reduce unneeded and/or unnecessarily costly services (25, 38). This generic definition incorporates the full spectrum of managed care models in use (see below). Managed care arrangements can also enable Medicaid programs to simultaneously introduce restrictions on free access to care, incorporate utilization management techniques, and, in some cases, use financial incentives to achieve cost containment and ensure availability of care. The paradoxical assertion that *by restricting free access to care its availability can be ensured* was once one of the most controversial features of Medicaid managed care, but now is recognized as one of its major contributions.

EVOLUTION AND GROWTH

Medicaid beneficiaries could have been enrolled in managed care plans almost from the passage of Title XIX in 1965. However, by end of the first era of Medicaid managed care in 1981, total enrollment was approximately a quarter of a million out of nearly 20 million beneficiaries. Virtually all of this enrollment could be found in a small number of established HMOs in major metropolitan areas, such as the Health Insurance Plan of New York, Kaiser Permanente, Northwest Region, Group Health Association in Washington, DC, and Group Health Cooperative of Puget Sound. Participants included only AFDC adults and children who had voluntarily enrolled in these plans; they typically represented a small fraction of the plan's total enrollment, thereby diluting the impact of Medicaid's low rates on the plans (12).

This period also included the notorious scandals associated with California's ill-starred effort to enroll rapidly substantial numbers of beneficiaries in prepaid health plans (5, 15). Plans engaged in shoddy marketing practices, enrolled beneficiaries without delivery systems in place, failed to develop sufficient reserves to pay providers in the event of financial difficulties and a variety of other problems. The California experience is most notable because it left a residue of discredit on Medicaid managed care that persisted for more than a decade, and remains an experience frequently invoked by the most trenchant critics of current initiatives.

The second era began in 1981 with the passage of OBRA, which explicitly promoted state-level experimentation by allowing federal agencies to issue demonstration waivers (called 1115 waivers) to explore new financing and delivery arrangements to arrest spiraling costs (8). A series of major demonstrations was initiated by the Health Care Financing Administration (HCFA), including the Arizona Health Care Cost Containment System and the Medicaid Competition Demonstrations to produce planned, albeit disparate, variation that could be systematically evaluated (15). By the mid-1980s, several states sought and acquired a new set of "programmatic waivers" [called 1915 (b)] that continued and expanded this variation, though without some of the requirements for evaluation found in demonstration waivers (11). As shown in

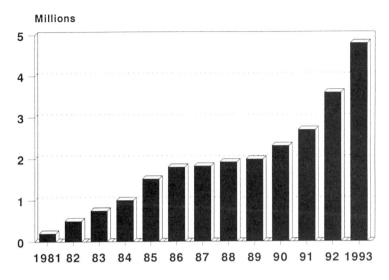

Growth in number of enrollees from 1981 to 1993 (18)

Figure 1   Medicaid managed care: 1981–1993

Figure 1, enrolled beneficiaries grew nearly tenfold by the end of the decade to 2.3 million.

The third era corresponds to the explosive growth in managed care in the private sector that has emerged in the 1990s (38). This growth has both reinforced Medicaid's efforts and created new opportunities as provider and consumer resistance to managed care has been surmounted. Whereas Medicaid, with its low payment rates, complex coverages, and extensive prior authorization, was once regarded as being a major hassle for providers, it no longer seems more burdensome than other managed care plans, which almost universally engage in these same activities. In addition, growing sophistication in program design and development among Medicaid agencies makes their managed care initiatives increasingly comparable to private sector efforts. Finally, because most credible health care reform proposals signal a central role for managed care plans, there is currently under way a major push to transform Medicaid to a baseline managed care program, at least for AFDC beneficiaries.

PROGRAM PROTOTYPES

A common rubric for managed care in Medicaid has proved as elusive and confusing as in the private sector. In part this reflects (*a*) the looseness with which initiatives have been characterized as managed care; (*b*) the distinctive terminology employed by the HCFA to classify programs based on its typology; and (*c*) the fact that many Medicaid programs did not fit under the generic classes of HMOs and PPOs. Some of the distinctiveness of Medicaid managed care programs appears to reflect the opportunistic nature of program development, given the financial, technical, and image constraints with which Medicaid agencies have entered the alternative service delivery arena.

An early effort by the authors to develop a useful classification scheme identified key program attributes that distinguished extant programs, though the empirical evidence at that time was scarce (23). This scheme was revisited several years later in the course of reviewing the best available research from 25 programs; three program prototypes were identified to facilitate synthesis and cross-program comparisons (26):

Type I: Fee-for-service primary care case management/gatekeeping
Type II: At-risk primary care case management/gatekeeping
Type III: Prepaid health plan enrollment

In each of these models, beneficiaries from covered eligibility classes enroll with a contracting provider (usually a primary care physician or clinic) or health plan that agrees to provide or authorize virtually all services and to be available to the enrollee on a 24-hour, 7-day per week basis. Providers could be primary care physicians, physician groups, or clinics. In some instances, enrollment was with the plan rather than with individually identifiable physicians. As noted earlier and discussed further in the conclusions, the vast majority of enrollees have been from the AFDC-related eligibility categories.

Traditionally, the first two program types have been mandatory enrollment, meaning that beneficiaries have to participate either by selecting or being assigned to a participating primary care provider. Prepaid health plan enrollment for Type III was voluntary in most instances (with notable exceptions in Arizona and Kansas City, Missouri), beneficiaries were offered an opportunity to enroll in participating HMOs or capitated prepaid health plans not licensed as HMOs. An increasing number of states have opted for mandatory enrollment models in HMOs in metropolitan areas such as Milwaukee, Minneapolis, Dayton, and more recently Sacramento.

The major differences between the prototypes relate to financial risk, scope of covered services, and the extent to which the models promote integration of service delivery. The fee-for-service gatekeeping model is clearly the least intrusive approach because it leaves intact the existing Medicaid payment and delivery systems, typically augmenting Medicaid fee-for-service payments with a case management fee of $2 to $3 per enrollee per month that is designed to compensate the physician for the administrative costs of gatekeeping duties. It focuses largely on promoting care coordination by the primary care provider through authorizing referral and ER contacts, but does not encourage providers either to form or join networks that are moving toward integrating systems. Its unobtrusiveness makes it a popular model in states with limited penetration of managed care plans and in rural states where few integrated systems have been available. Examples include the Michigan Physician Sponsor Plan, the Kentucky KenPAC program, and Virginia's MEDALLION program.

At the other extreme are the HMO/prepaid health plan enrollment programs that capitate a plan for most or all of the full scope of Medicaid-covered benefits. The shifting of risk to the plan creates incentives to develop integrating delivery systems as capitation is presumed to do for all commercial HMOs. From the standpoint of the Medicaid program, this strategy has special appeal as a means to obtain both predictability in expenditures and guaranteed savings. Thus savings are assured if the capitation rate is below the expected fee-for-service equivalent costs of the benefit package, and, not inconsequentially, if the plan enrolls a population that is fully representative of the group on which the rate has been set. The key presumption is that there will be plans willing to serve this population for this rate—an issue that continues to generate controversy and concern.

The middle category represents a diverse set of programs that rely largely on the care management technology of primary care gatekeeping, but attempt to use a variety of financial incentives such as partial capitation to primary care gatekeepers or the creation of pools of physicians who can be placed at varying degrees of risk for ancillary services, specialty, or hospital care. These arrangements commonly reflect an effort to promote networks of providers with some incentives to organize and integrate delivery of care in a less comprehensive fashion than that found in HMOs. For many providers this is a way to ease into prepayment. For Medicaid agencies it is a way to shift some financial risk to providers when there are insufficient numbers of pre-existing prepaid health plans with which to contract for the full scope of services. There are many of these program models in California (Santa Barbara and San Mateo have been operational for ten and seven years, respectively, and programs in Orange, Santa Cruz, and Solano counties are under development) and other western states where prepayment has gained wide acceptance among physicians.

It is instructive to re-examine the growth of Medicaid managed care from the vantage point of these prototypes (Figure 2). HMO enrollment grew substantially in the early 1980s and then leveled off, as the gatekeeper models became the faster-growing programs. This trend was due in part to adoption of managed care in second-wave states with little HMO capacity. By 1993, the proportion of enrollees in HMOs was about 40 percent (2 million) of all managed care enrollees, with approximately 140 participating plans (19, 20). A detailed examination of participation suggested that over half of this enroll-

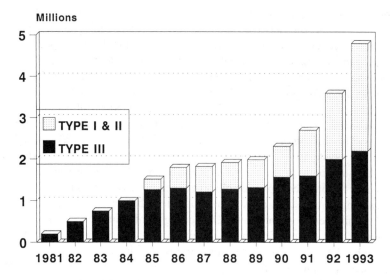

Growth in number of enrollees by program prototype (18)

Figure 2   Medicaid managed care: growth by type, 1981–1993

ment was in about 30 plans, and that most HMOs had a small number of enrollees. However, HMO interest in enrolling Medicaid beneficiaries has clearly picked up in the past two years. This interest is due to renewed state efforts to promote participation and the goal of many HMOs to prepare for health care reform, which is likely to drive many beneficiaries into the plans. But growth in gatekeeper programs has also remained strong, particularly as states interested in achieving statewide managed care coverage have opted for mixed, multiple-model initiatives, as noted in Figure 3.

KEY OPERATIONAL ISSUES

The early literature on Medicaid managed care (2, 10, 22) chronicled the challenges faced by Medicaid agencies in overcoming obstacles to obtaining waivers, meeting the resource and skill demands, customizing programs to local delivery systems, defusing provider resistance, and responding to bene- ficiary and advocacy opposition, especially to the restriction on freedom-of- choice. It is notable how far states have come in developing proficiency in each of these areas and the extent of collateral learning that has been diffused among the states (21, 34). As suggested earlier, the widespread acceptance of managed care in the population as a whole has been a major contributor to

STATE	PROGRAM TYPE(S)	ENROLLMENT
California	Type II,III	680000
Massachusetts	Type I,II,III	470000
Arizona	Type III	395000
Michigan	Type I,II,III	387000
Florida	Type I,III	383000
Kentucky	Type I	304000
Maryland	Type I,III	296000
Pennsylvania	Type II,III	243000
New York	Type II,III	193000
Ohio	Type III	159000
Colorado	Type I,III	129000
Illinois	Type I,III	124000
Wisconsin	Type III	120000

June 1993 enrollment and program types for largest programs (18)

Figure 3   States with largest enrollments, June 1993.

reducing obstacles, and the accumulated research and evaluation evidence has offered useful guidance to late entrants.

Program management has been another area where state agencies have demonstrated greater sophistication. The near-legendary problems in developing information systems to support managed care (23, 36) have been largely overcome. In the early 1980s, states did not know what data to collect or what technology to use to obtain information to monitor access, use, quality, and cost. Likewise, enrollment and marketing challenges, which stymied many first-generation programs, have been overcome and late entrants have drawn heavily from the knowledge and experience accumulated by pioneering states (21, 34). For example, the serious problems of assigning beneficiaries who fail to make a choice in mandatory enrollment programs are now handled quite smoothly by computer matching algorithms that take into consideration prior service contact, physician specialty, and geographic proximity. Oversight of marketing materials and practices by state agencies has been routinized to reduce the likelihood of reoccurrence of some of the pernicious practices noted in California in the 1970s (5).

State agencies have developed more understanding of and expertise in the setting of capitation rates and contract terms with prepaid programs. However, rate adequacy remains an area of considerable sensitivity and contention give what is often a low Medicaid payment base from which to start. Disputes over the adequacy of capitation rates depend not only on previous payment generosity but also on the extent to which managed care principles have diffused to the private sector payors in which the Medicaid managed care program is operating. States that have originally had low payment rates often cannot get existing health plans to agree to take Medicaid patients. The comment of an anonymous Medicaid director from one such state is instructive: "Given the capitation rate we are prepared to pay, we wouldn't want to do business with any plan that would be willing to accept it." In other states, where payment levels start out closer to private fee-for-service rates, states have less trouble. Regardless of the original payment baseline, states particularly committed to increasing access to certain types of services (such as obstetrical, orthopedic, psychiatric care) often find ways. In states such as California and Washington, for example, health plans have increased payment for obstetrical care to private sector managed care levels and have financed such payment enhancements with hospital efficiencies. How high payments must go depends on the extent of competition in the area. In spite of such success stories, it remains a HCFA policy that capitation rates in Medicaid managed care cannot exceed what would have been paid out under fee-for-service Medicaid. This underscores the fact that prepayment has the effect of dramatizing what in most but not all states has been the extraordinary inadequacy of Medicaid fees. A related and emerging issue is that as states continue to move to managed care, appropriate fee-for-service comparison groups used for rate setting will disappear and thus necessitate the development of new techniques. Neither the HCFA administration nor individual states have yet proposed well accepted solutions to this problem.

Traditionally, rates are set as a fraction (typically 95%) of the fee-for-service equivalent. Capitation of primary care physicians coupled with good utilization management on their part has led to better payment than they would have obtained under fee-for-service Medicaid. Indeed, in some California locales primary care payment under Medicaid managed care is comparable to private managed care. However, because of poor payment rate, access to specialists, especially in Type I and Type II programs, remains an issue. Specialists who remain compensated at traditional fee-for-service Medicaid rates continue to fail to participate. In the California Type II programs, for example, obstetrics, orthopedics, psychiatry, and neurology chronically remain underrepresented.

Biased selection also remains a concern. The problem arises because actuaries have been unable to predict precisely which Medicaid beneficiaries will select to enroll voluntarily in prepaid plans. Moreover, in mandatory programs enrollees may not distribute themselves evenly in terms of health status and risk, and thus selection bias can occur among plans and the technology to adjust for this adequately has yet to be developed. Finally, as in the private sector, there is a remaining concern that states will ratchet down payment rates if the plans make what they consider to be inordinate profits.

The oversight of contracted plan performance remains underdeveloped in most states, especially in terms of plan efforts to assure the quality of their services. A major joint initiative of HCFA, the states, and the Kaiser Family Foundation is to pilot a program called the Quality Assurance Reform Initiative (18), which is designed to assist states to issue and oversee guidelines to bolster quality assurance at the prepaid plan level. This effort corresponds closely to parallel efforts in the private sector regarding HMO accreditation and the development and dissemination of joint plan-industry performance indicators (31).

PROGRAM IMPACTS

The evidence of the impact of Medicaid managed care on program expenditures, beneficiary use, access, satisfaction, and quality of care has accumulated slowly and unevenly. This unevenness is due partly to the variety of models in place and to the enormous variation in the rigor with which studies have been conducted. This latter point was well-chronicled by Hurley, Freund & Paul who reported on the cost and use performance of Medicaid managed care programs in 25 evaluations (26).

The methodological problems for assessing the impacts of managed care programs in Medicaid are not necessarily distinct from those encountered in studies of private sector programs. In fact, some of the well-financed federal and foundation-sponsored programs are among the most comprehensive and exacting studies available on managed care (6, 12, 29, 36). Likewise, despite serious limitations in using Medicaid claims data for evaluation purposes, the uniformity and completeness of these data (for fee-for-service programs, at least) have yielded useful findings of cost and use impacts when coupled with a sound research/evaluation design. But many state-sponsored program evaluations are bedeviled by the fact they were done as part of a waiver-renewal application to demonstrate to federal officials both cost effectiveness and absence of adverse impact on access. Thus, many studies are either cursory or skewed to reflect favorably on the program; they sometimes employ dubious assumptions to ensure a conclusion of program savings without adverse effects.

Cost Effects

One review noted that 25 programs, despite their limitations, reported cost savings ranging from 5 to 15 percent (26). The source of these savings varied by program type. In the HMO enrollment program (Type III) the savings were achieved by contracting with plans to provide the benefit package at a rate 5 to 10 percent below the fee-for-service equivalent. Further research is needed to ascertain how the plans achieve their cost savings to live within these capitation rates, namely, whether they come from reductions in utilization or in the cost of service inputs, or a combination of both. Likewise, there is little up-to-date information on differences among HMO plan types (12). Finally, a persistent problem for all analyses of cost impacts has been that the most rigorous studies were conducted in the early years of implementation when effects were not stabilized and may be attributable to confusion and other perturbations. Longitudinal research of mature programs is needed to ascertain whether initial impacts intensify or dissipate over time, either of which is plausible, due to learning and/or gaming effects.

A crucial and oft-neglected issue for voluntary HMO enrollment programs has been the impact of selection bias. The two best studies, conducted by the RAND Corporation (29) using elegant research designs, yielded mixed results. One plan experienced profound favorable selection, meaning that the capitation rate grossly overpaid the HMO. The other study found adverse selection for the plan, of a smaller order of magnitude. However, both managed care programs were small in enrollment, and the experiences are unlikely to be replicated. Just how subtle this selection bias can be was demonstrated in an evaluation of a voluntary enrollment program in Ohio (Research Triangle Institute, unpublished information). This study showed that the prolonged delay in HMO enrollment for new eligibles resulted in childbirth occurring for nearly all new eligibles during the pre-enrollment window when care was paid by fee-for-service. Because the HMO rates were based on the assumption that delivery would occur during enrollment, this delay resulted in temporally biased selection effects distinctly favorable to the plans. Mandatory programs that rapidly enroll new beneficiaries avoid this temporal bias, as well as the bias due to voluntary choice of plans over traditional Medicaid.

How do cost savings of Type I and Type II programs compare with those from Type III models? The cost savings of the gatekeeper programs seem to be generally comparable to those in the HMOs, but these must be earned by actually reducing expenditures through improved care coordination, substitution of less costly care, reduced use of the emergency department for nonurgent care, and some reductions in inpatient use. Programs that pay a case management fee must pay for it out of savings. Many primary care gatekeepers see the case management fee as simply an overdue fee increase. These savings also seem to be more easily attained in urban areas where ER use and self-referral to specialists are prevalent. Although little is known about rural-based managed care initiatives in Medicaid (and in the private sector), it is likely that impacts are attenuated given the limited numbers of providers, more stable primary care relationships, and emergency rooms that offer more limited service and are less accessible to geographically dispersed beneficiaries.

Utilization Effects

The impacts on use referred to above have been widely observed, especially sharp reductions in inappropriate ER use (24). This reduction appears to be due to self-diversion rather than to denial of care by hospitals, which are highly sensitive to anti-dumping regulations, and to the greater likelihood that beneficiaries with a primary care case manager will call for information and reassurance in lieu of visiting an ER. However, Medicaid managed care programs have had uneven effects in reducing hospital use and increasing primary care physician service use.

The gatekeeper programs (and possibly the HMO programs, though little internal evidence is available for analysis) seem to have promoted greater use of primary care physicians, including substitution of primary for specialty care. Method of payment appears to influence this pattern: Fee-for-service programs may actually increase use of primary care services, whereas at-risk programs seem to encourage substitution effects. In both instances, more care is concentrated with primary care physicians, which improves care coordination and the potential for better continuity. However, virtually no studies using episodes of care have yet directly examined changes in care continuity.

Reduced inpatient use has been reported commonly, though it is difficult to attribute the reduction explicitly to gatekeeper effects, because these programs typically are accompanied by other utilization management initiatives, like preadmission certification and concurrent review. Because most enrollees are from the AFDC adult and child categories, impacts on use of inpatient services are constrained since more than two thirds of inpatient stays are for obstetrical care.

Access and Satisfaction

The impacts on access are dependent on whether impediments to access existed prior to the implementation of managed care. These programs provide a contractually based guarantee of access to a primary care provider, so preexisting constraints on access are overcome. Interestingly, beneficiaries sometimes express perceptions that access is limited, especially direct access to specialists, which is one of the goals of the program. But objective measures of access such as off-hour availability, telephone accessibility to a primary care physician, and wait/travel times tend to show improved access notwithstanding these perceptions (12). This improvement probably reflects the overall adjustment that all consumers—Medicaid and non-Medicaid—are experiencing in obtaining care from organized managed care delivery systems that restrict freedom of choice.

A related finding is that dissatisfaction with enrollment-based systems may be subject to misinterpretation. In a detailed study of five gatekeeper-based programs in which enrollees reported lower satisfaction relative to matched comparison groups of fee-for-service Medicaid beneficiaries, a supplemental analysis was conducted to see if persons whose prior regular source of care became their gatekeeper expressed dissatisfaction with enrollment (25). The findings indicated that these persons did not have lower satisfaction relative to the comparison group, but that persons whose gatekeeper was a new physician were significantly less satisfied. This study suggested that dissatisfaction was not engendered by restriction on choice, but rather by the dislocational consequences of having an unfamiliar physician play the gatekeeper role for them, criticism lodged also against private-sector gatekeeper programs.

Quality

Studies of the impact of Medicaid managed care on quality have been few and very limited (14). There are some indications that these programs have not experienced the improvements expected from enrollment in coordinated care and/or capitated delivery systems. Some studies have found that immunization levels continue to be disappointingly low among enrollees, prenatal care is not delivered more promptly or thoroughly, and birth-outcomes are not detectably better (4, 17). A recent study by Lurie et al (30) demonstrated that there were no adverse impacts on health status for enrollees in the first year of enrollment; however, neither was quality detectably improved.

These disappointing findings may seem surprising in light of assertions of the superiority of managed care delivery systems. This discrepancy might reflect that these initiatives may not be aggressive or intrusive enough to alter either care-seeking by or service provision to special-need populations. Poorer outcomes of pregnancy may be due to social factors beyond the control of Medicaid. However, these programs can be criticized for not aggressively seeking coordination with housing, social service, WIC, and food stamp programs. Another explanation could be that managed care systems are not being required by diligent oversight of contract performance to make new, additional efforts to reach out and engage these beneficiaries. And still others could respond that Medicaid administrators' historical inattentiveness to quality over its quarter century of existence stands in sharp contrast to administrators' expectations that managed care plans can and must outperform the baseline fee-for-service system. Additionally, evidence from qualitative studies of the implementation of Medicaid managed care programs strongly suggests that there often is a troubling lack of coordination between community-based agencies and contracted health plans. One frequent example is the lack of coordination between health departments or other providers responsible for the Early, Periodic, Screening Diagnosis, and Treatment Program (EPSDT) for children and health plans. Immunizations and other service provided by EPSDT often are "carved out" of a health plans capitation rate. As a result, children go without immunizations unless strong linkage arrangements are made with community public health agencies or primary care physicians provide immunizations to their enrollees free of charge. Strong linkages should be developed and enforced or else services provided by community public health agencies should be folded into capitation rates. Irrespective of which position one adopts, the scarcity of good, sound evidence about the impact on quality of programs now serving almost 10 million beneficiaries is reason for significant concern.

CONTEMPORARY CONSEQUENCES OF EXPANDED MANAGED CARE

Managed care in Medicaid is rapidly becoming the mainstream model for care, especially for AFDC-related beneficiaries, after more than a decade as merely a so-called alternative delivery system. Major initiatives now under way in California, New York, Texas, Tennessee, and elsewhere indicate that by the end of the 1990s, the number of enrollees could double to 10 million or more, over half of all AFDC beneficiaries. All metropolitan areas in California are now embarking on mandatory managed care programs, and New York has plans to enroll half of all of its Medicaid beneficiaries in a variety of managed care models. As noted below, health reform initiatives may fundamentally alter the structure, if not the existence, of Medicaid. In the meantime, several important developments are emerging because of the rise to predominance of managed care in Medicaid. Many of these issues transcend the bounds of Medicaid and will have implications for any health reform efforts.

MULTIPLE MODELS   One major development is further adoption by states of multiple models of managed care to afford them the flexibility to take their programs statewide. Thus, HMO enrollment strategies can be pursued in earnest in metropolitan areas, whereas primary care gatekeeper models, with or without risk, are implemented in rural areas. In addition, states with baseline primary care case management programs are beginning to offer HMOs as "opt out" options to foster competition among models and to permit HMOs to participate without having to absorb massive numbers of new members. Whether this type of voluntary enrollment results in selection bias will merit close attention, though the restriction on choice now in the baseline Medicaid program could reduce this bias. Similarly, health reform proposals that seek to channel citizens into HMOs, while allowing them to opt out into other models of care, will also promote selection effects that have to be monitored.

DESTABILIZATION OF TRADITIONAL MEDICAID PROVIDERS   Mandatory enrollment programs are provoking widespread challenges because they effectively
exclude providers who do not, or choose not to, qualify to participate as
gatekeepers or in prepaid health plan networks. Exclusive contracting exacer-
bates many tensions already being felt by traditional providers of Medicaid
services because of competitive market pressures. These providers include
indigenous community physicians with large Medicaid practices, public health
departments, federally qualified health centers, and community mental health
centers, as well as public and academic medical centers that have grown reliant
on special Medicaid reimbursement through the disproportionate share hospital
(DSH) program (which increases Medicaid payments to hospitals who care
for disproportionately high proportions of the uninsured). Members of these
groups have had to agonize over whether and how they could participate in
Medicaid managed care prototypes, based on the design of their respective
state's program and the eligible groups that the program covered.

Traditional inner-city physicians, who have been the bulwark of Medicaid
services in many metropolitan areas, may be reluctant to join plans or are
disinterested in becoming a primary care gatekeeper. But they risk loss of
major blocs of business if they pass on opportunities to participate or are
excluded from contracting networks. Local health departments that may have
long-standing traditions of well-child clinics, immunization services, and Early
Periodic Screening Diagnosis and Treatment (EPSDT) screening programs,
are confronted with the need either to develop round-the-clock coverage arrangements to qualify as primary care gatekeepers or, even more exactingly,
to develop the capacity to function as a prepaid health plan. In some instances
they even may be required to participate as a risk-bearing provider in the
network of a prepaid plan. Community mental health centers may find themselves in similar situations, if states opt to include special groups such as the
severely mentally ill. For hospitals that are currently reliant on DSH payments
to cross-subsidize care to the indigent, failure to sponsor or join managed care
networks can mean the loss of Medicaid inpatient volume and the higher
payments that they bring to the hospitals. Whether such providers can compete
successfully under a competition-based reform strategy is an open topic.

NEW OPPORTUNITIES/RISKS FOR MEDICAID AS ACTIVE PURCHASER   Medicaid
agencies are discovering the leverage that they now possess in buying care,
by being able to steer large volumes of enrollees to selected providers and
plans, just as aggressive private purchasers have discovered through their
experience with managed care. The potential jeopardy for relationships with
traditional providers has been noted above. But the increasingly competitive
environment has made the Medicaid beneficiary more attractive to providers
and plans, especially those who historically have not been responsive to this

population. Moreover, some states are beginning to extract important participation concessions from provider groups and plans. One approach has been to
set, as a condition of licensure or other regulatory consideration, the requirement that plans enroll Medicaid beneficiaries up to some specified level. Other
states are now setting, as a condition to enroll state employees under their
health benefit plan, the requirement that providers must also care for other
beneficiaries sponsored by the state, namely Medicaid-eligibles.

There are risks for Medicaid programs that attempt to deviate too far from
the mainstream managed care models by allowing the participation of new
forms of plans/provider networks that may be less comprehensive and accountable than HMOs. Such plans may not be subject to state insurance regulation
for licensure and solvency requirements; thus the onus for their oversight may
end up in Medicaid agencies that are not well-suited for this new responsibility.
This type of development is especially likely in states with immature managed
care markets. Medicaid agencies trying to accelerate development through
contracting with emergent or evolving plans invite possible risk and failure
that could set back managed care expansions in states already facing important
obstacles.

SCHIZOPHRENIC ROLES FOR STATES   A number of the emerging issues cited
above reflect a more basic problem for Medicaid agencies as they try to
transform themselves into predominantly or exclusively managed care programs. This transformation is challenging in the same ways that commercial
insurance companies and Blue Cross have discovered, but it is more problematic for state agencies because of their multiple and sometimes conflicting
missions.

The desire to act as a prudent purchaser of services on behalf of Medicaid
beneficiaries is a strong one, given the financially besieged status of state
budgets that have seen Medicaid grow at the expense of every other service
financed by state revenues. Gold aptly describes Medicaid as the "Pac Man
of state government" seemingly consuming all other programs in its path (16).
But aggressive purchasing policies quickly conflict with other state roles
including maintainer of the provider safety net for the uninsured, who will not
disappear until universal coverage is achieved. Thus, many local health departments and DSH providers are working assiduously to deflect or delay the
consequences of aggressive purchasing behavior as embedded in Medicaid
managed care.

Indigenous providers, many of whom are minority physicians serving predominantly minority and geographically or socially isolated populations, are
petitioning for protection against the near-certain jeopardy that managed care
represents for them. State agencies must wrestle with whether to accommodate
them, encourage and support their efforts to form their own managed care

plans and networks, or direct them to join existing or emergent plans and networks with which Medicaid wishes to contract. This dilemma invariably leads to delicate and complex negotiations against a backdrop of political, economic, and ethnic tensions.

Finally, the fact that Medicaid has become a back-door financier of public personal health (clinical services), mental health, and social services during a period when it has represented the only major source of new revenues to these service sectors raises the stakes dramatically when Medicaid agencies seek to alter their buying habits and align with new provider systems. The difficulty of reversing this so-called "medicaidization" (9) becomes apparent when state legislators recognize that they are expected to replace foregone federal matching dollars captured through Medicaid with state dollars to maintain their medical schools, personal health services in local health departments, and many social service agencies. Once again, the vague promise of health reform and its prospects of universal coverage are not sufficient to attenuate the crises that are already occurring in financially beleaguered states.

TOWARD HEALTH REFORM: MEDICAID MANAGED CARE—THE NEXT GENERATION

By mid-1994 there were numerous proposals for national health reform before Congress, with a wide variety of prescriptions for addressing Medicaid and its future. None of them is likely to be passed immediately or, if passed, to be implemented expeditiously, so it is a reasonable assumption that the rapid evolution of Medicaid managed care will continue, given the central role managed care plays in most serious reform proposals. Several important trends are likely to unfold while the nation awaits a more massive restructuring of its health care system.

CONVERTING ALL MODELS TO PREPAYMENT   Although much of the recent growth in managed care enrollment has come through fee-for-service gatekeeper programs, these programs must be transitioned toward prepaid models. This will be necessary because Medicaid must conform with private sector trends that are embracing capitation and risk-sharing with providers and plans; otherwise, Medicaid will remain one of the last fee-for-service payers. Continuing to send providers mixed or ambiguous signals via payment methods will inhibit the development of integrated delivery systems for a major segment of the population. The desire to convert to prepayment will be intensified if the federal government finds it necessary and/or expedient to limit the level of its financial support and participation in Medicaid, and thus shifts more of the risk of cost increases to the states. The states will have to find a way to transmit this risk to plans and providers. Developing models that convert fee-for-service systems to prepayment and make them applicable across disparate markets will be a major challenge for Medicaid agencies, but one they will have to face.

EXTENDING MANAGED CARE TO NON-AFDC BENEFICIARIES   The simple economics of Medicaid demand attention to making managed care models more inclusive. Most experience to date has been with the approximately 70 percent of eligibles (the AFDC-related) who consume only 30 percent of program expenditures (28), with the exception of long-standing programs in California and Minnesota. The aged, blind, disabled populations on the one hand and the distinctive and important institutionally based populations on the other, who together consume the other 70 percent of expenses, have remained excluded from Medicaid managed care; little progress has been made to date in finding models that will appropriately serve them. In part, this reflects the lack of care-management technology for these groups given that primary care–case management seems insufficient to manage their multiple medical, social, and developmental needs. Existing HMOs have had little experience with and apparent interest in extending their delivery systems to serve these special populations. However, Medicaid managed care is likely paving the way for service to all non-AFDC Medicaid populations.

The non-AFDC population itself includes several distinct subgroups with disparate and often highly specialized needs, for which a single model will never be robust enough. The populations of many of these subgroups reflect wide variation in expected expenditures, complicating the development of stable cost estimates that would be the basis for the prepaid rates, which are essential to give provider organizations sufficient flexibility to develop customized delivery plans. Finally, the policies and programs developed by Medicaid agencies for these populations and their advocacy groups originate in different sections of the agencies. These multifaceted policies and programs differ qualitatively in their scope and goals from the more limited role of financing of health care for the AFDC beneficiary populations. In every instance, these issues and obstacles will apply to any health care reform initiative that seeks to mainstream special-need populations.

IMPROVING PLAN MONITORING AND OVERSIGHT   Perhaps the single most important contribution of managed care in Medicaid to date is the fact that the 5 million enrollees have a guarantee of access to a contractually obligated provider who must be available to them on a 24-hour, 7-day per week basis. The other 25 million beneficiaries enjoy no such guarantee. But that guarantee alone does not ensure that plans will offer clinically appropriate services of high quality. Medicaid agencies, like most other buyers of managed care services, have had difficulties in extracting from plans assurances and indicators of a commitment to quality performance and quality improvement. Pre-payment, contracting with plans rather than directly with providers, and limited availability of performance data all complicate quality assurance efforts, which in truth have not been diligently performed in the fee-for-service era either.

The potential for problems—and thus need for greater vigilance—is inten-sified for Medicaid. Historically low payment rates on which prepaid rates are based raise the vivid specter of underservice. These low rates have attracted to Medicaid some providers whose performance under fee-for-service, which encourages excessive use, has been suspect; the reversal of incentives could elicit behaviors that might not be in the beneficiary's best interest. Benefici-aries, by definition, lack the financial means to go "out of network" to obtain desired care. Legitimate concerns exist about the geographical, cultural, and linguistic accessibility of prepaid health plans whose traditional members have not been economically disadvantaged or drawn from ethnic minorities. Finally, the special medical needs of these populations, such as early intervention programs for child health or outreach-based prenatal care services, may de-mand services and practitioners lacking in both new and existing prepaid plans.

The performance of Medicaid agencies will have to be like that of the health alliance/purchasing cooperatives envisioned in several of the leading health reform proposals. They will have to evaluate plans systematically for their capacity to serve special-need populations against objective measures of ac-cessibility and availability. Standards of cultural competence and sensitivity must be established and enforced. The specification of supplemental service needs such as transportation and outreach for prenatal care will be another major oversight area. And standards for contractor performance in crucial areas like marketing, consumer satisfaction, and health outcomes will have to be monitored and enforced aggressively. Many states are already moving in this direction. There is near-universal recognition that this is an area where much progress can and must be made.

ADDRESSING ROLE OF AND IMPACT ON SAFETY NET PROVIDERS   Continued progress in expanding Medicaid managed care will require confronting the problem of potentially adverse effects for "safety net providers." This issue has been discussed above. Its pertinence to the next generation of initiatives is that major efforts will be required to allow for transition of these providers into managed care plans and networks at the same pace as Medicaid adopts managed care as its mainstream model of service delivery. It may be difficult for Medicaid to contribute directly to fostering this provider readiness. In its absence, however, Medicaid agencies will find it hard to proceed with their managed care expansions. Resistance will come from the providers and their supporters within and outside of state government. Moreover, Medicaid agen-cies themselves often see many of these providers as their natural allies and may be reluctant to contract with new private plans of questionable commitment and staying power, should the "Medicaid line of business" prove less lucrative than desired.

Aaron & Schwartz have described the goal of managed competition as "the ruthless elimination of unjustified activities" in the health care sector (1). Safety net providers must understand that a competitive environment will threaten them with elimination and force them to justify their activities and indeed their very existence. Some may respond by seeking to be cordoned off from competitive forces, but this seems unlikely to succeed and is of dubious value if universal coverage ultimately arrives and these providers must respond to consumer demands to maintain their natural constituencies. More constructively, such providers would be wise to avail themselves of the opportunities presented by Medicaid managed care initiatives to begin a transition to prepaid, integrated systems, either as sponsors or network members.

BLENDING MEDICAID AND UNINSURED INTO A SINGLE-PURCHASER PROGRAM
For states like Arizona, Kentucky, Maryland, Oregon, and Washington that have committed to developing statewide managed care networks for enrolling all AFDC beneficiaries, the apparatus is in place to offer access to this same network to uninsured populations—if financing can be found. Some states will work toward a single-purchaser program by incrementally expanding Medicaid eligibility to draw in more of the uninsured. Others will finance this process with other state-only funds, or perhaps with some premium contribution from the working poor. Still others will attempt the controversial Tennessee Tenn-Care approach of obtaining a waiver that, in essence, converts Medicaid to a block grant program. The waiver granted effective January 1, 1994, allowed the state to use federal and state dollars to cover statewide a Medicaid and non-Medicaid population with a modified Medicaid benefits package through managed care plans.

The logic of blending these groups is obvious. They have similar health needs and there is fluidity in movement between the two groups. In a typical state, 30 percent of the AFDC population turns over yearly. Medicaid and uninsured programs often rely on the same providers, some of whom are now using Medicaid payments, meager as they may be, to cross-subsidize their services to the uninsured. The efforts invested in ensuring that plans meet the conditions of serving Medicaid beneficiaries can be applied directly to serving the uninsured. Substantial leverage can be mobilized by combining these groups and then used to extract price concession from providers, especially if they may not be receiving payments for the uninsured. Pooling purchasing power offers real promise. Research by Bice & Wintringham shows that providing stable enrollment of such groups in managed care will reduce cost, but without stabilization (e.g. enrollees moving in and out of managed care with eligibility) managed care costs are higher than fee-for-service (3).

CONCLUSION

There have been many changes from the early days of Medicaid managed care when great anxiety was expressed about the potentially adverse consequences of restricting freedom-of-choice and contracting with providers who had incentives to skimp on care. These concerns have not been validated based on more than a decade of expanding experience. Our current notions about prepayment and enrollment suggest that reduction in (nonessential) care may be desirable, or at least necessary, for everyone, not just Medicaid beneficiaries.

Medicaid managed care appears to have improved the ability of Medicaid programs to obtain better value for their expenditures. Thus, a troubled program has been made better in detectable ways, in large measure because managed care obtains guarantees of accessibility to providers and has the potential to improve the accountability of these providers. But as delivery system reform, managed care does not address Medicaid's severe financing problems, which are likely to persist so long as financing of programs and services for the poor are segregated from financing for other beneficiary groups. The iron law of Medicaid that "you don't get what you don't pay for" will continue to apply in its managed care manifestations, as it has in its fee-for-service version.

Any *Annual Review* chapter, as well as any article cited in an *Annual Review* chapter, may be purchased from the Annual Reviews Preprints and Reprints service.
1-800-347-8007; 415-259-5017; email: arpr@class.org

Literature Cited

1. Aaron H, Schwartz W. 1993. Managed competition: little cost containment without budget limits. *Health Aff.* 12: 204–16 (Suppl.)
2. Anderson M, Fox P. 1987. Lessons learned from medicaid managed care approaches. *Health Aff.* 6:70–86
3. Bice TW, Wintringham K. 1985. Effects of turnover on use: Medicaid beneficiaries in a health maintenance organization. *Group Health J.* 6(1):12–18
4. Carey T, Weis K, Homer C. 1991. Prepaid versus traditional medicaid plans: lack of effect on pregnancy outcomes and prenatal care. *Health Serv. Res.* 26: 165–81
5. Chavkin D, Treseder A. 1977. California's prepaid health plans: can the patient be saved? *Hastings Law J.* 28: 685–760
6. Davidson S, Fleming G, Holhen M, Manheim L, Shapiro B, Werner S. 1988. *Physician Reimbursement and Continuing Care Under Medicaid: A Demonstration (The Children's Medicaid Program).* Elk Grove, IL: Am. Acad. Pediatr.
7. Davis K, Schoen C. 1978. *Health and the War on Poverty.* Washington, DC: Brookings Inst.
8. Dobson A, Moran D, Young G. 1992. The role of federal waivers in the health policy process. *Health Aff.* 11:72–94
9. Fosset J. 1993. Medicaid and health reform: the case of New York. *Health Aff.* 12:95–110

10. Freund D. 1984. *Medicaid Reform: Four Studies of Case Management.* Washington, DC: Am. Enterprise Inst.

11. Freund D, Lewit E. 1993. Managed health care for children and pregnant women: promises and pitfalls. *The Future of Children* 3:92–123

12. Freund D, Neuschler E. 1986. Overview of medicaid capitation and case management initiatives. *Health Care Financ. Rev.* 8:21–30 (Suppl.)

13. Freund D, Rossiter L, Fox P, Meyer J, Hurley R, et al. 1989. Evaluation of the medicaid competition demonstrations. *Health Care Financ. Rev.* 11:81–97

14. Freund DA, Hurley RE. 1987. Managed care in medicaid: selected issues in program origins, designs, and research. *Annu. Rev. Public Health* 8:137–63

15. Galblum T, Trieger S. 1982. Demonstrations of alternative delivery systems under medicare and medicaid. *Health Care Financ. Rev.* 3:1–12

16. Gold S. 1993. The state budget context: how medicaid fits in. In *Medicaid Financing Crisis,* ed. D Rowland, J Feder, A Salganicoff, pp. 133–54. Washington, DC: Am. Assoc. Adv. Sci.

17. Goldfarb NI, Hillman AL, Eisenberg JM, Kelley MA, Cohen AV, Dellheim M. 1991. Impact of medicaid mandatory case management program on prenatal care and birth outcomes. *Med. Care* 29:64–71

18. Health Care Financ. Admin. Medicaid Bur. 1993. *A Health Care Quality Improvement System for Medicaid Managed Care. A Guide for States.* Washington, DC: USDHS

19. Health Care Financ. Admin. Medicaid Bur. 1993. *Medicaid Managed Care Enrollment Report.* Washington, DC: USDHHS

20. Health Care Financ. Admin. Medicaid Bur. 1993. *National Summary of State Medicaid Managed Care Programs.* Washington, DC: USDHHS

21. Heinen L, Fox P, Anderson M. 1990. Findings from the medicaid competition demonstrations: a guide for states. *Health Care Financ. Rev.* 11:55–67

22. Hurley R. 1986. Status of the medicaid competition demonstrations. *Health Care Financ. Rev.* 8:65–75

23. Hurley R, Freund D. 1988. A typology of medicaid managed care. *Med. Care* 26:764–74

24. Hurley R, Freund D, Paul J. 1993. *Medicaid Managed Care: Lessons for Policy and Program Development.* Ann Arbor, MI: Health Admin.

25. Hurley R, Freund D, Taylor D. 1989.

Emergency room use and primary care case management: evidence from four medicaid demonstration programs. *Am. J. Public Health* 79:843–47

26. Hurley R, Gage B, Freund D. 1992. Rollover effects in gatekeeper programs: cushioning the impact of restricted choice. *Inquiry* 28:375–84

27. Kaiser Comm. Future Medicaid. 1992. *Medicaid at the Crossroads.* Menlo Park, CA: Kaiser Family Found.

28. Kaiser Comm. Future Medicaid. 1993. *The Medicaid Cost Explosion: Causes and Consequences.* Menlo Park, CA: Kaiser Family Found.

29. Leibowitz A, Buchanan J, Mann J. 1992. A randomized trial to evaluate the effectiveness of a medicaid HMO. *J. Health Econ.* 11:235–57

30. Lurie N, Christianson J, Finch M, Moscovice I. 1994. The effects of capitation on health and functional status of the medicaid elderly. *Ann. Intern. Med.* 120:506–11

31. O'Kane M. 1993. Outside accreditation of managed care plans. In *The Managed Care Handbook,* ed. P Kongstvedt. Gaithersburg, MD: Aspen

32. Omenn GS. 1987. Lessons from a fourteen-state study of Medicaid. *Health Aff.* (Spring) 188–22

33. Research Triangle Institute. 1992. *Evaluation of the Ohio Medicaid Voluntary Enrollment Program.* Research Triangle Park, NC: Research Triangle Institute. Unpublished

34. Riley T, Coburn A, Kilbreth B. 1990. *Medicaid Managed Care: The State of the Art. A Guide for States.* Portland, ME: Natl. Acad. State Health Policy

35. Rowland D, Feder J, Salganicoff A, eds. 1993. *The Medicaid Crisis: Balancing Responsibilities, Priorities, and Dollars.* Washington, DC: Am. Assoc. Adv. Sci.

36. SRI Int. 1989. *Evaluation of the Arizona Health Care Cost Containment System: Final Report.* Contract No. HCFA-500-83-0027. Palo Alto, CA: SRI Int.

37. Stevens R, Stevens R. 1974. *Welfare Medicine in America.* New York: Free Press

38. Sullivan C, Miller M, Feldman R, Dowd B. 1992. Employer sponsored health insurance in 1991. *Health Aff.* 11:172–86

39. US Gen. Acc. Off. 1993. *Medicaid: States Turn to Managed Care to Improve Access and Control Costs.* GAO/HRD 93–86. Washington, DC

40. Wilensky G, Rossiter L. 1991. Coordinated care and public programs. *Health Aff.* 10:62–67

SUBJECT INDEX

CUMULATIVE INDEXES

CONTRIBUTING AUTHORS, VOLUMES 7–16

CHAPTER TITLES, VOLUMES 7–16

ENVIRONMENTAL AND OCCUPATIONAL HEALTH